BEFORE WE ARE BORN

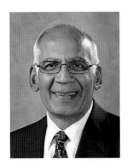

T.V.N. (VID) PERSAUD

Dr. Persaud was the recipient of the Henry Gray/Elsevier Distinguished Educator Award in 2010—"the American Association of Anatomists' highest honor in recognition of sustained excellence and leadership in human anatomy education"; the **Honored Member Award of the American Association of Clinical Anatomists (2008)** for "his distinguished career and significant contributions to the field of clinically relevant anatomy, embryology, and the history of anatomy"; and the **J.C.B. Grant Award of the Canadian Association of Anatomists (1991)** "in recognition of meritorious service and outstanding scholarly accomplishments in the field of anatomical sciences." In 2010 Professor Persaud was inducted as a **Fellow of the American Association of Anatomists**. The rank of Fellow "honors distinguished AAA members who have demonstrated excellence in science and in their overall contributions to the medical sciences." In 2003 Dr. Persaud was a recipient of the **Queen Elizabeth II Golden Jubilee Medal**, presented by the Government of Canada for "significant contribution to the nation, the community, and fellow Canadians."

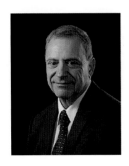

MARK G. TORCHIA

Dr. Mark G. Torchia was the recipient of the distinguished **Inaugural Governor General Award for Innovation** which "recognize(s) and celebrate(s) outstanding Canadian individuals, teams and organizations—trailblazers and creators who contribute to our country's success, who help shape our future and who inspire the next generation." Dr. Torchia is also a **Manning Principle Prize Laureate (2015)**, which recognizes "leaders and visionaries who are positively impacting the Canadian economy while improving the human experience in its various dimensions around the world." He is also a recipient of the **Norman and Marion Bright Memorial Medal and Award** for "individuals who have made an outstanding contribution to chemical technology" and the **TIMEC Medical Device Champion Award**. Dr. Torchia continues to engage learners at all levels through outreach opportunities and formal curricula. He has been nominated for MMSA teaching awards since their initiation and most recently received the **Award for Teaching Excellence** 2016 from the Rady Faculty of Health Sciences, University of Manitoba.

Eleventh Edition

BEFORE WE ARE BORN:

ESSENTIALS OF EMBRYOLOGY AND BIRTH DEFECTS

T.V.N. (Vid) Persaud, MD, PhD, DSc, FRCPath (Lond.), FAAA

Professor Emeritus and Former Head
Department of Human Anatomy and Cell Science,
Professor of Pediatrics and Child Health,
Associate Professor of Obstetrics, Gynecology, and
Reproductive Sciences
Max Rady College of Medicine, Rady Faculty of
Health Sciences;
Faculty of Medicine
University of Manitoba
Winnipeg, Manitoba, Canada

Mark G. Torchia, MSc, PhD

Associate Professor
Department of Surgery,
Associate Professor
Department of Human Anatomy and Cell Sciences
Max Rady College of Medicine, Rady Faculty of
Health Sciences;
Vice-Provost (Teaching and Learning
University of Manitoba
Winnipeg, Manitoba, Canada

ELSEVIER

Elsevier
1600 John F. Kennedy Blvd.
Ste 1800
Philadelphia, PA 19103-2899

BEFORE WE ARE BORN: ESSENTIALS OF EMBRYOLOGY AND
BIRTH DEFECTS, ELEVENTH EDITION

ISBN: 978-0-443-11697-1

Notice

Practitioners and researchers must always rely on their own experience and knowledge in evaluating and using any information, methods, compounds or experiments described herein. Because of rapid advances in the medical sciences, in particular, independent verification of diagnoses and drug dosages should be made. To the fullest extent of the law, no responsibility is assumed by Elsevier, authors, editors or contributors for any injury and/or damage to persons or property as a matter of products liability, negligence or otherwise, or from any use or operation of any methods, products, instructions, or ideas contained in the material herein.

Previous editions copyrighted 2020, 2016, 2013, 2008, 2003, 1998, 1993, 1989, 1983 and 1974.

Content Strategist: Jeremy Bowes
Content Development Specialist: Nicholas Henderson
Publishing Services Manager: Deepthi Unni
Senior Project Manager: Beula Christopher
Senior Book Designer: Margaret Reid

Printed in India

Last digit is the print number: 9 8 7 6 5 4 3 2 1

For Gisela
My lovely wife and best friend, for her endless support and patience; our three children—Indrani, Sunita, and Rainer (Ren)—and grandchildren (Brian, Amy, and Lucas).
—T.V.N. (Vid) Persaud

For Eddie James, Kitt Miko, and Flynn Henryk, the "Torchia brothers"
Our dear grandsons and little rays of sunshine; my amazing wife Barbara, our children Muriel and Erik, and their spouses Caleb and Sarah—thank you for your support, encouragement, laughs, and love.
—Mark G. Torchia

For Our Students and Their Teachers
To our students: We hope you will enjoy reading this book; increase your understanding of human embryology; pass all of your exams; and be excited and well prepared for your careers in patient care, research, and teaching, or whatever the future holds. You will remember some of what you hear, much of what you read, more of what you see, and almost all of what you experience.
To their teachers: May this book be a helpful resource to you and your students.
We appreciate the numerous constructive comments we have received over the years from both students and teachers. Your remarks have been invaluable to us in improving this book.

List of Contributors

CONTRIBUTORS

David D. Eisenstat, MD, MA, FRCPC, FRACP
Professor
Department of Paediatrics
University of Melbourne;
Director
Children's Cancer Centre
The Royal Children's Hospital Melbourne;
Group Leader, Neuro-Oncology
Stem Cell Medicine
Murdoch Children's Research Institute
Parkville, Victoria, Australia
Adjunct Professor
Departments of Medical Genetics, Pediatrics and Oncology
University of Alberta
Edmonton, Alberta, Canada
Chapter 20: The Cellular and Molecular Basis of Development

Jeffrey Theodore Wigle, BSc(H), PhD
Professor
Department of Biochemistry and Medical Genetics
University of Manitoba;
Principal Investigator
Institute of Cardiovascular Sciences
St. Boniface Hospital Research Centre
Winnipeg, Manitoba, Canada
Chapter 20: The Cellular and Molecular Basis of Development

CLINICAL REVIEWERS

Alison M. Elliott, PhD, MS, CGC
Associate Professor
Department of Medical Genetics,
Faculty of Medicine
University of British Columbia;Investigator
BC Children's and Women's Health Research Institutes;
Lead: Gen. COUNSEL
Vancouver, British Columbia, Canada

Michael Narvey, MD, FRCPC, FAAP
Section Head
Neonatal Medicine, Health Sciences Centre and St.
   Boniface Hospital;
Associate Professor of Pediatrics and Child Health
Max Rady College of Medicine, Rady Faculty of Health
   Sciences
University of Manitoba
Winnipeg, Manitoba, Canada

FIGURES AND IMAGES (SOURCES)

We are grateful to the following colleagues for the clinical images they have given us for this book and also for granting us permission to use figures from their published works:

Steve Ahing, DDS (Retired)
Division of Oral Diagnosis and Radiology, Faculty of Dentistry, Department of Pathology, University of Manitoba, Winnipeg, Manitoba, Canada
Fig. 18.10B–D

Franco Antoniazzi, MD, and Vassilios Fanos, MD
Department of Pediatrics, University of Verona, Verona, Italy
Fig. 19.3

Volker Becker, MD[†]
Pathologisches Institut der Universität, Erlangen, Germany
Figs. 8.12 and 8.14

Been, MD, M. Shuurman, MD, and S. Robben, MD
Maastricht University Medical Centre, Maastricht, The Netherlands
Fig. 11.6B

David Bolender, MD
Department of Cell Biology, Neurobiology, and Anatomy, Medical College of Wisconsin, Milwaukee, Wisconsin
Fig. 15.13A

Peter C. Brugger, MD, PhD
Associate Professor/Privat Dozent, Center for Anatomy and Cell Biology, Medical University of Vienna, Vienna, Austria
Cover image (MRI of breech fetus)

Jack C.Y. Cheng, MD
Department of Orthopaedics and Traumatology, The Chinese University of Hong Kong, Hong Kong, China
Fig. 15.18

Albert E. Chudley, MD, FRCPC, FCCMG
Department of Pediatrics and Child Health, Section of Genetics and Metabolism, Children's Hospital, University of Manitoba, Winnipeg, Manitoba, Canada
Figs. 5.12, 10.13, 10.30, 12.17A and B, 12.24, 13.13, 13.26, 15.24, 15.25, 15.26, 16.10, 16.11, 16.23, 17.14, 19.4, 19.5, 19.6, 19.7, 19.9, 19.10, 19.12, and 19.14A

Blaine M. Cleghorn, DMD, MSc
Department of Dental Clinical Sciences Faculty of Dentistry, Dalhousie University, Halifax, Nova Scotia, Canada
Fig. 18.10A

Heather Dean, MD, FRCPC
Department of Pediatrics and Child Health, University of Manitoba, Winnipeg, Manitoba, Canada
Figs. 13.17, 13.25, and 19.13

[†]Decased

Marc Del Bigio, MD, PhD, FRCPC
Department of Pathology (Neuropathology), University of Manitoba, Winnipeg, Manitoba, Canada
Figs. 15.10, 16.22, and 16.26

João Carlos Fernandes Rodrigues, MD
Servico de Dermatologia, Hospital de Desterro, Lisbon, Portugal
Fig. 18.3

Gary Geddes, MD
Family Physician, Legacy Emanuel Medical Center Lake Oswego, Oregon
Fig. 15.13B

Barry H. Grayson, MD, and Bruno L. Vendittelli, MD
New York University Medical Center, Institute of Reconstructive Plastic Surgery, New York, New York
Fig. 10.31

Jean Hay, MSc[†]
University of Manitoba, Winnipeg, Manitoba, Canada
Fig. 7.4

Lyndon M. Hill, MD
Magee-Women's Hospital, Pittsburgh, Pennsylvania, USA
Fig. 12.5

Klaus V. Hinrichsen, MD
Medizinische Fakultät, Institut für Anatomie, Ruhr-Universität Bochum, Bochum, Germany
Figs. 10.2 and 10.24

Evelyn Jain, MD, FCFP
Breastfeeding Clinic, Calgary, Alberta, Canada
Fig. 10.22

John A. Jane, Sr. MD
Department of Neurological Surgery, University of Virginia Health System, Charlottesville, Virginia
Fig. 15.11A and 15.11B

Dagmar K. Kalousek, MD
Department of Pathology, University of British Columbia, Children's Hospital, Vancouver, British Columbia, Canada
Figs. 12.12A and 13.10

James Koenig, MD, FRCPC
Department of Radiology, Health Sciences Centre, Winnipeg, Manitoba, Canada
Fig. 14.28D

Wesley Lee, MD
Department of Obstetrics and Gynecology, Division of Fetal Imaging, William Beaumont Hospital, Royal Oak, Michigan
Fig. 16.12A

Deborah Levine, MD, FACR
Department of Radiology, Obstetric and Gynecologic Ultrasound, Beth Israel Deaconess Medical Center, Boston, Massachusetts
Figs. 7.5B and 16.12B, and cover image (MRI of 27-week fetus)

Mina Leyder, MD
Universitair Ziekenhuis Brussels, Brussels, Belgium
Fig. 14.19

E.A. (Ted) Lyons, OC, MD, FRCPC, FACR
Departments of Radiology, Obstetrics & Gynecology, and
Human Anatomy and Cell Science, Division of Ultrasound,
Health Sciences Centre, University of Manitoba, Winnipeg,
Manitoba, Canada
*Figs. 4.6B, 5.1, 5.10, 6.6, 7.1, 7.9, 8.4, and 12.17C and D,
and cover image (ultrasound of 9-week fetus)*

Maulik S. Patel, MD
Consultant Pathologist, Surat, India; Radiopaedia.org
Fig. 5.13

Martin H. Reed, MD, FRCPC
Department of Radiology, University of Manitoba and
Children's Hospital, Winnipeg, Manitoba, Canada
Fig. 12.23

Gregory J. Reid, MD, FRCSC
Department of Obstetrics, Gynecology, and
Reproductive Sciences, University of Manitoba, Women's
Hospital, Winnipeg, Manitoba, Canada
Fig. 14.9

Michael and Michele Rice
Fig. 7.6

Prem S. Sahni, MD
Formerly of the Department of Radiology, Children's
Hospital, Winnipeg, Manitoba, Canada

Gerald S. Smyser, MD
Formerly of the Altru Health System, Grand Forks, North
Dakota
Figs. 10.17, 15.11C, and 17.13

Pierre Soucy, MD, FRCSC
Division of Pediatric Surgery, Children's Hospital of
Eastern Ontario, Ottawa, Ontario, Canada
Figs. 10.10 and 10.11

Alexandra Stanislavsky, MD
Department of Radiology, Mercy Hospital for Women,
Royal Melbourne Hospital, Melbourne, Victoria, Australia;
Radiopaedia.org
Fig. 12.12B

Richard Shane Tubbs, PhD, and W. Jerry Oakes, MD
Department of Pediatric Neurosurgery, Children's
Hospital, Birmingham, Alabama
Fig. 16.24

Edward O. Uthman, MD
Clinical Pathologist, Memorial Hermann Katy Hospital
Houston/Richmond, Texas
Fig. 5.3C

Elspeth H. Whitby, BSc, MB, ChB (Hons), FFDRCSI
Academic Unit of Reproductive and Developmental
Medicine, Department of Academic Pathology, University
of Sheffield, Sheffield, England, United Kingdom
Fig. 16.25

Nathan E. Wiseman, MD, FRCSC
Department of Surgery, Section of Pediatric and
Cardiothoracic Surgery, Children's Hospital, University of
Manitoba, Winnipeg, Manitoba, Canada
Figs. 9.8B, 9.8C, and 12.15

Preface

Before We Are Born has been in print for more than 48 years. This concise work is based on our larger book, *The Developing Human: Clinically Oriented Embryology, 11th Edition*.

The 11th edition of *Before We Are Born* has been completely updated to reflect the current understanding of clinical human embryology. It provides the essentials of normal and abnormal development. As in earlier editions, *clinically oriented materials* are highlighted in green color (often called clinical **green boxes**). Every chapter has been revised thoroughly to reflect new research findings and their clinical significance, as well as new understanding of the developmental biology.

This edition follows the official *international list of embryological terms* (*Terminologia Embryonica*, 2013). It is important that physicians, nurses, physician assistants, dentists, physical and occupational therapists, other health professionals, scientists, and students in the health professions throughout the world use the same name for each structure.

We have included numerous **new color photographs** of embryos, fetuses (normal and abnormal), neonates (newborns), and children. There are also many new *diagnostic images*: ultrasound, computed tomography scans, and magnetic resonance imaging studies of embryos and fetuses.

An important feature of this book is the **Clinically Oriented Questions**, which appear at the end of each chapter. In addition, available through Elsevier's *eBooks+* website,

there are many helpful **clinical case studies** and questions with answers and explanations. These will benefit students preparing for USMLE Step 1 and similar examinations.

Accompanying this 11th edition of *Before We Are Born* is an innovative set of **18 full-color animations** that will assist students in learning the complexities of embryological development. These animations are available at *eBooks+*. High-resolution animations are available to teachers for their lectures if they have adopted this book or *The Developing Human* (consult your Elsevier representative). When one of the animations is especially relevant to the book's text, an **icon** ▶ has been added in the margin.

The **teratology** (studies concerned with birth defects) section has been updated because the study of abnormal development is required for understanding the causes of birth defects and how these may be prevented. *Molecular aspects of developmental biology* have been highlighted throughout the book, especially in areas that appear promising for clinical medicine and future research. Moreover, Chapter 20 is devoted exclusively to more detailed information related to the cellular and molecular basis of embryonic development.

T.V.N. (Vid) Persaud
Mark G. Torchia

Acknowledgments

Many colleagues and students have made invaluable contributions to this 11th edition of *Before We Are Born*. We are indebted to the following colleagues (listed alphabetically) for either critical reviewing of chapters, making suggestions for improvement of this book, or providing some of the new figures:

Dr. Steve Ahing (Retired), Division of Oral Diagnosis and Radiology, Faculty of Dentistry, Department of Pathology, University of Manitoba, Winnipeg, Manitoba, Canada; Dr. Albert E. Chudley, Department of Pediatrics and Child Health, Section of Genetics and Metabolism, Children's Hospital, University of Manitoba, Winnipeg, Manitoba, Canada; Dr. Blaine M. Cleghorn, Department of Dental Clinical Sciences, Faculty of Dentistry, Dalhousie University, Halifax, Nova Scotia, Canada; Dr. Frank Gaillard, Department of Radiology, Royal Melbourne Hospital, Melbourne, Victoria, Australia; Dr. Boris Kablar, Department of Medical Neuroscience, Dalhousie University, Halifax, Nova Scotia, Canada; Dr. Peeyush Lala, Department of Anatomy and Cell Biology, Schulich School of Medicine and Dentistry, Western University, London, Ontario, Canada; Dr. Deborah Levine, Department of Radiology, Obstetric and Gynecologic Ultrasound, Beth Israel Deaconess Medical Center, Harvard University, Boston, Massachusetts; Dr. Marios Loukas, St. George's University, St. George's, Grenada; Dr. Bernard J. Moxham, Cardiff School of Biosciences, Cardiff University, Cardiff, Wales, United Kingdom; Dr. Drew Noden, Cornell University College of Veterinary Medicine, Ithaca, New York; Dr. Shannon Perry, School of Nursing, San Francisco State University, San Francisco, California; Dr. Gregory J. Reid, Department of Obstetrics, Gynecology, and Reproductive Sciences, University of Manitoba, Women's Hospital, Winnipeg, Manitoba, Canada; Dr. J. Elliott Scott, Departments of Oral Biology and Human Anatomy and Cell Science, University of Manitoba, Winnipeg, Manitoba, Canada; Dr. Brad Smith, University of Michigan, Ann Arbor, Michigan; Dr. Gerald S. Smyser, formerly of the Altru Health System, Grand Forks, North Dakota; Dr. Richard Shane Tubbs, Departments of Neurosurgery, Neurology, and Structural & Cellular Biology, Tulane University School of Medicine, New Orleans, Louisiana; Dr. Edward O. Uthman, Clinical Pathologist, Memorial Hermann Katy Hospital, Houston/Richmond, Texas; and Dr. Michael Wiley, Division of Anatomy, Department of Surgery, Faculty of Medicine, University of Toronto, Toronto, Ontario. The new illustrations were prepared by Hans Neuhart, President of the Electronic Illustrators Group in Fountain Hills, Arizona.

The collection of animations of developing embryos was produced in collaboration with Dr. David L. Bolender, Associate Professor, Department of Cell Biology, Neurobiology, and Anatomy, Medical College of Wisconsin, Milwaukee, Wisconsin. We would like to thank him for his efforts in design and in-depth review, as well as his invaluable advice. Our special thanks go to Ms. Carol Emery for skillfully coordinating the project. The animations have been enhanced with narration—we thank the Elsevier St. Louis Multimedia Department.

At Elsevier, we are indebted to Mr. Jeremy Bowes, Senior Content Strategist, and Mr. Nicholas Henderson, Content Specialist, as well as Priyashree Srikanth (Project Manager/ MPS Limited) and Beula Christopher (Senior Project Manager/ Health Consultant Management) for their invaluable insights and unstinting support in the preparation of this 11th edition of the book. Finally, we thank the entire Elsevier production team for bringing this book to completion. This new edition of *Before We Are Born* is the result of their dedication and technical expertise.

T.V.N. (Vid) Persaud
Mark G. Torchia

Get the Most Out of *Before We Are Born*, 11th Edition!

Included in your purchase is a rich variety of **BONUS content** to enhance the printed book and your learning. Look out for this icon ▶ indicating where there is directly related electronic material. Benefit from:

- **18 superb animations, now with new expert voiceovers**—to guide you through key embryology concepts:

Animation Title	Associated Chapter(s)	Animation Title	Associated Chapter(s)
Fertilization	2, 3	Gastrointestinal Tract	12
Blastocyst	3, 4	Urinary System	12, 13
Implantation	4	Reproductive System	13
Gastrulation	5	Heart	14
Folding of the Embryo	6	Vascular System	14
Body Cavities	9, 14	Limb Development	15
Pharyngeal Apparatus	10	The Nervous System	15, 16
Face and Palate	10	Development of the Eyes	17
Respiratory System	11	Development of the Ears	17

- **USMLE-style MCQs, explanations**—to help check your understanding and prepare for exams

  Don't miss out on this wealth of extra content—see the inside front cover for your access instructions!

TRIBUTE TO DR. KEITH LEON MOORE

At the age of 94 years, Dr. Keith Leon Moore passed away. He authored several anatomy and embryology textbooks, which not only won numerous awards but also were translated into many languages. Truly an international icon in the field of anatomy, Dr. Moore's books had a tremendous impact on generations of students and on medical education.

Dr. Moore had been the recipient of many prestigious awards and recognitions. He was the recipient of the **inaugural Henry Gray/Elsevier Distinguished Educator Award in 2007**—the American Association of Anatomists' (AAA) highest award for excellence in human anatomy education at the medical/dental, graduate, and undergraduate levels of teaching; the **Honored Member Award of the American Association of Clinical Anatomists (1994)** for significant contributions to the field of clinically relevant anatomy; and the **J.C.B. Grant Award of the Canadian Association of Anatomists (1984)** "in recognition of meritorious service and outstanding scholarly accomplishments in the field of anatomical sciences." In 2008 Dr. Moore was inducted as a **Fellow of the American Association of Anatomists**, which honors distinguished AAA members who have demonstrated excellence in science and in their overall contributions to the medical sciences. In 2012 Dr. Moore received an **Honorary Doctor of Science** degree from The Ohio State University and the University of Western Ontario in 2015, as well as the **Queen Elizabeth II Diamond Jubilee Medal** honoring significant contributions and achievements by Canadians, and the **Benton Adkins Jr. Distinguished Service Award** for an outstanding record of service to the American Association of Clinical Anatomists.

Dr. Moore's lifelong contributions as a medical educator in the anatomical sciences will stand as a lasting legacy.

Dr. Keith Leon Moore (1925–2019)

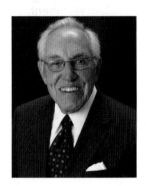

Contents

Introduction to Human Development

1

Human development begins at fertilization when an **oocyte** (ovum) from a female is fertilized by a **sperm** (spermatozoon) from a male and becomes a single-celled **zygote**. Development involves molecular and cellular changes that transform the zygote into a multicellular human being. **Embryology** is concerned with the origin and development of a human being from a zygote to birth. The stages of development before birth are shown in Fig. 1.1.

IMPORTANCE OF AND ADVANCES IN EMBRYOLOGY

The study of prenatal stages and mechanisms of human development helps us understand the normal relationships of adult body structures and the causes of **birth defects** (congenital anomalies). *(NOTE: In many sections of this textbook, rates of incidence or prevalence of a particular birth defect or disorder are provided. These numbers are estimates based on the best available data at the time; the actual values are highly dependent on many factors such as maternal characteristics, genetics, geography, and race.)* Much of the modern practice of obstetrics involves applied or clinical embryology. Because some children have birth defects, such as spina bifida or congenital heart disease, the significance of embryology is readily apparent to pediatricians. Advances in surgery, especially in procedures involving the prenatal and pediatric age groups, have made knowledge of human development more clinically significant. Fundamental research carried out in the area of early human embryology made in vitro fertilization a reality and led to assisted human reproduction and hope for infertile couples.

Rapid advances in molecular biology have led to the use of sophisticated techniques (e.g., **genomic technology**, **chimeric models**, **transgenics**, **organoids**, and **stem cell manipulation**) in research laboratories to explore such diverse issues as the genetic regulation of morphogenesis, the temporal and regional expression of specific genes, and the mechanisms by which cells are committed or differentiate to form the various parts of the embryo.

Development begins at fertilization (see Fig. 1.1, first week). The **embryonic period** covers the first 8 weeks of development of an embryo. The **fetal period** begins in the ninth week. Examination of the timetable shows that the most externally visible advances occur during the third to eighth weeks.

The critical role of genes, **signaling molecules**, receptors, and other molecular factors in regulating embryonic development is rapidly being delineated. In 1995 Edward B. Lewis, Christiane Nüsslein-Volhard, and Eric F. Wieschaus were awarded the **Nobel Prize** in Physiology or Medicine for their discovery of genes that control embryonic development. Such discoveries are contributing to a better understanding of the causes of spontaneous abortion and birth defects.

Robert G. Edwards (1925–2013) and Patrick Steptoe (1913–88) pioneered one of the most revolutionary developments in the history of human reproduction: the technique of in vitro fertilization. Their studies resulted in the birth of Louise Brown, the first "test tube baby," in 1978. Edwards was awarded the Nobel Prize in 2010.

In 1997 Ian Wilmut and colleagues were the first to produce a mammal (a sheep dubbed **Dolly**) by cloning using the technique of somatic cell nuclear transfer. Since then, other animals have been cloned successfully from cultured, differentiated adult cells. Interest in human cloning has generated considerable debate because of social, ethical, and legal implications. Moreover, there is concern that cloning may result in an increase in the number of newborns with birth defects and serious diseases.

Human embryonic stem cells are pluripotent and capable of developing into diverse cell types. The isolation and culture of human embryonic and other stem cells hold great promise for the development of molecular therapies.

DESCRIPTIVE TERMS

The body descriptions of an adult are based on the *anatomical position*; the body is erect, the upper limbs are at the sides, and the palms are directed anteriorly (Fig. 1.2A). The descriptive terms of position, direction, and planes used for *embryos* are shown in Fig. 1.2B–E. In describing development, it is necessary to use words denoting the position of one part relative to another or to the body as a whole. For example, the vertebral column develops in the dorsal part of the embryo, and the sternum is in the ventral part of the embryo.

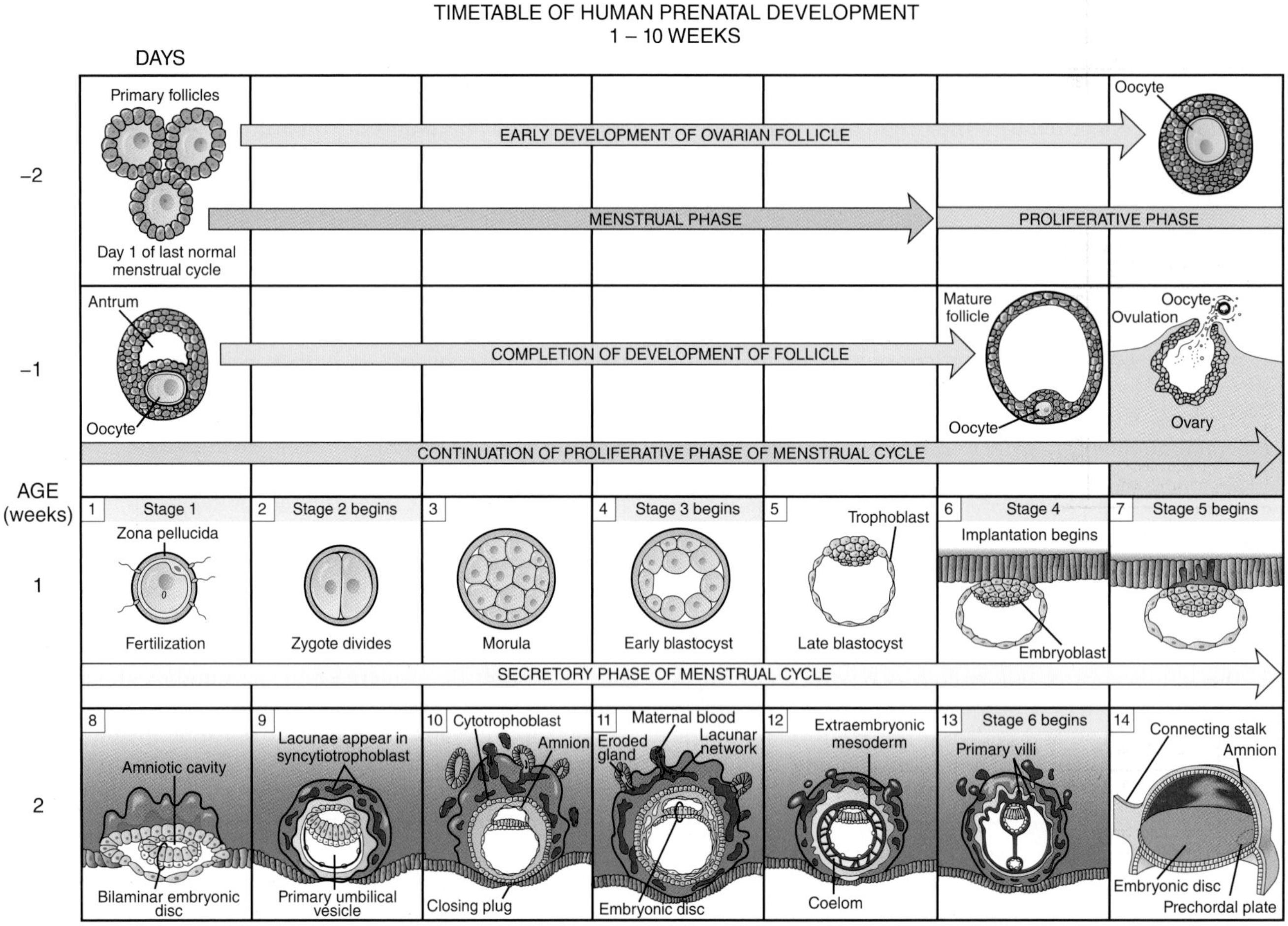

Fig. 1.1 Early stages of human development. An ovarian follicle containing an oocyte, ovulation, and phases of the menstrual cycle are shown.

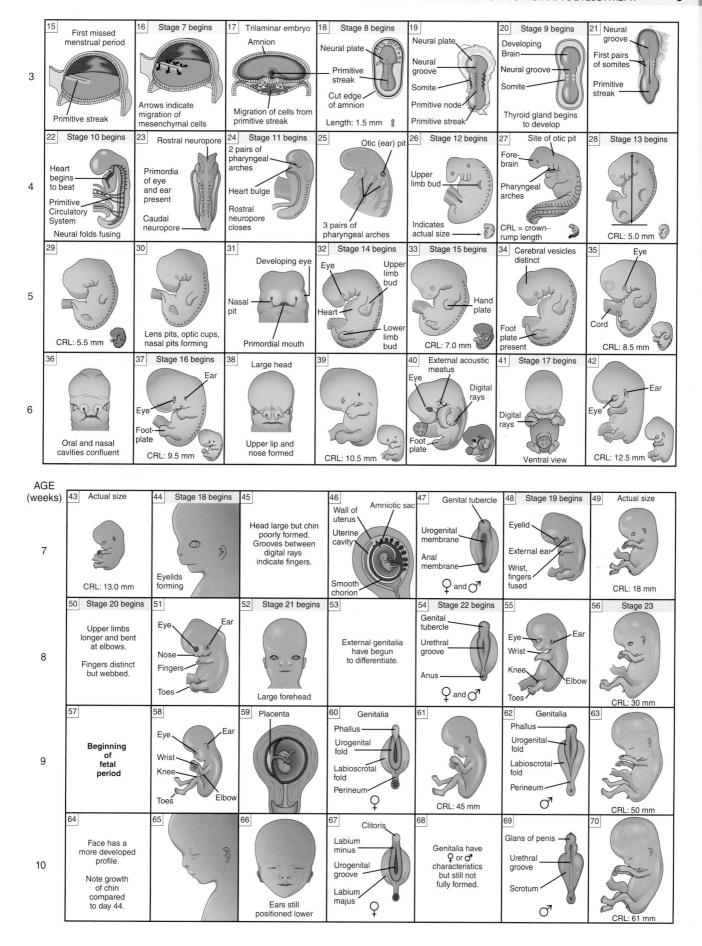

Fig. 1.1 Cont'd

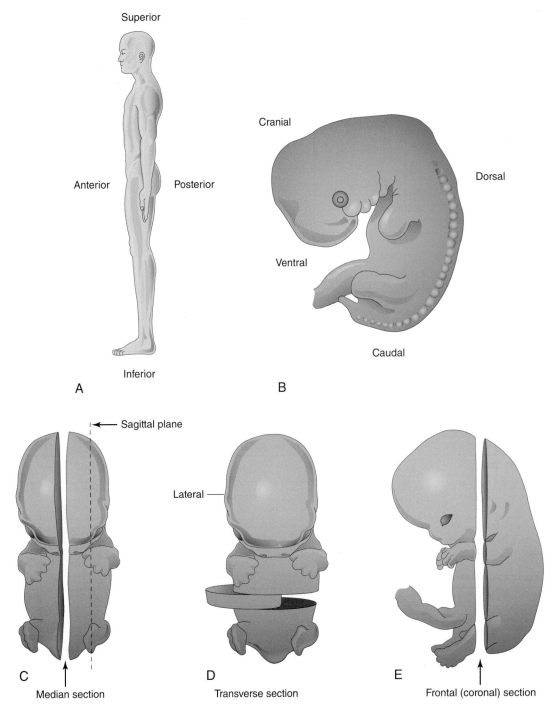

Fig. 1.2 Illustrations of descriptive terms of position, direction, and planes of the body. (A) Lateral view of an adult in the anatomical position. (B) Lateral view of a 5-week embryo. (C and D) Ventral views of a 6-week embryo. The median plane is an imaginary vertical plane of section that passes longitudinally through the body, dividing it into right and left halves. A sagittal plane refers to any plane parallel to the median plane. A transverse plane refers to any plane that is at right angles to both the median and frontal planes. (E) Lateral view of a 7-week embryo. A frontal (coronal) plane is any vertical plane that intersects the median plane at a right angle and divides the body into front (anterior or ventral) and back (posterior or dorsal) parts.

CLINICALLY ORIENTED QUESTIONS

1. Why do we study human embryology? Does it have any practical value in medicine and other health sciences?

2. Physicians date a pregnancy from the first day of the last normal menstrual period, but the embryo does not start to develop until approximately 2 weeks later (see Fig. 1.1). Why do physicians use this method?

The answers to these questions are at the back of this book.

Human Reproduction 2

Puberty begins when secondary sex characteristics appear and humans become functionally capable of procreation, usually between the ages of 8 to 13 years in females and 9 to 14 years in males. **Menarche** (first menstrual period) may occur as early as 8 years. Puberty in females and males is largely completed by the age of 16 years.

REPRODUCTIVE ORGANS

Reproductive organs produce and transport germ cells (gametes) from the gonads (testes or ovaries) to the site of fertilization in the uterine tube (Fig. 2.1).

FEMALE REPRODUCTIVE ORGANS

VAGINA

The **vagina** serves as the excretory passage for menstrual fluid, receives the penis during sexual intercourse, and forms the inferior part of the **birth canal**—the cavity of the uterus and vagina (see Fig. 2.1A).

UTERUS

The **uterus** is a thick-walled, pear-shaped organ (Fig. 2.2A and B) that consists of two main parts:

- The **body**, the expanded superior two-thirds
- The **cervix**, the cylindrical inferior third

The **fundus of the uterus** is the rounded part of the uterine body that lies superior to the orifices of the uterine tubes. The **body of the uterus** narrows from the fundus to the **isthmus**, the constricted region between the body and the **cervix** (see Fig. 2.2A). The lumen of the cervix, the **cervical canal**, has a constricted opening, the **os** (ostium), at each end. The **internal os** communicates with the cavity of the body of the uterus, whereas the **external os** communicates with the vagina. Walls of the uterine body consist of three layers:

- **Perimetrium**, a thin external peritoneal layer
- **Myometrium**, a thick smooth muscle layer
- **Endometrium**, a thin internal layer

At the peak of its development, the endometrium is 4 to 5 mm thick. During the luteal (secretory) phase of the menstrual cycle (see Fig. 2.8), three layers of the endometrium can be distinguished microscopically (see Fig. 2.2C) into the following:

- A compact layer, consisting of densely packed connective tissue around the neck of the uterine glands

- A spongy layer, composed of edematous connective tissue containing the dilated, tortuous bodies of the uterine glands
- A basal layer, containing the blind ends of the uterine glands

The compact and spongy layers—the **functional layer**—disintegrate and are shed at menstruation and after *parturition* (childbirth). The basal layer has its own blood supply and is not cast off during menstruation.

UTERINE TUBES

The **uterine tubes** extend laterally from the **horns of the uterus** (see Fig. 2.2A). Each tube opens into a horn at its proximal end and into the peritoneal cavity at its distal end. The uterine tube is divided into the following parts: **infundibulum, ampulla, isthmus,** and **uterine part**. The tubes carry oocytes from the ovaries and sperms to the fertilization site in the ampulla (see Fig. 2.2B). The uterine tube is lined with cilia and, together with the muscular contractions of the tube, conveys the dividing zygote to the uterine cavity.

OVARIES

The **ovaries** are almond-shaped reproductive glands that are located close to the lateral wall of the pelvis on each side of the uterus. The ovaries produce **oocytes** (see Fig. 2.5). When released from the ovary at **ovulation**, the secondary oocyte passes into one of the uterine tubes. These tubes open into the uterus, which protects and nourishes the embryo and fetus until birth. The ovaries also produce estrogen and progesterone, the hormones responsible for the development of secondary sex characteristics and the regulation of pregnancy.

FEMALE EXTERNAL SEX ORGANS

The female external sex organs are known as the **vulva** (Fig. 2.3). The **labia majora** conceals the **vaginal orifice**, the opening of the vagina. Inside these labia are two smaller folds of mucous membrane, the **labia minora**. The **clitoris**, a small erectile organ, is situated at the superior junction of these folds. The vagina and urethra open into the **vestibule** (cleft between the labia minora). The vaginal orifice varies with the condition of the **hymen**, a fold of mucous membrane that surrounds the orifice (see Fig. 2.3).

MALE REPRODUCTIVE ORGANS

The male reproductive organs (see Fig. 2.1B) include the **penis, testes, epididymis, ductus deferens (vas deferens),**

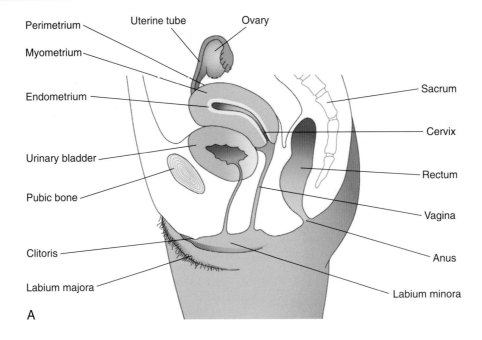

A

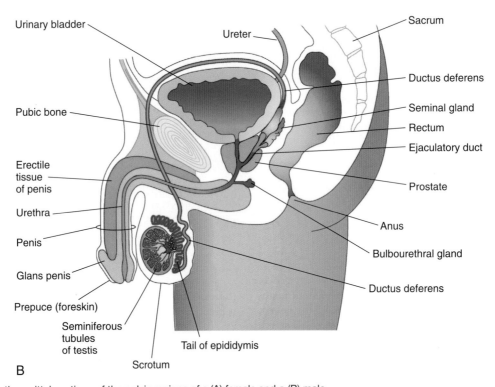

B

Fig. 2.1 Schematic sagittal sections of the pelvic regions of a (A) female and a (B) male.

prostate, seminal glands, bulbourethral glands, ejaculatory ducts, and urethra. The oval **testes** (testicles) are located in the cavity of the **scrotum**. Each **testis** consists of many highly coiled **seminiferous tubules** that produce sperms. Immature sperms pass from the testis into a single, complexly coiled tube, the **epididymis**, where they are stored. From the epididymis, the **ductus deferens** carries sperms to the ejaculatory duct. This duct descends into the pelvis, where it fuses with the ducts of the seminal glands to form the **ejaculatory duct**, which enters the urethra.

The urethra leads from the urinary bladder through the penis to the outside of the body. Within the penis, **erectile tissue** surrounds the urethra. During sexual excitement, this tissue fills with blood, causing the penis to become erect. **Semen** (ejaculate) consists of sperms mixed with seminal fluid produced by the seminal glands, bulbourethral glands, and prostate.

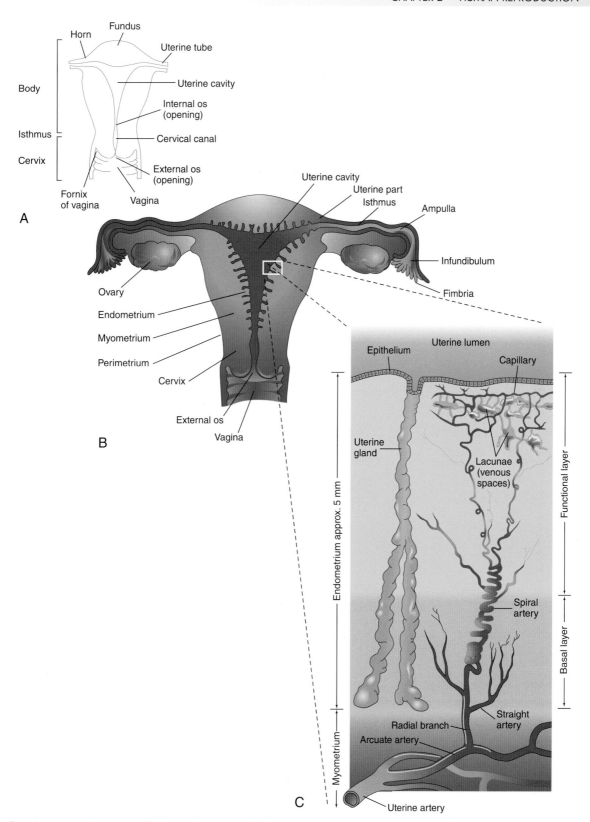

Fig. 2.2 Female reproductive organs. (A) Parts of the uterus. (B) Diagrammatic frontal (coronal) section of the uterus, uterine tubes, and vagina. The ovaries are also shown. (C) Enlargement of the area outlined in B. The functional layer of the endometrium is sloughed off during menstruation and following parturition.

GAMETOGENESIS

The sperms and oocytes are highly specialized gametes—**germ cells** (Fig. 2.4). Each of these cells contains half the number of required chromosomes (i.e., 23 instead of 46). The number of chromosomes is reduced during a special type of cell division—**meiosis**. This type of cell division occurs only during **gametogenesis** (formation of germ cells). In males, this process is termed **spermatogenesis**; in females, it is **oogenesis** (Fig. 2.5).

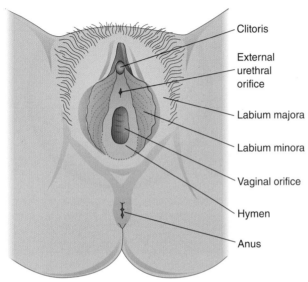

Fig. 2.3 External female genitalia. The labia are spread apart to show the external urethral and vaginal orifices.

MEIOSIS

Meiosis consists of two meiotic cell divisions (Fig. 2.6), during which the chromosome number of the germ cells is reduced to half (23, the **haploid** number) of the number in other cells in the body (46, the **diploid** number).

During the first meiotic division **homologous chromosomes** (one from each parent) pair during prophase and then separate during **anaphase**, with one representative of each pair randomly going to each pole of the **meiotic spindle**. The spindle connects to the chromosome at the **centromere** (see Fig. 2.6B). At this stage, they are **double chromatid chromosomes**. The X and Y chromosomes are not homologs; however, they have homologous segments at the tips of their short arms. They pair in these regions only. By the end of the first meiotic division, each new cell formed (**secondary spermatocyte** or **secondary oocyte**) has the haploid chromosome number of double chromatid chromosomes; therefore each cell contains half the number of chromosomes of the preceding cell (primary spermatocyte or primary oocyte). This **disjunction**, of paired homologous chromosomes is the physical basis of segregation, or separation, of allelic genes during meiosis.

The second meiotic division follows the first division, without a normal interphase (i.e., without an intervening step of DNA replication). Each double chromatid chromosome divides, and each half, or **chromatid**, is randomly drawn to a different pole of the meiotic spindle; thus the haploid number (23) of chromosomes is retained. Each daughter cell formed by meiosis has the reduced haploid number of chromosomes, with one representative of each chromosome pair (now a single chromatid chromosome).

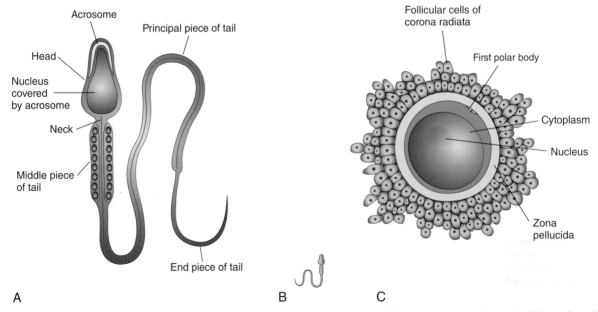

Fig. 2.4 Male and female gametes (germ cells). (A) The parts of a human sperm (×1250). The head, composed mostly of the nucleus, is partly covered by the acrosome, an organelle containing enzymes. (B) A sperm drawn to approximately the same scale as the oocyte. (C) The human secondary oocyte (×200) is surrounded by the zona pellucida and corona radiata.

NORMAL GAMETOGENESIS

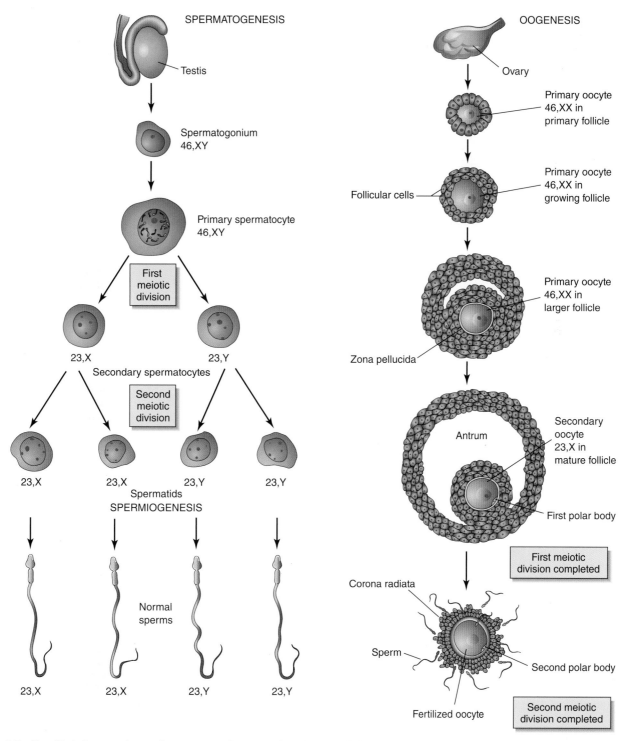

Fig. 2.5 Simplified diagram of normal gametogenesis: conversion of germ cells into gametes. The illustrations compare spermatogenesis and oogenesis. Oogonia are not shown in this figure because they differentiate into primary oocytes before birth. The chromosome complement of the germ cells is shown at each stage. The number designates the total number of chromosomes, including sex chromosome(s) (shown after the comma). Note: (1) After the two meiotic divisions, the diploid number of chromosomes, 46, is reduced to the haploid number, 23; (2) four sperms form from one primary spermatocyte, whereas only one secondary oocyte results from maturation of a primary oocyte; and (3) the cytoplasm is conserved during oogenesis to form one large cell, the oocyte.

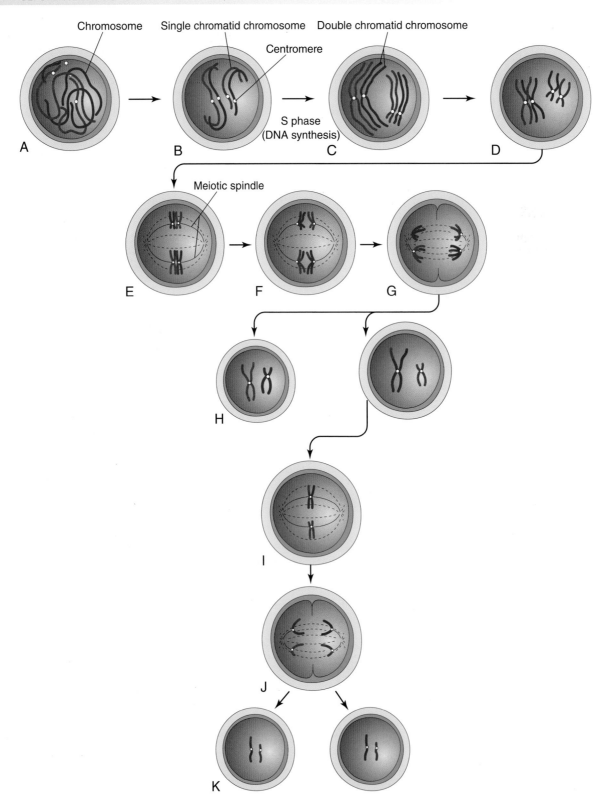

Fig. 2.6 Diagrammatic representation of meiosis. Two chromosome pairs are shown. (A–D) Stages of prophase of the first meiotic division. The homologous chromosomes approach each other and pair; each member of the pair consists of two chromatids. Observe the single crossover in one pair of chromosomes, resulting in the interchange of chromatid segments. (E) Metaphase. The two members of each pair become oriented on the meiotic spindle. (F) Anaphase. (G) Telophase. The chromosomes migrate to opposite poles. (H) Distribution of parental chromosome pairs at the end of the first meiotic division. (I–K) Second meiotic division, which is similar to mitosis, except that the cells are haploid.

Meiosis:

- Provides for *constancy of the chromosome number* from generation to generation by reducing the chromosome number from diploid to haploid, thereby producing haploid gametes.
- Allows *random assortment of maternal and paternal chromosomes* between the gametes.
- Relocates segments of maternal and paternal chromosomes by *crossing over of chromosome segments*, which "shuffles" the genes and produces a recombination of genetic material.

SPERMATOGENESIS

Before puberty, **spermatogonia** (primordial sperms) remain dormant in the seminiferous tubules of the testes from the late fetal period. At puberty they begin to increase in number. After several mitotic cell divisions, the sperms grow and undergo gradual changes that transform them into **primary spermatocytes**—the largest germ cells in the seminiferous tubules (see Fig. 2.5). Each primary spermatocyte subsequently undergoes a reduction division—the first meiotic division—to form two haploid **secondary spermatocytes**, which are approximately half the size of primary spermatocytes (see Fig. 2.5). Subsequently, the secondary spermatocytes undergo a second meiotic division to form four haploid **spermatids**, which are approximately half the size of secondary spermatocytes. The spermatids are gradually transformed into four **mature sperms** during a process known as **spermiogenesis** (see Fig. 2.5).

During spermiogenesis, the nucleus of the spermatid condenses and the **acrosome** forms (see Fig. 2.4A). The acrosome contains enzymes that facilitate the sperm's penetration of the oocyte zona pellucida (see Fig. 3.1). When spermiogenesis is complete, sperms enter the lumina of the **seminiferous tubules** (see Fig. 2.1B). The sperms then move to the **epididymis**, where they are stored and become functionally mature. Spermatogenesis requires approximately 2 months for completion. It is regulated by testosterone signaling through androgens in the Sertoli cells. Spermatogenesis normally continues throughout the reproductive life of a male.

When ejaculated, the mature sperms are free-swimming, actively motile cells consisting of a **head** and a **tail** (see Fig. 2.4A). The **neck** of the sperm is the junction between the head and tail. The head of the sperm, forming most of the bulk of the sperm, contains the nucleus. The anterior two-thirds of the head are covered by the **acrosome**, a cap-like organelle containing enzymes that facilitate sperm penetration during fertilization. The tail provides the motility of the sperm, assisting with its transport to the site of fertilization in the ampulla of the uterine tube. The tail of the sperm consists of three parts: middle piece, principal piece, and end piece. The middle piece contains the energy-producing **mitochondria**, which fuel the lashing movements of the tail. Hox *genes influence microtube dynamics at the molecular level in shaping the head of the sperm and in the formation of the tail.*

OOGENESIS

Oogenesis refers to the sequence of events by which **oogonia** (primordial oocytes) are transformed into primary **oocytes**. The maturation process begins during the fetal period; however, it is not completed until after puberty. During early fetal life, oogonia proliferate by mitosis and enlarge to form **primary oocytes** (see Fig. 2.5). At birth, all primary oocytes have completed prophase of the first meiotic division (see Fig. 2.6). The oocytes remain in prophase until puberty. Shortly before ovulation, a primary oocyte completes the **first meiotic division**. Unlike the corresponding stage of spermatogenesis, the division of cytoplasm is unequal (see Fig. 2.5). The **secondary oocyte** receives almost all the cytoplasm, whereas the **first polar body** receives very little, causing it to degenerate after a short time. At **ovulation**, the nucleus of the secondary oocyte begins the second meiotic division but progresses only to the metaphase.

If the secondary oocyte is fertilized by a sperm, the second meiotic division is completed, and a **second polar body** is formed (see Fig. 2.5). The secondary oocyte released at ovulation is surrounded by a covering of amorphous material—the **zona pellucida**—and a layer of follicular cells—the **corona radiata** (see Fig. 2.4C). The **secondary oocyte** is large, being just visible to the unaided eye.

Up to 2 million primary oocytes are usually present in the ovaries of a neonate. Most of these oocytes regress during childhood so that, by puberty, no more than 40,000 remain. Of these, only *approximately 400 oocytes mature into secondary oocytes and are expelled at ovulation* (see Fig. 2.5).

COMPARISON OF MALE AND FEMALE GAMETES

Compared with sperms, the oocytes are massive, are immotile, and have an abundance of cytoplasm (see Fig. 2.4B and C). In terms of sex chromosome constitution, **there are two kinds of sperms** (see Fig. 2.5): 22 autosomes plus either an X sex chromosome (i.e., 23,X) or a Y sex chromosome (i.e., 23,Y). **There is only one kind of secondary oocyte**: 22 autosomes plus an X sex chromosome (i.e., 23,X). *The difference in sex chromosome complement forms the basis of primary sex determination.*

Abnormal Gametogenesis

During gametogenesis, homologous chromosomes sometimes fail to separate—**nondisjunction**—and as a result, some gametes have 24 chromosomes and others only 22 (Fig. 2.7). If a gamete with 24 chromosomes unites with a normal one with 23 chromosomes, a zygote with 47 chromosomes results, as occurs in neonates with **Down syndrome** (see Fig. 19.4). This condition is called **trisomy** because of the presence of three representatives of a particular chromosome instead of the usual two. If a gamete with only 22 chromosomes unites with a normal gamete, a zygote with 45 chromosomes results. This condition—**monosomy**—occurs because only one representative of the particular chromosomal pair is present. Monosomic blastocysts usually fail to implant; most embryos and fetuses with monosomy will die.

ABNORMAL GAMETOGENESIS

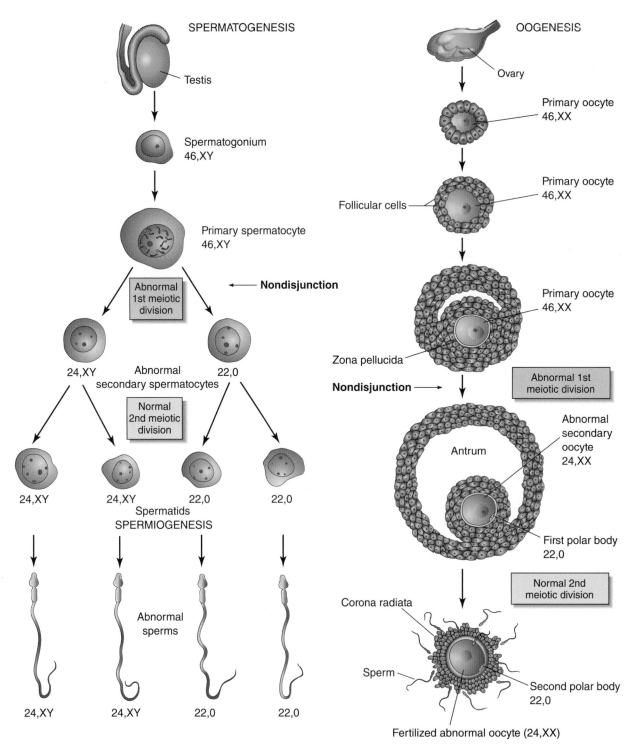

Fig. 2.7 Abnormal gametogenesis. The illustrations show how nondisjunction, an error in cell division, results in an abnormal chromosome distribution in gametes. Although nondisjunction of sex chromosomes is illustrated, a similar defect may occur during the division of autosomes (any chromosomes other than sex chromosomes). When nondisjunction occurs during the first meiotic division of spermatogenesis, one secondary spermatocyte contains 22 autosomes plus an X and a Y chromosome, whereas the other one contains 22 autosomes and no sex chromosome. Similarly, nondisjunction during oogenesis may give rise to an oocyte with 22 autosomes and two X chromosomes (as shown) or one with 22 autosomes and no sex chromosome.

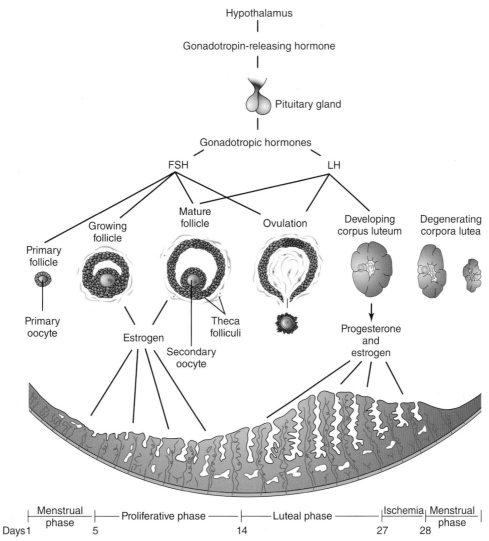

Fig. 2.8 Illustrations of the interrelationships among the hypothalamus, pituitary gland, ovaries, and endometrium. One complete menstrual cycle and the beginning of another are shown. *FSH*, Follicle-stimulating hormone; *LH*, luteinizing hormone.

FEMALE REPRODUCTIVE CYCLES

Beginning at menarche (first menstrual period), females undergo monthly reproductive cycles regulated by the **hypothalamus**, **pituitary gland**, and **ovaries** (Fig. 2.8). These cycles prepare the reproductive system for pregnancy. **Gonadotropin-releasing hormone** is synthesized by neurosecretory cells in the hypothalamus. It stimulates the release of two hormones (gonadotropins), which are produced by the anterior pituitary and act on the ovaries:

- **Follicle-stimulating hormone (FSH)** stimulates the development of ovarian follicles and the production of **estrogen** by the follicular cells.
- **Luteinizing hormone (LH)** serves as the "trigger" for ovulation and stimulates the follicular cells and corpus luteum to produce **progesterone**.

Estrogen and progesterone also produce the growth of the endometrium.

OVARIAN CYCLE

FSH and LH produce cyclic changes in the ovaries (development of ovarian follicles, ovulation, and formation of the corpus luteum), collectively known as the **ovarian cycle**. During each cycle, FSH promotes the growth of several primary follicles (Fig. 2.9; also see Fig. 2.8); however, only one of them usually develops into a mature follicle and ruptures, expelling its oocyte (Fig. 2.10).

FOLLICULAR DEVELOPMENT

Development of an ovarian follicle (see Figs. 2.8 and 2.9) is characterized by:

- Growth and differentiation of a primary oocyte
- Proliferation of follicular cells
- Formation of the zona pellucida
- Development of a connective tissue capsule surrounding the follicle—**theca folliculi**. Thecal cells are believed to produce an **angiogenic factor** that promotes the growth of blood vessels that provide nutritive support for follicular development.

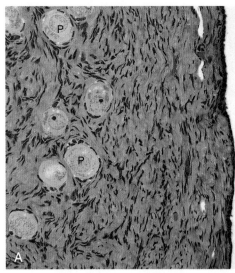
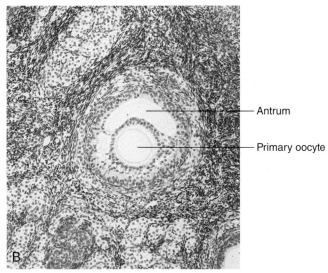

Fig. 2.9 Photomicrographs of sections from adult human ovaries. (A) Light micrograph of the ovarian cortex demonstrating primordial follicles (*P*), which are primary oocytes surrounded by follicular cells (×270). (B) Light micrograph of a secondary follicle. Observe the primary oocyte and antrum containing the follicular fluid (×132). From Gartner LP, Hiatt JL: *Color textbook of histology*, ed 2, Philadelphia, 2001, Saunders.

OVULATION

The **follicular cells** divide actively, producing a stratified layer around the oocyte (see Fig. 2.9A and B). Subsequently, fluid-filled spaces appear around the follicular cells, which coalesce to form a single cavity, the **antrum**, containing **follicular fluid** (see Fig. 2.9B). When the antrum forms, the ovarian follicle is called a **secondary follicle**. The primary oocyte is surrounded by follicular cells—the **cumulus oophorus**—that project into the enlarged antrum. The follicle continues to enlarge and soon forms a bulge on the surface of the ovary. A small oval, avascular spot, the **stigma**, soon appears on this bulge (see Fig. 2.10A). Before ovulation, the secondary oocyte and some cells of the cumulus oophorus detach from the interior of the distended follicle (see Fig. 2.10B).

Ovulation follows within 24 to 36 hours of a surge of LH production. This surge is elicited by a continuous high estrogen level in the blood (produced by granulosa cells), activating more frequent GnHR pulsing (Fig. 2.11). LH also appears to cause the stigma to rupture, expelling the secondary oocyte along with the follicular fluid (see Fig. 2.10D). Plasmins and matrix metalloproteinases also appear to have some control over stigma rupture.

The expelled secondary oocyte is surrounded by the **zona pellucida**, an acellular glycoprotein coat, and one or more layers of follicular cells, which are radially arranged to form the **corona radiata** and cumulus oophorus (see Fig. 2.4C).

Mittelschmerz and Ovulation

A variable amount of abdominal pain—*mittelschmerz*—accompanies ovulation in some females. Mittelschmerz may be used as a secondary **sign of ovulation**; however, there are better primary indicators, including slight elevation of basal body temperature, fertile cervical mucus, and change in the cervical position.

Anovulation and Hormones

Sometimes ovulation does not occur because of the inadequate release of gonadotropins. Anovulation is a common cause of infertility. In some situations, ovulation can be induced by the administration of **gonadotropins** or an ovulatory agent, resulting in the maturation of several ovarian follicles and multiple ovulations. The incidence of multiple pregnancies may increase when ovulation is induced.

Anovulatory Menstrual Cycles

In anovulatory cycles, the endometrial changes are minimal; the proliferative endometrium develops as usual, but ovulation does not occur and no **corpus luteum** forms (see Fig. 2.8). Consequently, the endometrium does not progress to the **luteal phase**; it remains in the proliferative phase until menstruation begins. The estrogen in **oral contraceptives**, with or without **progesterone**, suppresses ovulation by acting on the hypothalamus and pituitary gland; this inhibits secretion of gonadotropin-releasing hormone, FSH, and LH.

CORPUS LUTEUM

Shortly after ovulation, the ovarian follicle collapses (see Fig. 2.10D). Under the influence of LH, the walls of the follicle develop into a glandular structure, the **corpus luteum**, which secretes primarily progesterone and some estrogen. If the oocyte is fertilized, the corpus luteum enlarges to form a **corpus luteum of pregnancy** and increases its hormone production. Degeneration of the corpus luteum is prevented by **human chorionic gonadotropin** (hCG) produced by the developing placenta (see Chapter 4).

If the oocyte is not fertilized, the corpus luteum degenerates 10 to 12 days after ovulation (see Fig. 2.8). It is then called a **corpus luteum of menstruation**. The degenerated

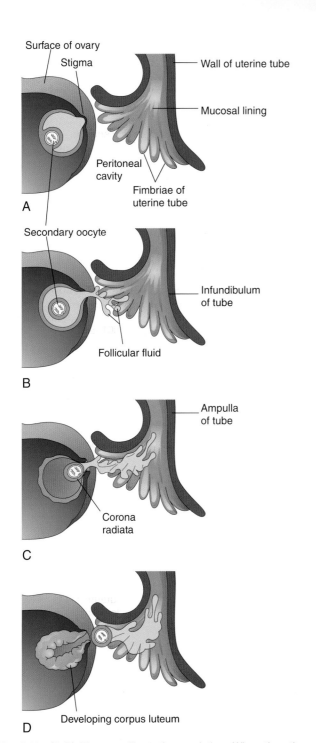

Fig. 2.10 (A–D) Diagrams illustrating ovulation. When the stigma ruptures, the secondary oocyte is expelled from the ovarian follicle with the follicular fluid. After ovulation, the wall of the follicle collapses.

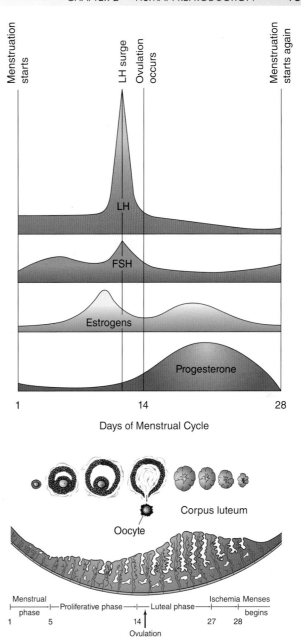

Fig. 2.11 Blood levels of various hormones during the menstrual cycle. Follicle-stimulating hormone (*FSH*) stimulates the ovarian follicles to develop and produce estrogens. The level of estrogens rises to a peak just before the luteinizing hormone (*LH*) surge induces ovulation. Ovulation normally occurs approximately 24 to 36 hours after the LH surge. If fertilization does not occur, the blood levels of circulating estrogens and progesterone fall. This hormone withdrawal causes the endometrium to regress and menstruation to start again.

corpus luteum is subsequently transformed into white scar tissue in the ovary, forming the **corpus albicans**.

MENSTRUAL CYCLE

The cycle is the period of time during which the oocyte matures, is ovulated, and enters the uterine tube (see Figs. 2.10D and 2.11). Estrogen and progesterone produced by

the ovarian follicles and corpus luteum cause **cyclic changes in the endometrium** of the uterus. These monthly changes in the uterine lining constitute the **menstrual cycle**. The average cycle length is 28 days (ranging from 23 to 35 days). Day 1 of the cycle corresponds to the day on which menstruation begins.

PHASES OF MENSTRUAL CYCLE

The cycle is divided into three main phases for descriptive purposes only (see Fig. 2.11). In actuality, *the menstrual cycle is a continuous process;* each phase gradually passes into the next one. The cycles normally continue until the permanent cessation of the menses; **menopause** usually occurs between the ages of 48 and 55 years.

Menstrual Phase

The first day of menstruation is the beginning of the menstrual phase. The functional layer of the uterine wall is sloughed off and discarded with the menstrual flow, which usually lasts for 4 to 5 days. The menstrual flow (menses) consists of varying amounts of blood combined with small pieces of endometrial tissue. After menstruation, the eroded endometrium is thin (see Figs. 2.8 and 2.11).

Proliferative Phase

This phase, lasting approximately 9 days, coincides with the growth of the ovarian follicles and is controlled by estrogen secreted by the follicles. There is a two- to threefold increase in the thickness of the endometrium during this time (see Fig. 2.8). Early during this phase, the surface epithelium of the endometrium regenerates. The glands increase in number and length, and the spiral arteries elongate (see Fig. 2.2B and C).

Luteal Phase

The luteal (secretory) phase, lasting approximately 13 days, coincides with the formation, function, and growth of the **corpus luteum** (see Fig. 2.8). The progesterone produced by the corpus luteum stimulates the glandular epithelium to secrete a glycogen-rich, mucoid material. The **uterine glands** become wide, tortuous, and saccular (see Fig. 2.2C). The endometrium thickens because of the influence of progesterone and estrogen from the corpus luteum and the increase in fluid in the connective tissue (see Fig. 2.8).

If fertilization does not occur:

- The corpus luteum degenerates.
- Estrogen and progesterone levels decrease, and the endometrium undergoes ischemia.
- Menstruation occurs.

Ischemia of the **spiral arteries** occurs by constriction resulting from the decrease in the secretion of progesterone (see Fig. 2.2C). Hormone withdrawal also results in the stoppage of glandular secretions, a loss of interstitial fluid, and a marked shrinking of the endometrium. As the spiral arteries constrict for longer periods, **stasis** (stagnation of blood and other fluids) and patchy ischemic **necrosis** in the superficial tissues occur. Eventually, the rupture of vessel walls follows, and blood seeps into the surrounding connective tissue. Small pools of blood form and break through the endometrial surface, resulting in bleeding into the uterus and vagina.

As small pieces of the endometrium detach and pass into the uterine cavity, the torn ends of the spiral arteries bleed into the uterine cavity, resulting in an accumulated loss of 20 to 80 mL of blood. Over 3 to 5 days, the entire compact layer and most of the spongy layer of the endometrium are discarded.

If fertilization occurs:

- Cleavage of the zygote and formation of the blastocyst occur.

- The blastocyst begins to implant on approximately the sixth day of the luteal phase (see Fig. 4.1A).
- hCG maintains secretion of estrogens and progesterone by the corpus luteum.
- The luteal phase continues, and menstruation does not occur.

The menstrual cycles cease during pregnancy, and the endometrium passes into a **pregnancy phase**. With the termination of pregnancy, the ovarian and menstrual cycles resume after a variable amount of time.

TRANSPORTATION OF GAMETES

OOCYTE TRANSPORT

During ovulation, the fimbriated end of the uterine tube comes in close proximity to the ovary (see Fig. 2.10A). The finger-like processes of the tube—**fimbriae**—move back and forth over the ovary. The sweeping action of the fimbriae and the fluid currents produced by them "sweep" the secondary oocyte into the funnel-shaped **infundibulum** of the uterine tube (see Figs. 2.2B and 2.10B). The oocyte passes into the **ampulla** of the tube (see Fig. 2.10B and D), primarily as a result of waves of peristalsis—movements of the wall of the tube characterized by alternate contraction and relaxation.

SPERM TRANSPORT

During ejaculation, sperms are rapidly transported from their storage in the **epididymis** to the urethra by peristaltic contractions of the **ductus deferens** (see Fig. 2.1B). Sperms and secretions from the seminal glands, prostate, and bulbourethral glands form the semen (ejaculate). The number of sperms ejaculated ranges from 200 to 600 million. The sperms pass slowly through the cervical canal by the movements of their tails (see Fig. 2.4A). Vesiculase, an enzyme produced by the seminal glands, coagulates some of the semen and forms a **cervical plug** in the external os that may prevent the backflow of semen into the vagina. At the time of ovulation, the amount of cervical mucus increases and becomes less viscid, making it more favorable for sperm transport. Prostaglandins in the semen stimulate uterine motility and help to move the sperms through the uterus to the site of fertilization in the **ampulla** of the uterine tube (see Figs. 2.2B and 2.10C).

The sperms move 2 to 3 mm per minute. They move slowly in the acidic environment of the vagina but more rapidly in the alkaline environment of the uterus. Approximately 200 sperms reach the ampulla for fertilization.

Sperm Counts

Semen analysis is an important part of evaluating patients for infertility. Sperms account for less than 5% of the volume of semen. The remainder of the ejaculate consists of secretions of the seminal glands (60%), prostate (30%), and bulbourethral glands (5%). The ejaculate of normal males usually contains more than 100 million sperms per milliliter of semen. Although there is much variation in individual cases, males whose semen contains a minimum of 20 million sperms per milliliter, or 50 million in the total specimen, are probably fertile. A male with fewer than 10 million sperms per milliliter is likely to be sterile, especially when the specimen contains immotile and abnormal sperms. For potential fertility, at least 40% of the sperms should be motile after 2 hours and some should be motile after 24 hours. Male infertility may result from endocrine disorders, abnormal spermatogenesis, reduced levels of seminal plasma proteins, or obstruction of a genital duct (e.g., the ductus deferens). Male infertility is found in approximately 60% of involuntarily childless couples. Computer-assisted sperm morphometric analysis and fluorescence probes provide a more objective and rapid assessment of the ejaculate. Guidelines for semen analysis are provided in the World Health Organization Laboratory Manual for the Examination and Processing of Human Semen, 6th edition, 2021.

Vasectomy

An effective method of contraception in males is **vasectomy**—excision of a segment of the ductus deferens (Fig. 2.1B). Eighty percent of males have no sperm detected at the time of the 3-month postvasectomy semen test; the amount of seminal fluid is the same as before the procedure.

MATURATION OF SPERMS

Freshly ejaculated sperms are unable to fertilize oocytes. They must undergo a period of conditioning—**capacitation**—lasting approximately 7 hours. During this period, a glycoprotein coat and seminal proteins are removed from the **acrosome**, which partly covers the nucleus of the sperm (see Fig. 2.4A). *Capacitation and acrosome reaction are regulated by src kinase, a tyrosine kinase.* Capacitated sperms show no morphological changes, but they exhibit increased activity. Sperms are usually capacitated in the uterus or the uterine tubes by substances (including interleukin-6) secreted by these organs.

VIABILITY OF OOCYTES AND SPERMS

Oocytes in the uterine tube are usually fertilized within 12 hours of ovulation. In vitro observations have shown that oocytes cannot be fertilized after 24 hours, and they degenerate shortly thereafter. Most sperms do not survive for more than 24 hours in the female genital tract. Some sperms are captured in folds of the mucosa of the cervix and are gradually released into the cervical canal and pass through the body of the uterus into the uterine tubes. Semen and oocytes can be frozen and stored for many years to be used in assisted reproduction.

CLINICALLY ORIENTED QUESTIONS

1. There have been reports of a female who claimed that she menstruated throughout her pregnancy. How could this happen?

2. If a female forgets to take an oral contraceptive and then takes two doses, is she likely to become pregnant?

3. What is *coitus interruptus*? Is it an effective method of birth control?

4. What is the difference between spermatogenesis and spermiogenesis?

5. Is an intrauterine device a contraceptive? Explain.

The answers to these questions are at the back of this book.

First Week of Human Development

3

Development begins at fertilization, when a sperm penetrates an oocyte to form a zygote. A zygote is a highly specialized, totipotent cell—a cell with the ability to differentiate into any type of cell. It contains chromosomes and genes derived from the mother and father. The zygote divides many times and is progressively transformed into a multicellular human being through cell division, migration, growth, and differentiation (see Fig. 1.1, first week).

FERTILIZATION

The usual site of fertilization is in the **ampulla** of the **uterine tube** (see Fig. 2.2B). If the oocyte is not fertilized, it slowly passes along the tube into the cavity of the uterus, where it degenerates. Fertilization is a complex sequence of coordinated physical and molecular events (Fig. 3.1) that begins with the contact between a sperm and an oocyte (Fig. 3.2). Fertilization ends with the intermingling of maternal and paternal chromosomes at the **metaphase** of the first mitotic division of the **zygote** (see Fig. 2.6). Carbohydrate- and protein-binding molecules on the surface of the **gametes** (oocyte or sperm) are involved in sperm **chemotaxis** (movement of cells), gamete recognition, and in the process of fertilization (see Fig. 3.1).

PHASES OF FERTILIZATION

The phases of fertilization follow (Fig. 3.3; also see Fig. 3.2):

- *Passage of a sperm through the corona radiata of the oocyte.* Dispersal of the follicular cells of the corona radiata results mainly from the action of the enzyme hyaluronidase, which is released from the acrosome of the sperm. Tubal mucosal enzymes also appear to assist hyaluronidase. Additionally, movements of the tail of the sperm are important during penetration of the **corona radiata**.
- *Penetration of the zona pellucida.* The formation of a pathway through the **zona pellucida** for the sperm results from the action of enzymes released from the acrosome. The proteolytic enzyme acrosin, as well as esterases and neuraminidase, appears to cause lysis of the zona pellucida, thereby forming a path for the sperm to follow to the oocyte.
- *Fusion of the plasma cell membranes of the oocyte and sperm.* Once fusion occurs, the contents of cortical granules from the oocyte are released into the perivitelline space, between the oocyte and zona pellucida, resulting in changes in the zona pellucida. These changes prevent other sperms from entering. The cell membranes break down at the area of

fusion. The head and tail of the sperm then enter the cytoplasm of the oocyte, but the plasma membrane and mitochondria of the sperm remain behind (see Figs. 3.2 and 3.3A). Sperm phospholipase C-zeta causes calcium concentration changes, triggering cell cycling in the egg.

- *Completion of the second meiotic division of the oocyte.* The oocyte completes the second meiotic division and forms a **mature oocyte** and a second polar body (see Fig. 3.3A). The nucleus of the mature oocyte becomes the female pronucleus.
- *Formation of the male pronucleus.* Within the cytoplasm of the oocyte, the sperm chromatin undergoes decondensation to form the male pronucleus. The tail of the sperm degenerates (see Fig. 3.3B). During growth, the male and female pronuclei replicate their DNA (see Fig. 3.3C).
- *Breakdown of the pronuclear membranes.* Condensation of the chromosomes, arrangement of the chromosomes for mitotic cell division, and the first cleavage division of the zygote occur (Figs. 3.3D and 3.4A). The combination of 23 chromosomes in each pronucleus results in a zygote with 46 chromosomes.

RESULTS OF FERTILIZATION

Fertilization:

- Stimulates the secondary oocyte to complete the second meiotic division, producing the second polar body (Fig. 3.3A)
- Restores the normal diploid number of chromosomes (46) in the zygote
- Results in variation of the human species through mingling of maternal and paternal chromosomes
- Determines the chromosomal sex of the embryo; an X-bearing sperm produces a female embryo and a Y-bearing sperm produces a male embryo
- Causes metabolic activation of the oocyte, which initiates cleavage of the zygote.

The zygote is genetically unique because half of its chromosomes come from the mother and half are derived from the father. This mechanism forms the basis for **biparental inheritance** and variation in the human species. Meiosis allows independent assortment of maternal and paternal chromosomes among the germ cells. Crossing over of chromosomes, by relocating segments of the maternal and paternal chromosomes, "shuffles" the genes, thereby producing a recombination of genetic material (see Fig. 2.6). The term **conceptus** refers to the entire products of conception, which include the embryo from fertilization onward and its membranes (e.g., placenta).

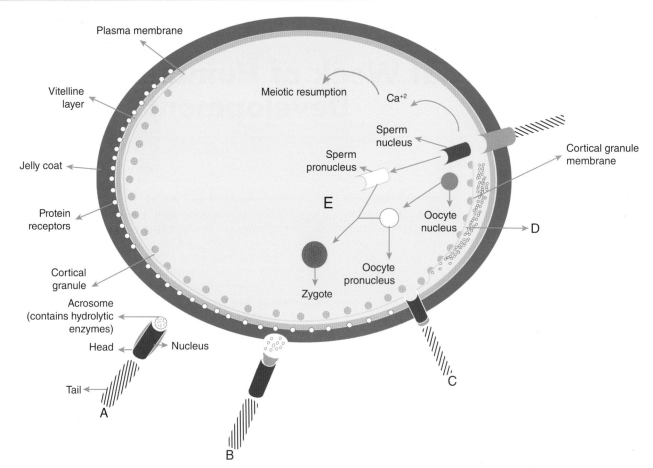

Fig. 3.1 The events taking place in fertilization. (A) Sperm preparation–capacitation: Molecules (resact, speract) secreted from the oocyte orient and stimulate sperm (guanylate cyclase). (B) Acrosome reaction: release of hydrolytic enzymes. The sperm via SED1 protein is connected to ZP3. (C) Fusion of sperm with the plasma membrane of the oocyte: sperm pre-acrosin binds to ZP2. Proteins of sperm IZUMO, ADAMs 1, ADAMs 2, ADAMs 3, and CRISP1 bind to receptors on the oocyte (Juno, integrins, CD9, CD81). Other molecules identified as playing roles in gamete fusion are as follows: trypsin-like acrosin, spermosin, SPAM1, HYAL5, and ACE3. (D) Cortical reaction: Ca^{+2} release/wave of Ca^{+2} and formation of fertilization cone. Enzymes released by cortical granules digest sperm receptors ZP2 and ZP3 (blocking polyspermy). (E) Sperm chromatin decondensation to form the male pronucleus: The oocyte nucleus completes the second meiosis and eliminates the second polar body. *From Georgadaki K, Khoury N, Spandidos D, Zoumpourlis V: The molecular basis of fertilization (review), Int J Mol Med 38:979–986, 2016.*

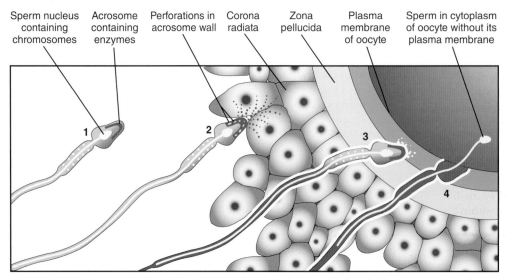

Fig. 3.2 Acrosome reaction and sperm penetration of an oocyte. 1: Sperm during capacitation. 2: Sperm undergoing the acrosome reaction. 3: Sperm forming a path through the zona pellucida. 4: Sperm entering the cytoplasm of the oocyte.

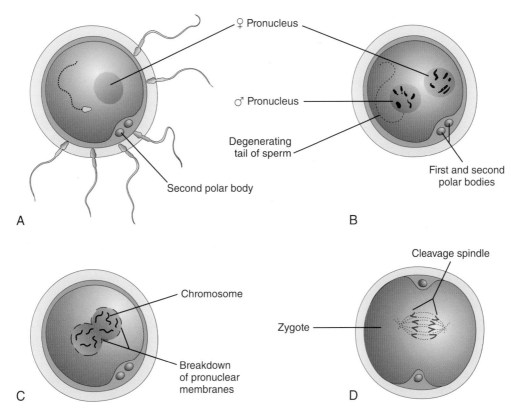

Fig. 3.3 Illustrations of fertilization. (A) A sperm has entered the oocyte and the second meiotic division has occurred, resulting in the formation of a mature oocyte. The nucleus of the oocyte is now the female pronucleus. (B) The sperm head has enlarged to form the male pronucleus. (C) The pronuclei are fusing. (D) The zygote has formed; it contains 46 chromosomes.

CLEAVAGE OF ZYGOTE

Cleavage consists of repeated mitotic divisions of the zygote, resulting in a rapid increase in the number of cells—**blastomeres**. Division of the zygote begins approximately 30 hours after fertilization (see Fig. 1.1). The blastomeres become smaller with each cleavage division (see Fig. 3.4A–D). During cleavage, the zygote is still surrounded by the zona pellucida.

After the eight-cell stage, the blastomeres change their shape and tightly align themselves against each other—**compaction**. This phenomenon may be mediated by cell surface adhesion glycoproteins and the formation of adherens junctions. Compaction permits greater cell-to-cell interaction and is a prerequisite for segregation of the internal cells that form the inner cell mass (see Fig. 3.4E). This also leads to the development of polarization of each blastomere with an apical and a basolateral domain. When there are 12 to 32 blastomeres, the conceptus is called a **morula**.

The inner cells of the morula—the **embryoblast** or **inner cell mass**—are surrounded by a layer of flattened blastomeres that form the trophoblast. *Hippo signaling is an essential factor in segregating the inner cell mass from the trophoblast.* An immunosuppressant protein—the **early pregnancy factor**—is secreted by the trophoblastic cells and appears in the maternal serum within 24 to 48 hours after implantation.

FORMATION OF BLASTOCYST

Shortly after the morula enters the uterus (about 4 days after fertilization), uterine fluid passes through the zona pellucida to form a fluid-filled space—the **blastocystic cavity**—inside the morula (see Fig. 3.4E). As fluid increases in the cavity, the blastomeres are separated into two parts:

- The **trophoblast**, the thin outer cells that give rise to the embryonic part of the placenta
- The **embryoblast**, a discrete group of blastomeres that is the primordium of the embryo

During this stage of development—**blastogenesis**—the conceptus is called a **blastocyst**. The embryoblast now projects into the **blastocystic cavity**, and the trophoblast forms the wall of the blastocyst (see Fig. 3.4E and F). After the blastocyst has floated in the uterine fluid for approximately 2 days, the zona pellucida degenerates and disappears. Shedding of the zona pellucida has been observed in vitro. The shedding permits the blastocyst to increase rapidly in size. While floating freely in the uterine cavity, the blastocyst derives nourishment from secretions of the uterine glands.

Approximately 6 days after fertilization, the blastocyst attaches to the endometrial epithelium (Fig. 3.5A). As soon as it attaches to the epithelium, the trophoblast starts to proliferate rapidly and differentiate into two layers (see Fig. 3.5B):

- The **cytotrophoblast**, the inner layer of cells
- The **syncytiotrophoblast**, the outer layer consisting of a multinucleate protoplasmic mass formed by the fusion of cells.

The finger-like processes of the syncytiotrophoblast extend through the endometrial epithelium and invade the

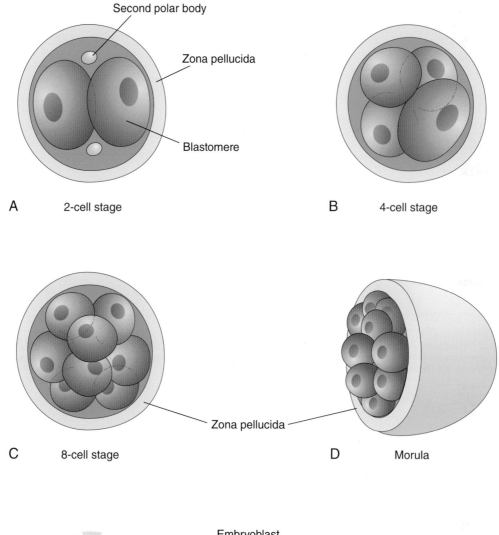

Second polar body

Zona pellucida

Blastomere

A   2-cell stage

B   4-cell stage

Zona pellucida

C   8-cell stage

D   Morula

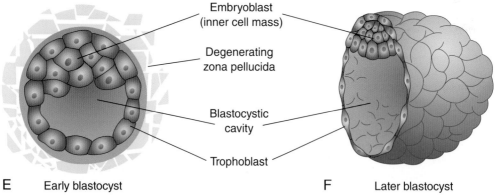

Embryoblast
(inner cell mass)

Degenerating
zona pellucida

Blastocystic
cavity

Trophoblast

E   Early blastocyst

F   Later blastocyst

Fig. 3.4 Illustrations showing cleavage of the zygote and formation of the blastocyst. (A–D) show various stages of cleavage. The period of the morula begins at the 12- to 32-cell stage and ends when the blastocyst forms. (E and F) show sections of blastocysts. The zona pellucida disappears by the late blastocyst stage (5 days). Although cleavage increases the number of blastomeres, note that each of the daughter cells is smaller than the parent cells. As a result, there is no increase in the size of the developing embryo until the zona pellucida degenerates. The blastocyst then enlarges considerably (E and F).

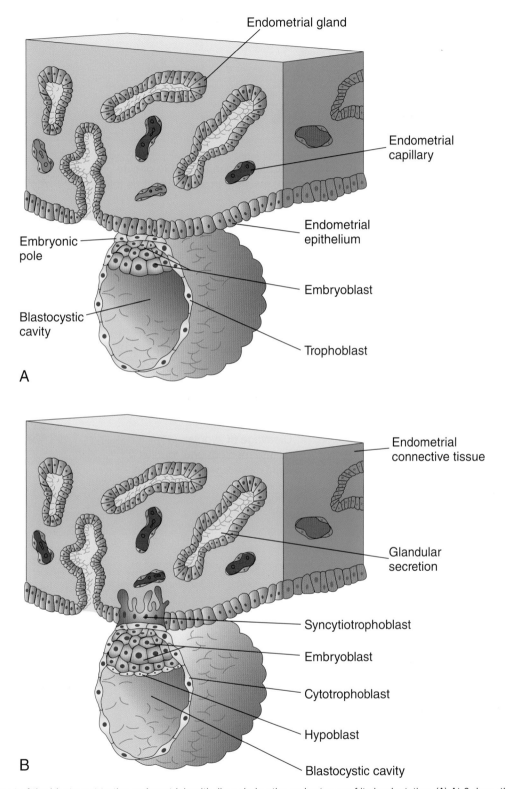

Fig. 3.5 Attachment of the blastocyst to the endometrial epithelium during the early stages of its implantation. (A) At 6 days, the trophoblast is attached to the endometrial epithelium at the embryonic pole of the blastocyst. (B) At 7 days, the syncytiotrophoblast has penetrated the epithelium and has started to invade the endometrial connective tissue.

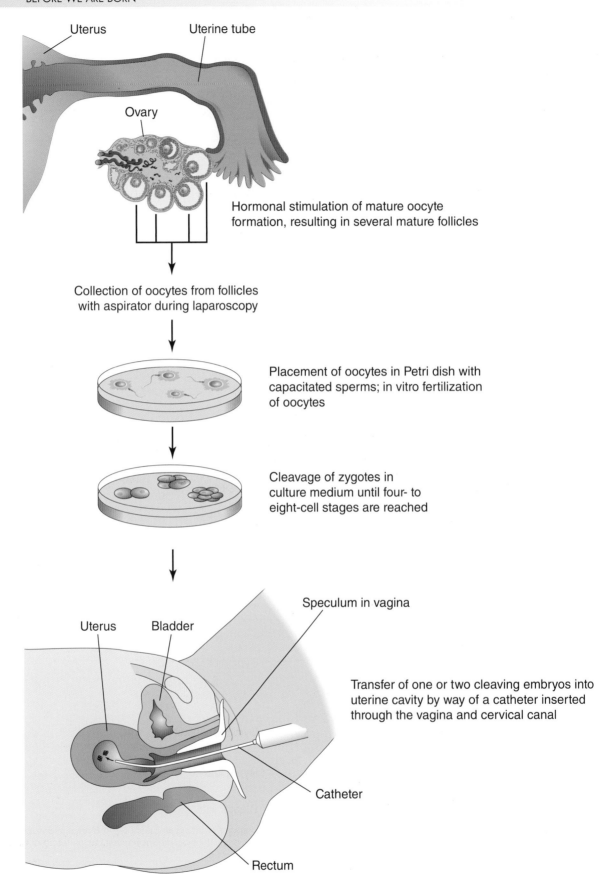

Uterus   Uterine tube

Ovary

Hormonal stimulation of mature oocyte formation, resulting in several mature follicles

Collection of oocytes from follicles with aspirator during laparoscopy

Placement of oocytes in Petri dish with capacitated sperms; in vitro fertilization of oocytes

Cleavage of zygotes in culture medium until four- to eight-cell stages are reached

Speculum in vagina

Uterus   Bladder

Transfer of one or two cleaving embryos into uterine cavity by way of a catheter inserted through the vagina and cervical canal

Catheter

Rectum

Fig. 3.6 In vitro fertilization and embryo transfer procedures.

endometrial connective tissue. By the end of the first week, the blastocyst is superficially implanted in the compact layer of the endometrium and is deriving its nourishment from the eroded maternal tissues. The highly invasive syncytiotrophoblast rapidly expands adjacent to the embryoblast—the **embryonic pole** (see Fig. 3.5A). The syncytiotrophoblast produces proteolytic enzymes that erode the maternal tissues, enabling the blastocyst to "burrow" into the endometrium. At the end of the first week, a cuboidal layer of cells, called the **hypoblast**, appears on the surface of the embryoblast, facing the blastocystic cavity (see Fig. 3.5B). Decidual cells also help control the depth of penetration of the syncytiotrophoblast.

Preimplantation Diagnosis of Genetic Disorders

In couples with inherited genetic disorders, preimplantation genetic diagnosis is carried out to determine the genotype of the embryo and select a chromosomally healthy embryo for transfer to the mother. The indications for preimplantation genetic diagnosis include single-gene disorders, single mutations, translocations, and subchromosomal and other genetic abnormalities. Preimplantation genetic screening of all 23 chromosomes in older or infertile patients is carried out to secure an embryo with a normal karyotype that can be transferred and produce a healthy baby. The presence of cell-free fetal DNA in the maternal plasma of pregnant females, advances in genomic medicine, and newly introduced technologies have transformed the practice of preimplantation genetic diagnosis.

In Vitro Fertilization and Embryo Transfer

The process of in vitro fertilization (IVF) of oocytes and the transfer of either the dividing zygotes or a blastocyst into the uterus have provided an opportunity for many couples who are infertile. The first of these IVF babies was born in 1978. The steps involved in IVF and embryo transfer are summarized in Fig. 3.6. The incidence of multiple pregnancies is higher with IVF than when pregnancy results from normal ovulation. The incidence of spontaneous abortion of transferred embryos is also higher with IVF.

The technique of **intracytoplasmic sperm injection** involves injecting a sperm directly into the cytoplasm of the mature oocyte. This procedure is invaluable in cases of infertility resulting from blocked uterine tubes or *oligospermia* (reduced number of sperms).

Abnormal Embryos and Spontaneous Abortions

Many early embryos abort spontaneously. The early implantation stages of the blastocyst are critical periods of development that may fail to occur because of inadequate production of progesterone and estrogen by the corpus luteum (see Fig. 2.8). Clinicians occasionally see a patient whose last menstrual period was delayed by several days and whose last menstrual flow was unusually profuse. Very likely, such patients have had an early spontaneous abortion. *The overall early spontaneous abortion rate is believed to be 50% to 70% with clinically recognized rates of 25% to 30%.* Early spontaneous abortions occur for a variety of reasons, an important one being the presence of **chromosomal abnormalities**.

CLINICALLY ORIENTED QUESTIONS

1. Although females do not commonly become pregnant after they are 48 years old, very elderly males may still be fertile. Why is this? Is there an increased risk of Down syndrome or other congenital anomalies in the child when the father is older than 50 years of age?

2. Are there oral contraceptives for males? If not, what is the reason?

3. Is a polar body ever fertilized? If so, does the fertilized polar body give rise to a viable embryo?

4. What is the most common cause of spontaneous abortion during the first week of development?

5. When referring to a zygote, do the terms *cleavage* and *mitosis* mean the same thing?

6. How is the zygote nourished during the first week?

7. Is it possible to determine the sex of a cleaving zygote developing in vitro? If so, what medical reasons would there be for doing so?

The answers to these questions are at the back of this book.

Second Week of Human Development

Implantation of the blastocyst is completed during the second week of development. Cellular and molecular changes occur in the blastocyst, producing a **bilaminar embryonic disc** composed of two layers, the epiblast and hypoblast (Fig. 4.1A).

The **embryonic disc** gives rise to germ layers that form all the tissues and organs of the embryo. Extraembryonic structures forming during the second week include the amniotic cavity, amnion, **umbilical vesicle**, connecting stalk, and chorionic sac.

The molecular mechanisms of implantation involve synchronization between the invading blastocyst and a receptive endometrium. The window of implantation is relatively brief, 2 to 3 days, during which bone morphogenetic proteins (BMPs) are expressed in the endometrium and are essential for fertilization. The microvilli of endometrial cells, cell adhesion molecules (integrins), cytokines, prostaglandins, hormones (human chorionic gonadotropin [hCG] and progesterone), growth factors, cell–cell and cell–extracellular matrix communication enzymes (matrix metalloproteinase and protein kinase A), and Wnt signaling pathways play a role in making the endometrium receptive. Implantation is also modulated by tumor necrosis factor-alpha, an inflammatory cytokine, secreted by endometrial cells. These cells help to modulate the depth of penetration of the syncytiotrophoblast, which reaches a maximum at 9 to 12 weeks.

Implantation of the blastocyst is completed during the second week and normally occurs in the endometrium, usually superiorly in the posterior wall of the uterus. The actively erosive syncytiotrophoblast invades the endometrial connective tissue that supports the uterine capillaries and glands. As this occurs, the blastocyst slowly embeds itself in the endometrium. Syncytiotrophoblastic cells from this region displace endometrial cells in the central part of the implantation site. The endometrial cells undergo **apoptosis** (a form of programmed cell death), which facilitates implantation. Proteolytic enzymes produced by the syncytiotrophoblast are involved in this process. The uterine connective tissue cells around the implantation site become loaded with glycogen and lipids. Some of these cells—**decidual cells**—degenerate adjacent to the penetrating syncytiotrophoblast. The syncytiotrophoblast engulfs these degenerating cells, providing a rich source of embryonic nutrition. As the blastocyst implants, more trophoblast contacts the endometrium and continues to differentiate into two layers (see Fig. 4.1A):

- The cytotrophoblast, a layer of mononucleated cells that is mitotically active. It forms new trophoblastic cells that migrate into the increasing mass of syncytiotrophoblast, where they fuse and lose their cell membranes.

- The syncytiotrophoblast, a rapidly expanding, multinucleated mass in which no cell boundaries are discernible.

The syncytiotrophoblast produces a hormone, **human chorionic gonadotropin (hCG)**, that enters the maternal blood in the lacunae in the syncytiotrophoblast (see Fig. 4.1B). hCG maintains the development of spiral arteries in the myometrium and formation of the syncytiotrophoblast. It also forms the basis for most pregnancy tests. Highly sensitive assays are available for detecting hCG before the end of the second week.

FORMATION OF AMNIOTIC CAVITY, EMBRYONIC DISC, AND UMBILICAL VESICLE

As implantation of the blastocyst progresses, the embryoblast is transformed into a flattened, almost circular, bilaminar plate of cells—the **embryonic disc**—consisting of two layers (Fig. 4.2B; see also Fig. 4.1B):

- The pluripotent **epiblast**, the thicker layer, consisting of high, columnar cells related to the amniotic cavity
- The **hypoblast**, the thinner layer, consisting of small, cuboidal cells adjacent to the exocoelomic cavity

Concurrently, a small cavity appears in the embryoblast, which is the primordium of the **amniotic cavity** (see Fig. 4.1A). Soon, amnioblasts (amniogenic or amnion-forming cells) separate from the epiblast and organize to form a thin membrane, the **amnion**, which encloses the amniotic cavity.

The **epiblast** forms the floor of the amniotic cavity and is continuous peripherally with the amnion. The **hypoblast** forms the roof of the **exocoelomic cavity** and is continuous with the cells that migrated from the hypoblast to form the **exocoelomic membrane**. This membrane surrounds the blastocystic cavity and lines the internal surface of the cytotrophoblast.

The **exocoelomic membrane and cavity** soon become modified to form the **primary umbilical vesicle**. The embryonic disc then lies between the amniotic cavity and primary umbilical vesicle (see Fig. 4.1B). The outer layer of cells from the umbilical vesicle endoderm forms a layer of loosely arranged connective tissue, the **extraembryonic mesoderm** (see Fig. 4.1B).

As the amnion, embryonic disc, and primary umbilical vesicle form, **lacunae** (small spaces) appear in the syncytiotrophoblast (see Figs. 4.1B and 4.2). The lacunae are soon filled with a mixture of maternal blood from ruptured endometrial capillaries and cellular debris from eroded uterine

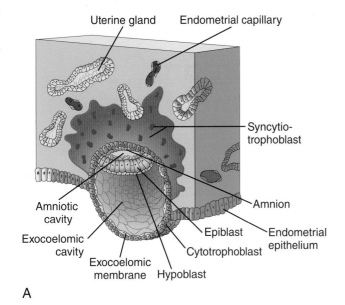

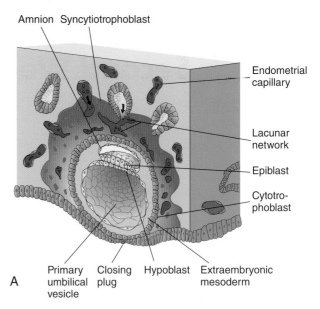

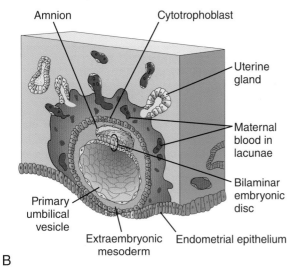

Fig. 4.1 Implantation of blastocyst. The actual size of the conceptus is approximately 0.1 mm. (A) Illustration of a section of a partially implanted blastocyst (approximately 8 days after fertilization). Note the slit-like amniotic cavity. (B) Illustration of a section through a blastocyst at approximately 9 days.

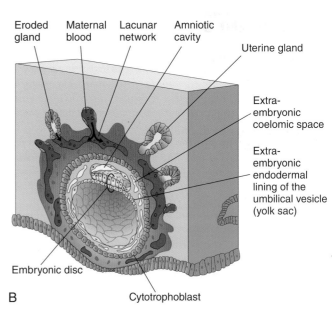

Fig. 4.2 Illustration of sections of two implanted blastocysts at 10 days (A) and 12 days (B).

glands. The fluid in the lacunae passes to the embryonic disc by diffusion. The communication of the eroded uterine vessels with the lacunae represents the beginning of the **primordial uteroplacental circulation**. When maternal blood flows into the lacunae, oxygen and nutritive substances become available to the extraembryonic tissues over the large surface of the syncytiotrophoblast. Oxygenated blood passes into the lacunae from the **spiral endometrial arteries** in the endometrium (see Fig. 2.2C); deoxygenated blood is removed from the lacunae through endometrial veins.

The 10-day conceptus is completely embedded in the endometrium (see Fig. 4.2A). For approximately 2 more days, there is a defect in the endometrial epithelium that is filled by a **closing plug**, a fibrinous coagulum of blood. By day 12, an almost completely regenerated uterine epithelium covers the closing plug (see Fig. 4.2B).

As the conceptus implants, the endometrial connective tissue cells undergo a transformation—the **decidual reaction**—resulting from cyclic adenosine monophosphate and progesterone signaling. The endometrial cells swell because of the accumulation of glycogen and lipid in their cytoplasm, and they are then called **secretory decidual cells**. The primary function of the decidual reaction is to provide an immunologically privileged site for the conceptus.

In the 12-day embryo, adjacent syncytiotrophoblastic lacunae have fused to form **lacunar networks** (see Fig. 4.2B), the primordia of the intervillous space of the placenta (see Chapter 8). The endometrial capillaries around the implanted embryo become congested and dilated to form sinusoids, which are thin-walled terminal vessels larger than ordinary capillaries. The syncytiotrophoblast then erodes the **sinusoids** and maternal blood flows into the lacunar networks. The degenerated endometrial stromal cells and glands, together with the maternal blood, provide a rich source of material for embryonic nutrition. Growth of the bilaminar embryonic disc is slow compared with the growth of the trophoblast.

As changes occur in the trophoblast and endometrium, the extraembryonic mesoderm increases and isolated **extraembryonic coelomic spaces** appear within it (see Fig. 4.2B). These spaces rapidly fuse to form a large, isolated cavity, the **extraembryonic coelom** (Fig. 4.3A). This fluid-filled cavity surrounds the amnion and umbilical vesicle, except where they are attached to the **chorion** by the **connecting stalk**. As the extraembryonic coelom forms, the primary umbilical vesicle decreases in size and a smaller, **secondary umbilical vesicle** forms (see Fig. 4.3B). During formation of the secondary umbilical vesicle, a large part of the **primary umbilical vesicle** is pinched off. The umbilical vesicle may have a role in the processing and selective transfer of nutritive materials from coelomic fluid to the embryonic disc.

DEVELOPMENT OF CHORIONIC SAC

The end of the second week is characterized by the appearance of **primary chorionic villi** (Fig. 4.4A and C; see also Fig. 4.3A). Proliferation of the cytotrophoblastic cells produces cellular extensions that grow into the overlying syncytiotrophoblast. The cellular projections form primary chorionic villi, the first stage in the development of the chorionic villi of the placenta. The extraembryonic coelom splits the extraembryonic mesoderm into two layers (see Fig. 4.3A):

- The *extraembryonic somatic mesoderm*, which lines the trophoblast and covers the amnion
- The *extraembryonic splanchnic mesoderm*, which surrounds the umbilical vesicle.

The growth of these cytotrophoblastic extensions is believed to be induced by the underlying **extraembryonic somatic mesoderm**. The extraembryonic somatic mesoderm and the two layers of trophoblast form the **chorion**. The chorion forms the wall of the chorionic sac (see Fig. 4.3A). The embryo, amniotic sac, and umbilical vesicle are suspended in the **chorionic cavity** by the connecting stalk (see Figs. 4.3B and 4.4B). Transvaginal ultrasonography (endovaginal sonography) is used to measure the diameter of the chorionic sac. This measurement is valuable for evaluating early embryonic development and pregnancy outcome.

IMPLANTATION SITES OF BLASTOCYSTS

Blastocysts usually implant in the uterine endometrium in the superior part of the body of the uterus, slightly more often on the posterior than on the anterior wall of the uterus (Fig. 4.5). Implantation of a blastocyst can be detected by ultrasonography at the end of the second week (Fig. 4.6).

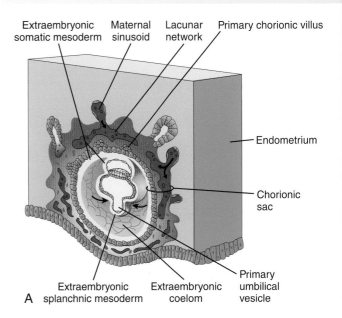

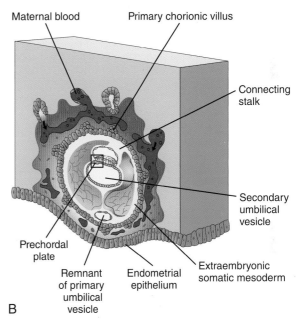

Fig. 4.3 Sections of implanted embryos. (A) At 13 days. Note the decrease in the relative size of the primary umbilical vesicle and the appearance of primary chorionic villi. (B) At 14 days. Note the newly formed secondary umbilical vesicle.

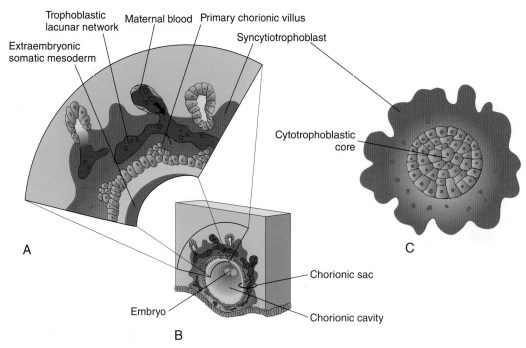

Fig. 4.4 (A) Illustration of a section of the wall of the chorionic sac. (B) Illustration of a 14-day conceptus showing the chorionic sac and the chorionic cavity. (C) Transverse section through a primary chorionic villus.

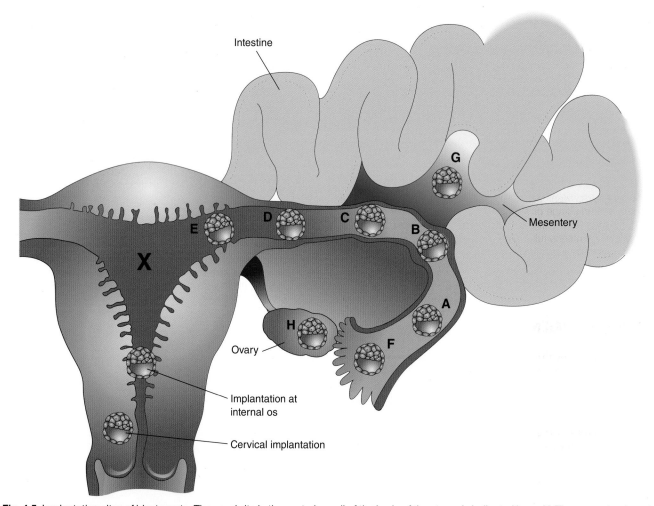

Fig. 4.5 Implantation sites of blastocysts. The usual site in the posterior wall of the body of the uterus is indicated by an X. The approximate order of frequency of ectopic implantations is indicated alphabetically (A, most common, H, least common). (A–F) Tubal pregnancies, (G) abdominal pregnancy, and (H) ovarian pregnancy. Tubal pregnancies are the most common type of ectopic pregnancy. Although appropriately included with uterine pregnancy sites, a cervical pregnancy is often considered to be an ectopic pregnancy.

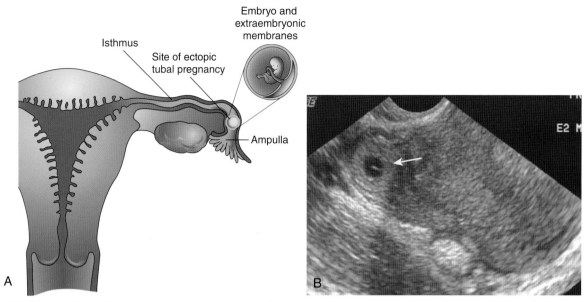

Fig. 4.6 (A) Coronal section of the uterus and uterine tube illustrating an ectopic pregnancy in the ampulla of the uterine tube. (B) Endovaginal axial scan of the uterine fundus and isthmic portion of the right uterine tube. The ring-like mass is a 4-week ectopic chorionic (gestational) sac in the tube *(arrow)*. **Source:** B, Courtesy E.A. Lyons, MD, Department of Radiology, Health Sciences Centre, University of Manitoba, Winnipeg, Manitoba, Canada.

Extrauterine Implantation Sites

Blastocysts sometimes implant outside the uterus. These implantations result in **ectopic pregnancies**; 95% to 98% of ectopic implantations occur in the uterine tubes, most often in the ampulla and isthmus (see Fig. 2.2B; see Fig. 4.6A and B). **Ectopic tubal pregnancy** occurs in 1% to 2% of pregnancies in North America. A tubal pregnancy has the usual signs and symptoms of pregnancy; however, additional symptoms such as abdominal pain (from distention of the uterine tube), abnormal bleeding, or irritation of the pelvic peritoneum may also occur.

The causes of tubal pregnancy are often related to factors that delay or prevent transport of the cleaving zygote to the uterus (e.g., blockage of the uterine tube). Ectopic tubal pregnancies may be managed medically with methotrexate, but rupture of the uterine tube and hemorrhage into the peritoneal cavity will require surgical intervention.

Inhibition of Implantation

The administration of progestins or antiprogestins (morning-after pills) for several days, beginning shortly after unprotected intercourse, prevents ovulation and may affect implantation of the blastocyst.

Using an **intrauterine device** (IUD) is a safe, reversible, and reliable method for the prevention of pregnancy. It is inserted into the uterus through the vagina, and the cervix usually interferes with implantation by causing a local inflammatory reaction. Although typically used as a primary contraceptive, IUDs may also be used for emergency contraception. Some IUDs contain slow-release progesterone, which interferes with the development of the endometrium by inhibiting critical molecular factors. Copper-based IUDs appear to inhibit migration of sperm in the tube, whereas long-term releasing levonorgestrel-based IUDs affect fertilization and also alter endometrial development.

CLINICALLY ORIENTED QUESTIONS

1. What is meant by the term *implantation bleeding*? Is this the same as *menses* (menstrual fluid)?

2. Can a drug taken during the first 2 weeks of pregnancy cause abortion of the embryo?

3. Can an ectopic pregnancy occur in a female who has an intrauterine device?

4. Can a blastocyst that implants in the abdomen develop into a full-term fetus?

The answers to these questions are at the back of this book.

Third Week of Human Development

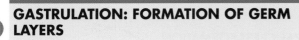

Rapid development of the embryo from the trilaminar embryonic disc during the third week is characterized by:

- Appearance of the primitive streak
- Development of the notochord
- Differentiation of three germ layers.

The third week of development occurs during the week of the first missed menstrual period, that is, 5 weeks LNMP (last normal menstrual period). Cessation of menstruation is often the first indication that a female may be pregnant. At approximately 5 weeks LNMP a normal pregnancy can be detected with transvaginal ultrasonography (Fig. 5.1).

GASTRULATION: FORMATION OF GERM LAYERS

Gastrulation is the process by which the bilaminar embryonic disc is converted into a **trilaminar embryonic disc** (Fig. 5.2A–H). Each of the three germ layers (**ectoderm, endoderm, and mesoderm**) of the embryonic disc gives rise to specific tissues and organs (see Fig. 6.4).

Gastrulation is the beginning of **morphogenesis**—development of body form and structure of various organs and parts of the body. It begins with the formation of the **primitive streak** (see Fig. 5.2B and C).

PRIMITIVE STREAK

At the beginning of the third week, the primitive streak appears on the dorsal aspect of the embryonic disc (see Fig. 5.2B). This thickened linear band results from the proliferation and migration of cells of the epiblast to the median plane of the embryonic disc (see Fig. 5.2D). As soon as the primitive streak appears, it is possible to identify the embryo's craniocaudal axis (cranial and caudal ends), dorsal and ventral surfaces, and right and left sides. As the primitive streak elongates by the addition of cells to its caudal end, its cranial end proliferates to form the **primitive node** (see Fig. 5.2E and F). Concurrently, a narrow **primitive groove** develops in the primitive streak that ends in a small depression in the primitive node, the **primitive pit** (see Fig. 5.2F).

Under the influence of various embryonic growth factors, including *bone morphogenetic protein signaling*, epiblast cells migrate through the **primitive groove** to become endoderm and mesoderm, a loose network of embryonic connective tissue known as mesenchyme (Fig. 5.3B and C; also see Fig. 5.2H) that forms the supporting tissues of the embryo. Mesenchymal cells have the potential to proliferate and differentiate into diverse types of cells, such as fibroblasts,

chondroblasts, and osteoblasts. *Recent studies indicate that signaling molecules (nodal factors) of the transforming growth factor-β superfamily, CDHI and FST, BMPs, SOX 17, SNAI2 genes, and other signaling molecules have been detected in the embryonic germ layers and induce the formation of mesoderm. The mesodermal progenitor cells are activated by Hox gene signaling, which is regulated by Tbx16 genes.*

The primitive streak actively forms mesoderm until the early part of the fourth week; thereafter, its production slows down. The streak diminishes in relative size and becomes an insignificant structure in the sacrococcygeal region of the embryo (Fig. 5.4A–D).

NOTOCHORDAL PROCESS AND NOTOCHORD

Some mesenchymal cells migrate cranially from the primitive node and pit, forming a median cellular cord, the **notochordal process (notochord)** (Fig. 5.5A–C; also see Figs. 5.2G and 5.4B–D). This process soon acquires a lumen, the **notochordal canal** (see Fig. 5.5C and D). The notochord grows cranially between the ectoderm and endoderm until it reaches the **prechordal plate**, a small, circular area of cells that is an important organizer of the head region (see Fig. 5.2C). The rod-like notochord can extend no farther because the prechordal plate is firmly attached to the overlying ectoderm. Fused layers of ectoderm and endoderm form the **oropharyngeal membrane** (Fig. 5.6C), located at the future site of the oral cavity (mouth).

Mesenchymal cells from the primitive streak and the notochordal process migrate laterally and cranially between the ectoderm and endoderm until they reach the margins of the embryonic disc. These mesenchymal cells are continuous with the extraembryonic mesoderm that covers the amnion and the umbilical vesicle (see Fig. 5.2D and F). Some cells from the primitive streak migrate cranially on each side of the notochordal process and around the prechordal plate. They meet cranially to form the cardiogenic mesoderm in the **cardiogenic area**, where the **heart primordium** begins to develop at the end of the third week (see Fig. 5.9B). Caudal to the primitive streak, there is a circular area—the **cloacal membrane**—that indicates the future site of the anus (see Fig. 5.5A and D).

The **notochord**:

- Defines the axis of the embryo and gives it some rigidity
- Serves as the basis for the development of the axial skeleton (such as the bones of the head and vertebral column)
- Indicates the future site of the vertebral bodies

.The **vertebral column** forms around the notochord, which extends from the oropharyngeal membrane to the

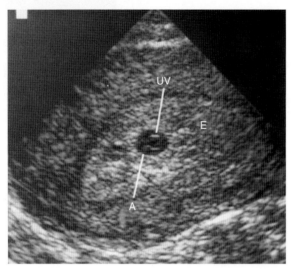

Fig. 5.1 Endovaginal ultrasonogram of a conceptus 3 weeks after conception implanted in the posterior endometrium, showing the umbilical vesicle. The endometrium completely surrounds the conceptus. *A*, Amnion; *UV*, umbilical sac; *E*, endometrium. Courtesy E.A. Lyons, MD, Professor of Radiology, and Obstetrics and Gynecology, and Anatomy, Health Sciences Centre and University of Manitoba, Winnipeg, Manitoba, Canada.

primitive node. The notochord degenerates and disappears as the bodies of the vertebrae form, but parts of it persist as the **nucleus pulposus** of each intervertebral disc. The notochord functions as the primary inductor in the early embryo. It induces the overlying embryonic ectoderm to thicken and form the **neural plate** (see Figs. 5.4B and C and 5.6A–C), the primordium of the central nervous system.

ALLANTOIS

The **allantois** appears on approximately day 16 as a small diverticulum from the caudal wall of the umbilical vesicle into the **connecting stalk** (see Figs. 5.5B–D and 5.6B). The allantois is involved with early blood formation and is associated with the urinary bladder as well. The blood vessels of the allantois become the umbilical arteries and veins.

NEURULATION: FORMATION OF THE NEURAL TUBE

16 Neurulation includes the formation of the neural plate and neural folds and closure of these folds to form the neural tube. These processes are completed by the end of the fourth week, when closure of the **caudal neuropore** occurs (see Fig. 6.11A and B).

NEURAL PLATE AND NEURAL TUBE

As the notochord develops, it induces the overlying embryonic ectoderm over it to thicken and form an elongated **neural plate** of thickened neuroepithelial cells, the neuroectoderm, which gives rise to the **central nervous system (CNS)—the brain and spinal cord** and other structures such as the retina. At first, the neural plate corresponds

in length to the underlying *notochord*. It appears cranial to the primitive node and dorsal to the notochord and the mesoderm adjacent to it (see Fig. 5.4B). As the notochord elongates, the neural plate broadens and eventually extends cranially as far as the *oropharyngeal membrane* (see Fig. 5.4C). Eventually, the neural plate extends beyond the notochord.

On approximately day 18, the neural plate invaginates along its central axis to form a median longitudinal **neural groove** that has **neural folds** on each side (see Fig. 5.6F and G). The neural folds are particularly prominent at the cranial end of the embryo and are the first signs of brain development (Fig. 5.7C). By the end of the third week, the neural folds have begun to move together and fuse, converting the neural plate into the **neural tube, the primordium of the brain vesicles and spinal cord** (Figs. 5.7F and 5.8). Neural tube formation is a complex cellular and multifactorial process involving genes and extrinsic and mechanical factors (see Chapter 16). The neural tube soon separates from the surface ectoderm as the neural folds meet (see Fig. 5.8E). The free edges of the ectoderm fuse so that this layer becomes continuous over the neural tube and the back of the embryo. Subsequently, the surface ectoderm differentiates into the epidermis of the skin. Neurulation is completed during the fourth week (see Chapter 6).

NEURAL CREST FORMATION

As the neural folds fuse to form the neural tube, some neuroectodermal cells lying along the crest of each neural fold lose their epithelial affinities and attachments to neighboring cells (see Fig. 5.8A–C). As the neural tube separates from the surface ectoderm, these **neural crest cells** migrate dorsolaterally on each side of the neural tube. They form a flattened irregular mass, the **neural crest**, between the neural tube and the overlying surface ectoderm (see Fig. 5.8D and E). The neural crest soon separates into right and left parts that migrate in a wave to the dorsolateral aspects of the neural tube (see Fig. 5.8F). Neural crest cells also migrate widely within the mesenchyme guided by signaling molecules, such as ephrins. Neural crest cells differentiate into various cell types (see Fig. 6.4), including the spinal ganglia and the ganglia of the autonomic nervous system. The ganglia of cranial nerves V, VII, IX, and X are partially derived from neural crest cells. Neural crest cells also form the sheaths of the peripheral nerves and the pia mater and arachnoid mater (see Chapter 16).

DEVELOPMENT OF SOMITES

16

As the notochord and neural tube form, the intraembryonic mesoderm on each side proliferates to form a thick, longitudinal column of **paraxial mesoderm** (see Figs. 5.6G and 5.7B). Each column is continuous laterally with the **intermediate mesoderm**, which gradually thins into a layer of **lateral mesoderm**. The lateral mesoderm is continuous with the extraembryonic mesoderm that covers the umbilical vesicle and amnion (see Fig. 4.3B). Toward the end of the third week, the **paraxial mesoderm** differentiates and begins to divide into paired **somites**, on each side of the developing

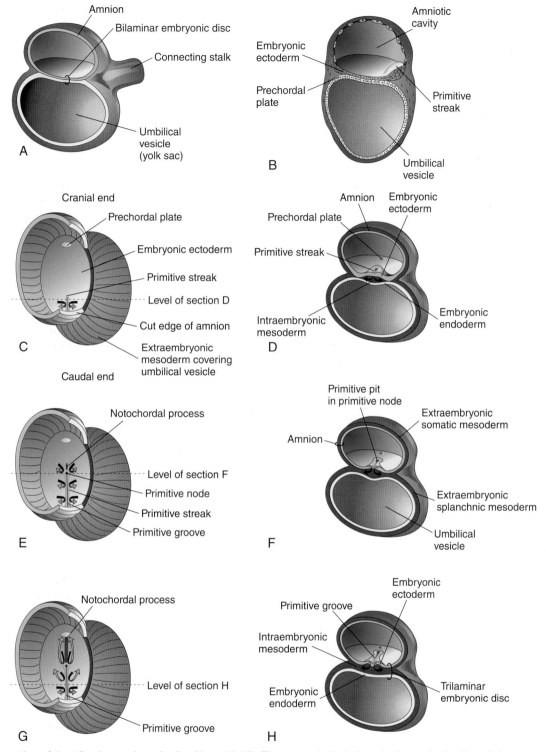

Fig. 5.2 Formation of the trilaminar embryonic disc (days 15–16). The *arrows* indicate invagination and migration of the mesenchymal cells between the ectoderm and the endoderm. (A, B, C, D, F, and H) Transverse sections through the embryonic disc at the levels indicated. (C, E, and G) Dorsal views of the embryonic disc early in the third week, exposed by removal of the amnion.

neural tube (see Fig. 5.7C and E). The somites form distinct surface elevations on the embryo and appear somewhat triangular on transverse section (see Fig. 5.7D and F). Because the somites are so prominent during the fourth and fifth weeks, they are used as one of several criteria for determining an embryo's age (see Table 6.1).

The first pair of somites appears at the end of the third week (see Fig. 5.7C) near the cranial end of the notochord. Subsequent pairs form in a craniocaudal sequence. By day 32, approximately 38 to 39 somites can be found. Somites give rise to most of the **axial skeleton**, the associated musculature, and to the adjacent dermis of the skin.

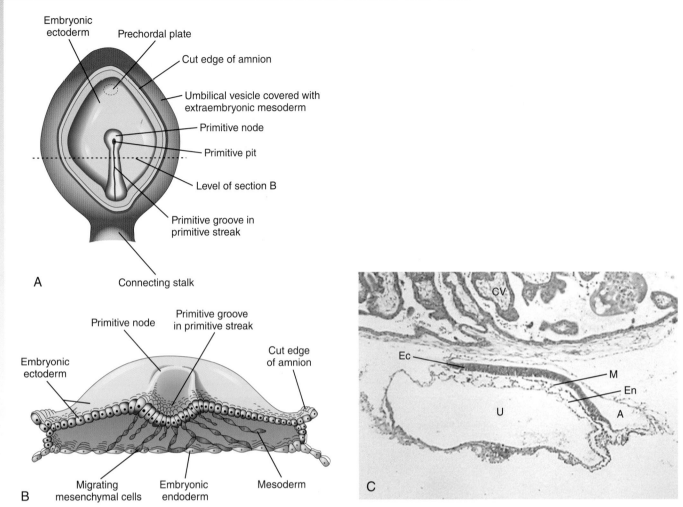

Fig. 5.3 (A) Dorsal view of a 16-day embryo. The amnion has been removed to expose the embryonic disc. (B) Illustration of the cranial half of the embryonic disc during the third week. The disc has been cut transversely to show the migration of mesenchymal cells from the primitive streak to form the mesoblast that soon organizes to form the intraembryonic mesoderm. (C) Sagittal section of a trilaminar embryo showing ectoderm (Ec), mesoderm (M), and endoderm (En). Also visible are the amniotic sac (A), the umbilical vesicle (U), and chorionic villi (CV). C, Courtesy Dr. E. Uthman, Houston/Richmond, Texas.

Somite formation from the paraxial mesoderm is preceded by the expression of the forkhead transcription factors Fox C1 and C2. The craniocaudal segmental pattern of the somites is regulated by the Delta–Notch (Delta 1 and Notch 1) signaling pathway. A molecular oscillator, or clock, has been proposed as the mechanism responsible for the orderly sequencing of the somites. The size and shape of somites are determined by cell–cell interactions. TBX6, a member of the T-box gene family, plays an important role in somitogenesis.

DEVELOPMENT OF INTRAEMBRYONIC COELOM

The intraembryonic coelom (body cavity) first appears as small, isolated, **coelomic spaces** in the lateral intraembryonic mesoderm and cardiogenic (heart-forming) mesoderm (see Fig. 5.7A–D). These spaces coalesce to form a single,

horseshoe-shaped cavity—the **intraembryonic coelom** (see Fig. 5.7E and F). The coelom divides the lateral mesoderm into two layers (see Fig. 5.7F):

- A somatic, or parietal (**somatopleure**), layer that is continuous with the extraembryonic mesoderm covering the amnion
- A splanchnic, or visceral (**splanchnopleure**), layer that is continuous with the extraembryonic mesoderm covering the umbilical vesicle.

The somatic mesoderm and overlying embryonic ectoderm form the embryonic body wall (see Fig. 5.7F), whereas the splanchnic mesoderm and the underlying embryonic endoderm form the wall of the gut. During the second month, the intraembryonic coelom is divided into three body cavities: **pericardial cavity, pleural cavities**, and **peritoneal cavity** (see Chapter 9).

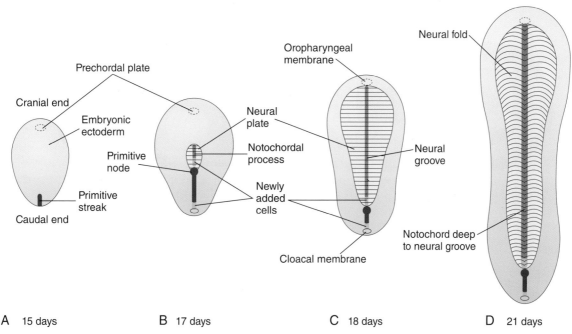

Fig. 5.4 (A–D) Dorsal views of the embryonic disc, showing how it lengthens and changes shape during the third week. The primitive streak lengthens by the addition of cells at its caudal end; the notochordal process lengthens by the migration of cells from the primitive node. At the end of the third week, the notochordal process is transformed into the notochord.

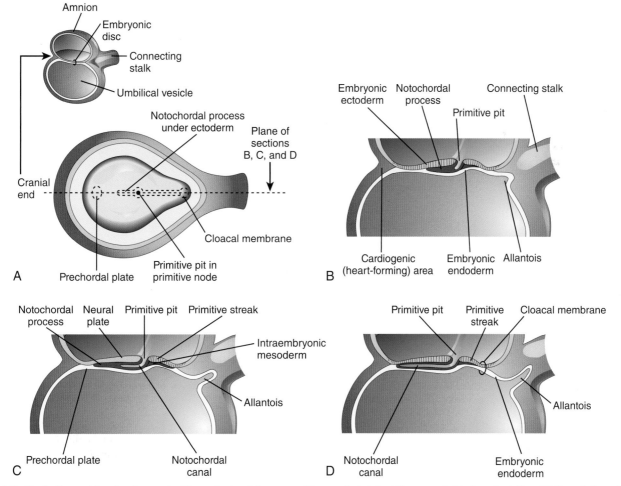

Fig. 5.5 Illustrations of the development of the notochordal process. The small sketch at the upper left is for orientation. (A) Dorsal view of the embryonic disc (at approximately 16 days), exposed by removal of the amnion. The notochordal process is shown as if it were visible through the embryonic ectoderm. (B–D) Median sections, at the same plane as shown in A, illustrating successive stages in the development of the notochordal process and canal. The stages shown in C and D occur at approximately 18 days.

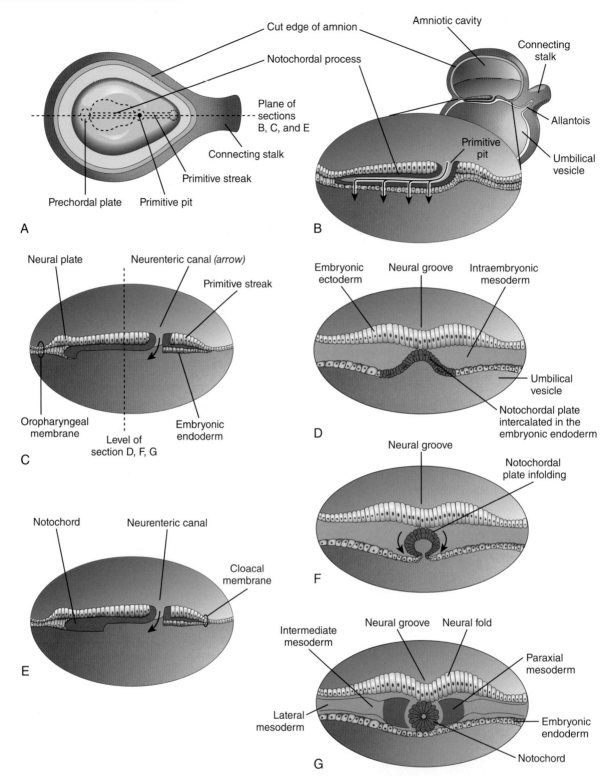

Fig. 5.6 Development of the notochord by transformation of the notochordal process. (A) Dorsal view of the embryonic disc (at approximately 18 days), exposed by removing the amnion. (B) Three-dimensional median section of the embryo. (C and E), Similar sections of slightly older embryos. (D, F and G) Transverse sections of the trilaminar embryonic disc shown in C and E.

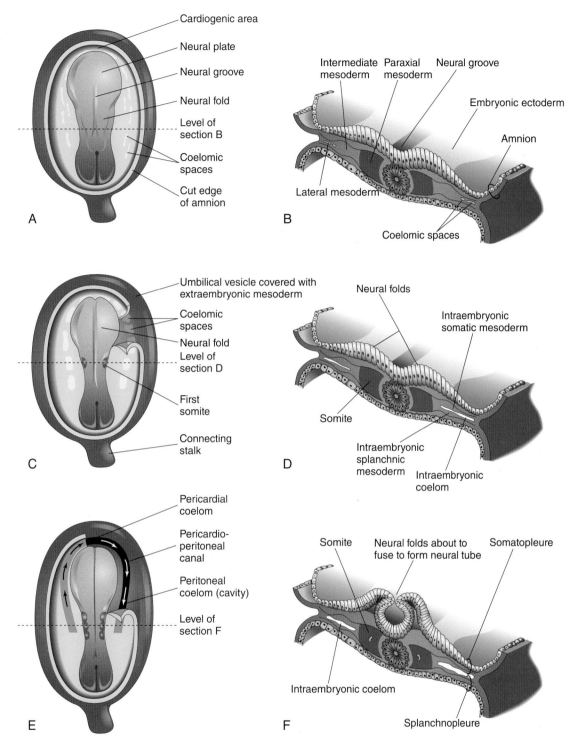

Fig. 5.7 Illustrations of embryos 19 to 21 days old, illustrating the development of the somites and the intraembryonic coelom. (A,C, and E) Dorsal view of the embryo, exposed by removal of the amnion. (B, D, and F) Transverse sections through the embryonic disc at the levels shown. (A) A presomite embryo of approximately 18 days. (C) An embryo of approximately 20 days, showing the first pair of somites. A portion of the somatopleure on the right has been removed to show the isolated coelomic spaces in the lateral mesoderm. (E) A three-somite embryo (approximately 21 days old), showing the horseshoe-shaped intraembryonic coelom, exposed on the right by removal of part of the somatopleure.

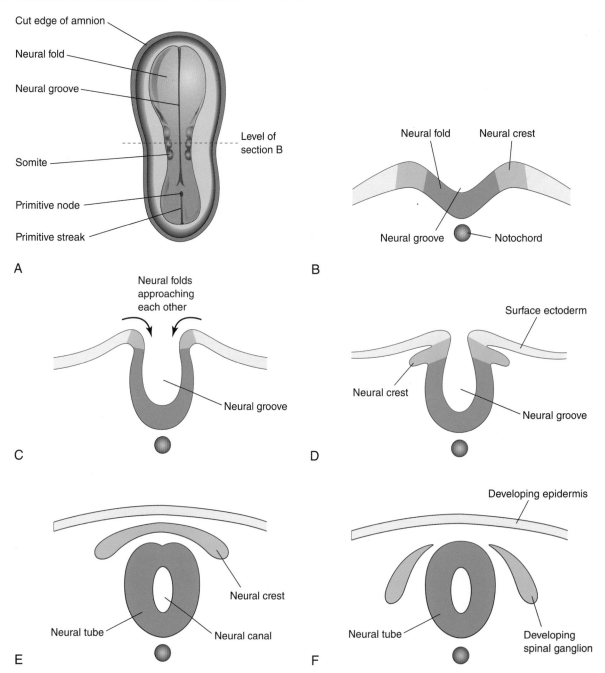

Fig. 5.8 (A–F) Diagrammatic transverse sections through progressively older embryos, illustrating the formation of the neural groove, neural tube, and neural crest up to the end of the fourth week.

EARLY DEVELOPMENT OF CARDIOVASCULAR SYSTEM

At the end of the second week, embryonic nutrition is obtained from the maternal blood by diffusion through the extraembryonic coelom and umbilical vesicle. The early formation of the cardiovascular system correlates with the urgent need for the transportation of oxygen and nourishment to the embryo from the maternal circulation through the chorion. At the beginning of the third week, blood vessel formation, or **vasculogenesis**, begins in the extraembryonic mesoderm of the umbilical vesicle, connecting stalk, and chorion. Vasculogenesis begins in the chorion (Fig. 5.9A and B). Blood vessels develop approximately 2 days later. At the end of the third week, a **primordial uteroplacental circulation** has developed (Fig. 5.10).

VASCULOGENESIS AND ANGIOGENESIS

Blood vessel formation in the embryo and the extraembryonic membranes during the third week may be summarized as follows (see Fig. 5.9C–F):

Vasculogenesis:

- Mesenchymal cells differentiate into endothelial cell precursors, or **angioblasts**, that aggregate to form isolated

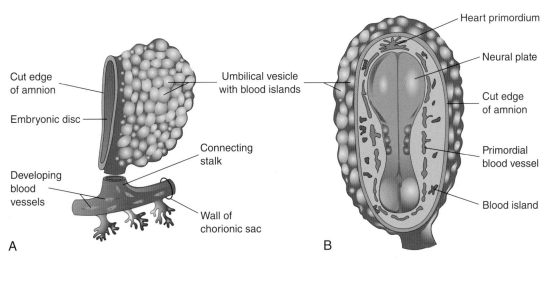

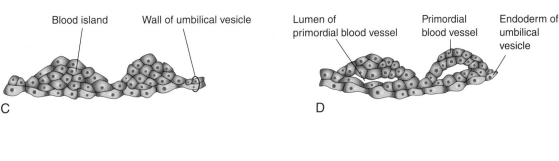

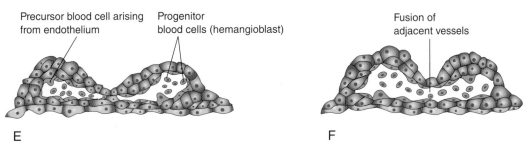

Fig. 5.9 Successive stages in the development of blood and blood vessels. (A) The umbilical vesicle (yolk sac) and a portion of the chorionic sac (at approximately 18 days). (B) Dorsal view of the embryo exposed by removing the amnion. (C–F) Sections of blood islands, showing progressive stages in the development of blood and blood vessels.

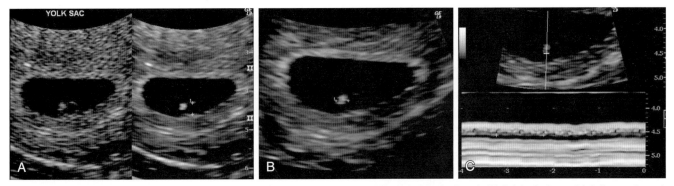

Fig. 5.10 Endovaginal scan of a 4-week embryo. (A) A 2-mm secondary umbilical vesicle (*calipers*). (B) Bright (echogenic) 2.4-mm, 4-week embryo (*calipers*). (C) Cardiac activity of 116 beats/min demonstrated with motion mode. *Calipers* used to encompass two beats. Courtesy E.A. Lyons, MD, Professor of Radiology, and Obstetrics and Gynecology, and Anatomy, Health Sciences Centre and University of Manitoba, Winnipeg, Manitoba, Canada.

angiogenic cell clusters known as **blood islands** (see Fig. 5.9B and C).

- Small cavities appear within the blood islands by the confluence of intercellular clefts.
- Angioblasts flatten to form endothelial cells that arrange themselves around the cavities in the blood islands to form the primordial endothelium.
- The endothelium-lined cavities soon fuse to form networks of endothelial channels. *Anastomosis of these primordial blood vessels is spatially regulated by Flt 1 (VEGFR1) signaling.*

Angiogenesis:

- Vessels sprout by endothelial budding into adjacent non-vascularized areas and fuse with other vessels forming communicating channels..

Blood cells develop from hematopoietic stem cells or hemangiogenic endothelium of blood vessels as they grow on the umbilical vesicle and allantois at the end of the third week (see Fig. 5.9E and F). Blood formation (**hematogenesis**) does not begin within the embryo until the fifth week. This process occurs first in various parts of the embryonic mesenchyme, chiefly the liver, and later in the spleen, bone marrow, and lymph nodes. Fetal and adult erythrocytes are also derived from hematopoietic progenitor cells (**hemangioblasts**). The mesenchymal cells that surround the primordial endothelial blood vessels differentiate into muscular and connective tissue elements of the vessels.

The **heart and great vessels** form from mesenchymal cells in the heart primordium, or **cardiogenic area** (see Figs. 5.7A and 5.9B). Paired, endothelium-lined channels—endocardial **heart tubes**—develop during the third week and fuse to form a **primordial heart tube**. The tubular heart joins with blood vessels in the embryo, connecting stalk, chorion, and umbilical vesicle to form a **primordial cardiovascular system** (Fig. 5.11C). By the end of the third week, blood is flowing and the heart begins to beat on day 21 or 22. The cardiovascular system is the first organ system to reach a primitive functional state. The embryonic heartbeat can be detected by Doppler ultrasonography during the fourth week, approximately 6 weeks after the last normal menstrual period (see Fig. 5.10).

DEVELOPMENT OF CHORIONIC VILLI

Shortly after the **primary chorionic villi** appear at the end of the second week, they begin to branch. Early in the third week, mesenchyme grows into the primary villi, forming a core of loose mesenchymal tissue (Fig. 5.11A and B). The villi at this stage—**secondary chorionic villi**—cover the entire surface of the chorionic sac (see Fig. 5.9A and B). Some mesenchymal cells in the villi soon differentiate into both capillaries and blood cells (see Fig. 5.11C and D). When capillaries are present, the villi are called **tertiary chorionic villi**.

The capillaries in the chorionic villi fuse to form **arteriocapillary networks**, which soon become connected with the embryonic heart through vessels that differentiate from the mesenchyme of the chorion and connecting stalk. By the end of the third week, embryonic blood begins to flow slowly through the capillaries in the chorionic villi. Oxygen

and nutrients in the maternal blood plasma in the **intervillous space** diffuse through the walls of the villi and enter the embryo's blood (see Fig. 5.11C). Carbon dioxide and waste products diffuse from blood in the fetal capillaries through the wall of the villi into the maternal blood. Concurrently, cytotrophoblastic cells of the chorionic villi proliferate and extend through the syncytiotrophoblast to form a **cytotrophoblastic shell**, which gradually surrounds the chorionic sac and attaches it to the endometrium (see Fig. 5.11C).

Villi that attach to the maternal tissues through the cytotrophoblastic shell are called **stem chorionic villi** (anchoring villi). The villi that grow from the sides of the stem villi are **branch chorionic villi** (terminal villi). It is through the walls of the branch villi that the main exchange of material between the blood of the mother and the embryo takes place. The branch villi are bathed in continually changing maternal blood in the intervillous space (see Fig. 5.11C).

Sacrococcygeal Teratoma

Remnants of the primitive streak may persist and give rise to a tumor known as a **sacrococcygeal teratoma** (Fig. 5.12). Because it is derived from pluripotent primitive streak cells, the tumor contains tissues derived from all three germ layers in incomplete stages of differentiation. Sacrococcygeal teratomas are the most common tumors in newborn infants and have an incidence of approximately 1 in 35,000 neonates. Female infants are mostly affected. These tumors are usually surgically excised promptly, and the prognosis is good as a majority are benign. The mortality of fetuses diagnosed antenatally with sacrococcygeal teratoma is approximately 30%, including pregnancy termination; excluding termination, the mortality is approximately 10% to 15%.

Abnormal Neurulation

Disturbance of neurulation may result in severe abnormalities of the brain and spinal cord (see Chapter 16). **Neural tube defects** are among the most common congenital anomalies. Available evidence suggests that the primary disturbance affects the neuroectoderm. Failure of the neural folds to fuse and form the neural tube in the brain region results in meroencephaly or holoencephaly, and in the lumbar region, spina bifida cystica (see Fig. 16.9).

Abnormal Growth of Trophoblast

Sometimes the embryo dies and the chorionic villi do not become vascularized to form tertiary villi. These degenerating villi may form cystic swellings, called **hydatidiform moles** (Fig. 5.13). These moles exhibit variable degrees of trophoblastic proliferation and produce excessive amounts of human chorionic gonadotropin. In 3% to 5% of such cases, these moles develop into malignant trophoblastic lesions, called **choriocarcinomas**. These tumors invariably metastasize by way of the blood to various sites, such as the lungs, vagina, liver, bone, intestine, and brain. Choriocarcinomas are generally sensitive to chemotherapy with survival over 90%.

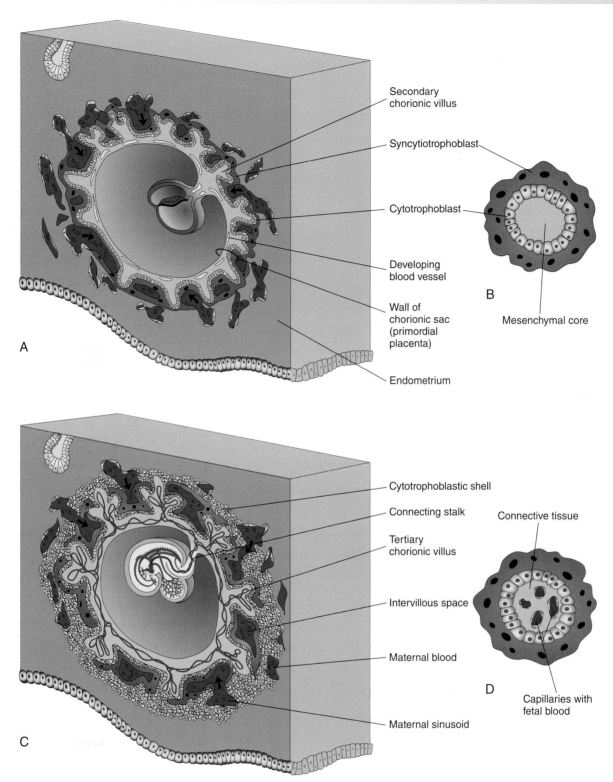

Fig. 5.11 Illustrations of the development of the secondary chorionic villi into the tertiary chorionic villi. (A) Sagittal section of an embryo (at approximately 16 days). (B) Section of a secondary chorionic villus. (C) Section of an embryo (at approximately 21 days). (D) Section of a tertiary chorionic villus. By the end of the third week, a primordial uteroplacental circulation has developed.

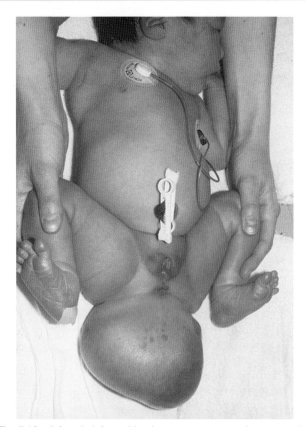

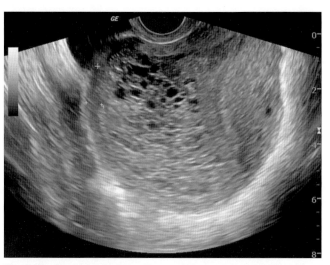

Fig. 5.13 Ultrasound image demonstrating a complete hydatidiform mole. Note numerous small cystic spaces. The "cluster of grapes sign" is a typical feature of a molar pregnancy. Courtesy Dr. Maulik S. Patel and Dr. Frank Gaillard, Radiopaedia.com.

Fig. 5.12 A female infant with a large sacrococcygeal teratoma that developed from remnants of the primitive streak. Courtesy A.E. Chudley, MD, Section of Genetics and Metabolism, Department of Pediatrics and Child Health, Children's Hospital, University of Manitoba, Winnipeg, Manitoba, Canada.

CLINICALLY ORIENTED QUESTIONS

1. Can drugs and other agents cause birth defects in the embryo if they are present in the mother's blood during the third week? If so, what organs would be most susceptible?

2. Are there increased risks for the embryo associated with pregnancies in females older than 40 years of age? If so, what are they?

The answers to these questions are at the back of this book.

Fourth to Eighth Weeks of Human Development

All major structures of the body are established during the fourth to eighth weeks. The three germ layers (ectoderm, mesoderm, and endoderm) formed during gastrulation give rise to the primordia of all tissues and organs (Fig. 6.1). The cells of each germ layer divide, migrate, aggregate, and differentiate in rather precise patterns as they form the various organ systems (organogenesis).

By the end of this period, the main organ systems have begun to develop. Exposure of embryos to **teratogens** (e.g., drugs and viruses) during this period may cause **major birth defects** (see Chapter 19). As the tissues and organs form, the shape of the embryo changes so that, by the eighth week, the embryo has a distinctly human appearance.

 ## FOLDING OF EMBRYO

A significant event in the establishment of body form is the folding of the trilaminar embryonic disc into a somewhat cylindrical-shaped embryo (Fig. 6.2). Folding results from the rapid growth of the embryo, particularly the brain and spinal cord. Folding at the cranial and caudal ends and at the sides of the embryo occurs simultaneously. Concurrently, a relative constriction occurs at the junction of the embryo and the umbilical vesicle. Head and tail folds cause the cranial and caudal regions to move ventrally as the embryo elongates (see Fig. 6.2A_2–D_2).

Reconstructions made of the surface ectoderm and all organs and cavities within human embryos at representative stages of development have revealed new findings on the movements that occur from one stage to the next. Movement is caused by biokinetic forces acting on specific tissues. This has been shown to take place simultaneously at every level of magnification from the cell membrane all the way to the surface of the embryo. The movements and forces bring about genetically controlled differentiation that begins on the outside of the cell and then moves to the inside to react with the nucleus.

HEAD AND TAIL FOLDS

By the beginning of the fourth week, the neural folds in the cranial region form the **primordium of the brain**. The developing forebrain grows cranially beyond the oropharyngeal membrane and overhangs the developing heart. Concomitantly, the **primordial heart** and the **oropharyngeal membrane** move onto the ventral surface of the embryo (Fig. 6.3).

Folding of the caudal end of the embryo results primarily from the growth of the distal part of the neural tube, the **primordium of the spinal cord**. As the embryo grows, the tail region projects over the **cloacal membrane**, the future site of the anus (Fig. 6.4B). During folding, part of the endodermal germ layer is incorporated into the embryo as the **hindgut** (see Fig. 6.4C). The terminal part of the hindgut soon dilates to form the **cloaca** (see Fig. 6.4C). The **connecting stalk** (primordium of the umbilical cord) is now attached to the ventral surface of the embryo, and the **allantois**—an endodermal diverticulum of the umbilical vesicle—is partially incorporated into the embryo (see Figs. 6.2D_2 and 6.4C).

LATERAL FOLDS

Folding of the sides of the developing embryo results from the growth of the **somites**, which produce right and left **lateral folds** (see Fig. 6.2A_3–D_3). The lateral abdominal body wall folds toward the median plane, rolling the edges of the embryonic disc ventrally and forming a roughly cylindrical embryo. During lateral (longitudinal) folding, a part of the endoderm of the umbilical vesicle is incorporated into the embryo as the **foregut**, the primordium of the pharynx (see Fig. 6.3C). The foregut lies between the brain and heart, and the oropharyngeal membrane separates the foregut from the **stomodeum**, the primordium of the mouth. As the abdominal wall forms by fusion of the lateral folds, part of the endoderm germ layer is incorporated into the embryo as the **midgut**.

Initially, there is a wide connection between the midgut and the umbilical vesicle (see Fig. 6.2C_2). After lateral folding, the connection is reduced to an **omphaloenteric duct** (see Fig. 6.2C_2). As the **umbilical cord** forms from the connecting stalk, ventral fusion of the lateral folds reduces the region of communication between the intraembryonic and extraembryonic coelomic cavities (see Fig. 6.2C_2). As the amniotic cavity expands and obliterates most of the **extraembryonic coelom**, the amnion forms the epithelial covering of the umbilical cord (see Fig. 6.2D_2).

CONTROL OF EMBRYONIC DEVELOPMENT

Embryonic development results from genetic programs in the chromosomes. Most developmental processes depend on a precisely coordinated interaction of genetic and environmental factors. Specific genes and signaling factors guide differentiation and ensure synchronized development, such as tissue interactions, regulated migration of cells, controlled proliferation, and apoptosis (programmed cell death). Each system of the body has its own developmental

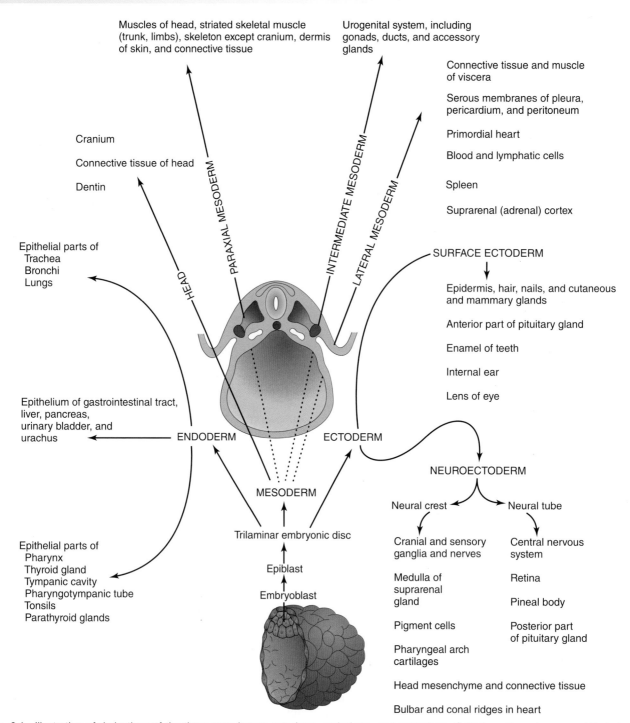

Fig. 6.1 Illustration of derivatives of the three germ layers: ectoderm, endoderm, and mesoderm. Cells from these layers contribute to the formation of different tissues and organs; for example, the endoderm forms the epithelial lining of the gastrointestinal tract and the mesoderm gives rise to connective tissues and muscles.

pattern, and morphogenesis is regulated by complex molecular pathways.

Embryonic development is essentially a process of growth and increasing complexity of structure and function. **Growth is achieved by mitosis**, together with the production of extracellular matrices, whereas complexity is achieved through morphogenesis and differentiation. The cells that make up the tissues of very early embryos are **pluripotential**; that is, depending on the circumstances, they are able to

follow more than one pathway of development. This broad developmental potential becomes progressively restricted as tissues acquire the specialized features necessary for increased sophistication of structure and function. Such restriction presumes that choices must be made to achieve tissue diversification.

Most evidence indicates that these choices are determined not as a consequence of cell lineage, but rather in response to cues from the immediate surroundings, including the

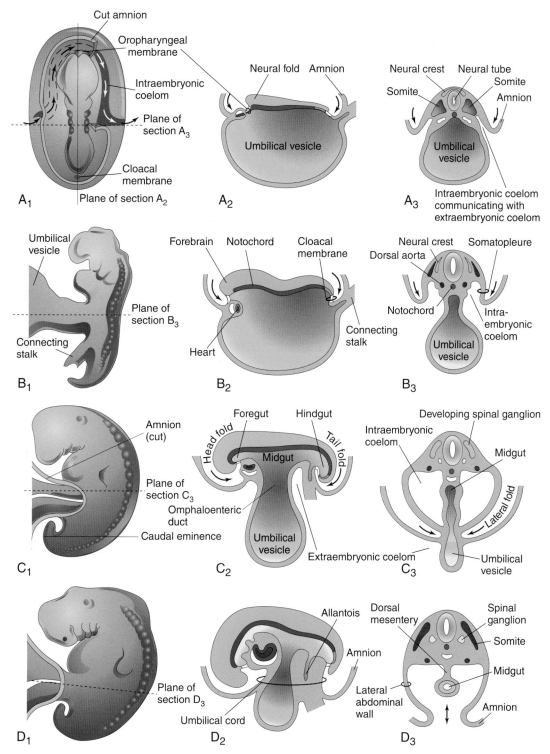

Fig. 6.2 Folding of embryos during the fourth week. (A_1) Dorsal view of an embryo early in the fourth week. Three pairs of somites are visible. The continuity of the intraembryonic coelom and extraembryonic coelom is shown on the right side by removing a part of the embryonic ectoderm and mesoderm. (B_1, C_1, and D_1) Lateral views of embryos at 22, 26, and 28 days, respectively. (A_2, B_2, C_2, and D_2) Sagittal sections at the plane shown in (A_1). (A_3, B_3, C_3, and D_3) Transverse sections at the levels are indicated in A_1 to D_1.

adjacent tissues. As a result, the architectural precision and coordination that are often required for the normal function of an organ appear to be achieved by the interaction of its constituent parts during development.

The interaction of tissues during development is a recurring theme in embryology. The interactions that lead to a change in the course of development of at least one of the interactants are called **inductions**. Numerous examples

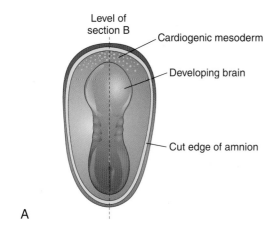

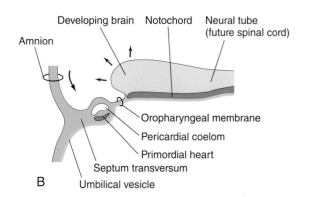

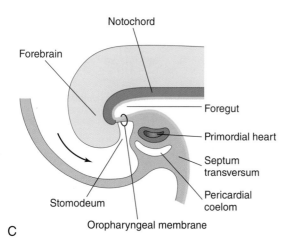

Fig. 6.3 Folding of the cranial end of the embryo. (A) Dorsal view of an embryo at 21 days. (B) Sagittal section of the cranial part of the embryo at the plane in (A), showing the ventral movement of the heart. (C) Sagittal section of an embryo at 26 days. Note that the septum transversum, heart, pericardial coelom, and oropharyngeal membrane have moved to the ventral surface of the embryo.

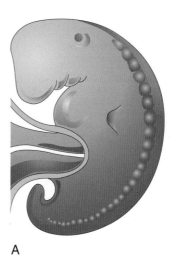

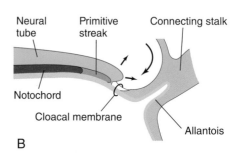

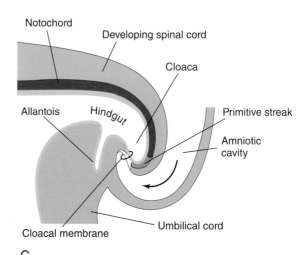

Fig. 6.4 Folding of caudal end of the embryo. (A) Lateral view of a 4-week embryo. (B) Sagittal section of the caudal part of the embryo at the beginning of the fourth week. (C) Similar section at the end of the fourth week. Note that part of the umbilical vesicle is incorporated into the embryo as the hindgut and that the terminal part of the hindgut has dilated to form the cloaca. Observe also the change in position of the primitive streak, allantois, cloacal membrane, and connecting stalk.

of inductive interactions can be found in the scientific literature; for example, during the development of the eye, the optic vesicle induces the development of the lens from the surface ectoderm of the head. When the optic vesicle is absent, the eye does not develop. Moreover, if the optic vesicle is removed and placed in association with a surface ectoderm that is not usually involved in eye development, lens formation can be induced. Clearly then, the development of a lens depends on the ectoderm acquiring an association with a second tissue. In the presence of the neuroectoderm of the optic vesicle, the surface ectoderm of the head follows a pathway of development that it would not otherwise have taken. Similarly, many of the morphogenetic tissue movements that play such important roles in shaping the embryo also provide for the changing tissue associations that are fundamental to *inductive tissue interactions.*

The fact that one tissue can influence the developmental pathway adopted by another tissue presumes that a signal passes between the two interactants. Analysis of the molecular defects in mutant animal strains that show abnormal tissue interactions during embryonic development and studies of the development of embryos with targeted pathogenic variants (gene mutations) have begun to reveal the molecular mechanisms of induction. The mechanism of signal transfer appears to vary with the specific tissues involved. In some cases, the signal appears to take the form of a diffusible molecule that passes from the inductor to the reacting tissue. In other instances, the message appears to be mediated through a nondiffusible extracellular matrix that is secreted by the inductor and that comes into contact with the reacting tissue. In other cases, the signal appears to require physical contact between the inducing tissue and the responding tissue. Regardless of the mechanism of intercellular transfer involved, the signal is translated into an intracellular message that influences the gene-regulatory network of the responding cells.

To be competent to respond to an inducing stimulus, the cells of the reacting system must express the appropriate receptor for the specific inducing signal molecule, the components of the particular intracellular signal transduction pathway, and the transcription factors that mediate the particular response. Experimental evidence suggests that the acquisition of competence by the responding tissue is often dependent on its previous interactions with other tissues. For example, the lens-forming response of the head ectoderm to the stimulus provided by the optic vesicle appears to be dependent on a previous association of the head ectoderm with the anterior neural plate (see Chapter 20).

ESTIMATION OF EMBRYONIC AGE

Estimates of the age of embryos recovered after spontaneous abortion, for example, are determined from their external characteristics and measurements of their length (Table 6.1). However, *size alone may be an unreliable criterion* because some embryos undergo a progressively slower rate of growth before death. **Greatest Length (GL)** is used to measure embryos in the third and early fourth weeks (Fig. 6.5A). **Crown–rump length (CRL)** is used to estimate the age of older embryos (see Fig. 6.5B and C). **Crown–heel length** is sometimes measured during weeks 14 to 18 (see Fig. 6.5D). The *Carnegie Embryonic Staging System* is used internationally for comparison of embryonic age and development (see Table 6.1).

Ultrasonographic Examination of Embryos

Most females seeking obstetric care have at least one ultrasonographic examination during their pregnancy for one or more of the following reasons:

- Estimation of gestational age for confirmation of clinical dating
- Evaluation of embryonic growth when intrauterine growth restriction is suspected
- Guidance during chorionic villus or amniotic fluid sampling
- Suspected ectopic pregnancy
- Possible uterine abnormality
- Detection of birth defects

The size of an embryo in a pregnant woman can be estimated using ultrasonographic measurements. Transvaginal or endovaginal ultrasonography permits accurate measurement of crown–rump length in early pregnancy (Fig. 6.6).

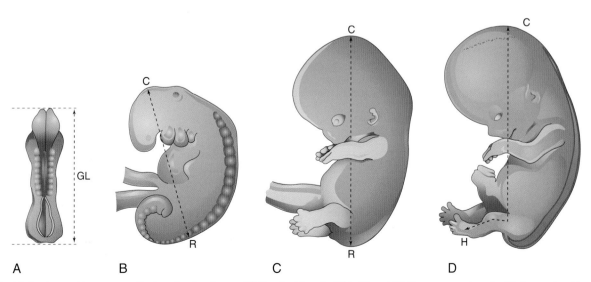

Fig. 6.5 Methods used to measure the length of embryos. (A) Greatest length *(GL)*. (B) and (C) Crown–rump length. (D) Crown–heel length.

Table 6.1   Criteria for Estimating Developmental Stages in Human Embryos

Age (Days)	Figure Reference	Carnegie Stage	Number of Somites	Length (mm)[a]	Main External Characteristics[b]
20–21	6.2A₁	9	1–3	1.5–3.0	Flat embryonic disc. Deep neural groove and prominent neural folds. Head fold is evident.
22–23	6.8A and C	10	4–12	2.0–3.5	Embryo is straight or slightly curved. Neural tube is forming or has formed opposite somites, but is widely open at the rostra l and caudal neuropores. The first and second pairs of pharyngeal arches are visible.
24–25	6.9A	11	13–20	2.5–4.5	Embryo is curved owing to head and tail folds. Rostral neuropore is closing. Otic placodes are present. Optic vesicles have formed.
26–27	6.7B 6.10A	12	21–29	3.0–5.0	Upper limb buds appear. Rostral neuropore is closed. Caudal neuropore is closing. Three pairs of pharyngeal arches are visible. Heart prominence is distinct. Otic pits are present.
28–30	6.6 6.11A	13	30–35	4.0–6.0	Embryo has C-shaped curve. Caudal neuropore is closed. Four pairs of pharyngeal arches are visible. Lower limb buds appear. Otic vesicles are present. Lens placodes are distinct.
31–32	6.12A	14	[c]	5.0–7.0	Lens pits and nasal pits are visible. Optic cups are present.
33–36		15		7.0–9.0	Hand plates have formed; digital rays are present. Lens vesicles are present. Nasal pits are prominent. Cervical sinuses are visible.
37–40		16		8.0–11.0	Foot plates have formed. Pigment is visible in the retina. Auricular hillocks are developing.
41–43	6.13A	17		11.0–14.0	Digital rays are clearly visible on hand plates. Auricular hillocks outline the future auricle of the external ear. Cerebral vesicles are prominent.
44–46		18		13.0–17.0	Digital rays are clearly evident on foot plates. Elbow region is visible. Eyelids are forming. Notches are between the digital rays in the hands. Nipples are visible.
47–48		19		16.0–18.0	Limbs extend ventrally. Trunk is elongating and straightening. Midgut herniation is prominent.
49–51		20		18.0–22.0	Upper limbs are longer and are bent at the elbows. Fingers are distinct but webbed. Notches are between the digital rays in the feet. Scalp vascular plexus appears.
52–53		21		22.0–24.0	Hands and feet approach each other. Fingers are free and longer. Toes are distinct but webbed. Stubby caudal eminence (tail) is present.
54–55		22		23.0–28.0	Toes are free and longer. Eyelids and auricles of the external ears are more developed.
56	6.14A	23		27.0–31.0	Head is more rounded. External genitalia still have an undifferentiated appearance. Midgut herniation is still present. Caudal eminence has disappeared.

[a]The embryonic lengths indicate the usual range. In stages 9 and 10, the measurement is greatest length; in subsequent stages, crown–rump measurements are given.

[b]Based on O'Rahilly R, Müller F: *Developmental stages in human embryos*, Washington, DC, 1987, Carnegie Institute of Washington; and Gasser RF: *Digitally reproduced embryonic morphology DVDs. Computer imaging laboratory, cell biology and anatomy*, New Orleans, LA, 2002–2006, Louisiana State University Health Sciences Center.

[c]At this stage and subsequent stages, the number of somites is difficult to determine and so is not a useful criterion.

HIGHLIGHTS OF THE FOURTH TO EIGHTH WEEKS

The criteria for estimating developmental stages in human embryos are listed in Table 6.1.

FOURTH WEEK

Major changes in body form occur during the fourth week. Earlier, the embryo is almost straight. In the fourth week, the somites produce conspicuous surface elevations and the **neural tube** is open at the rostral and caudal neuropores (Figs. 6.7A and 6.8C and D). By 24 days, the **pharyngeal arches** had appeared (see Fig. 6.7A–C). The embryo is now slightly curved because of the head and tail folds. *The early heart produces a large ventral prominence and pumps blood* (Figs. 6.9 and 6.10). The rostral neuropore is closing by 24 days (see Fig. 6.9B).

At 26 days, the **forebrain** produces a prominent elevation of the head and the long, curved **caudal eminence** is present (see Fig. 6.10B). At 28 days, **upper limb buds** are recognizable

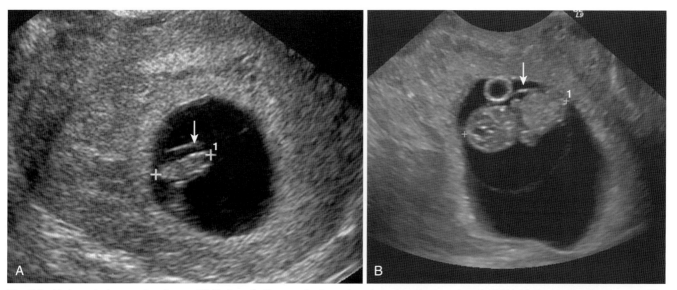

Fig. 6.6   Endovaginal scan of embryos. (A) Endovaginal scan of a 5-week embryo (crown–rump length [CRL] 10 mm *[calipers]*) surrounded by the amniotic membrane *(arrow)*. (B) Coronal scan of a 7-week embryo (CRL 22 mm *[calipers]*). Amnion seen anterior *(arrow)*. Umbilical vesicle (yolk sac) anterior. Courtesy E.A. Lyons, MD, Professor of Radiology and Obstetrics and Gynecology, Health Sciences Centre and University of Manitoba, Winnipeg, Manitoba, Canada.

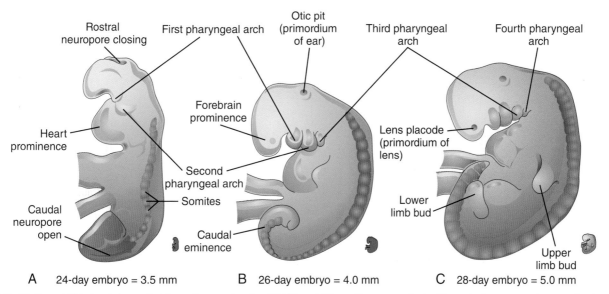

Fig. 6.7   (A, B, and C) Lateral views of older embryos, showing 16, 27, and 33 somites, respectively. The rostral neuropore is normally closed by 25 to 26 days, and the caudal neuropore is usually closed by the end of the fourth week.

as small swellings on the ventrolateral body walls (Fig. 6.11A and B). At 26 days, the **otic pits** (primordia of internal ears) are also visible (see Fig. 6.10B). Ectodermal thickenings called **lens placodes**, indicating the future lenses of the eyes, are visible on the sides of the head. The fourth pair of pharyngeal arches and the **lower limb buds** are visible by the end of the fourth week (Fig. 6.12; also see Fig. 6.7C), and the **caudal neuropore** is usually closed (see Fig. 6.10). Rudiments of many organ systems, especially the cardiovascular system, are established.

FIFTH WEEK

Changes in body form are minor during the fifth week compared with those that occurred during the fourth week. *Growth of the head exceeds that of other regions* (see Fig. 6.12A and B), which is caused mainly by the rapid development of the brain and facial prominences. The face soon contacts the heart prominence. The **mesonephric ridges** indicate the site of the mesonephric kidneys (see Fig. 6.12B),

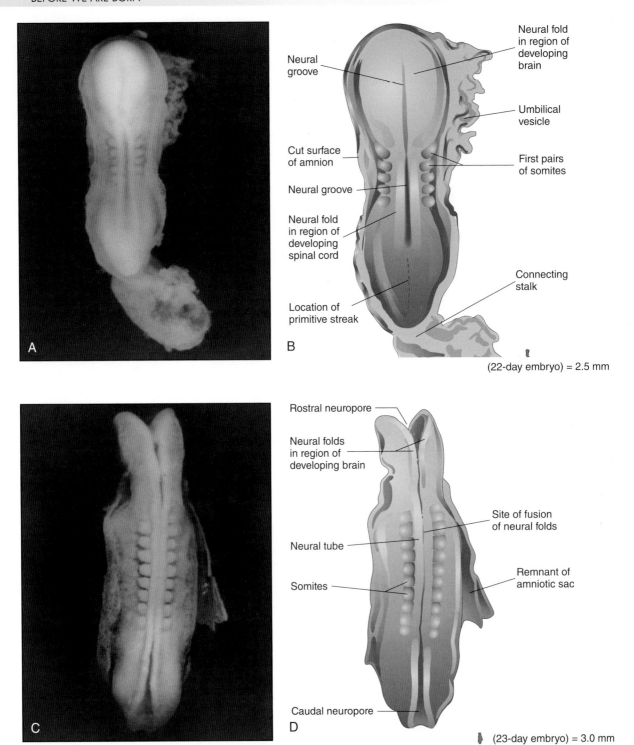

Fig. 6.8 (A) Dorsal view of a five-somite embryo at Carnegie stage 10, approximately 22 days. Observe the neural folds and neural groove. The neural folds in the cranial region have thickened to form the primordium of the brain. (B) Drawing of the structures shown in (A). Most of the amniotic and chorionic sacs have been cut away to expose the embryo. (C) Dorsal view of an older embryo at Carnegie stage 10, approximately 23 days. The neural folds have fused opposite the somites to form the neural tube (primordium of spinal cord in this region). The neural tube is in open communication with the amniotic cavity at the cranial and caudal ends through the rostral and caudal neuropores, respectively. (D) Diagram of the structures shown in (C). The amniotic fluid provides a buoyant medium that supports the delicate tissues of the early embryo.

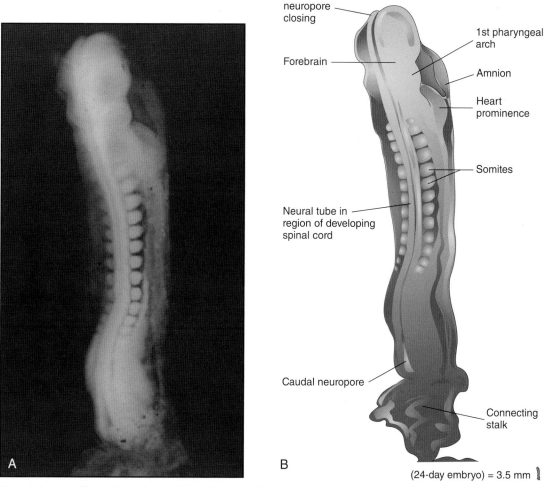

Fig. 6.9   (A) Dorsal view of a 13-somite embryo at Carnegie stage 11, approximately 24 days. The rostral neuropore is closing, but the caudal neuropore is wide open. (B) Illustration of the structures shown in (B). The embryo is curved because of the folding of cranial and caudal ends.

the primordia of the permanent kidneys (see Fig. 6.12A and B).

SIXTH WEEK

Embryos in the sixth week show spontaneous movements, such as twitching of the trunk and limbs, and show reflex responses to touch. The primordia of the fingers—the **digital rays**—begin to develop in the hand plates (Fig. 6.13A and B). Development of the lower limbs occurs 4 to 5 days later than that of the upper limbs.

Several small swellings—**auricular hillocks**—develop and contribute to the formation of the **auricle** of the external ear. The eyes are now obvious largely because retinal pigment has formed. The head is much larger relative to the trunk and is bent over the large heart prominence. This head position results from bending in the cervical (neck) region. During the sixth week, the intestines enter the

extraembryonic coelom in the proximal part of the umbilical cord. This **herniation** is a normal event in the embryo, occurring because the abdominal cavity is too small at this stage to accommodate the rapidly growing intestines (see Fig. 12.11C).

SEVENTH WEEK

The limbs undergo considerable change during the seventh week. Notches appear between the digital rays in the **hand plates**, partially separating the future digits. Communication between the primordial gut and the umbilical vesicle is now reduced to a relatively slender duct, the omphaloenteric duct (see Fig. 6.2C$_2$).

EIGHTH WEEK

By the beginning of the eighth week, the digits of the hand are distinct but noticeably webbed (see Fig. 6.13B).

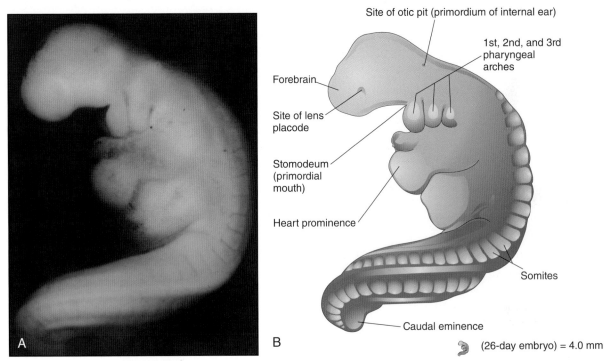

Fig. 6.10 (A) Lateral view of a 27-somite embryo at Carnegie stage 12, approximately 26 days. The embryo is curved, especially its tail-like caudal eminence. Observe the lens placode (primordium of lens of the eye). The otic pit indicates early development of the internal ear. (B) Illustration of the structures shown in (A). The rostral neuropore is closed, and three pairs of pharyngeal arches are present. A, From Nishimura H, Semba H, Tanimura T, Tanaka O: *Prenatal development of the human with special reference to craniofacial structures: an atlas*, Washington, DC, 1977, National Institutes of Health.

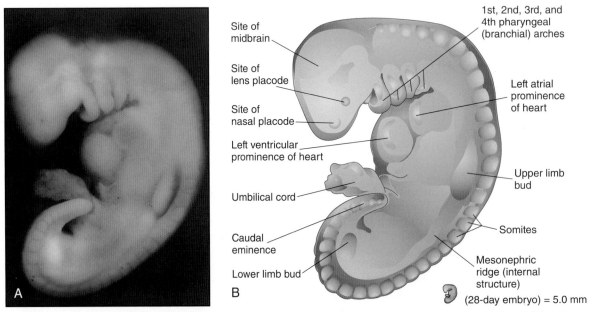

Fig. 6.11 (A) Lateral view of an embryo at Carnegie stage 13, approximately 28 days. The primordial heart is large and is divided into a primordial atrium and a ventricle. The rostral and caudal neuropores are closed. The mesonephric ridge indicates the site of the mesonephric kidney, an interim functional kidney. (B) Drawing indicating the structures shown in (A). The embryo has a characteristic C-shaped curvature, four pharyngeal arches, and upper and lower limb buds. A, From Nishimura H, Semba H, Tanimura T, Tanaka O: *Prenatal development of the human with special reference to craniofacial structures: an atlas*, Washington, DC, 1977, National Institutes of Health.

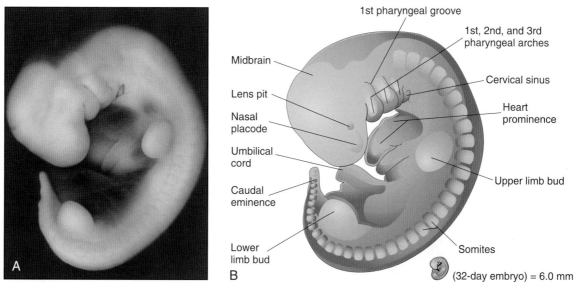

Fig. 6.12   (A) Lateral view of an embryo at Carnegie stage 14, approximately 32 days. The second pharyngeal arch has overgrown the third arch, forming the *cervical sinus*. (B) Illustration of the structures shown in (A). A, From Nishimura H, Semba H, Tanimura T, Tanaka O: *Prenatal development of the human with special reference to craniofacial structures: an atlas*, Washington, DC, 1977, National Institutes of Health.

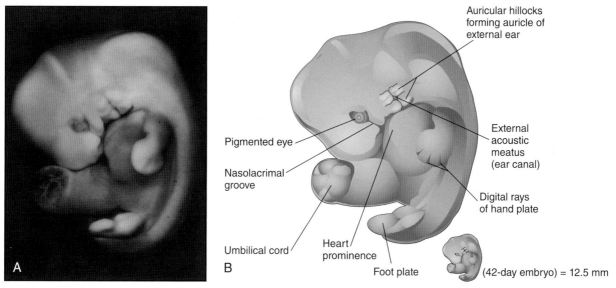

Fig. 6.13   (A) Lateral view of an embryo at Carnegie stage 17, approximately 42 days. Digital rays are visible in the hand plate, indicating the future site of the digits (fingers). (B) Illustration of the structures shown in (A). The eye, auricular hillocks, and external acoustic meatus are now obvious. From Moore KL, Persaud TVN, Shiota K: *Color atlas of clinical embryology*, ed 2, Philadelphia, 2000, Saunders.

Notches are clearly visible between the digital rays of the feet. The **scalp vascular plexus** has appeared and forms a characteristic band around the head. At the end of the fetal period, the digits have lengthened and are separated (Fig. 6.14A and B). *Coordinated limb movements first occur during this week.* Primary ossification begins in the femur. All evidence of the tail-like caudal eminence had disappeared by the end of the eighth week. The hands and feet each approach each other ventrally. At the end of the eighth

week, the head is still disproportionately large, constituting almost half of the embryo (see Fig. 6.14). The neck region is established, and the eyelids begin to unite by epithelial fusion. The intestines are still in the proximal portion of the umbilical cord (see Fig. 12.11C). The auricles of the external ears begin to assume their final shape but are still low-set on the head. Although sex differences exist in the appearance of the external genitalia, they are not distinctive enough to permit accurate sex identification.

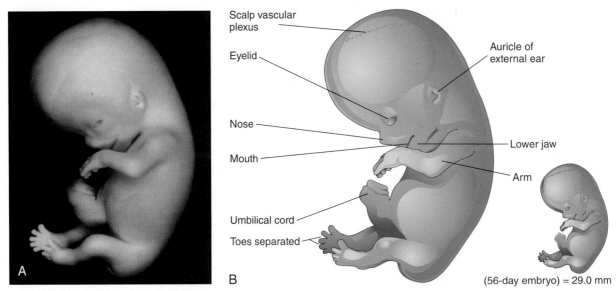

Fig. 6.14   (A) Lateral view of an embryo at Carnegie stage 23, approximately 56 days (end of embryonic period). (B) Illustration of the structures shown in (A). A, From Nishimura H, Semba H, Tanimura T, Tanaka O: *Prenatal development of the human with special reference to craniofacial structures: an atlas*, Washington, DC, 1977, National Institutes of Health.

CLINICALLY ORIENTED QUESTIONS

1. There is little apparent difference between an 8-week embryo and a 9-week fetus. Why do embryologists give them different names?

2. When does the embryo become a human being?

3. Can the sex of embryos be determined by ultrasonography? What other methods can be used to determine sex?

The answers to these questions are at the back of this book.

Fetal Period 7

THE NINTH WEEK TO BIRTH

The fetal period is concerned primarily with body growth and tissue differentiation. The rate of body growth during the fetal period is rapid, and fetal weight gain is phenomenal during the terminal weeks (Table 7.1). Ultrasonographic measurements of the **crown–rump length (CRL)** are often used to determine fetal size and probable age (Fig. 7.1). The intrauterine period may be divided into days, weeks, or months (Table 7.2), but confusion arises if it is not stated whether the age is calculated from the last normal menstrual period (LNMP) or from the **fertilization age**. *Unless otherwise stated, fetal age in this book is calculated from the estimated time of fertilization and months refers to calendar months.* Clinically, the gestational period is divided into **three trimesters**, each lasting 3 months. Various measurements and external characteristics are useful for estimating fetal age (see Table 7.1).

HIGHLIGHTS OF FETAL PERIOD

There is no formal staging system for the fetal period; however, it is helpful to consider the main changes that occur during the period of 9 to 38 weeks.

NINE TO TWELVE WEEKS

At the beginning of the ninth week, the head constitutes half of the CRL of the fetus (see Fig. 7.1). Growth in body length accelerates rapidly so that, by the end of 12 weeks, the CRL has almost doubled (see Table 7.1). Ossification begins in the cranium between 9 and 11 weeks, first in the complex occipital bone.

At 9 weeks, the face is broad, the eyes are widely separated, the ears are low set, and the eyelids are fused. Early in the ninth week, the legs are short and the thighs are relatively small. By the end of 12 weeks, the upper limbs have almost reached their final relative lengths, but the lower limbs are still slightly shorter than their final relative lengths.

The *external genitalia* of males and females are not fully developed until the end of the 12th week. Intestinal coils are clearly visible in the proximal end of the umbilical cord until the middle of the 10th week. By the 11th week, the intestines have returned to the abdomen (Fig. 7.2). Urine formation begins between the 9th and 12th weeks, and urine is discharged through the urethra into the amniotic cavity and added to the amniotic fluid. The fetus reabsorbs some of this fluid after swallowing it. Fetal waste products in the blood are transferred to the maternal circulation by passing across the placental membrane (see Chapter 8).

THIRTEEN TO SIXTEEN WEEKS

Growth is very rapid during this period (Figs. 7.3 and 7.4; see Table 7.1). By 16 weeks, the head is relatively small compared with that of the 12-week fetus, and the lower limbs have lengthened. **Coordinated limb movements** begin by the 14th week, but they are too slight to be felt by the mother. However, these movements are visible during ultrasonographic examinations.

By the beginning of the 16th week, the developing bones are clearly visible on ultrasound images. **Slow eye movements** occur at 14 weeks. Scalp hair patterning is also determined during this period. By 16 weeks, the ovaries are differentiated and contain primordial ovarian follicles that have **oogonia** (primordial germ cells). The eyes face anteriorly rather than anterolaterally.

SEVENTEEN TO TWENTY WEEKS

Growth slows down during this period, but the fetus still increases its CRL by approximately 50 mm (Fig. 7.5; see also Fig. 7.3 and Table 7.1). Fetal movements—**quickening**—are commonly felt by the mother. The skin is now covered with **vernix caseosa** consisting of dead epidermal cells and a fatty secretion from the fetal sebaceous glands. The vernix caseosa protects the delicate fetal skin from abrasions, chapping, and hardening that could result from exposure to the amniotic fluid. Fetuses are usually completely covered with fine, downy hair—**lanugo**—that helps hold the vernix on the skin.

Eyebrows and head hair are also visible. **Brown fat** forms during weeks 17 to 20 and is the site of heat production, particularly in the neonate. This specialized adipose tissue, found chiefly at the neck, posterior to the sternum, produces heat by oxidizing fatty acids.

By 18 weeks, the **uterus** is formed and canalization of the vagina has begun. By 20 weeks, the testes have begun to descend, but they are still located on the posterior abdominal wall.

TWENTY-ONE TO TWENTY-FIVE WEEKS

Substantial weight gain occurs during this period, and the fetus is better proportioned. The skin is usually wrinkled, more translucent, and pink to red colored because blood is visible in the capillaries. At 21 weeks, rapid eye movements begin, and startle eye blinks have been reported at 22 to 23 weeks. Fingernails are present by 24 weeks. Also by 24 weeks, the secretory epithelial cells (type II pneumocytes) in the interalveolar walls of the lung have begun to secrete

57

Table 7.1   Criteria for Estimating Fertilization Age During the Fetal Period

Age (Weeks)	Crown–Rump Length (mm)[a]	Foot Length (mm)[a]	Fetal Weight (g)[b]	Main External Characteristics
Previable Fetus				
9	50	7	8	Eyelids are closing or have closed. Head is rounded. External genitalia are still not distinguishable as male or female. Intestinal herniation is present.
10	61	9	14	Intestine is in the abdomen. Early fingernail development.
12	87	14	45	Sex is distinguishable externally. Well-defined neck.
14	120	20	110	Head is erect. Lower limbs are well developed. Early toenail development.
16	140	27	200	Auricles of the ears stand out from the head.
18	160	33	320	Vernix caseosa covers the skin. Fetal movement (quickening) is felt by the mother.
20	190	39	460	Head and body hair (lanugo) are visible.
Viable Fetus[c]				
22	210	45	630	Skin is wrinkled and red.
24	230	50	820	Fingernails are present. Lean body.
26	250	55	1000	Eyes are partially open. Eyelashes are present.
28	270	59	1300	Eyes are open. Most fetuses have scalp hair. Skin is slightly wrinkled.
30	280	63	1700	Toenails are present. Body is filling out. Testes are descending.
32	300	68	2100	Fingernails extend to fingertips. Skin is smooth.
36	340	79	2900	Body is usually plump. Lanugo is almost absent. Toenails extend to the toe tips. Flexed limb; firm grasp.
38	360	83	3400	Prominent chest; breasts protrude. Testes in the scrotum or palpable in the inguinal canals. Fingernails extend beyond fingertips.

[a]These measurements are averages, and dimensional variations increase with age.

[b]These weights refer to fetuses that have been fixed for approximately 2 weeks in 10% formalin. Fresh specimens usually weigh approximately 5% less.

[c]There is no sharp limit of development, age, or weight at which a fetus automatically becomes viable or beyond which survival is ensured, but experience has shown that it is uncommon for an infant to survive if its weight is less than 500 g or if its fertilization age or developmental age is less than 22 weeks.

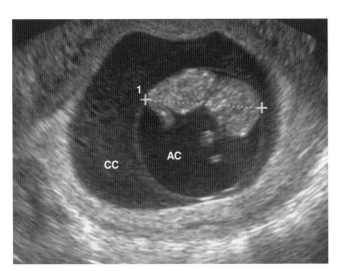

Fig. 7.1 Endovaginal scan of a 9-week fetus with a crown–rump length of 41.7 mm *(calipers)*. Chorionic cavity *(CC)* has low-level echoes normally, whereas the amniotic cavity *(AC)* is echo-free. Courtesy E.A. Lyons, MD, Professor of Radiology, and Obstetrics and Gynecology, and Anatomy, University of Manitoba, Health Sciences Centre, Winnipeg, Manitoba, Canada.

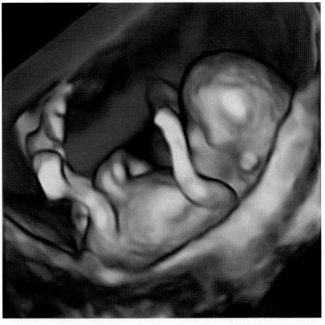

Fig. 7.2 A transvaginal 3D ultrasound (with superficial rendering) of an 11-week fetus. Note it is relatively large head. The limbs are fully developed. An auricle of the ear can also be observed on the left lateral aspect of the head.

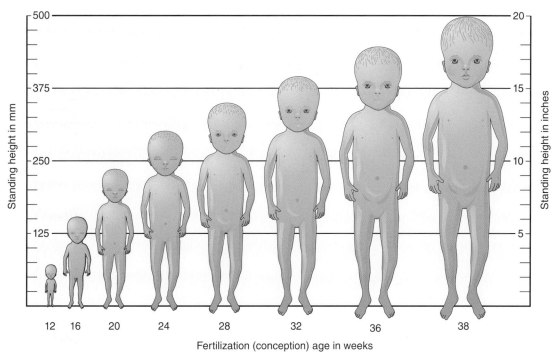

Fig. 7.3   Diagram drawn to scale illustrating the changes in size of human fetuses.

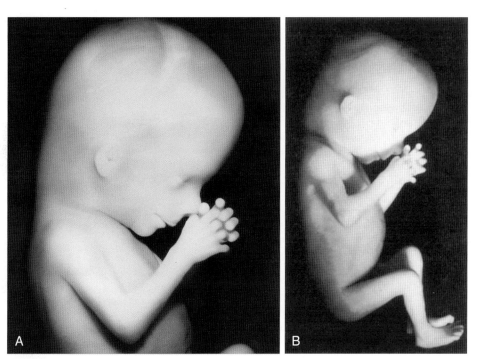

Fig. 7.4   A 13-week fetus. (A) An enlarged photograph of the head and shoulders (×2). (B) Actual size. Courtesy Jean Hay, late, Associate Professor, University of Manitoba, Winnipeg, Manitoba, Canada.

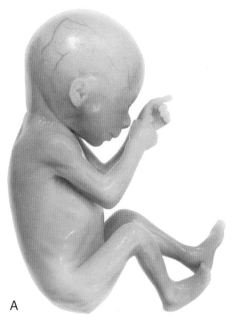
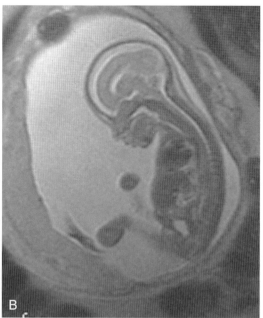

Fig. 7.5 (A) A 17-week fetus (actual size). Fetuses at this age are unable to survive if born prematurely, mainly because the respiratory system is immature. (B) Magnetic resonance imaging scan of an 18-week-old normal fetus (20 weeks' gestational age). A, From Moore KL, Persaud TVN, Shiota K: *Color atlas of clinical embryology*, ed 2, Philadelphia, 2000, Saunders. B, Courtesy Deborah Levine, MD, Director of Obstetric and Gynecologic Ultrasound, Department of Radiology, Beth Israel Deaconess Medical Center, Boston, MA.

Table 7.2   Comparison of Gestational Time Units

	Calendar			Lunar
Reference Point	Days	Weeks	Months	Months
Fertilization	266	38	8.75	9.5
Last normal menstrual period	280	40	9.25	10

surfactant, a surface-active lipid that maintains the patency of the developing alveoli of the lungs (see Chapter 11). A 22- to 25-week fetus born prematurely may survive initially if given intensive care support; however, the fetus may die because its respiratory system is still immature. Fetuses born before 26 weeks of gestation have a high risk of neurodevelopmental (functional) disability.

TWENTY-SIX TO TWENTY-NINE WEEKS

During this period, fetuses usually survive if born prematurely and given intensive care because the lungs have developed sufficiently to provide adequate gas exchange. In addition, the central nervous system has matured to the stage at which it can direct rhythmic breathing movements and control body temperature. The highest neonatal mortality occurs in low-birth-weight infants weighing 2500 g or less. The eyelids are open at 26 weeks, and lanugo and head hair are well developed. Toenails are visible, and considerable subcutaneous fat is now present, smoothing out many of the skin wrinkles.

THIRTY TO THIRTY-EIGHT WEEKS

The pupillary light reflex of the eyes can be elicited at 30 weeks. Usually, by the end of this period, the skin is pink

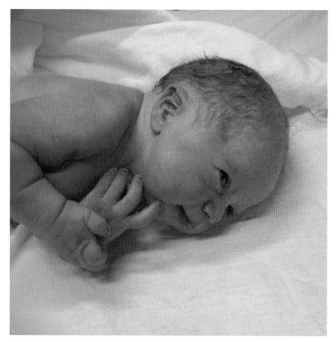

Fig. 7.6 A healthy male neonate at 36 weeks' gestational age. Courtesy Michael and Michele Rice.

and smooth, and the upper and lower limbs have a chubby appearance. Fetuses born at 32 weeks usually survive. Fetuses at 35 weeks have a firm grasp and exhibit a spontaneous orientation to light. As term approaches (37–38 weeks), the nervous system is sufficiently mature to carry out some integrative functions. Most fetuses during this "finishing period" are plump (Fig. 7.6). At 36 weeks, the circumferences of the head and abdomen are approximately equal (Fig. 7.7).

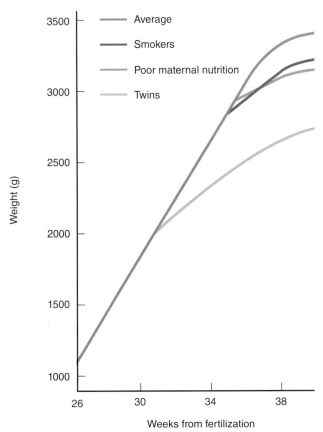

Fig. 7.7 Graph showing the rate of fetal growth during the last trimester. After 36 weeks, the average growth rate deviates from the straight line. The decline, particularly after full term (38 weeks), probably reflects inadequate fetal nutrition caused by placental changes. Other factors affecting fetal growth rate (smoking, maternal malnutrition, and twins) are also shown. Modified from Gruenwald P: Growth of the human fetus. I. Normal growth and its variation, *Am J Obstet Gynecol* 94:1112, 1966.

Fig. 7.8 Full-term female neonate weighing 3.3 kg (7.2 lb). Note the fatty vernix caseosa covering part of her body.

Most fetuses weigh approximately 3400 g at term (Fig. 7.8). A fetus adds approximately 14 g of fat daily during the last weeks of gestation.

EXPECTED DATE OF DELIVERY

The expected date of delivery of a fetus is 266 days, or 38 weeks, after fertilization (see Table 7.2). Approximately 60% are born on or before the expected date of birth.

FACTORS INFLUENCING FETAL GROWTH

The fetus requires substrates for growth and production of energy. Gases and nutrients pass freely to the fetus from the mother through the **placental membrane** (see Chapter 8). **Glucose** is a primary source of energy for fetal metabolism and growth; **amino acids** are also required. **Insulin** is required for the metabolism of glucose and is secreted by the fetal pancreas. Insulin, human growth hormone, and some small polypeptides (e.g., insulin-like growth factor I) are believed to stimulate fetal growth.

Many factors—maternal, fetal, and environmental—may affect prenatal growth. In general, factors operating throughout pregnancy tend to produce intrauterine growth restriction (IUGR) and small neonates, whereas factors operating during the last trimester usually produce underweight neonates with normal length and head size (see Fig. 7.7).

Neonates resulting from twin, triplet, and other multiple pregnancies usually weigh considerably less than infants resulting from a single pregnancy (see Fig. 7.7). It is evident that the total requirements of two or more fetuses exceed the nutritional supply available from the placenta during the third trimester.

Repeated cases of IUGR in one family indicate that recessive genes may be the cause of the abnormal growth. Placental genes and structural and numeric chromosomal aberrations have also been shown to be associated with cases of restricted fetal growth. IUGR is more common in underdeveloped or developing countries.

Lower birth weight is a risk factor for many adult diseases, including hypertension, diabetes, and cardiovascular disease. Higher birth weight resulting from gestational diabetes is associated with adult obesity and diabetes.

PROCEDURES FOR ASSESSING FETAL STATUS

ULTRASONOGRAPHY

Ultrasonography is the primary imaging modality in the evaluation of the fetus because of its wide availability, quality of images, low cost, and lack of known adverse effects (Fig. 7.9). Placental and fetal size, multiple births, abnormalities of placental shape, and abnormal presentations can also be determined. Many structural anomalies can also be detected prenatally by ultrasonography.

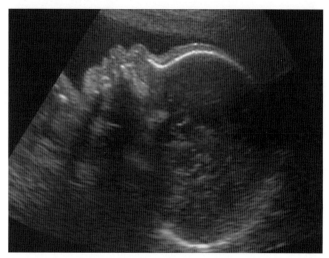

Fig. 7.9 Ultrasonogram (axial scan) of a 25-week fetus showing the facial profile. Courtesy E.A. Lyons, MD, Professor of Radiology, Obstetrics and Gynecology, and Anatomy, University of Manitoba, Health Sciences Centre, Winnipeg, Manitoba, Canada.

DIAGNOSTIC AMNIOCENTESIS

Diagnostic amniocentesis is a common invasive prenatal diagnostic procedure (Fig. 7.10A) typically performed at 13 to 16 weeks (15–18 weeks LNMP). For prenatal diagnosis, amniotic fluid is sampled by the insertion of a needle through the mother's anterior abdominal and uterine walls and into the amniotic sac. A syringe is then attached to the needle, and amniotic fluid containing shed fetal cells for genetic analysis is withdrawn. The procedure is relatively devoid of risk (0.5% spontaneous abortion), especially when performed by an experienced physician using ultrasonography as a guide for outlining the position of the fetus and placenta.

CHORIONIC VILLUS SAMPLING

Biopsy of chorionic villi (see Fig. 7.10B) is performed to detect chromosomal abnormalities, inborn errors of metabolism, and X-linked disorders through genetic analysis. Chorionic villus sampling is typically carried out between 8 and 10 weeks (10–12 weeks LNMP). The rate of fetal loss is approximately 1%. The major advantage of chorionic villus sampling over amniocentesis is that it allows fetal chromosomal sampling to be performed several weeks earlier.

PERCUTANEOUS UMBILICAL CORD BLOOD SAMPLING

Fetal blood samples may be obtained from the umbilical vein by **percutaneous umbilical cord blood sampling (PUBS)**. Ultrasonographic scanning is used to outline the location of the vessels. PUBS is often performed at approximately 16 weeks (18 weeks LNMP). With a normal fetus, the loss of pregnancy rate is approximately 1.3%. Beyond genetics

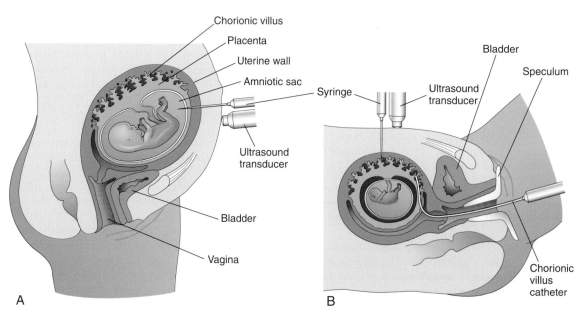

Fig. 7.10 (A) Illustration of the technique of amniocentesis. Using ultrasonographic guidance, a needle is inserted through the mother's abdominal and uterine walls into the amniotic sac. A syringe is attached, and amniotic fluid is withdrawn for diagnostic purposes. (B) Illustration of chorionic villus sampling. Two sampling approaches are shown—one through the anterior abdominal wall and amniotic sac using a needle, and one through the vagina and cervical canal using a malleable chorionic villus catheter.

testing, the blood can also be analyzed to detect infection and blood disorders such as thrombocytopenia.

MAGNETIC RESONANCE IMAGING

When fetal treatment, such as surgery, is planned, computed tomography and **magnetic resonance imaging (MRI)** may be used. MRI has the advantage of not using ionizing radiation and can produce images with very high tissue resolution. These imaging studies can provide additional information about a fetal abnormality detected by ultrasound.

FETAL MONITORING

Continuous fetal heart rate monitoring in high-risk pregnancies is routine and provides information about the oxygenation of the fetus. **Fetal distress**, as indicated by an abnormal heart rate or rhythm, suggests that the fetus is in jeopardy.

ALPHA-FETOPROTEIN ASSAY

Alpha fetoprotein (AFP), a glycoprotein that is synthesized in the fetal liver and umbilical vesicle, escapes from the fetal circulation into the amniotic fluid in fetuses with open neural tube defects, such as spina bifida with myeloschisis (see Chapter 19). AFP can also enter the amniotic fluid from open ventral wall defects, as occurs with gastroschisis and omphalocele (see Chapter 13). AFP is formed at the end of the first trimester and begins to decrease by the third trimester of pregnancy. It can also be measured in maternal serum.

NONINVASIVE PRENATAL DIAGNOSIS

Trisomy 21 is the most commonly known of the chromosomal disorders, and children born with this condition have varying degrees of intellectual disability. Noninvasive screening for trisomy 21 is based on the isolation of fetal cells in maternal blood and the detection of cell-free fetal DNA and RNA. Compared with amniocentesis and chorionic villus biopsy, the results are available earlier, and there are fewer complications.

NEONATAL PERIOD

The **neonatal period** pertains to the first 4 weeks after birth. The early neonatal period is from birth to 7 days. The late neonatal period is from 7 to 28 days. The umbilical cord usually drops off 7 to 8 days after birth, at the end of the early neonatal period.

The neonate is not a "miniature adult," and an extremely preterm infant is not the same as a full-term infant. Usually, a neonate loses about 10% of its birth weight over the 3 to 4 days after birth, owing to the loss of excess extracellular fluid and discharge of **meconium**, the first greenish intestinal material ejected from the rectum.

When the neonate's hand is touched, it will usually grasp a finger. If the mother holds the baby close to her chest, the baby will search (root) for her breast to find the nipple and feed. Neonates are born with full visual capacity to see objects and colors about 8 to 15 inches away; however, they are extremely nearsighted. A gentle stroke on the baby's cheek makes the baby turn toward the touch with its mouth open.

CLINICALLY ORIENTED QUESTIONS

1. Do mature embryos move at all? Can a first-trimester fetus move its limbs? If so, can the mother feel her baby kicking at this time?

2. Some reports suggest that vitamin supplementation around the time of conception will prevent neural tube defects, such as spina bifida. Is there scientific proof to support this statement?

3. Can the needle injure the fetus during amniocentesis? Is there a risk of inducing an abortion or causing maternal or fetal infection?

The answers to these questions are at the back of this book.

Placenta and Fetal Membranes   **8**

The fetal part of the placenta and fetal membranes separates the embryo or fetus from the **endometrium**—the inner mucous layer of the uterine wall. The chorion, amnion, umbilical vesicle, and allantois constitute the **fetal membranes**. The vessels in the umbilical cord connect the placental circulation with the fetal circulation.

PLACENTA

The placenta is the primary site of nutrient and gas exchange between the mother and fetus. The placenta is a **fetomaternal organ** that has two components:

- A **fetal part** that develops from part of the chorionic sac
- A **maternal part** that is derived from the endometrium

.The placenta and umbilical cord form a transport system for substances passing between the mother and fetus. Nutrients and oxygen pass from the maternal blood through the placenta to the fetal blood, and waste materials and carbon dioxide pass from the fetal blood through the placenta to the maternal blood. The placenta and fetal membranes perform the following functions and activities: protection, nutrition, respiration, excretion of waste products, and hormone production. Shortly after birth, the placenta and fetal membranes are expelled from the uterus as the **afterbirth**.

DECIDUA

The decidua is the endometrium of the uterus in a pregnant woman. It is the functional layer of the endometrium that separates from the remainder of the uterus after **parturition** (childbirth). The three regions of the decidua are named according to their relation to the implantation site (Fig. 8.1):

- **Decidua basalis**—the part of the decidua deep to the conceptus that forms the maternal part of the placenta
- **Decidua capsularis**—the superficial part of the decidua overlying the conceptus
- **Decidua parietalis**—the remaining intervening parts of the decidua.

In response to increasing **progesterone** levels in the maternal blood, the connective tissue cells of the decidua enlarge to form pale-staining **decidual cells**. These cells enlarge as glycogen, and lipids accumulate in their cytoplasm. The cellular and vascular changes in the decidua that result from pregnancy are referred to as the **decidual reaction**. Many decidual cells degenerate near the chorionic sac in the region of the syncytiotrophoblast and, together

with maternal blood and uterine secretions, provide a rich source of nutrition for the embryo. Decidual regions, clearly recognizable during antenatal ultrasonography, are important in diagnosing early pregnancy.

DEVELOPMENT OF PLACENTA

Early placental development is characterized by the rapid proliferation of the trophoblast and development of the chorionic sac and chorionic villi. By the end of the third week, the anatomic structures necessary for physiological exchanges between the mother and embryo have formed. By the end of the fourth week, a complex vascular network develops in the placenta, allowing maternal–embryonic exchanges of gases, nutrients, and metabolic waste products.

Chorionic villi cover the entire chorionic sac until the beginning of the eighth week (Fig. 8.2). As this sac grows, the villi associated with the decidua capsularis are compressed, reducing the blood supply to them. These villi soon degenerate, producing a relatively avascular bare area, the **smooth chorion** (see Fig. 8.1D). As these villi disappear, others associated with the decidua basalis rapidly increase in number, branch profusely, and enlarge (Fig. 8.3). This bushy part of the chorionic sac is the **villous chorion** or **chorion frondosum** (Fig. 8.4; see also Fig. 8.1E).

Homeobox (HLX, MSX2, *and* DLX3) *and other genetic factors expressed on the trophoblast and blood vessels induce trophoblast invasion and help regulate the development of the placenta.*

Ultrasonography of Chorionic Sac

The size of the chorionic sac is useful in determining the gestational age of embryos in patients with uncertain menstrual histories. The growth of the chorionic sac is extremely rapid between the 5th and 10th weeks of development. Modern ultrasound imaging devices permit detection of the chorionic sac when it has a median diameter of 2 to 3 mm (see Fig. 8.4). Chorionic sacs with this diameter indicate a gestational age of approximately 18 days after fertilization.

FETOMATERNAL JUNCTION

The villous chorion is attached to the decidua basalis by the **cytotrophoblastic shell**, the external layer of trophoblastic cells on the maternal surface of the placenta (Fig. 8.5). The

65

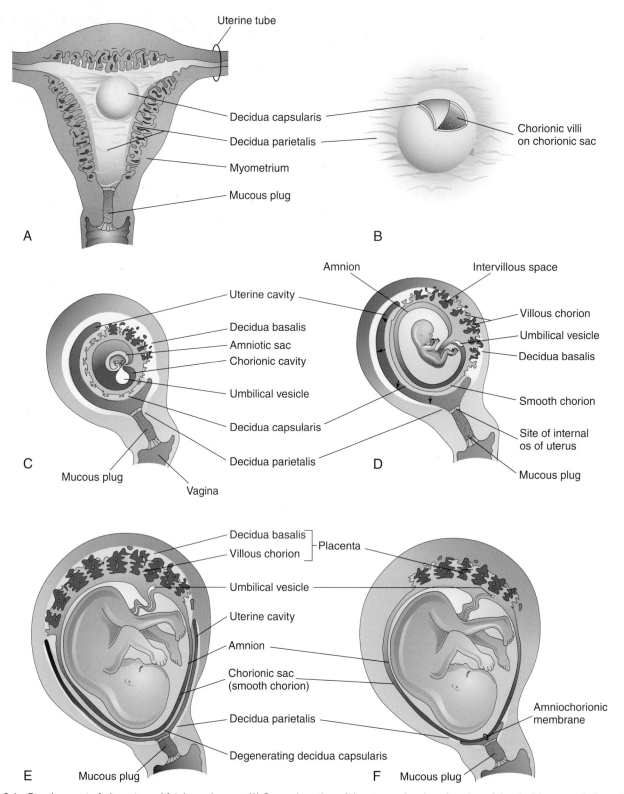

Fig. 8.1   Development of placenta and fetal membranes. (A) Coronal section of the uterus showing elevation of the decidua capsularis and the expanding chorionic sac at 4 weeks. (B) Enlarged illustration of the implantation site. The chorionic villi were exposed by cutting an opening in the decidua capsularis. (C–F) Sagittal sections of the gravid (pregnant) uterus from the 5th to 22nd weeks, showing the changing relationship of the fetal membranes to the decidua. (F) The amnion and chorion are fused with each other and with the decidua parietalis, thereby obliterating the uterine cavity.

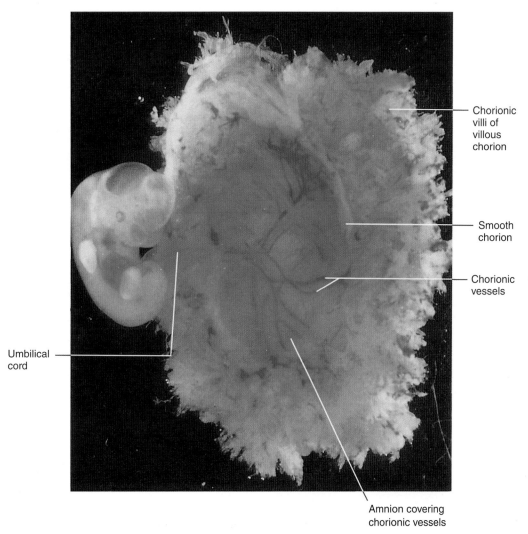

Chorionic villi of villous chorion

Smooth chorion

Chorionic vessels

Umbilical cord

Amnion covering chorionic vessels

Fig. 8.2 Lateral view of a spontaneously aborted embryo at Carnegie stage 14, approximately 32 days. The chorionic and amniotic sacs have been opened to show the embryo.

chorionic villi attach firmly to the decidua basalis through the cytotrophoblastic shell and anchor the chorionic sac to the decidua basalis. **Endometrial arteries and veins** pass freely through gaps in the cytotrophoblastic shell and open into the **intervillous space** (see Fig. 8.5).

The shape of the placenta is determined by the persistent area of chorionic villi (see Fig. 8.1F). Usually, this is a circular area, giving the placenta a discoid shape. As the chorionic villi invade the decidua basalis during placental formation, decidual tissue is eroded to enlarge the intervillous space. This erosion produces several wedge-shaped areas of decidua—**placental septa**—that project toward the **chorionic plate** (see Fig. 8.5). The placental septa divide the fetal part of the placenta into irregular convex areas—**cotyledons** (see Fig. 8.3). Each cotyledon consists of two or more **stem villi** and many **branch villi**.

The decidua capsularis, the layer overlying the implanted chorionic sac, forms a capsule over the external surface of the sac (see Fig. 8.1A–D). As the conceptus enlarges, the decidua capsularis bulges into the uterine cavity and becomes greatly attenuated. Eventually, parts

of the decidua capsularis make contact and fuse with the decidua parietalis, thereby slowly obliterating the uterine cavity (see Fig. 8.1E and F). By 22 to 24 weeks, reduced blood supply to the decidua capsularis causes it to degenerate and disappear.

INTERVILLOUS SPACE

The large intervillous space of the placenta contains maternal blood (see Fig. 4.1B), and it results from the coalescence and enlargement of the **lacunar networks**. The intervillous space is divided into compartments by the **placental septa**; however, free communication occurs between the compartments because the septa do not reach the chorionic plate (see Fig. 8.5), the part of the chorion associated with the placenta. Maternal blood enters the intervillous space from the **spiral arteries** in the decidua basalis (see Fig. 8.5); these arteries pass through gaps in the cytotrophoblastic shell and discharge blood into the intervillous space. Trophoblastic cells invade the spiral arteries and create plugs within the arteries. These plugs allow only maternal plasma to enter

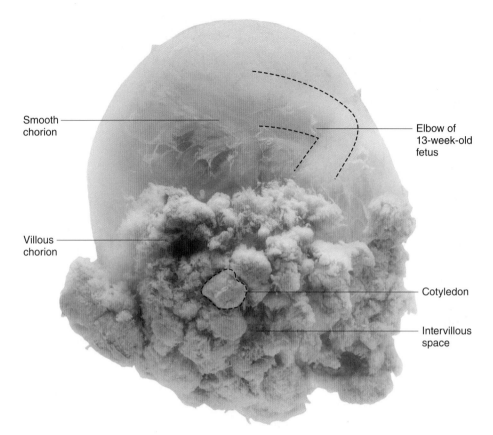

Smooth chorion

Elbow of 13-week-old fetus

Villous chorion

Cotyledon

Intervillous space

Fig. 8.3 A human chorionic sac containing a 13-week fetus that aborted spontaneously. The villous chorion is where chorionic villi persist and form the fetal part of the placenta. In situ, the cotyledons were attached to the decidua basalis, and the intervillous space was filled with maternal blood.

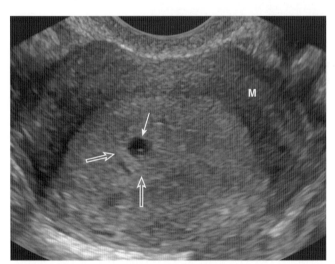

M

Figure 8.4 Endovaginal axial scan of a gravid uterus showing a 3-week chorionic sac (*arrow*) in the posterior endometrium (decidua). There is a bright (echogenic) ring of chorionic villi (*open arrows*) around the sac. *M,* Myometrium. Courtesy E.A. Lyons, MD, Professor of Radiology, Obstetrics and Gynecology, and Anatomy, University of Manitoba, Health Sciences Centre, Winnipeg, Manitoba, Canada.

the intervillous space. As a result, a net negative oxygen gradient is created; it has been shown that elevated oxygen levels during the early stages of development can cause complications such as spontaneous abortion and preeclampsia. However, by 11 to 14 weeks, as the plugs begin to break down, maternal whole blood begins to flow and oxygen concentrations increase. This intervillous space is drained by endometrial veins that also penetrate the cytotrophoblastic shell. The numerous branch villi, arising from stem villi, are continuously showered with maternal blood as it circulates through the intervillous space. The blood in this space carries oxygen and nutritional materials that are necessary for fetal growth and development. The maternal blood also contains fetal waste products, such as carbon dioxide, salts, and products of protein metabolism.

AMNIOCHORIONIC MEMBRANE

The amniotic sac enlarges faster than the chorionic sac. As a result, the amnion and smooth chorion soon fuse to form the **amniochorionic membrane** (see Fig. 8.1F). This composite membrane fuses with the decidua capsularis and, after the disappearance of this part of the decidua, adheres to the decidua parietalis. *It is the amniochorionic membrane that ruptures during labor.* Preterm early rupture of this membrane is the most common event leading to premature labor. When the amniochorionic membrane ruptures, the amniotic fluid escapes through the cervix and vagina.

PLACENTAL CIRCULATION

The many branch chorionic villi of the placenta provide a large surface area where materials (e.g., oxygen and

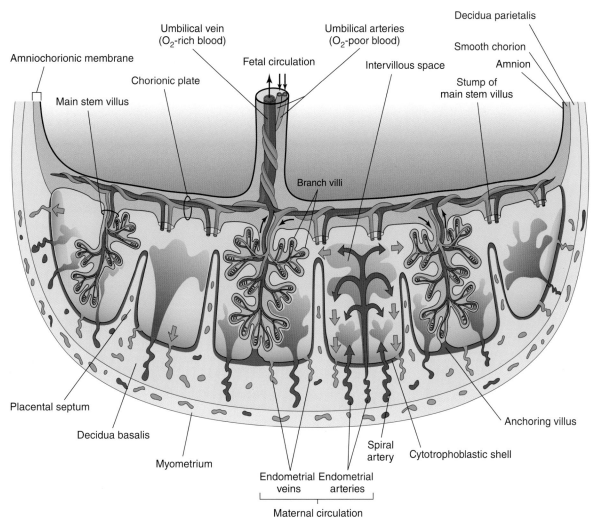

Fig. 8.5 Illustration of a transverse section through a full-term placenta, showing (1) the relation of the villous chorion (fetal part of placenta) to the decidua basalis (maternal part of the placenta); (2) the fetal placental circulation; and (3) the maternal–placental circulation. Maternal blood flows into the intervillous spaces in funnel-shaped spurts from the spiral arteries, and exchanges occur with the fetal blood as the maternal blood flows around the branch villi. The inflowing arterial blood pushes venous blood out of the intervillous space and into the endometrial veins. Note that the umbilical arteries carry poorly oxygenated fetal blood (shown in *blue*) to the placenta and that the umbilical vein carries oxygenated blood (shown in *red*) to the fetus. Only one stem villus is shown in each cotyledon, but the stumps of those that have been removed are indicated. *Arrows* indicate direction of maternal (*red* and *blue*) and fetal (*black*) blood flow.

nutrients) are exchanged across the very thin **placental membrane** interposed between the fetal and maternal circulations (Fig. 8.6B and C). It is through the branch villi that the main exchange of material between the mother and the fetus takes place.

FETOPLACENTAL CIRCULATION

Poorly oxygenated blood leaves the fetus and passes through the **umbilical arteries** (Fig. 8.7; see also Fig. 8.5). At the attachment of the umbilical cord to the placenta, these arteries divide into a number of radially disposed **chorionic arteries** that branch freely in the **chorionic plate** before entering the chorionic villi (see Fig. 8.5). The blood vessels form an extensive **arteriocapillary-venous system** within the chorionic villi (see Fig. 8.6A), which brings the fetal blood extremely close to the maternal blood (see Fig. 8.7). This system provides a very large surface area for the exchange of metabolic and gaseous products between the maternal and fetal blood.

The well-oxygenated fetal blood in the fetal capillaries passes into thin-walled veins that follow the chorionic arteries to the site of attachment of the umbilical cord, where they converge to form the **umbilical vein**. This large vessel carries oxygen-rich blood to the fetus (see Fig. 8.5).

Bidirectional transfer of blood cells (fetal–maternal) does occur, although the mechanisms are not well understood. Maternal **microchimerism** has been detected in up to 50% of umbilical cord blood samples at the time of birth and includes T memory and B cells. Fetal microchimerism also occurs and is detected in the mother's blood more commonly in cases of preeclampsia. The long-term consequences of these microchimerisms continue to be investigated.

MATERNAL–PLACENTAL CIRCULATION

The maternal blood enters the intervillous space through 80 to 100 **spiral endometrial arteries** in the decidua basalis (see Fig. 8.5). The entering blood is at considerably higher pressure than that in the intervillous space, so the blood

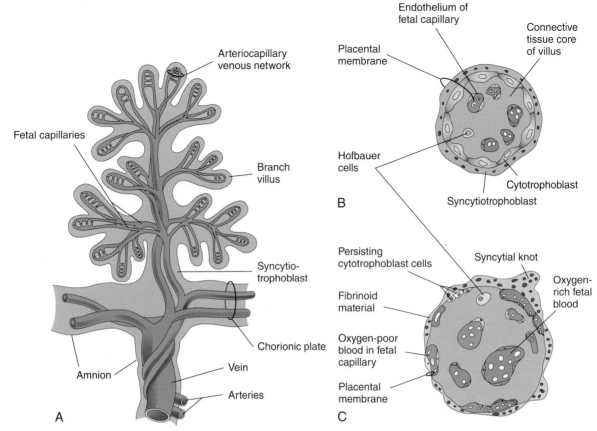

Fig. 8.6 (A) Illustration of a stem chorionic villus showing its arteriocapillary-venous system. The arteries carry poorly oxygenated fetal blood and waste products from the fetus, whereas the vein carries oxygenated blood and nutrients to the fetus. (B and C) Sections through a branch villus at 10 weeks' gestation and at full term, respectively. The placental membrane, composed of extrafetal tissues, separates the maternal blood in the intervillous space from the fetal blood in the capillaries in the villi. Note that the placental membrane becomes very thin at full term. Hofbauer cells (B) are believed to be phagocytic cells.

spurts toward the **chorionic plate**. As the pressure dissipates, the blood flows slowly around the branch villi, allowing an exchange of metabolic and gaseous products with the fetal blood. The blood eventually returns through the endometrial veins to the maternal circulation (see Fig. 8.7). The reduction in uteroplacental circulation results in **fetal hypoxia** and **intrauterine growth restriction**. The intervillous space of the mature placenta contains approximately 150 mL of blood that is replenished three or four times each minute.

PLACENTAL MEMBRANE

The membrane consists of the extrafetal tissues that separate maternal and fetal blood. Until about 20 weeks, the placental membrane consists of four layers (see Fig. 8.6B and C): syncytiotrophoblast, cytotrophoblast, connective tissue of the villus, and endothelium of the fetal capillaries. After the 20th week, microscopic changes occur in the branch villi that result in the cytotrophoblast becoming attenuated in many villi. Fetal macrophages (Hofbauer cells) present in the villi play an essential role in the formation and function of the placenta (see Fig. 8.6B).

Eventually, cytotrophoblastic cells disappear over large areas of the villi, leaving only thin patches of syncytiotrophoblast. As a result, the placental membrane at full term consists of only three layers in most places (see Fig. 8.6C). In some areas, the placental membrane becomes markedly thin. At these sites, the syncytiotrophoblast comes into direct contact with the endothelium of the fetal capillaries to form a **vasculosyncytial placental membrane**.

Only a few substances, endogenous or exogenous, are unable to pass through the placental membrane. In this regard, the membrane acts as a true barrier only when the molecule or organism has a certain size, configuration, and charge. *Most drugs and other substances in the maternal plasma pass through the placental membrane and are found in the fetal plasma* (see Fig. 8.7). During the third trimester, numerous nuclei in the syncytiotrophoblast of the villi aggregate to form **syncytial knots**—nuclear aggregations (see Fig. 8.6C). These knots regularly break off and are carried from the intervillous space into the maternal circulation. Some knots may lodge in the capillaries of the maternal lungs, where they are rapidly destroyed by local enzyme action. Toward the end of pregnancy, **fibrinoid material** forms on the surfaces of villi (see Fig. 8.6C).

FUNCTIONS OF PLACENTA

The placenta has many functions:

- Metabolism
- Transport of gases, nutrients, drugs, and infectious agents
- Protection by maternal antibodies
- Excretion of waste products
- Endocrine synthesis and secretion (e.g., human chorionic gonadotropin [hCG])

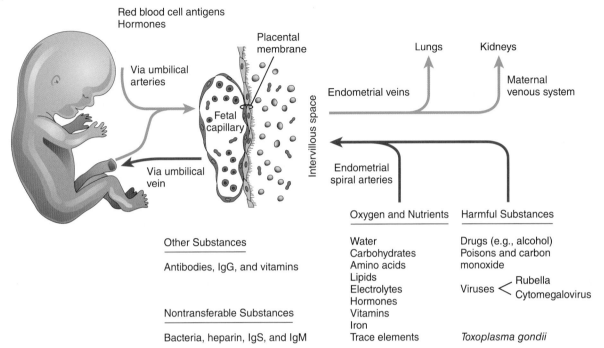

Waste Products

Carbon dioxide, water,
urea, uric acid, bilirubin

Other Substances

Red blood cell antigens
Hormones

Placental membrane

Via umbilical arteries

Fetal capillary

Intervillous space

Via umbilical vein

Lungs   Kidneys

Endometrial veins   Maternal venous system

Endometrial spiral arteries

Other Substances

Antibodies, IgG, and vitamins

Nontransferable Substances

Bacteria, heparin, IgS, and IgM

Oxygen and Nutrients

Water
Carbohydrates
Amino acids
Lipids
Electrolytes
Hormones
Vitamins
Iron
Trace elements

Harmful Substances

Drugs (e.g., alcohol)
Poisons and carbon monoxide

Viruses ⟨ Rubella
        Cytomegalovirus

Toxoplasma gondii

Fig. 8.7 Transport across the placental membrane. The extrafetal tissues, across which the transport of substances between the mother and fetus occurs, collectively constitute the placental membrane. *IgG*, Immunoglobulin G; *IgM*, immunoglobulin M; *IgS*, immunoglobulin S.

Placental Metabolism

The placenta synthesizes glycogen, cholesterol, and fatty acids, which serve as sources of nutrients and energy for the embryo or fetus. Many of the metabolic activities of the placenta are critical for two of its other major activities: transport and endocrine secretion. At term, these metabolic needs result in the placenta itself using 40% to 60% of the oxygen and glucose reaching the uterus.

Placental Transport

The large surface area of the placental membrane facilitates the transport of substances in both directions between the placenta and the maternal blood. Almost all materials are transported across the placental membrane by one of the following four main transport mechanisms: simple **diffusion, facilitated diffusion, active transport**, and **pinocytosis**.

Passive transport by simple diffusion is usually characteristic of substances moving from areas of higher to lower concentration until equilibrium is established. Facilitated diffusion requires a transporter but no energy. Active transport against a concentration gradient requires energy. This mechanism of transport may involve carrier molecules that temporarily combine with the substances to be transported. Pinocytosis is a form of endocytosis in which the material being engulfed is a small amount of extracellular fluid.

Some proteins are transferred very slowly through the placenta by pinocytosis.

Transfer of Gases. Oxygen and carbon dioxide cross the placental membrane by simple diffusion. *Interruption of oxygen transport for several minutes endangers the survival of the embryo or fetus.* The efficiency of the placental membrane approaches that of the lungs for gas exchange. The quantity of oxygen reaching the fetus is generally blood flow-limited rather than oxygen diffusion-limited. **Fetal hypoxia** results primarily from factors that diminish either uterine blood flow or fetal blood flow through the placenta. The placenta has a number of mechanisms that allow it to react to various situations including hypoxia so that the fetal effects can be minimized. Nitrous oxide, an inhalation analgesic and anesthetic, and carbon monoxide, an environmental toxin, readily cross the placenta.

Nutritional Substances. Nutrients constitute the bulk of substances transferred from the mother to the embryo or fetus. Water is rapidly exchanged by simple diffusion and in increasing amounts as pregnancy advances. Glucose produced by the mother and placenta is quickly transferred to the embryo or fetus by facilitated diffusion mediated primarily by GLUT-1 (glucose transporter 1)—an insulin-independent glucose carrier. Maternal cholesterol, triglycerides, and phospholipids are transferred. Although free fatty acids are transported, the amount transferred appears to be relatively small with a preference toward long-chain polyunsaturated fatty acids. Amino acids cross the placenta to the fetus in high concentrations by active transport. Vitamins cross the placental membrane and are essential for normal development. A maternal protein, **transferrin**, crosses the placental membrane and carries iron to the embryo or fetus. The placental surface contains special receptors for this protein.

Hormones. Protein hormones such as insulin and pituitary hormones do not reach the embryo or fetus in significant amounts, except for a slow transfer of **thyroxine** and **triiodothyronine**. Unconjugated steroid hormones cross the placental membrane relatively freely. **Testosterone** and certain synthetic progestins also cross the placenta (see Chapter 19).

Electrolytes. These compounds are freely exchanged in significant quantities, each at its own rate. When a mother receives intravenous fluids with electrolytes, they also pass to the fetus and affect the fetal water and electrolyte status.

Drugs and Drug Metabolites. Most drugs and drug metabolites cross the placenta by simple diffusion. Drugs taken by the mother can affect the embryo or fetus, directly or indirectly, by interfering with maternal or placental metabolism. Some drugs cause major birth defects (see Chapter 19). Most drugs used for the management of labor readily cross the placental membrane. Depending on the dose and timing in relation to delivery, these drugs may cause respiratory depression in the neonate. Neuromuscular blocking agents such as succinylcholine, which might be used during operative obstetrics, cross the placenta in only very small amounts. All sedatives and analgesics affect the fetus to some degree. Inhaled anesthetics can also cross the placental membrane and affect fetal breathing if used during parturition.

Infectious Agents. Cytomegalovirus, rubella, coxsackieviruses, and viruses associated with variola, varicella, measles, and poliomyelitis may pass through the placental membrane and cause fetal infection. In some cases, as with **cytomegalovirus** and the **rubella virus**, severe birth defects may result (see Chapter 19). *Treponema pallidum* can cause fetal syphilis, and *Toxoplasma gondii* can produce destructive changes in the brain and eyes of the fetus.

Placental Protection by Maternal Antibodies

The fetus produces only small amounts of antibodies because of its immature immune system. Some passive immunity is conferred on the fetus by placental transfer of maternal antibodies. Only **immunoglobulin G** is transferred across the placenta (receptor-mediated transcytosis). Beginning at approximately week 16, **maternal antibodies** confer fetal immunity for diseases such as **diphtheria, smallpox, and measles**; however, no immunity is acquired for **pertussis** or **varicella**.

Placental Excretion of Waste Products

Urea, a nitrogenous waste product, and uric acid pass through the placental membrane by simple diffusion.

Conjugated bilirubin, which is fat soluble, is easily transported by the placenta and is quickly removed.

Placental Endocrine Synthesis and Secretion

Using precursors derived from the fetus, the mother, or both, the syncytiotrophoblast of the placenta synthesizes protein and steroid hormones. **Protein hormones** synthesized by the placenta include the following:

- Human chorionic gonadotropin (hCG)
- Human chorionic somatomammotropin (human placental lactogen)
- Human chorionic thyrotropin
- Human chorionic corticotropin

.The glycoprotein **hCG**, similar to luteinizing hormone, is first secreted by the syncytiotrophoblast during the second week of development. The hCG maintains the corpus luteum, preventing the onset of menstrual periods. The concentration of hCG in the maternal blood and urine rises to a maximum by the eighth week and then declines. The placenta also plays a major role in the production of **steroid hormones** (i.e., progesterone and estrogens). Progesterone is essential for the maintenance of pregnancy. Other hormones produced include **relaxin** and **activin**.

Hemolytic Disease of the Neonate

Small amounts of fetal blood may pass into the maternal blood through microscopic breaks in the placental membrane. If the fetus is Rh-positive and the mother is Rh-negative, the fetal cells may stimulate the formation of an anti-Rh antibody by the mother's immune system. This antibody passes to the fetal blood and causes hemolysis of fetal Rh-positive blood cells and anemia in the fetus. Some fetuses with **hemolytic disease of the neonate**, or **fetal erythroblastosis**, do not make a satisfactory intrauterine adjustment. They may die unless delivered early or given intraperitoneal or intravenous transfusions of packed Rh-negative blood cells to maintain them until after birth. Hemolytic disease of the neonate is relatively uncommon now because $Rh_0(D)$ immune globulin given to the mother usually prevents the development of this disease in the fetus.

UTERINE GROWTH DURING PREGNANCY

The uterus of a nonpregnant woman is positioned in the pelvis. It increases in size during pregnancy to accommodate the growing fetus. As the uterus enlarges, it increases in weight and its walls become thinner. During the first trimester, the uterus expands out of the pelvic cavity, and by 20 weeks, it usually reaches the level of the umbilicus. By 28 to 30 weeks, the uterine fundus reaches the epigastric region.

PARTURITION

Parturition (childbirth) is the process during which the fetus, placenta, and fetal membranes are expelled from the mother (Fig. 8.8). **Labor** is the sequence of uterine contractions that result in dilation of the uterine cervix and delivery

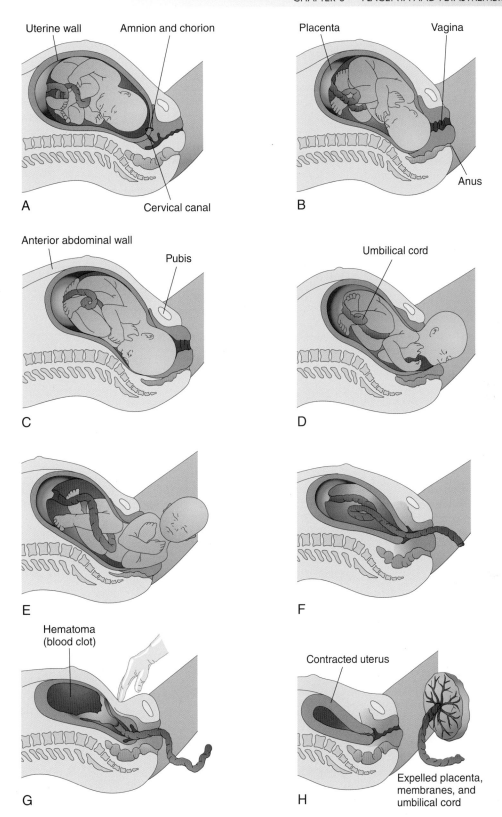

Fig. 8.8   Illustrations of parturition (childbirth). (A and B) The cervix is dilating during the first stage of labor. (C–E) The fetus is passing through the cervix and vagina during the second stage of labor. (F and G) As the uterus contracts during the third stage of labor, the placenta folds and pulls away from the uterine wall. Separation of the placenta results in bleeding and the formation of a large hematoma (mass of blood). Pressure on the abdomen facilitates placental separation. (H) The placenta is expelled, and the uterus contracts.

of the fetus and placenta from the uterus. The factors that trigger labor are not completely understood, but several hormones are related to the initiation of contractions. The fetal hypothalamus secretes **corticotropin-releasing hormone**, stimulating the pituitary gland to produce **adrenocorticotropic hormone (ACTH)**. ACTH causes the suprarenal cortex to secrete **cortisol**, which is involved in the synthesis of **estrogens**.

Peristaltic contractions of the uterine smooth muscle are elicited by **oxytocin**, which is released by the maternal neurohypophysis of the pituitary gland. This hormone is administered clinically when it is necessary to induce labor. Oxytocin also stimulates the release of **prostaglandins** that, in turn, stimulate myometrial contractility by sensitizing the myometrial cells to oxytocin. Estrogens also increase myometrial contractile activity and stimulate the release of oxytocin and prostaglandins. The connective tissue of the cervix is also altered to allow for softening and dilation.

STAGES OF LABOR

Labor is a continuous process; however, for clinical purposes, it is divided into three stages:

- **Dilation** begins with progressive dilation of the cervix (see Fig. 8.8A and B) and ends with complete dilation (10 cm) of the cervix. During this phase, regular **contractions of the uterus occur** less than 10 minutes apart. The average duration of the first stage is approximately 12 hours for **primiparous women** (first delivery) and approximately 7 hours for multiparous women (who have delivered previously).
- **Expulsion** begins when the cervix is fully dilated and ends with delivery of the fetus (see Fig. 8.8C–E). During this stage, the fetus descends through the cervix and vagina. As soon as the fetus is outside the mother, it is called a neonate. The average duration of this stage is 50 minutes for primiparous women and 20 minutes for multiparous women.
- **Placental separation** begins as soon as the fetus is born and ends with the expulsion of the placenta and fetal membranes (see Fig. 8.8F–H). A **hematoma** forms deep in the placenta and separates it from the uterine wall. The placenta and fetal membranes are then expelled. Contractions of the uterus constrict the spiral arteries, preventing excessive uterine bleeding. The duration of this stage is approximately 15 minutes. A retained or **adherent placenta**—one not expelled within 1 hour of delivery—is a cause of **postpartum uterine hemorrhage**.

PLACENTA AND FETAL MEMBRANES AFTER BIRTH

The placenta usually has a discoid shape, with a diameter of 15 to 20 cm and a thickness of 2 to 3 cm (Fig. 8.9). The margins of the placenta are continuous with the ruptured amniotic and chorionic sacs.

VARIATIONS IN THE PLACENTAL SHAPE

As the placenta develops, chorionic villi usually persist only where the villous chorion is in contact with the decidua basalis (see Fig. 8.1E and F). When villi persist elsewhere, several variations in placental shape occur, such as **accessory placenta** (Fig. 8.10). Examination of the placenta, prenatally by ultrasonography or postnatally by gross and microscopic study, may provide clinical information about the causes of placental dysfunction, intrauterine growth restriction, fetal distress and death, and neonatal illness. Postnatal placental examination can also determine whether the expelled placenta is intact. Retention of cotyledons or an accessory placenta in the uterus causes postpartum uterine hemorrhage.

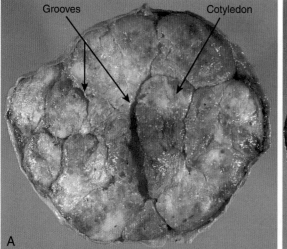 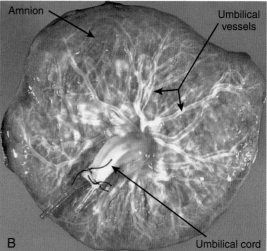

Fig. 8.9 Placentas and fetal membranes after birth are shown to be approximately one-third of their actual size. (A) Maternal surface, showing cotyledons and grooves around them. Each convex cotyledon consists of a number of main stem villi with their many branch villi. The grooves were occupied by the placental septa when the maternal and fetal parts of the placenta were together (see Fig. 8.5). (B) Fetal surface showing blood vessels running in the chorionic plate deep to the amnion and converging to form the umbilical vessels at the attachment of the umbilical cord.

Placental Abnormalities

Abnormal adherence of the chorionic villi to the myometrium of the uterine wall is called **placenta accreta** (Fig. 8.11). When chorionic villi penetrate the myometrium all the way to the perimetrium (peritoneal covering), the abnormality is called **placenta percreta**. Third-trimester bleeding is the most common presenting sign of these placental abnormalities. After birth, the placenta does not separate from the uterine wall, and attempts to remove it may cause severe hemorrhage that is difficult to control. When the blastocyst implants close to or overlying the internal os of the uterus, the abnormality is called **placenta previa**. Late-pregnancy bleeding can result from this placental abnormality. In such cases, the fetus is delivered by cesarean section because the placenta blocks the cervical canal. Magnetic resonance imaging and ultrasonography are used for imaging the placenta in various clinical situations.

Absence of Umbilical Artery

In approximately 1 in 200 neonates, only one umbilical artery is present (Fig. 8.12), a condition that may be associated with chromosomal and fetal abnormalities. Absence of an umbilical artery is accompanied by a 15% to 20% incidence of cardiovascular anomalies in the fetus. Absence of an artery results from either agenesis or degeneration of this vessel early in development.

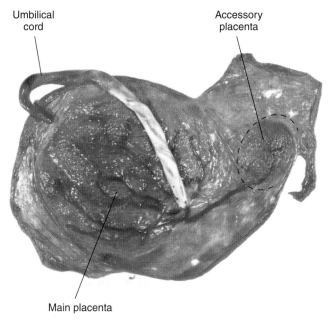

Fig. 8.10 Maternal surface of a full-term placenta and an accessory placenta. The umbilical cord is attached to the edge of the fetal surface of the placenta.

MATERNAL SURFACE OF PLACENTA

The cobblestone appearance of the maternal surface of the placenta is produced by slightly bulging villous areas—the **cotyledons**—which are separated by grooves formerly occupied by placental septa (see Fig. 8.9A).

FETAL SURFACE OF PLACENTA

The umbilical cord usually attaches near the center of the fetal surface, and its epithelium is continuous with the amnion adhering to the chorionic plate of the placenta (see Fig. 8.9B), giving the fetal surface a smooth texture. The chorionic vessels radiating to and from the umbilical cord are visible through the transparent amnion. The umbilical vessels branch on the fetal surface, forming the chorionic vessels, which enter the chorionic villi (see Fig. 8.5).

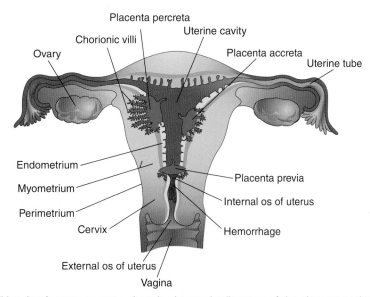

Fig. 8.11 Placental abnormalities. In **placenta accreta**, there is abnormal adherence of the placenta to the myometrium (muscle layer). In **placenta percreta**, the placenta has penetrated the full thickness of the myometrium. In **placenta previa**, the placenta overlies the internal os of the uterus, blocking the cervical canal.

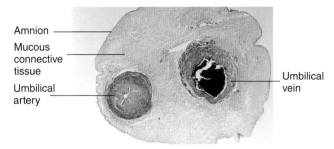

Fig. 8.12 Transverse section of the umbilical cord. Note that the cord is covered by a single-layered epithelium derived from the enveloping amnion. It has a core of mucous connective tissue. Observe also that the cord has one umbilical artery and one vein. Usually, there are two arteries. *Courtesy V. Becker, Professor, Pathologisches Institut der Universität, Erlangen, Germany.*

UMBILICAL CORD

The attachment of the cord to the placenta is usually near the center of the fetal surface of the placenta (Fig. 8.9B), but it may attach at other locations (see Fig. 8.10). The cord is usually 1 to 2 cm in diameter and 30 to 90 cm in length (see Fig. 8.10). Doppler ultrasonography and magnetic resonance imaging may be used for prenatal diagnosis of the position and structural abnormalities of the cord. Long cords have a tendency to prolapse through the cervix or to coil around the fetus. Prompt recognition of **prolapse of the cord** is important because, during delivery, it may be compressed between the presenting body part of the fetus and the mother's bony pelvis, causing **fetal anoxia**.

The umbilical cord usually has two arteries and one vein surrounded by mucoid connective tissue (**Wharton jelly**). Because the umbilical vessels are longer than the cord, twisting and bending of the cord is common. The cord frequently forms loops, producing false knots that are of no significance; however, in approximately 1% of pregnancies, true knots form in the umbilical cord. These may tighten and cause fetal death secondary to fetal anoxia (Fig. 8.13C). In most cases, the knots form during labor as a result of the fetus passing through a loop of the cord. Because these knots are usually loose, they have no clinical significance. Simple looping of the cord around the fetus occasionally occurs. In approximately one-fifth of all deliveries, the cord is loosely looped around the neck without causing increased fetal risk.

AMNION AND AMNIOTIC FLUID

The amnion forms a membranous **amniotic sac** that surrounds the embryo and later the fetus; the sac contains **amniotic fluid** (see Fig. 8.13). As the amnion enlarges, it gradually obliterates the chorionic cavity and forms the epithelial covering of the umbilical cord (see Fig. 8.13A and B). Amniotic fluid plays a major role in fetal growth and development. Initially, the cells of the amnion secrete some amniotic fluid. Most of the fluid is derived from maternal tissue by diffusion across the amniochorionic membrane from the decidua parietalis (see Fig. 8.5). Later, there is diffusion of fluid through the chorionic plate from blood in the intervillous space of the placenta.

Before **keratinization** of the fetal skin occurs, a major pathway for the passage of water and solutes in tissue fluid from the fetus to the amniotic cavity is through the skin. Fluid is also secreted by the fetal respiratory and gastrointestinal tracts and enters the amniotic cavity. Beginning in the 11th week, the fetus contributes to the amniotic fluid by expelling urine into the amniotic cavity. By 19 to 20 weeks, urine is the greatest source of amniotic fluid, as the skin begins to undergo keratinization and no longer supports diffusion.

The water content of amniotic fluid changes every 3 hours. Large amounts of water pass through the amniochorionic membrane into the maternal tissue fluid and into the uterine capillaries. An exchange of fluid with fetal blood also occurs through the umbilical cord and at the site where the amnion adheres to the chorionic plate on the fetal surface of the placenta (see Figs. 8.5 and 8.9B); thus amniotic fluid is in balance with the fetal circulation.

Amniotic fluid is swallowed by the fetus and absorbed by its respiratory and digestive tracts. It has been estimated that, during the final stages of pregnancy, the fetus swallows up to 400 mL of amniotic fluid daily. The fluid is absorbed by the gastrointestinal tract and passes into the fetal bloodstream. The waste products then cross the placental membrane and enter the maternal blood in the intervillous space. Excess water in the fetal blood is excreted by the fetal kidneys and returned to the amniotic sac through the fetal urinary tract.

Virtually all of the fluid in the amniotic cavity is water, in which undissolved material, such as desquamated fetal epithelial cells, is suspended. Amniotic fluid contains approximately equal portions of dissolved organic compounds and inorganic salts. Half of the organic constituents are protein; the other half is composed of carbohydrates, fats, enzymes, hormones, and pigments. As pregnancy advances, the composition of the amniotic fluid changes as fetal urine is added. Because fetal urine enters the amniotic fluid, fetal enzyme systems, amino acids, hormones, and other substances can be studied by examining the fluid removed by amniocentesis. Studies of cells in the amniotic fluid permit the detection of chromosomal abnormalities.

Disorders of Amniotic Fluid Volume

A low volume of amniotic fluid—**oligohydramnios**—results, in some cases, from placental insufficiency, with diminished placental blood flow. Preterm rupture of the amniochorionic membrane is the most common cause of oligohydramnios. In the presence of **renal agenesis**, the lack of fetal urine in the amniotic fluid is the main cause of oligohydramnios. A similar decrease in amniotic fluid occurs with obstructive **uropathy** (urinary tract obstruction). Complications of oligohydramnios include fetal abnormalities such as pulmonary hypoplasia, facial defects, and limb defects.

A high volume of amniotic fluid is termed **polyhydramnios**. Most cases (60%) of polyhydramnios are idiopathic; 20% of cases are caused by maternal factors, whereas 20% are fetal in origin. Polyhydramnios may be associated with severe anomalies of the central nervous system, such as **meroencephaly** (see Chapter 16). With other birth defects, such as esophageal atresia, amniotic fluid accumulates because it cannot pass to the fetal stomach and the intestines for absorption.

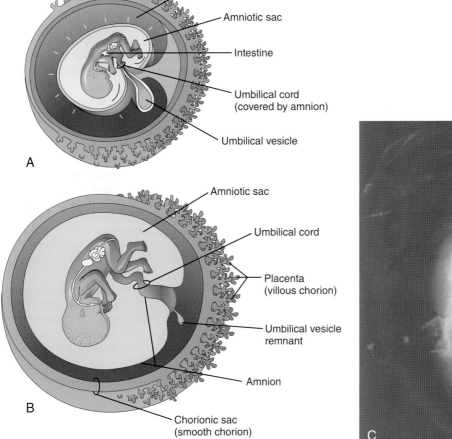

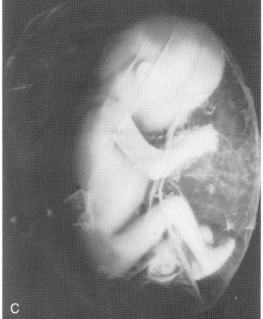

Fig. 8.13 Illustrations of how the amnion enlarges, fills the chorionic sac, and envelops the umbilical cord. Observe that part of the umbilical vesicle is incorporated into the embryo as the primordial gut. Formation of the fetal part of the placenta and degeneration of the chorionic villi are also shown. (A) At 10 weeks. (B) At 20 weeks. (C) A 12-week fetus within its amniotic sac (actual size). The fetus and its membranes aborted spontaneously. It was removed from its chorionic sac with the amniotic sac intact.

SIGNIFICANCE OF AMNIOTIC FLUID

The embryo floats freely in the amniotic sac. Amniotic fluid has critical functions in the development of the embryo and fetus:

- Permits uniform external growth of the embryo
- Protects and acts as a barrier to infection
- Permits fetal lung development
- Prevents adherence of the amnion to the embryo
- Cushions the embryo against injuries by distributing impacts that the mother may receive
- Helps control embryonic body temperature by maintaining a relatively constant temperature
- Enables the fetus to move freely, thereby aiding muscular development (e.g., in the limbs)
- Assists in maintaining homeostasis of fluid and electrolytes.

UMBILICAL VESICLE

The umbilical vesicle can be observed sonographically early during the fifth week of gestation. At 32 days, the umbilical

vesicle is large (see Fig. 8.1C). By 10 weeks, the umbilical vesicle has shrunk to a pear-shaped remnant approximately 5 mm in diameter (see Fig. 8.13A). By 20 weeks, the umbilical vesicle is very small (see Fig. 8.13B).

SIGNIFICANCE OF THE UMBILICAL VESICLE

The umbilical vesicle has several roles:

- **Transfer of nutrients** to the embryo during the second and third weeks before the uteroplacental circulation is established.
- **Blood cells** develop first in the well-vascularized, extraembryonic mesoderm covering the wall of the umbilical vesicle beginning in the third week (see Chapter 5) and continue to develop there until hematopoietic activity begins in the liver during the sixth week.
- During the fourth week, the dorsal part of the umbilical vesicle is incorporated into the embryo as the **primordial gut** (see Fig. 6.1). Its endoderm, derived from the epiblast, gives rise to the epithelium of the trachea, bronchi, lungs, and alimentary canal.

- **Primordial germ cells** appear in the endodermal lining of the wall of the umbilical vesicle in the third week and subsequently migrate to the developing gonads—testis or ovary (see Chapter 13). The cells differentiate into spermatogonia in males and oogonia in females.

ALLANTOIS

The allantois is not functional in human embryos; however, it is important for three reasons:

- **Blood cell formation** occurs in its wall during the third to fifth weeks of development.
- Its blood vessels become the **umbilical vein and arteries**.
- The intraembryonic portion of the allantois runs from the umbilicus to the urinary bladder, with which it is continuous (see Fig. 13.11E). As the bladder enlarges, the allantois involutes to form a thick tube, the **urachus** (see Fig. 13.11G). After birth, the urachus becomes a fibrous cord, the median umbilical ligament, which extends from the apex of the urinary bladder to the umbilicus.

Premature Rupture of Fetal Membranes

Premature rupture of the amniochorionic membrane is the most common event leading to premature labor and delivery and the most common complication resulting in oligohydramnios. Loss of amniotic fluid removes the major protection the fetus has against infection. Rupture of the membrane may cause various fetal birth defects that constitute the **amniotic band syndrome**, or *amniotic band disruption complex* (Fig. 8.14). These birth defects are associated with a variety of abnormalities, ranging from constriction of digits (fingers) to major scalp, craniofacial, and visceral defects. The cause of these defects is probably related to constriction by encircling amniotic bands (see Fig. 8.14).

MULTIPLE PREGNANCIES

Multiple pregnancies (gestations) are associated with higher risks of chromosomal anomalies, fetal morbidity, and fetal mortality than single gestations. The risks are progressively greater as the number of fetuses increases. In North America, twins naturally occur approximately once in every 85 pregnancies, triplets approximately once in every 90^2 pregnancies, quadruplets approximately once in every 90^3 pregnancies, and quintuplets approximately once in every 90^4 pregnancies.

TWINS AND FETAL MEMBRANES

Twins that originate from two zygotes are **dizygotic (DZ) twins**—fraternal twins (Fig. 8.15), whereas twins that originate from one zygote are **monozygotic (MZ) twins**—identical twins (Fig. 8.16). The fetal membranes and placentas vary according to the origin of the twins. Approximately two-thirds of twins are dizygotic, and the rate of DZ twinning increases with maternal age. The study of twins is important in human genetics because it is useful for comparing the effects of genes and environment on development. If an abnormal condition does not show a simple genetic pattern, comparison of its incidence in MZ and DZ twins may show that heredity is involved.

DIZYGOTIC TWINS

Because they result from the fertilization of two oocytes by two sperms, DZ twins may be of the same sex or different sexes. For the same reason, they are no more alike genetically than brothers or sisters born at different times. DZ twins always have two amnions and two chorions (see Fig. 8.15A), but the chorions and placentas may be fused (see Fig. 8.15B). DZ twinning shows a hereditary tendency. The recurrence risk in families with one set of DZ twins is approximately triple that of the general population. The incidence of DZ twinning shows considerable racial variation, ranging from 1 in 500 in Asian populations to 1 in 125 in white populations to as high as 1 in 20 in some African populations.

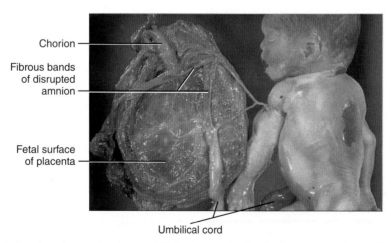

Fig. 8.14   A fetus with amniotic band syndrome, showing amniotic bands constricting the left arm. Courtesy V. Becker, Professor, Pathologisches Institut der Universität, Erlangen, Germany.

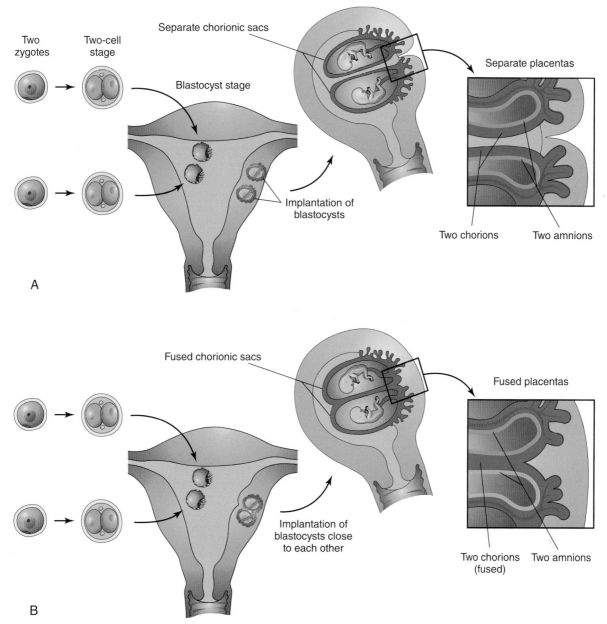

Fig. 8.15 Dizygotic twins developing from two zygotes. The relationship between the fetal membranes and placentas is shown for instances in which the blastocysts implant separately (A) and the blastocysts implant close together (B). In both cases, there are two amnions and two chorions.

MONOZYGOTIC TWINS

Because they result from the fertilization of one oocyte and develop from one zygote (see Fig. 8.16), MZ twins are of the same sex, their genomes are virtually identical and are similar in physical appearance. Differences between MZ twins result from epigenetic and environmental effects (Fig. 8.17). MZ twinning usually begins in the blastocyst stage, approximately at the end of the first week, and results from the division of the embryoblast into two embryonic primordia (see Fig. 8.16). Subsequently, two embryos, each in its own amniotic sac, develop within one chorionic sac and share a common placenta, a **monochorionic-diamniotic twin placenta**. Uncommonly, early separation of the embryonic blastomeres (e.g., during the two- to eight-cell stage) results in MZ twins with two amnions, two chorions, and two placentas that may or may not be fused (Fig. 8.18). In such cases, it is impossible to determine, from the membranes alone, whether the twins are monozygotic or dizygotic.

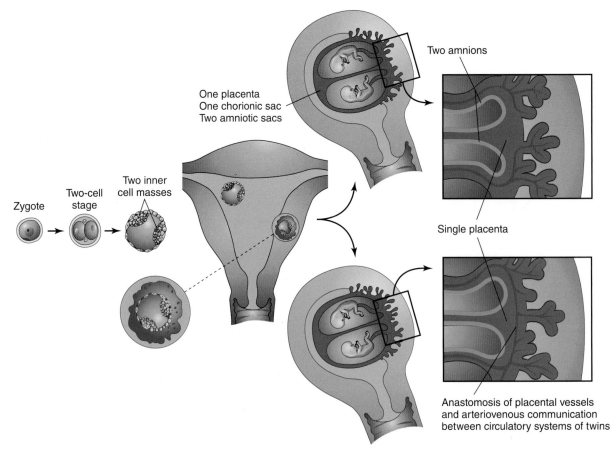

Fig. 8.16 Illustrations of how approximately 65% of monozygotic twins develop from one zygote by division of the inner cell mass. These twins always have separate amnions, a single chorionic sac, and a common placenta. If there is anastomosis of the placental vessels, one twin may receive most of the nutrition from the placenta (see Fig. 8.17).

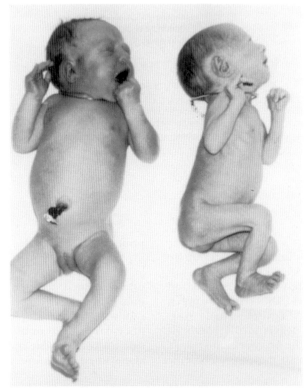

Fig. 8.17 Monozygotic, monochorionic-diamniotic twins. Note the wide discrepancy in size resulting from an uncompensated arteriovenous anastomosis of the placental vessels. Blood was shunted from the smaller twin to the larger one, producing the twin transfusion syndrome.

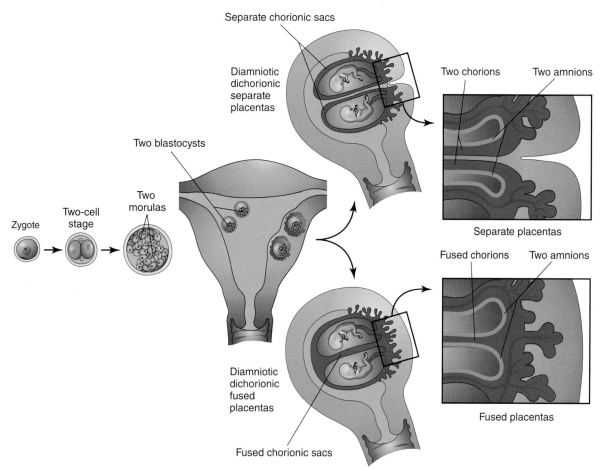

Fig. 8.18 Illustrations of how approximately 35% of monozygotic twins develop from one zygote. Separation of the blastomeres may occur at any point from the two-cell stage to the morula stage, producing two identical blastocysts. Each embryo subsequently develops its own amniotic and chorionic sacs. The placentas may be separate or fused. In most cases, there is a single placenta resulting from secondary fusion, whereas in fewer cases, there are two placentas. In the latter cases, examination of the placenta suggests that they are dizygotic twins. This explains why some monozygotic twins are incorrectly classified as dizygotic twins at birth.

Twin-to-Twin Transfusion Syndrome

Twin-to-twin transfusion syndrome occurs in approximately 10% to 15% of **monochorionic-diamniotic MZ twins**. Arterial blood may be preferentially shunted from one twin through unidirectional umbilical–placental arteriovenous anastomoses in the placenta into the venous circulation of the other twin. The donor twin is small, pale, and anemic (see Fig. 8.17), whereas the recipient twin is large and polycythemic (i.e., having a higher-than-normal red blood cell count). The placenta shows similar abnormalities; the part of the placenta supplying the anemic twin is pale, whereas the part supplying the polycythemic twin is dark red. In lethal cases, death results from anemia in the donor twin and from congestive heart failure in the recipient twin. Depending on the clinical situation, treatment, if possible, may include expectant management, delivery, amnioreduction, or fetoscopic laser photocoagulation of involved vessels.

Establishing Zygosity of Twins

Establishment of the zygosity of twins is important, particularly because of the introduction of tissue and organ transplantation (e.g., bone marrow transplants). **Twin zygosity** is now determined by molecular testing.

Late division of the early embryonic cells (i.e., division of the embryonic disc during the second week) results in MZ twins with one amniotic sac and one chorionic sac (1% of MZ twins). A **monochorionic-monoamniotic twin placenta** is associated with a fetal mortality rate approaching 50%. The umbilical cords are frequently so entangled that circulation of the blood through their vessels ceases, and one or both fetuses die.

Ultrasonography plays an important role in the diagnosis of twin pregnancies and the management of various conditions that may complicate MZ twinning, such as intrauterine growth restriction, intrauterine fetal distress, and premature labor.

OTHER TYPES OF MULTIPLE BIRTHS

Triplets may be derived from:

- One zygote and be identical
- Two zygotes consist of identical twins and a singleton
- Three zygotes may be of the same sex or of different sexes, in which case the infants are no more similar than infants from three separate pregnancies.

Similar combinations can occur in larger sets of multiple gestations.

Conjoined Twins

If the embryonic disc does not divide completely, various types of monozygote conjoined twins may form. The terminology used to describe the twins is based on the regions of the body that are attached; for example, **thoracopagus** indicates anterior union of the thoracic regions. In some cases, the twins are connected to each other by skin only or by cutaneous and other tissues, such as fused livers. Some conjoined twins can be separated successfully by surgery. The incidence of conjoined twins is 1 in 50,000 to 1 in 100,000 births.

CLINICALLY ORIENTED QUESTIONS

1. What is meant by the term *stillbirth*? Do older women have more stillborn infants?

2. A fetus was born dead, reportedly because of a "cord accident." What does this mean? Do these "accidents" always kill the infant? If not, what birth defects may be present?

3. What is the scientific basis of the home pregnancy tests that are sold in drugstores?

4. What is the proper name for what laypeople sometimes refer to as the *bag of water*? Does premature rupture of the "bag" induce the birth of the fetus? What is meant by a *dry birth*?

5. What does *fetal distress* mean? How is the condition recognized? What causes the distress?

6. Is twinning more common in older mothers? Is twinning hereditary?

The answers to these questions are at the back of this book.

Body Cavities, Mesenteries, and Diaphragm

9

By the fourth week of development, the **intraembryonic coelom**—the primordium of the body cavities—appears as a horseshoe-shaped cavity (Fig. 9.1A). The bend in this cavity at the cranial end of the embryo represents the future **pericardial cavity**, and its limbs indicate the future **pleural and peritoneal cavities**. The intraembryonic coelom provides room for the abdominal organs to develop and move during development. The distal part of each limb of the intraembryonic coelom is continuous with the **extraembryonic coelom** at the lateral edges of the embryonic disc (see Fig. 9.1B). Most of the midgut normally herniates through this communication into the umbilical cord. During lateral folding, the limbs of the coelom are brought together on the ventral aspect of the embryo (Fig. 9.2A–F).

EMBRYONIC BODY CAVITY

The **intraembryonic coelom** becomes three well-defined body cavities during the fourth week (see Figs. 9.2 and 9.4): a pericardial cavity, a pair of pericardioperitoneal canals connecting the pericardial and peritoneal cavities, and a large peritoneal cavity. These body cavities are lined by the mesothelium—a parietal wall derived from the somatic mesoderm and a visceral wall derived from the splanchnic mesoderm (Fig. 9.3E). The mesothelium forms the major portion of the peritoneum.

The peritoneal cavity is connected to the extraembryonic coelom at the umbilicus (Fig. 9.4C and D). The peritoneal cavity loses its connection with the extraembryonic coelom during the 10th week as the intestines return to the abdomen from the umbilical cord (see Chapter 12).

During the formation of the head fold, the heart and pericardial cavity are relocated ventrocaudally, anterior to the foregut (see Fig. 9.2A, B, D, and E). As a result, the pericardial cavity opens into the pericardioperitoneal canals, which pass dorsally to the foregut (see Fig. 9.4B and D). After embryonic folding, the caudal parts of the foregut, midgut, and hindgut are suspended in the peritoneal cavity from the dorsal abdominal wall by the **dorsal mesentery** (see Figs. 9.2F and 9.3B–E).

MESENTERIES

A mesentery is a double layer of peritoneum that begins as an extension of the visceral peritoneum that covers an organ. The mesentery connects the organ to the body wall and conveys its vessels and nerves. Transiently, the dorsal and ventral mesenteries divide the peritoneal cavity into the right and left halves (see Fig. 9.3C). The ventral mesentery soon disappears (see Fig. 9.3E), except where it is attached to the caudal part of the **foregut**. The peritoneal cavity then becomes a continuous space (see Figs. 9.3A and 9.4D). The arteries supplying the primordial gut—**celiac arterial trunk** (foregut), the **superior mesenteric artery** (midgut), and **inferior mesenteric artery** (hindgut)—pass between the layers of the dorsal mesentery (see Fig. 9.3C).

DIVISION OF EMBRYONIC BODY CAVITY

Each pericardioperitoneal canal lies lateral to the proximal part of the foregut (future esophagus) and dorsal to the **septum transversum**—a thick plate of mesoderm that occupies the space between the thoracic cavity and the omphaloenteric duct (see Fig. 9.4A and B).

The septum transversum is the primordium of the **central tendon of the diaphragm**. Partitions form in each pericardioperitoneal canal, separating the pericardial cavity from the pleural cavities and the pleural cavities from the peritoneal cavity (see Fig. 9.3A). Because of the growth of the **bronchial buds** (primordia of bronchi and lungs) into the pericardioperitoneal canals (Fig. 9.5A), a pair of membranous ridges is produced in the lateral wall of each canal. The cranial ridges—the **pleuropericardial folds**—are located superior to the developing lungs, and the caudal ridges—the **pleuroperitoneal folds**—are located inferior to the lungs.

PLEUROPERICARDIAL MEMBRANES

As the pleuropericardial folds enlarge, they form partitions that separate the pericardial cavity from the pleural cavities. These partitions—**pleuropericardial membranes**—contain the **common cardinal veins** (see Fig. 9.5A and B), which drain the venous system into the **sinus venosus** of the primordial heart (see Chapter 14). Initially, the bronchial buds are small relative to the heart and pericardial cavity (see Fig. 9.5). The buds grow laterally from the caudal end of the trachea into the pericardioperitoneal canals (future pleural canals). As the primordial **pleural cavities** expand ventrally around the heart, they extend into the body wall, splitting the mesenchyme into an outer layer that becomes the thoracic wall and an inner layer (pleuropericardial membrane) that becomes the fibrous pericardium, the outer layer of the pericardial sac that encloses the heart (see Fig. 9.5C and D).

The pleuropericardial membranes project into the cranial ends of the pericardioperitoneal canals (see Fig. 9.5B). With subsequent growth of the common cardinal veins, positional displacement of the heart, and expansion of the pleural cavities, the pleuropericardial membranes become mesentery-like folds extending from the lateral thoracic wall. By the seventh week, the pleuropericardial membranes fuse with the

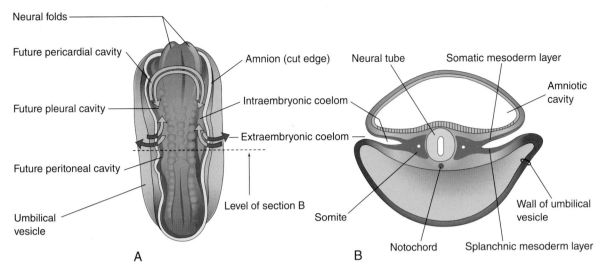

Fig. 9.1 (A) Dorsal view of a 22-day embryo, showing the outline of the horseshoe-shaped intraembryonic coelom. The amnion has been removed, and the coelom is shown as if the embryo were translucent. The continuity of the intraembryonic coelom and the communication of its right and left limbs with the extraembryonic coelom is indicated by *arrows*. (B) Transverse section through the embryo at the level shown in (A).

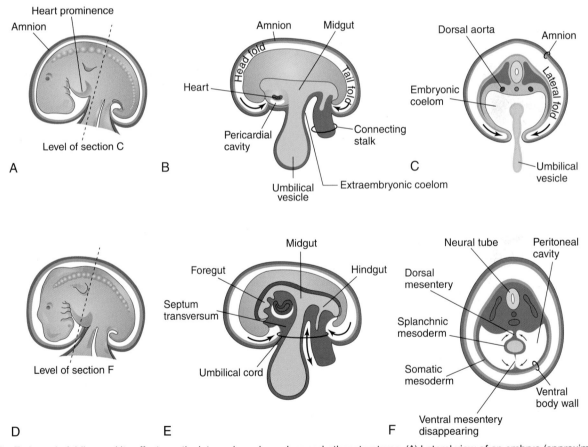

Fig. 9.2 Embryonic folding and its effects on the intraembryonic coelom and other structures. (A) Lateral view of an embryo (approximately 26 days). (B) Schematic sagittal section of the embryo, showing the head and tail folds. (C) Transverse section at the level shown in (A), indicating how fusion of the lateral folds gives the embryo a cylindrical form. (D) Lateral view of an embryo (approximately 28 days). (E) Schematic sagittal section of the embryo, showing the reduced communication between the intraembryonic and extraembryonic coeloms (*double-headed arrow*). (F) Transverse section, as indicated in (D), shows the formation of the ventral body wall and the disappearance of the ventral mesentery. The arrows indicate the junction of the somatic and splanchnic layers of the mesoderm. The somatic mesoderm will become the parietal peritoneum lining the abdominal wall, and the splanchnic mesoderm will become the visceral peritoneum covering the organs (e.g., stomach).

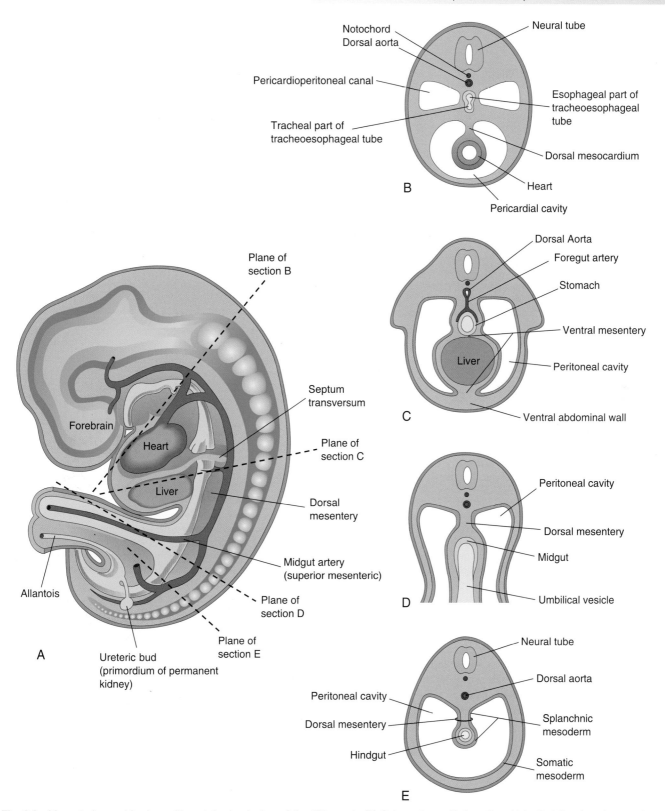

Fig. 9.3 Mesenteries and body cavities at the beginning of the fifth week. (A) Schematic sagittal section. Note that the dorsal mesentery serves as a pathway for the arteries that supply the developing gut. Nerves and lymphatics also pass between the layers of this mesentery. (B–E) Transverse sections through the embryo at the levels shown in (A). The ventral mesentery disappears except in the region of the terminal esophagus, stomach, and first part of the duodenum. Note that the right and left parts of the peritoneal cavity, which are separate in (C), are continuous in (E).

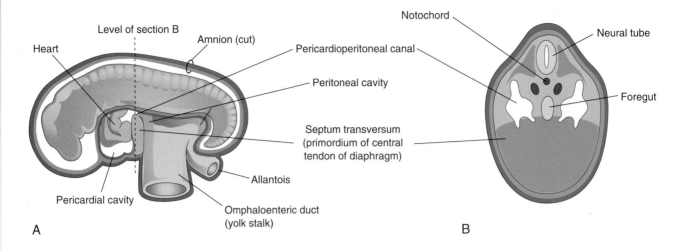

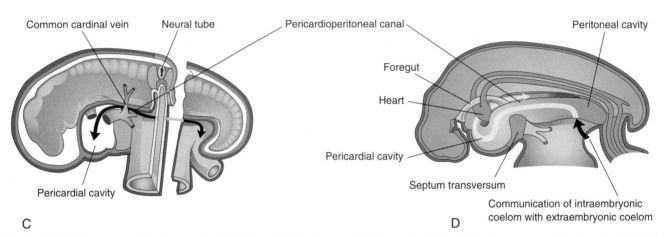

Fig. 9.4 Illustration of an embryo (approximately 24 days). (A) The lateral wall of the pericardial cavity has been removed to show the primordial heart. (B) Transverse section of the embryo, showing the relationship of the pericardioperitoneal canals to the septum transversum and foregut. (C) Lateral view of the embryo with the heart removed. The embryo has also been sectioned transversely to show the continuity of the intraembryonic and extraembryonic coeloms *(arrow)*. (D) Illustration of the pericardioperitoneal canals that arise from the dorsal wall of the pericardial cavity and pass on each side of the foregut to join the peritoneal cavity. The *arrow* shows the communication of the extraembryonic coelom with the intraembryonic coelom and the continuity of the intraembryonic coelom at this stage.

mesenchyme ventral to the esophagus, separating the pericardial cavity from the pleural cavities (see Fig. 9.5C). The primordial **mediastinum** consists of a mass of mesenchyme that separates the developing lungs (see Fig. 9.5D). The right pleuropericardial opening closes slightly earlier than the left one and produces a larger pleuropericardial membrane.

PLEUROPERITONEAL MEMBRANES

As the pleuroperitoneal folds enlarge, they project into the pericardioperitoneal canals. Gradually, the folds become membranous, forming the pleuroperitoneal membranes (Fig. 9.6B and C). Eventually, these membranes separate the pleural cavities from the peritoneal cavity. The pleuroperitoneal membranes are attached dorsolaterally to the abdominal wall and their crescentic free edges initially project into the caudal ends of the pericardioperitoneal canals.

During the sixth week, the pleuroperitoneal membranes extend ventromedially until their free edges fuse with the dorsal mesentery of the esophagus and the septum transversum (see Fig. 9.6C). This membrane separates the pleural cavities from the peritoneal cavity. Closure of the pleuroperitoneal

openings is completed by the migration of **myoblasts** (primordial muscle cells) into the pleuroperitoneal membranes (see Fig. 9.6D and E). The pleuroperitoneal opening on the right side closes slightly before the left one.

DEVELOPMENT OF DIAPHRAGM

The diaphragm is a dome-shaped musculotendinous partition that separates the thoracic and abdominal cavities. It is a composite structure that develops from four embryonic components (see Fig. 9.6):

- Septum transversum
- Pleuroperitoneal membranes
- Dorsal mesentery of esophagus
- Muscular ingrowth from lateral body walls.

SEPTUM TRANSVERSUM

This transverse septum, which is composed of mesodermal tissue, is the primordium of the **central tendon of the**

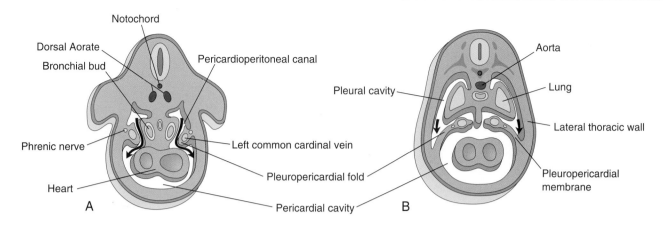

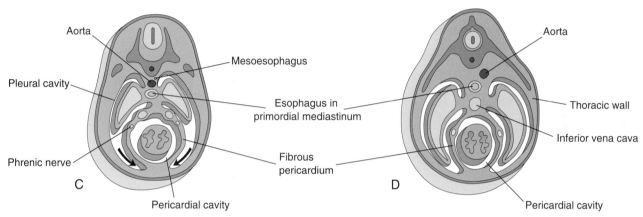

Fig. 9.5 Transverse sections through an embryo cranial to the septum transversum, showing successive stages in the separation of the pleural cavities from the pericardial cavity. Growth and development of the lungs, expansion of the pleural cavities, and formation of the fibrous pericardium are also shown. (A) At 5 weeks. The *arrows* indicate the communications between the pericardioperitoneal canals and the pericardial cavity. (B) At 6 weeks. The arrows indicate the development of the pleural cavities as they expand into the body wall. (C) At 7 weeks. Expansion of the pleural cavities ventrally (*arrows*) around the heart is evident. The pleuropericardial membranes are now fused in the median plane with each other and with the mesoderm ventral to the esophagus. (D) At 8 weeks. Continued expansion of the lungs and pleural cavities and the formation of the fibrous pericardium and the thoracic wall are shown.

diaphragm (see Fig. 9.6D and E). The septum transversum grows dorsally from the ventrolateral body wall and forms a semicircular shelf that separates the heart from the liver. After the head folds ventrally during the fourth week, the septum transversum forms a thick, incomplete connective tissue partition between the pericardial and abdominal cavities (see Fig. 9.4). The septum transversum expands and fuses with the mesenchyme ventral to the esophagus and the pleuroperitoneal membranes (see Fig. 9.6C).

PLEUROPERITONEAL MEMBRANES

These membranes fuse with the dorsal mesentery of the esophagus and the septum transversum (see Fig. 9.6C). This fusion completes the partition between the thoracic and abdominal cavities and forms the **primordial diaphragm**. The pleuroperitoneal membranes represent relatively small portions of the neonate's diaphragm (see Fig. 9.6E).

DORSAL MESENTERY OF ESOPHAGUS

The septum transversum and pleuroperitoneal membranes fuse with the dorsal mesentery of the esophagus. This

mesentery becomes the median portion of the diaphragm. The **crura of the diaphragm**—a pair of diverging muscle bundles that cross in the median plane anterior to the aorta (see Fig. 9.6E)—develop from myoblasts that grow into the dorsal mesentery of the esophagus.

MUSCULAR INGROWTH FROM LATERAL BODY WALLS

During the 9th to 12th weeks, the lungs and pleural cavities enlarge, "burrowing" into the lateral body walls (see Fig. 9.5). During this process, the tissue of the body wall is split into two layers:

- An external layer that becomes part of the definitive thoracic wall
- An internal layer that contributes to the peripheral parts of the diaphragm, external to the parts derived from the pleuroperitoneal membranes (see Fig. 9.6D and E).

Further extension of the developing pleural cavities into the lateral body walls forms the right and left **costodiaphragmatic recesses** (Fig. 9.7), establishing the characteristic dome-shaped configuration of the diaphragm.

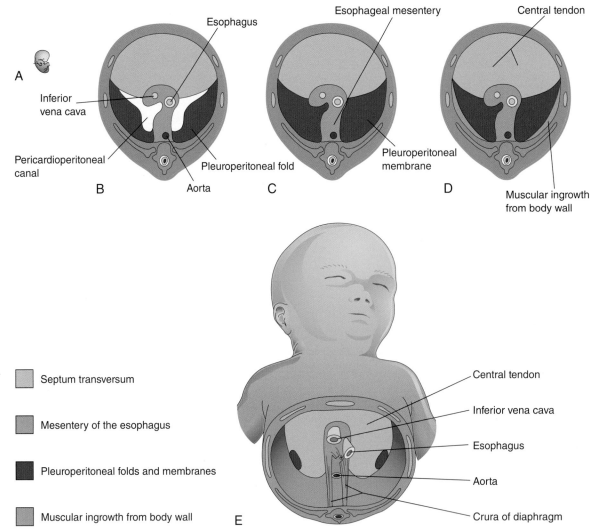

Septum transversum

Mesentery of the esophagus

Pleuroperitoneal folds and membranes

Muscular ingrowth from body wall

Fig. 9.6 Development of the diaphragm. (A) Lateral view of an embryo at the end of the fifth week (actual size), indicating the level of (B) to (D) sections. (B–E) show the developing diaphragm as viewed inferiorly. (B) Transverse section, showing the unfused pleuroperitoneal membranes. (C) Similar section at the end of the sixth week, after fusion of the pleuroperitoneal membranes with the other two diaphragmatic components. (D) Transverse section of a 12-week embryo, after ingrowth of the fourth diaphragmatic component from the body wall. (E) View of the diaphragm of a neonate, indicating the embryologic origin of its components.

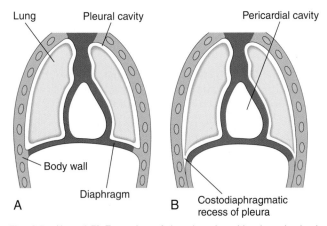

Fig. 9.7 (A and B) Extension of the pleural cavities into the body walls to form the peripheral parts of the diaphragm, the costodiaphragmatic recesses, and the characteristic dome-shaped configuration of the diaphragm.

POSITIONAL CHANGES AND INNERVATION OF THE DIAPHRAGM

During the fourth week of development, the septum transversum lies opposite the third to fifth **cervical somites**. During the fifth week, myoblasts from these somites migrate into the developing diaphragm, bringing their nerve fibers with them. Consequently, the **phrenic nerves** that supply motor innervation to the diaphragm arise from the ventral primary rami of the third, fourth, and fifth cervical spinal nerves, which join together on each side to form a phrenic nerve. The phrenic nerves also supply sensory fibers to the superior and inferior surfaces of the right and left domes of the diaphragm.

Rapid growth of the dorsal part of the embryo's body results in an apparent descent of the diaphragm. By the sixth week, the developing diaphragm is at the level of the thoracic somites. The phrenic nerves now have a descending course. By the beginning of the eighth week, the dorsal part of the diaphragm lies at the level of the first lumbar vertebra. The phrenic nerves in the embryo enter the diaphragm by passing through the pleuropericardial membranes. For this reason, the phrenic nerves subsequently lie on the fibrous pericardium of the heart, which is derived from the pleuropericardial membranes (see Fig. 9.5C and D). The costal border of the diaphragm receives sensory fibers from the lower intercostal nerves because of the origin of the peripheral part of the diaphragm from the lateral body walls (see Fig. 9.6D and E).

complex chromosomal abnormalities, copy number variations, specific gene mutations, and deletions, including Sonic hedgehog (Shh), signaling, HLX1, and zinc finger factor GATA6 pathways, have been implicated in cases of CDH. Ultrasonography and magnetic resonance imaging can provide a prenatal diagnosis of CDH.

Posterolateral Defect of Diaphragm

Posterolateral defect of the diaphragm is the only relatively common congenital anomaly involving the diaphragm (Fig. 9.8A). This defect occurs in approximately 1 in 3000 neonates and is associated with **congenital diaphragmatic hernia (CDH)**—herniation of abdominal contents into the thoracic cavity.

CDH can lead to life-threatening respiratory difficulties. CDH is the most common cause of **pulmonary hypoplasia**. If severe lung hypoplasia is present, some primordial alveoli may rupture, causing air to enter the pleural cavity (*pneumothorax*). Usually unilateral, CDH results from defective formation or fusion of the pleuroperitoneal membrane with the other three parts of the diaphragm (see Fig. 9.6B). This birth defect produces a large opening in the posterolateral region of the diaphragm. If a pleuroperitoneal canal is still open when the intestines return to the abdomen from the umbilical cord in the 10th week, some intestines and other viscera may pass into the thorax and compress the lungs. Often the stomach, spleen, and most of the intestines herniate (see Fig. 9.8B and C). The defect most commonly occurs in the left posterolateral portion of the diaphragm, less commonly in the anterior portion, and it is likely related to the earlier closure of the right pleuroperitoneal opening. Congenital diaphragmatic hernia may occur as isolated sporadic cases or as part of a syndrome. *Aneuploidy,*

Eventration of Diaphragm

In congenital **diaphragmatic eventration**, a type of CDH, half of the diaphragm has defective musculature, causing it to balloon into the thoracic cavity as an aponeurotic (membranous) sheet, forming a **diaphragmatic pouch**. Consequently, the abdominal viscera are displaced superiorly into the pocket-like outpouching of the diaphragm. This birth defect (1:2000 births) results from the failure of the muscular tissue from the body wall to extend into the pleuroperitoneal membrane on the affected side. Some cases of eventration of the diaphragm may be acquired, for example, due to phrenic nerve injury. Congenital diaphragmatic eventration may result in lung hypoplasia.

Retrosternal (Parasternal) Hernia

In this rare type of CDH (2% of all CDH cases), herniations may occur through the **sternocostal hiatus**, the opening for the superior epigastric vessels in the retrosternal area. The hiatus is located between the sternal and costal parts of the diaphragm. Herniation of the intestine into the pericardial sac may occur, or, conversely, part of the heart may descend into the peritoneal cavity in the epigastric region. Large birth defects are commonly associated with **body wall defects** in the umbilical region (e.g., omphalocele; see Chapter 12).

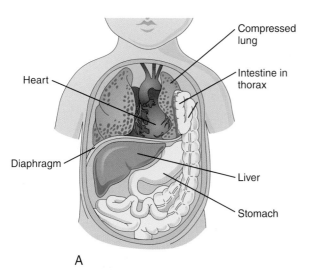 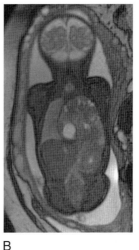 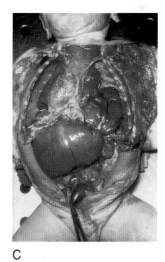

A   B   C

Fig. 9.8 (A) This "window view" overlooking the thorax and the abdomen shows the herniation of the intestine into the thorax through a posterolateral defect in the left side of the diaphragm. Note that the left lung is compressed and hypoplastic. (B) Magnetic resonance imaging of a third-trimester fetus demonstrating findings of congenital diaphragmatic hernia with evidence of herniated liver, bowel, and stomach. (C) Postmortem examination demonstrating a diaphragmatic hernia. Note the herniation of the stomach and small intestine into the thorax through a posterolateral defect in the left side of the diaphragm, similar to that shown in (A). Note that the heart is pushed to the right side of the thorax. *B, Courtesy Dr. Teresa Victoria, MD, PhD, and Dr. Monica Epelman, The Children's Hospital of Philadelphia, Pennsylvania; C, Dr. Nathan Wiseman, MD, FRCS, Department of Surgery, Max Radi College of Medicine, University of Manitoba.*

CLINICALLY ORIENTED QUESTIONS

1. Is it possible for an infant to be born with a defect that results in its stomach and liver being located in its chest? How might this occur?

2. A male neonate had respiratory distress and was diagnosed with CDH. Is this a common birth defect? What would determine whether this infant would survive? Can diaphragmatic defects be operated on before birth?

3. Do the lungs develop normally in infants who are born with a CDH?

4. A man underwent routine chest radiography approximately 1 year ago and was told that a small part of his small intestine was in his chest. Is it possible for him to have a CDH without being aware of it? Would his lung on the affected side be normal?

The answers to these questions are at the back of this book.

Pharyngeal Apparatus, Face, and Neck

PHARYNGEAL ARCHES

The **pharyngeal arches** begin to develop early in the fourth week as **neural crest cells** migrate into the future head and neck regions (see Fig. 6.4).

Initially, each pharyngeal arch consists of a core of mesenchyme and is covered externally by ectoderm and internally by endoderm (Fig. 10.1D and E). The first pair of arches, the primordium of the jaws, appears as surface elevations lateral to the developing pharynx. By the end of the fourth week, four pairs of arches are visible externally (see Fig. 10.1A). The fifth and sixth arches are rudimentary and are not visible on the surface of the embryo. The arches are separated from each other by the **pharyngeal grooves** (clefts). Like the arches, the grooves are numbered in a craniocaudal sequence. *The identity and fate of individual arches are determined by the migrating neural crest cells and the expression of Hox genes.*

The arches support the lateral walls of the primordial pharynx, which is derived from the cranial part of the foregut. The **stomodeum** (primordial mouth) initially appears as a slight depression of the surface ectoderm (see Fig. 10.1A). It is separated from the cavity of the primordial pharynx by a bilaminar membrane—the **oropharyngeal membrane**—composed of fused ectoderm and endoderm. The oropharyngeal membrane ruptures at approximately 26 days (see Fig. 10.1B and C), bringing the primordial pharynx and foregut into communication with the amniotic cavity. The arches contribute extensively to the formation of the face, nasal cavities, mouth, larynx, pharynx, and neck (Fig. 10.2; see Fig. 10.23).

The **first arch** develops two prominences (see Figs. 10.1B and 10.2): the smaller **maxillary prominence** and the larger **mandibular prominence**. The **second arch (hyoid)** makes a major contribution to the formation of the hyoid bone (see Fig. 10.4B).

PHARYNGEAL ARCH COMPONENTS

A typical arch has the following components (Fig. 10.3A and B):

- An *arch artery* (aortic arch artery) that arises from the truncus arteriosus of the primordial heart and courses around the primordial pharynx to enter the dorsal aorta
- A *cartilaginous rod* that forms the skeleton of the arch
- A *muscular component* that is the primordium of the muscles in the head and neck
- A *nerve* that supplies the mucosa and muscles derived from each arch

DERIVATIVES OF PHARYNGEAL ARCH ARTERIES

The transformation of the arch arteries into the adult arterial pattern of the head and neck is described in the section on the pharyngeal arch artery derivatives in Chapter 14.

DERIVATIVES OF PHARYNGEAL ARCH CARTILAGES

The dorsal end of the **first arch cartilage** becomes ossified to form two ossicles, the **malleus** and **incus** (Fig. 10.4 and Table 10.1). The middle section of the cartilage regresses, but its perichondrium forms the **anterior ligament of the malleus** and **sphenomandibular ligament** (see Fig. 10.4B). Ventral parts of the first arch cartilage form the horseshoe-shaped primordium of the **mandible**. Each half of the mandible forms lateral to and in close association with its cartilage. The cartilage disappears as the mandible develops around it by **intramembranous ossification** (see Chapter 15).

The dorsal end of the **second arch cartilage** contributes to the **stapes**, and the **styloid process** of the temporal bone. The part of the cartilage between the **styloid process** and the hyoid bone regresses; its perichondrium forms the **stylohyoid ligament**. The ventral end of the second arch cartilage ossifies to form the **lesser cornu** of the **hyoid bone**.

The **third arch cartilage** ossifies to form the greater cornu of the hyoid bone and the superior cornu of the thyroid cartilage. The **fourth and sixth arch cartilages** fuse to form the **laryngeal cartilages**, except for the epiglottis. The epiglottic and thyroid cartilages appear to develop from neural crest cells (see Fig. 10.21A–C). The cricoid cartilage develops from mesoderm.

DERIVATIVES OF PHARYNGEAL ARCH MUSCLES

The muscular components of the arches form various muscles in the head and neck; for example, the musculature of the first arch forms the **muscles of mastication** and others (Fig. 10.5 and Table 10.1).

DERIVATIVES OF PHARYNGEAL ARCH NERVES

Each arch is supplied by its own cranial nerve (CN). The **special visceral efferent (branchial)** components of the CNs supply muscles derived from the pharyngeal arches (Fig. 10.6A and Table 10.1). Because the mesenchyme from the pharyngeal arches contributes to the dermis and mucous membranes of the head and neck, these areas are supplied with the **special visceral afferent nerves**. The facial skin is supplied by the **trigeminal nerve** (CN V); however, only the caudal two branches (maxillary and mandibular) supply derivatives of the first pharyngeal arch (see Fig. 10.6B). CN V is the principal sensory nerve of the head and neck and is the motor nerve for the muscles of mastication. Its sensory

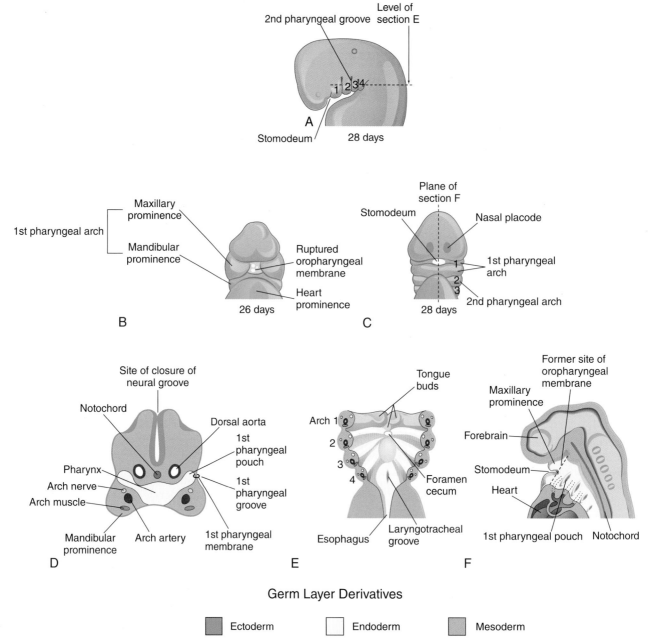

Germ Layer Derivatives

☐ Ectoderm   ☐ Endoderm   ☐ Mesoderm

Fig. 10.1 Illustrations of the pharyngeal apparatus. (A) Lateral view showing the development of four pharyngeal arches. (B and C) Ventral (facial) views showing the relationship of the pharyngeal arches to the stomodeum. (D) Frontal section through the cranial region of an embryo. (E) Horizontal section showing the arch components and the floor of the primordial pharynx. (F) Sagittal section of the cranial region of an embryo, showing the openings of the pharyngeal pouches in the lateral wall of the primordial pharynx.

branches innervate the face, teeth, and mucous membranes of the nasal cavities, palate, mouth, and tongue (see Fig. 10.6C). The **facial nerve** (CN VII), the **glossopharyngeal nerve** (CN IX), and the **vagus nerve** (CN X) supply the second, third, and caudal (fourth to sixth) arches, respectively. The superior laryngeal branch of the vagus nerve supplies the fourth arch, whereas its recurrent laryngeal branch supplies the sixth arch. The nerves of the second to sixth pharyngeal arches (see Fig. 10.6A) innervate the mucous membranes of the tongue, pharynx, and larynx (see Fig. 10.6C).

PHARYNGEAL POUCHES

The primordial pharynx widens cranially where it joins the stomodeum and narrows caudally, where it joins the esophagus (see Fig. 10.3A). The endoderm of the pharynx lines the internal aspects of the pharyngeal arches and passes into the **pharyngeal pouches** (Fig. 10.7A; see Fig. 10.1D and E). The pairs of pouches develop in a craniocaudal sequence between the arches. The first pair of pouches, for example, lies between the first and second pharyngeal arches. Four

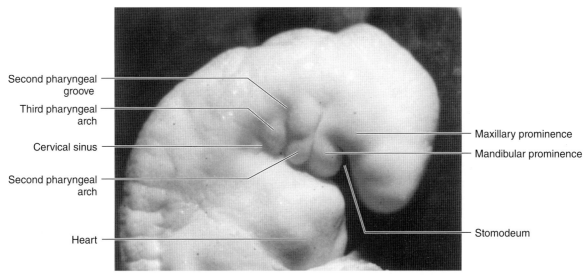

Second pharyngeal groove

Third pharyngeal arch

Cervical sinus

Second pharyngeal arch

Heart

Maxillary prominence

Mandibular prominence

Stomodeum

Fig. 10.2 A Carnegie stage 13, 4½-week human embryo. (Courtesy the late Professor Emeritus Dr. K.V. Hinrichsen, Medizinische Fakultät, Institut für Anatomie, Ruhr-Universität Bochum, Bochum, Germany.)

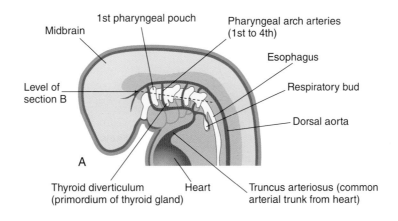

Midbrain

1st pharyngeal pouch

Pharyngeal arch arteries (1st to 4th)

Esophagus

Respiratory bud

Dorsal aorta

Level of section B

A

Thyroid diverticulum (primordium of thyroid gland)

Heart

Truncus arteriosus (common arterial trunk from heart)

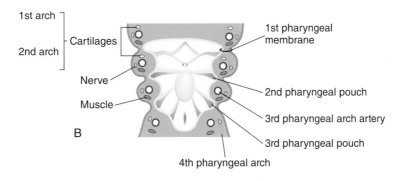

1st arch

2nd arch

Cartilages

Nerve

Muscle

B

1st pharyngeal membrane

2nd pharyngeal pouch

3rd pharyngeal arch artery

3rd pharyngeal pouch

4th pharyngeal arch

Germ Layer Derivatives

Ectoderm   Endoderm   Mesoderm

Fig. 10.3 (A) Illustration of the pharyngeal pouches and pharyngeal arch arteries. (B) Horizontal section through the embryo showing the floor of the primordial pharynx and illustrating the germ layer origin of the pharyngeal arch components.

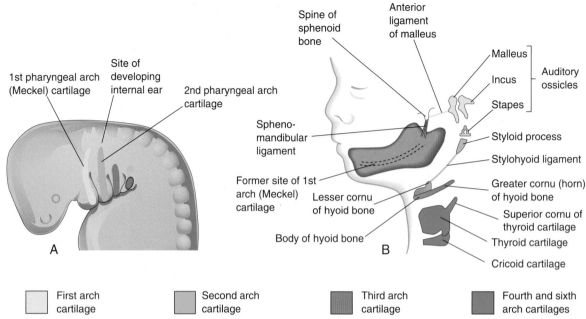

Fig. 10.4 (A) Schematic lateral view of the head, neck, and thoracic regions of a 4-week embryo, showing the location of the cartilages in the pharyngeal arches. (B) Similar view of a 24-week fetus showing the adult derivatives of the arch cartilages. Note that the mandible is formed by intramembranous ossification of mesenchymal tissue surrounding the first arch cartilage.

Table 10.1   Structures Derived From Pharyngeal Arch Components[a]

Arch	Nerve	Muscles	Skeletal Structures	Ligaments
First (mandibular)	Trigeminal[b] (CN V)	Muscles of mastication[c] Mylohyoid and anterior belly of digastric Tensor tympani Tensor veli palatini	Malleus Incus	Anterior ligament of malleus Sphenomandibular ligament
Second (hyoid)	Facial (CN VII)	Muscles of facial expression[d] Stapedius Stylohyoid Posterior belly of digastric	Stapes (portion) Styloid process Lesser cornu of hyoid bone	Stylohyoid ligament
Third	Glossopharyngeal (CN IX)	Stylopharyngeus	Greater cornu of hyoid bone Superior cornu of thyroid cartilage	
Fourth and sixth[e]	Superior laryngeal branch of vagus (CN X) Recurrent laryngeal branch of vagus (CN X)	Cricothyroid Levator veli palatini Constrictors of pharynx Intrinsic muscles of larynx Striated muscles of esophagus	Thyroid cartilage Cricoid cartilage Arytenoid cartilage Corniculate cartilage Cuneiform cartilage Hyoid bone body (via the hypobranchial eminence)	

CN, Cranial nerve.

[a]The derivatives of the pharyngeal arch arteries are described in Chapter 14.

[b]The ophthalmic division of the CN V does not supply any pharyngeal arch components.

[c]Temporalis, masseter, medial, and lateral pterygoids.

[d]Buccinator, auricularis, frontalis, platysma, and orbicularis oris and oculi.

[e]The fifth pharyngeal arch regresses. The cartilaginous components of the fourth and sixth arches fuse to form the cartilages of the larynx.

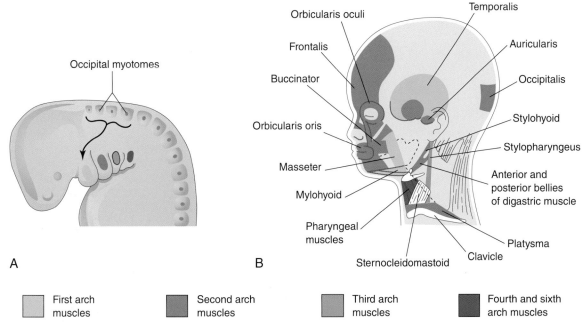

Fig. 10.5 (A) Lateral view of the head, neck, and thoracic regions of a 4-week embryo showing the muscles derived from the pharyngeal arches. The *arrow* shows the pathway taken by myoblasts from the occipital myotomes to form the tongue musculature. (B) The head and neck regions of a 20-week fetus, showing the muscles derived from the pharyngeal arches. Parts of the platysma and sternocleidomastoid muscles have been removed to show the deeper muscles. Note that myoblasts from the second arch migrate from the neck to the head, where they give rise to the muscles of facial expression. These muscles are supplied by the facial nerve (cranial nerve VII), the nerve of the second pharyngeal arch.

pairs of pouches are well defined. The endoderm of the pouches contacts the ectoderm of the pharyngeal grooves, and together they form the double-layered **pharyngeal membranes** (see Fig. 10.3B). *Retinoic acid, Wnt, and fibroblast growth factor (FGF) control the formation and differentiation of the pharyngeal pouches. Tbx2 gene expression in the pharyngeal pouch endoderm is essential for the formation of the pharyngeal arches. Sonic hedgehog (SHH) signaling in the pharyngeal pouch endoderm, in addition to the facial ectoderm and the neuroectoderm of the ventral forebrain, plays a critical role in the development of the face and cranium.*

DERIVATIVES OF PHARYNGEAL POUCHES

The **first pouch** gives rise to the **tubotympanic recess** (see Fig. 10.7B). The first pharyngeal membrane contributes to the formation of the **tympanic membrane** (eardrum) (see Fig. 10.7C). The cavity of the tubotympanic recess gives rise to the **tympanic cavity** and **mastoid antrum**. The connection of the tubotympanic *recess* with the pharynx forms the **pharyngotympanic tube** (auditory tube).

The **second pouch** is largely obliterated as the **palatine tonsil** develops (Fig. 10.8; see Fig. 10.7C). A part of this pouch remains as the **tonsillar sinus (fossa)**. The endoderm of the second pouch proliferates and grows into the underlying mesenchyme. The central parts of these buds break down, forming **tonsillar crypts**. The pouch endoderm forms the surface epithelium and the lining of the crypts. Lymphoid infiltration occurs approximately in the seventh month, whereas germinal centers are not apparent until the neonatal period.

The **third pouch** expands and develops a solid, bulbar, dorsal part and a hollow, elongate ventral part (see Fig. 10.7B). The connection between the pouch and pharynx is reduced to a narrow duct that soon degenerates. By the sixth week of development, the epithelium of each bulbar dorsal part begins to differentiate into an **inferior parathyroid gland**. The epithelium of the elongated ventral parts of the third pair of pouches proliferates, obliterating their cavities. These parts come together in the median plane to form the **thymus**. The primordia of the thymus and parathyroid glands lose their connections with the pharynx. Later, the inferior parathyroid glands separate from the thymus and lie on the dorsal surface of the thyroid gland, whereas the thymus descends into the superior mediastinum (see Figs. 10.7C and 10.8). The mesenchyme surrounding the thymic primordium is derived from neural crest cells.

The dorsal part of each **fourth pouch** develops into a **superior parathyroid gland**, which lies on the dorsal surface of the thyroid gland (see Fig. 10.7B). The parathyroid glands derived from the third pouches descend with the thymus and are carried to a more inferior position than the parathyroid glands that are derived from the fourth pouches (see Fig. 10.8). The elongated ventral part of each fourth pouch develops into the **hypobranchial eminence**, which fuses with the thyroid gland, giving rise to the **parafollicular cells (C cells)** of the thyroid gland. These cells produce **calcitonin**, a hormone involved in the regulation of calcium. C cells differentiate from **neural crest cells** that migrate from the pharyngeal arches into the fourth pair of pharyngeal pouches. *The parathormone, GATA3, Gcm2, Sox3, and FGF-signaling*

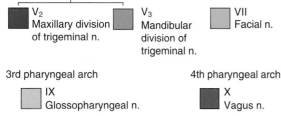

Fig. 10.6   (A) Lateral view of the head, neck, and thoracic regions of a 4-week embryo, showing the cranial nerves that supply the pharyngeal arches. (B) The head and neck regions of a 20-week fetus, showing the superficial distribution of the two caudal branches of the first arch nerve (cranial nerve V). (C) Sagittal section of the fetal head and neck, showing the deep distribution of the sensory fibers of the nerves to the teeth and mucosa of the tongue, pharynx, nasal cavity, palate, and larynx.

pathways, acting through FGF-receptor substrate 2, are involved in the development of the thymus and parathyroid glands.

PHARYNGEAL GROOVES

The head and neck regions of the embryo exhibit four grooves (clefts) on each side during the fourth and fifth weeks (see Fig. 10.1A). These grooves separate the pharyngeal arches externally. Only one pair of grooves contributes to structures; the first pair persists as the **external acoustic meatus** (ear canal) (see Fig. 10.7C). The other grooves lie in a slit-like depression—the **cervical sinus**—and are usually obliterated with it as the neck develops (see Fig. 10.7A and B).

Auricular Sinuses and Cysts

Small auricular sinuses and cysts are usually located in a triangular area of skin anterior to the auricle of the external ear (Fig. 10.9D); however, they may occur in other sites around the auricle or in its lobule (earlobe). Although some sinuses and cysts are remnants of the first pharyngeal groove, others represent ectodermal folds sequestered during the formation of the auricle from the auricular hillocks.

Cervical (Branchial)/Lateral Sinuses

Cervical sinuses are rare (1:10,000), uncommon, and almost all that open externally on the side of the neck result from failure of the second pharyngeal groove and cervical sinus to obliterate (Fig. 10.10A; see Fig. 10.9B). The sinus typically opens along the anterior border of the sternocleidomastoid muscle in the inferior third of the neck. Anomalies of the other grooves occur in approximately 5% of cases.

External cervical sinuses are commonly detected during infancy because of the discharge of mucous material from their orifices in the neck. These sinuses are bilateral in approximately 10% of cases and are commonly associated with auricular sinuses.

Internal cervical sinuses open into the pharynx and are very rare. Almost all of these sinuses result from the persistence of the proximal part of the second pharyngeal pouch, so they usually open into the tonsillar sinus or near the palatopharyngeal arch (see Fig. 10.9B and D).

Cervical (Branchial) Fistula

An abnormal canal that opens internally into the tonsillar sinus and externally on the side of the neck is a **cervical fistula**. This extremely rare birth defect results from the persistence of parts of the second pharyngeal groove and pouch (see Figs. 10.9C and D and 10.10B). The fistula ascends from its opening in the neck, through the subcutaneous tissue and platysma muscle, to reach the tonsillar sinus.

Germ Layer Derivatives

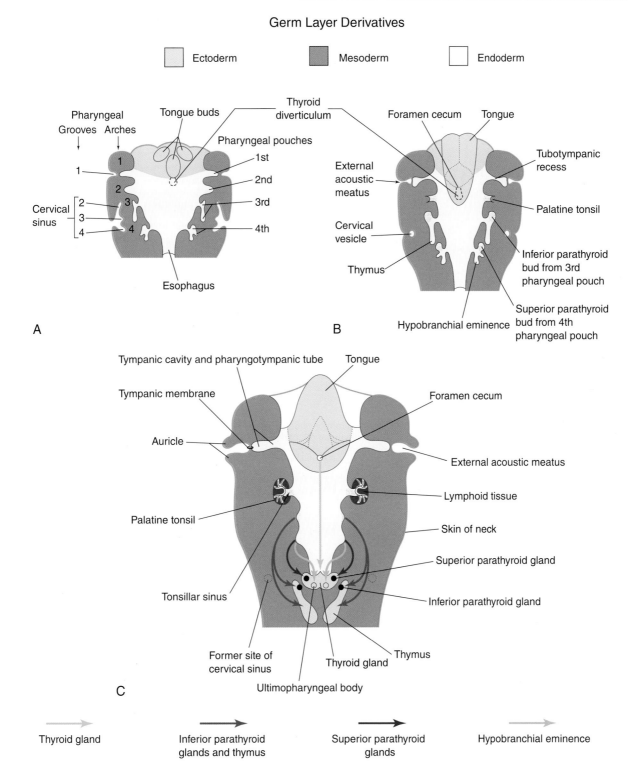

Ectoderm   Mesoderm   Endoderm

Fig. 10.7 Schematic horizontal sections of the embryo showing the adult derivatives of the pharyngeal pouches. (A) At 5 weeks. Note that the second pharyngeal arch grows over the third and fourth arches, burying the second to fourth pharyngeal grooves in the cervical sinus. (B) At 6 weeks. (C) At 7 weeks. Note the migration of the developing thymus, parathyroid, and thyroid glands into the neck.

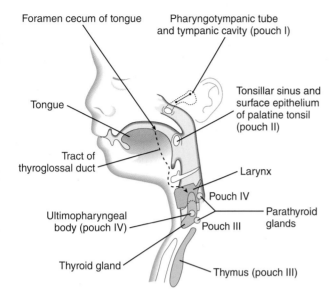

Fig. 10.8 A sagittal section of the head, neck, and upper thoracic regions of a 20-week fetus, showing the adult derivatives of the pharyngeal pouches and the descent of the thyroid gland into the neck.

Cervical (Branchial) Cysts

The third and fourth pharyngeal arches are buried in the cervical sinus (see Fig. 10.7A). Remnants of parts of the cervical sinus, the second groove, or both may persist and form a spherical or elongated cyst (see Fig. 10.9D). Cervical cysts often do not become apparent until late childhood or early adulthood, when they produce a slowly enlarging, painless swelling in the neck, usually along the anterior border of the sternocleidomastoid muscle or in the periauricular region (Fig. 10.11). The cysts enlarge because of the accumulation of fluid and cellular debris derived from the desquamation of their epithelial linings (Fig. 10.12). The incidence of cervical cysts is not well established as many cysts are asymptomatic.

Chondrocutaneous Branchial Remnants (Vestiges)

Normally, the pharyngeal arch cartilages disappear, except for the parts that form ligaments or bones; however, in unusual cases, cartilaginous or bony remnants of the pharyngeal arch cartilages appear under the skin on the side of the neck. These are usually found anterior to the inferior third of the sternocleidomastoid muscle (see Fig. 10.9D).

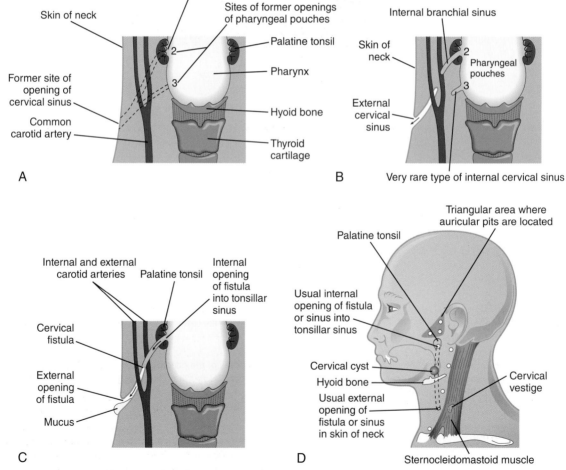

Fig. 10.9 (A) The adult pharyngeal and neck regions, indicating the former sites of openings of the cervical sinus and pharyngeal pouches (*2* and *3*). The *broken lines* indicate possible courses of cervical fistulas. (B) The embryologic basis for various types of cervical sinus. (C) Illustration of a cervical fistula resulting from the persistence of parts of the second pharyngeal groove and the second pharyngeal pouch. (D) Possible sites of cervical cysts and openings of the cervical sinuses and fistulas. A cervical vestige is also shown.

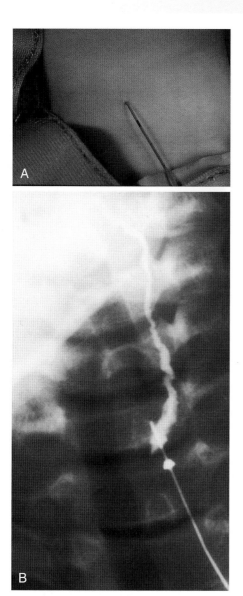

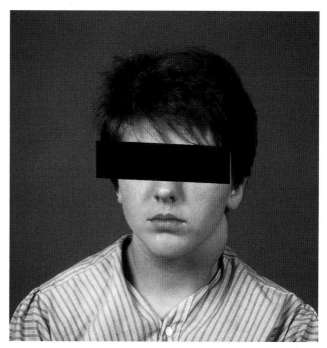

Fig. 10.11 A swelling in a boy's neck produced by a cervical cyst. These large cysts often lie free in the neck, just inferior to the angle of the mandible, but they may develop anywhere along the anterior border of the sternocleidomastoid muscle, as in this case. (Courtesy Dr. Pierre Soucy, Division of Paediatric Surgery, Children's Hospital of Eastern Ontario, Ottawa, Ontario, Canada.)

Fig. 10.10 (A) A child's neck showing a catheter inserted into the external opening of a cervical (branchial) sinus. The catheter allows definition of the length of the tract, which facilitates surgical excision. (B) A fistulogram of a complete cervical fistula. The radiograph was taken after the injection of a contrast medium to show the course of the fistula through the neck. (Courtesy Dr. Pierre Soucy, Division of Paediatric Surgery, Children's Hospital of Eastern Ontario, Ottawa, Ontario, Canada.)

First Pharyngeal Arch Syndrome

Abnormal development of the first pharyngeal arch results in various congenital anomalies of the eyes, ears, mandible, and palate that together constitute **first pharyngeal arch syndrome** (Fig. 10.13). This syndrome is believed to result from insufficient migration of neural crest cells into the first arch during the fourth week. There are two main clinical manifestations of first arch syndrome:

- **Treacher Collins syndrome** (mandibulofacial dysostosis) (1:50,000) is most often (80%–90%) caused by an autosomal-dominant gene defect (*TCOF1*) and results in underdevelopment of the zygomatic bones of the face—**malar hypoplasia**. Characteristic features of the syndrome include

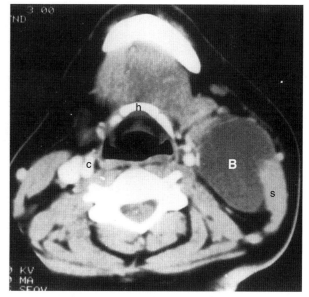

Fig. 10.12 A large cervical cyst *(B)* shown by computed tomography of the neck region of a female who had a "lump" in the neck, similar to that shown in Fig. 10.11. The low-density cyst is anterior to the right sternocleidomastoid muscle *(s)* at the level of the hyoid bone *(h)*. The normal appearance of the left carotid sheath *(c)* is shown for comparison with the compressed sheath on the right side. (From McNab T, McLennan MK, Margolis M: Radiology rounds, *Can Fam Physician* 41:1673, 1995.)

down-slanting palpebral fissures, birth defects of the lower eyelids, deformed external ears, and sometimes defects of the middle and internal ears.

- **Pierre Robin sequence** (1:10,000) consists of hypoplasia of the mandible, cleft palate, and defects of the eye and ear. Many cases of this syndrome are sporadic; however, some appear to have a genetic basis including defects in SOX9 enhancers. The proposed initiating defect is a small mandible (micrognathia), which results in posterior displacement of the tongue and obstruction to full closure of the palatine processes, resulting in a bilateral cleft palate (see Fig. 10.33).

PHARYNGEAL MEMBRANES

These membranes form where the epithelia of the grooves and pouches approach each other. The membranes appear in the floors of the grooves during the fourth week (see Figs. 10.1D and 10.3B). Only one pair of membranes contributes to the formation of adult structures; the first membrane is the primordium of the **tympanic membrane** (see Fig. 10.7C).

DEVELOPMENT OF THYROID GLAND

The **thyroid gland** is the first endocrine gland to develop. It begins to form approximately 24 days from a median endodermal thickening in the floor of the primordial pharynx. This thickening soon forms a small outpouching—the **thyroid primordium** (Fig. 10.14A). In addition, two lateral primordia from the fourth pouch (hypobranchial eminence) fuse together with the median outpouch, with the median contributing the majority of the **follicular cells** and the lateral contributing the **parafollicular cells (C cells)**. As the embryo and tongue grow, the developing thyroid gland repositions in the neck, passing ventral to the developing hyoid bone and the laryngeal cartilages. For a short time, it is connected to the tongue by the **thyroglossal duct** (see Fig. 10.14A and B). As a result of rapid cell proliferation, the lumen of the thyroid diverticulum soon obliterates and divides into right and left lobes, which are connected by the **thyroid isthmus** of the thyroid gland.

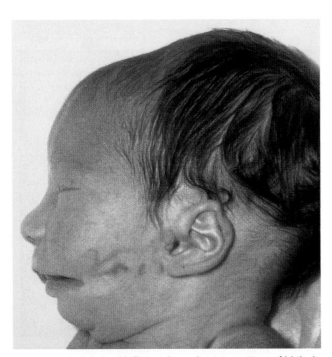

Fig. 10.13 An infant with first arch syndrome, a pattern of birth defects resulting from insufficient migration of the neural crest cells into the first pharyngeal arch. Note the deformed auricle of the external ear, preauricular appendage, defect in the cheek between the auricle and the mouth, hypoplasia of the mandible, and macrostomia (large mouth). (Courtesy Health Sciences Centre, Children's Hospital, Winnipeg, Manitoba, Canada.)

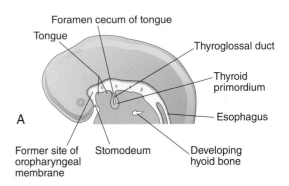

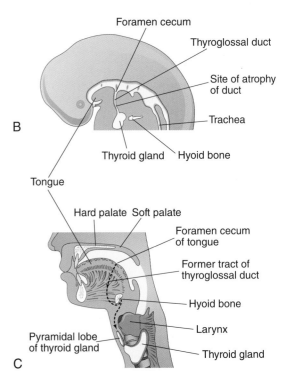

Fig. 10.14 Development of the thyroid gland. (A and B) Schematic sagittal sections of the head and neck regions at 5 and 6 weeks, showing successive stages in the development of the thyroid gland. (C) Similar section of an adult head and neck, showing the path taken by the thyroid gland during its embryonic descent (indicated by the former tract of the thyroglossal duct).

DiGeorge Syndrome

Infants with DiGeorge syndrome (22q11.2 deletion syndrome) (2.5–5:10,000) are born without a thymus (thymic dysplasia) and parathyroid glands. The disease is characterized by **congenital hypoparathyroidism** (hypocalcemia), increased susceptibility to infections from immune deficiency (defective T-cell function), palate abnormalities, micrognathia (airway obstruction due to retropositioned tongue), low-set notched ears, nasal clefts, and cardiac and renal abnormalities. DiGeorge syndrome, the most common of the microdeletion syndromes, occurs when the third and fourth pharyngeal pouches do not differentiate into the thymus and parathyroid glands. The facial birth defects result primarily from the abnormal development of the first pharyngeal arch components during the formation of the face and ears. Microdeletion inactivates the HIRA, UFDIL, and Tbx1 genes and causes neural crest cell defects *due to CXCR4 signaling errors*. The incidence of DiGeorge syndrome is 1 in 2000 to 4000 births.

Ectopic Parathyroid Glands

The pea-sized parathyroids are highly variable in number and location and may be found anywhere near or within the thyroid gland or the thymus (Fig. 10.15). The superior glands are more constant in position than the inferior ones. Occasionally, an inferior parathyroid gland does not descend and remains near the bifurcation of the common carotid artery. In other cases, it may accompany the thymus into the thorax.

In unusual cases, there may be more than four parathyroid glands. **Supernumerary parathyroid glands** probably result from the division of the primordia of the original glands. Absence of a parathyroid gland results from the failure of one of the primordia to differentiate or from atrophy of a gland early in development. Parathyroid gland tumors occur frequently and lead to increased parathyroid hormone secretion.

By 7 weeks, the thyroid gland has assumed its definitive shape and has usually reached its final site in the neck (see Fig. 10.14C). By this time, the **thyroglossal duct** has usually degenerated and disappeared. The proximal opening of the thyroglossal duct persists as a small pit—the **foramen cecum** in the dorsum of the tongue (see Fig. 10.7C). A **pyramidal lobe** of the thyroid gland extends superiorly from the isthmus in approximately 50% of people. This lobe may be attached to the hyoid bone by fibrous tissue, smooth muscle, or both.

Thyroglossal Duct Cysts and Sinuses

A remnant of the thyroglossal duct may often persist and form a cyst in the tongue or the anterior part of the neck, usually just inferior to the hyoid bone (Fig. 10.16). The prevalence is approximately 7% in the general population. The swelling produced by a **thyroglossal duct cyst** usually develops as a painless, progressively enlarging, and movable median mass (Fig. 10.17). The cyst

may contain some thyroid tissue. After infection of a cyst, perforation of the skin occurs in some cases, forming a **thyroglossal duct sinus** that usually opens in the median plane of the neck, anterior to the laryngeal cartilages (Fig. 10.18A).

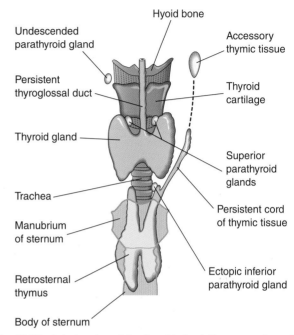

Fig. 10.15 Anterior view of the thyroid gland, thymus, and parathyroid glands, showing various possible congenital anomalies that may occur.

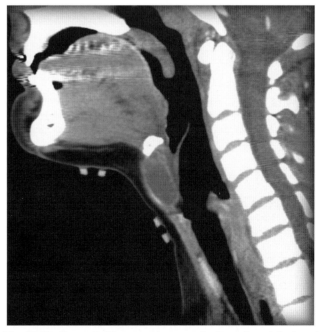

Fig. 10.16 Computed tomography scan of a thyroglossal duct cyst in a child. The cyst is located in the neck, anterior to the thyroid cartilage (see also Fig. 10.4B). (From Dr. Frank Gaillard, https://radiopaedia.org, with permission.)

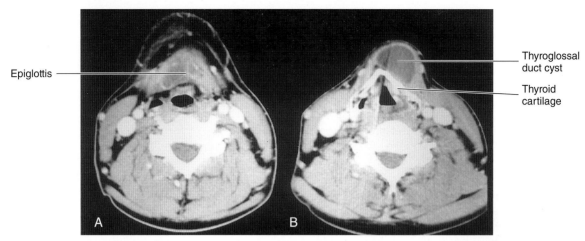

Fig. 10.17 Computed tomography scans. (A) The level of the thyrohyoid membrane and the base of the epiglottis. (B) The level of the thyroid cartilage, which is calcified. A thyroglossal duct cyst extends cranially to the margin of the hyoid bone. (Courtesy Dr. Gerald S. Smyser, Altru Health System, Grand Forks, North Dakota.)

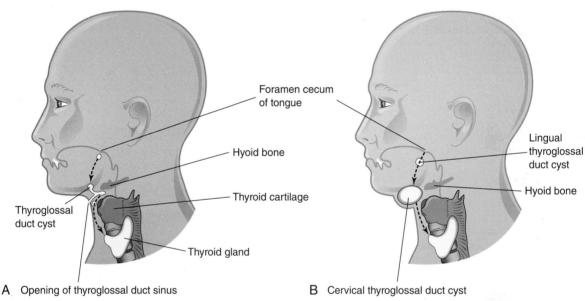

Fig. 10.18 (A) Illustration of the head and neck, showing the possible locations of thyroglossal duct cysts. A thyroglossal duct sinus is also illustrated. The *broken line* indicates the course taken by the duct during the descent of the developing thyroid gland from the foramen cecum to its final position in the anterior part of the neck. (B) Similar sketch showing lingual and cervical thyroglossal duct cysts. Most thyroglossal duct cysts are located just inferior to the hyoid bone.

Ectopic Thyroid Gland

Very rarely, an **ectopic thyroid gland** is located along the normal route of its descent from the tongue (see Fig. 10.14B). In 90% of cases, this is represented by **lingual thyroid glandular tissue**. Incomplete descent of the thyroid gland results in a **sublingual thyroid gland** that appears high in the neck, at or just inferior to the hyoid bone (Figs. 10.19 and 10.20). In 70% of cases an ectopic sublingual thyroid gland is the only thyroid tissue present.

It is clinically important to differentiate an ectopic thyroid gland from a thyroglossal duct cyst or accessory thyroid tissue to prevent *inadvertent surgical removal of the thyroid gland* because this ectopic gland may be the only thyroid tissue present. Failure to recognize the thyroid gland may leave the person permanently dependent on thyroid medication.

During the 11th week, **colloid** begins to appear in the **thyroid follicles**; thereafter, iodine concentration and the synthesis of thyroid hormones (THs) can be demonstrated. By 20 weeks, the levels of fetal thyroid-stimulating hormone and thyroxine begin to increase, reaching adult levels by 35 weeks. TH is required for brain development and is provided by the mother before fetal thyroid tissue is functioning.

DEVELOPMENT OF THE TONGUE

Myoblasts from the occipital somites and cranial neural crest cells contribute to the formation of the tongue. By the end of the fourth week, a median triangular elevation appears in the floor of the primordial pharynx, just rostral to the foramen cecum (Fig. 10.21A). The **median lingual swelling** (tongue bud) is the first indication of tongue development. Soon, two oval **lateral lingual swellings (distal tongue buds)** develop on each side of the median tongue swelling. The three lingual swellings result from the proliferation of mesenchyme in the ventromedial parts of the first pair of pharyngeal arches. The lateral lingual swellings rapidly increase in size, merge with each other, and overgrow the median tongue swelling.

The merged lateral swellings form the anterior two-thirds (oral part) of the tongue (see Fig. 10.21C). The plane of fusion of the lateral swellings is indicated superficially by the midline groove of the tongue and internally by the fibrous **lingual septum**. The median lingual swelling forms no recognizable part of the adult tongue.

Formation of the posterior third (pharyngeal part) of the tongue is indicated by two elevations that develop caudal to the foramen cecum (see Fig. 10.21A):

- The **copula** forms by fusion of the ventromedial parts of the second pair of pharyngeal arches.
- The **hypopharyngeal eminence** develops caudal to the copula from a cluster of mesenchymal cells in the ventromedial parts of the third and fourth pairs of pharyngeal arches.

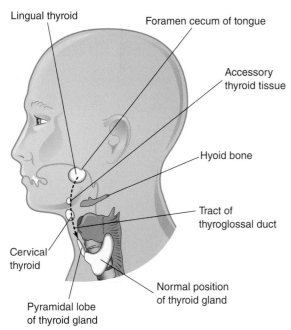

Fig. 10.19 Illustration of the head and neck showing the usual sites of ectopic thyroid tissue. The *broken line* indicates the path followed by the thyroid gland during its descent and the former tract of the thyroglossal duct.

Congenital Lingual Cysts and Fistulas

Cysts in the tongue may be derived from remnants of the thyroglossal duct (see Fig. 10.14A). They may enlarge and produce pharyngeal pain, dysphagia (difficulty in swallowing), or both. Fistulas may also arise as a result of the persistence of the lingual parts of the thyroglossal duct; such fistulas open through the **foramen cecum** into the oral cavity.

As the tongue develops, the copula is gradually overgrown by the hypopharyngeal eminence and disappears (see Fig. 10.21B and C). As a result, the pharyngeal part of the tongue develops from the rostral part of the **hypopharyngeal eminence**. The line of fusion of the anterior and posterior parts of the tongue is roughly indicated by a V-shaped groove—the

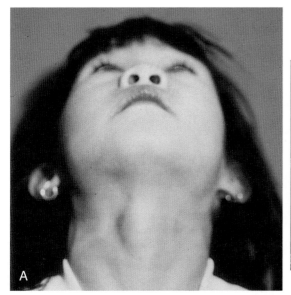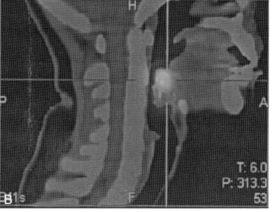

Fig. 10.20 (A) Sublingual thyroid mass in a 5-year-old girl. (B) Technetium-99m pertechnetate scan showing a sublingual thyroid gland (*) without evidence of functioning thyroid tissue in the anterior part of the neck. (From Leung AKC, Wong AL, Robson WLLM: Ectopic thyroid gland simulating a thyroglossal duct cyst: a case report, *Can J Surg* 38:87, 1995.)

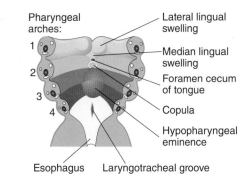

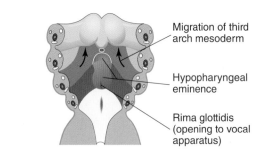

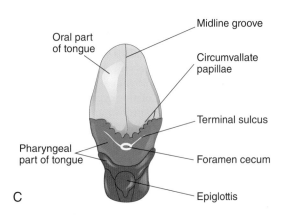

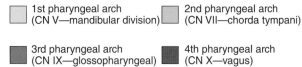

Pharyngeal Arch Derivatives of Tongue

☐ 1st pharyngeal arch
(CN V—mandibular division)

☐ 2nd pharyngeal arch
(CN VII—chorda tympani)

■ 3rd pharyngeal arch
(CN IX—glossopharyngeal)

■ 4th pharyngeal arch
(CN X—vagus)

Fig. 10.21 (A and B) Schematic horizontal sections through the pharynx, showing successive stages in the development of the tongue during the fourth and fifth weeks. (C) Drawing of an adult tongue, showing the pharyngeal arch derivation of the nerve supply of its mucosa (mucous membrane). *CN*, Cranial nerve.

terminal sulcus (see Fig. 10.21C). Cranial neural crest cells migrate into the developing tongue and give rise to its connective tissue and vasculature. Most of the tongue muscles are derived from myoblasts that migrate from the occipital somites (see Fig. 10.5A). The **hypoglossal nerve (CN XII)**

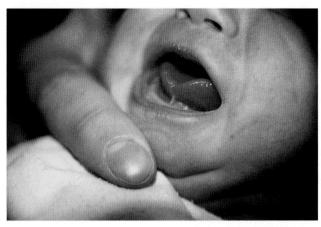

Fig. 10.22 An infant with ankyloglossia (tongue-tie). Note the short frenulum, which extends to the tip of the tongue. (Courtesy Dr. Evelyn Jain, Lakeview Breastfeeding Clinic, Calgary, Alberta, Canada.)

accompanies the myoblasts during their migration and innervates the tongue muscles as they develop. *The molecular mechanisms involved in the development of the tongue include myogenic regulating factors, the paired box genes Pax3 and Pax7, and the transforming growth factor-β (TGF-β), FGF, and SHH genes. For the formation of the connective tissue and blood vessels, Nf2 plays a critical role.*

Ankyloglossia

The lingual frenulum normally connects the inferior surface of the tongue to the floor of the mouth (Fig. 10.22). **Ankyloglossia** (tongue-tie) occurs in approximately 1 in 300 North American infants but is usually of no functional significance. The associated short frenulum usually stretches with time, making surgical correction of the anomaly unnecessary. In some neonates, ankyloglossia interferes with breastfeeding and may require frenotomy.

LINGUAL PAPILLAE AND TASTE BUDS

Lingual papillae appear by the end of the eighth week. The **vallate** and **foliate papillae** appear first, close to the terminal branches of the glossopharyngeal nerve (CN IX) (see Fig. 10.21C). The **fungiform** papillae appear later, near the terminations of the chorda tympani branch of the facial nerve. The numerous and thread-like **filiform papillae** develop during the early fetal period (10–11 weeks). They contain afferent nerve endings that are sensitive to touch.

Taste buds develop during weeks 11 to 13 by inductive interaction between the epithelial cells of the tongue and invading gustatory nerve cells from the chorda tympani, glossopharyngeal, and vagus nerves. **Facial responses** can be induced by bitter-tasting substances at 26 to 28 weeks, indicating that reflex pathways between taste buds and facial muscles are established by this stage.

NERVE SUPPLY OF TONGUE

The sensory supply to the mucosa of almost the entire anterior tongue (oral part) is from the lingual branch of the mandibular division of the trigeminal nerve (CN V), the nerve of the first pharyngeal arch (see Fig. 10.21C). Although the facial nerve is the nerve of the second pharyngeal arch, its chorda tympani branch supplies the taste buds in the anterior two-thirds of the tongue, except for the vallate papillae. Because the second arch component, the **copula**, is overgrown by the third arch component, the facial nerve does not supply any of the tongue mucosa, except for the taste buds in the anterior part of the tongue. The vallate papillae in the anterior tongue are innervated by the glossopharyngeal nerve (CN IX) of the third pharyngeal arch (see Fig. 10.21C). The posterior third of the tongue is innervated mainly by the glossopharyngeal nerve (CN IX) of the third pharyngeal arch. The superior laryngeal branch of the vagus nerve (CN X) of the fourth arch supplies a small area of the tongue anterior to the epiglottis (see Fig. 10.21C). All muscles of the tongue are supplied by the hypoglossal nerve (CN XII), except for the palatoglossus, which is supplied from the pharyngeal plexus by fibers arising from the vagus nerve.

DEVELOPMENT OF SALIVARY GLANDS

During the sixth and seventh weeks, the salivary glands begin as solid epithelial buds from the endoderm of the primordial oral cavity (see Fig. 10.6C). The buds undergo branching morphogenesis and grow into the underlying mesenchyme. The connective tissue in the glands is derived from neural crest cells. All parenchymal (secretory) tissue arises due to the proliferation of the oral epithelium.

The **parotid glands** appear early in the sixth week. They develop from buds that arise from the oral ectodermal lining near the angles of the stomodeum. The buds grow toward the ears, branching to form solid cords with rounded ends. Later, the cords canalize and become ducts in approximately 10 weeks. The rounded ends of the cords differentiate into acini. Secretions begin at 18 weeks. The capsule of the connective tissue develops from the surrounding mesenchyme.

The **submandibular glands** appear late in the sixth week. They develop from endodermal buds in the floor of the stomodeum. Solid cellular processes grow posteriorly, lateral to the developing tongue. Later, they branch and differentiate. Acini begin to form at 12 weeks, and secretory activity begins at 16 weeks. Growth of the submandibular glands continues after birth, with the formation of mucous acini. Lateral to the developing tongue, a linear groove forms that soon closes over to form the submandibular duct.

The **sublingual glands** appear in the eighth week, approximately 2 weeks later than the other salivary glands (see Fig. 10.6C). They develop from multiple endodermal epithelial buds in the **paralingual sulcus**. These buds branch and canalize to form 10 to 12 ducts that open independently into the floor of the mouth.

DEVELOPMENT OF THE FACE

The facial primordia appear around the stomodeum early in the fourth week (Fig. 10.23A). Facial development depends on the inductive influence of three organizing areas:

- Forebrain (which establishes a gradient of SHH factors)
- Frontonasal ectoderm
- Developing eye

The **five facial primordia** that appear as prominences around the stomodeum (see Fig. 10.23A) are the following:

- A frontonasal prominence (FNP)
- Paired maxillary prominences
- Paired mandibular prominences

The maxillary and mandibular prominences are derivatives of the first pair of pharyngeal arches. The prominences are produced by mesenchyme derived from HOX-negative neural crest cells that migrate into the arches during the fourth week of development. These cells are the major source of connective tissue components, including cartilage, bone, and ligaments in the facial and oral regions.

The FNP surrounds the ventrolateral part of the forebrain, which gives rise to the optic vesicles that form the eyes (Fig. 10.24; see Fig. 10.23A). The frontal part of the FNP forms the forehead; the nasal part of the FNP forms the rostral boundary of the stomodeum and nose. The **maxillary prominences** form the lateral boundaries of the stomodeum, and the **mandibular prominences** constitute the caudal boundary of the stomodeum (see Figs. 10.23A and 10.24). The lower jaw and the lower lip are the first parts of the face to form. They result from the merging of the medial ends of the mandibular prominences. The common "chin dimple" results from an incomplete fusion of the prominences.

By the end of the fourth week, bilateral oval thickenings of the surface ectoderm—**nasal placodes**—have developed on the inferolateral parts of the FNP (Fig. 10.25A and B; see also Fig. 10.24). Initially, these placodes are convex, but later, they are stretched to produce a flat depression in each placode. The mesenchyme in the margins of the placodes proliferates, producing horseshoe-shaped elevations—the medial and lateral **nasal prominences** (see Figs. 10.23B and 10.25D and E). As a result, the nasal placodes lie in depressions—**nasal pits** (see Figs. 10.23B and 10.25C and D). These pits are the primordia of the anterior nares (nostrils) and nasal cavities (see Fig. 10.25E).

The proliferation of mesenchyme in the maxillary prominences causes them to enlarge and grow medially toward each other and the nasal prominences (see Figs. 10.23B and C and 10.24). The medial migration of the maxillary prominences moves the medial nasal prominences toward the median plane and each other. *This process is regulated by the transcription factors such as PDGFRα, TGF-β, BMP, and Wnt genes.* Each lateral nasal prominence is separated from the maxillary prominence by a cleft called the **nasolacrimal groove** (see Fig. 10.23B).

By the end of the fifth week, the primordia of the auricle, **six auricular hillocks** (mesenchymal swellings), form around the first pharyngeal groove (three on each side), the primordium of the external acoustic meatus (ear canal). Initially, the external ears are positioned in the neck region; however, as the mandible develops, they are positioned to the side of the head at the level of the eyes (see Fig. 10.23B and C).

By the end of the sixth week, each maxillary prominence has begun to merge with the lateral nasal prominence along

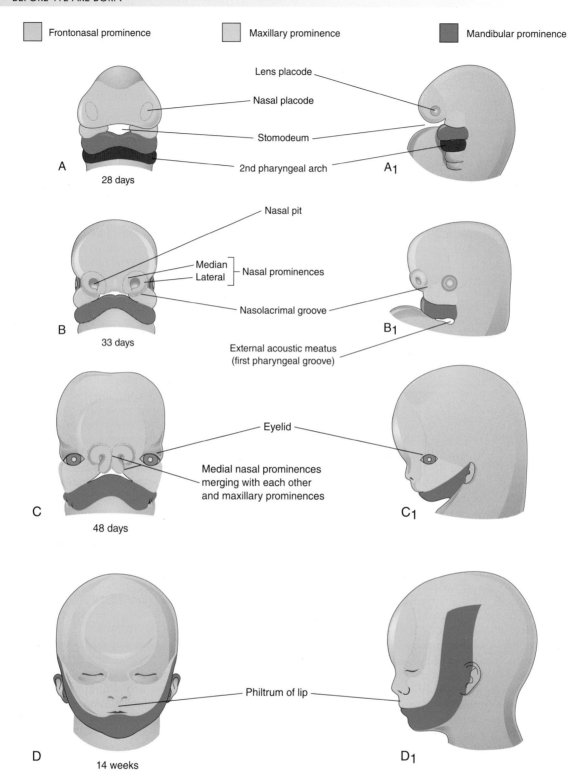

Fig. 10.23 (A–D₁) Diagrams illustrating progressive stages in the development of the human face.

the line of the nasolacrimal groove (Fig. 10.26A and B). This establishes continuity between the side of the nose, formed by the lateral nasal prominence, and the cheek region, formed by the maxillary prominence.

The **nasolacrimal duct** develops from a rod-like thickening of ectoderm in the floor of the **nasolacrimal groove**. This thickening gives rise to a solid epithelial cord that separates from the ectoderm and sinks into the mesenchyme. Later, as a result of **apoptosis**, this cord canalizes to form the nasolacrimal duct. The cranial end of this duct expands to form the **lacrimal sac**. In the late fetal period, the nasolacrimal duct drains into the inferior meatus in the lateral wall of

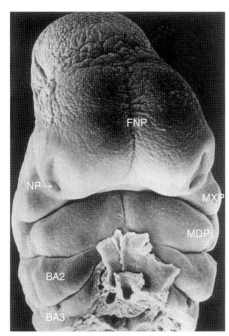

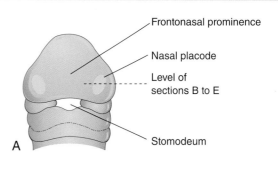

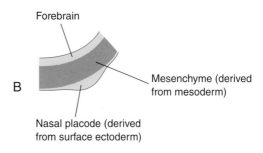

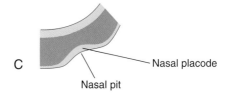

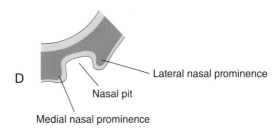

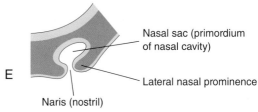

Fig. 10.24 Scanning electron micrograph of a ventral view of a human embryo at approximately 33 days (Carnegie stage 15; crown–rump length, 8 mm). Observe the prominent frontonasal prominence (*FNP*) surrounding the telencephalon (forebrain). Also observe the nasal pits (*NP*) located in the ventrolateral regions of the FNP. Medial and lateral nasal prominences surround these pits. The wedge-shaped maxillary prominences (*MXP*) form the lateral boundaries of the stomodeum. The fusing mandibular prominences (*MDP*) are located just caudal to the stomodeum. The second pharyngeal arch (*BA2*) is clearly visible and shows overhanging margins. The third pharyngeal arch (*BA3*) is also clearly visible. (From Hinrichsen K: The early development of morphology and patterns of the face in the human embryo, *Adv Anat Embryol Cell Biol* 98:1, 1985.)

Fig. 10.25 Progressive stages in the development of a human nasal sac (primordial nasal cavity). (A) Ventral view of an embryo at approximately 28 days. (B–E) Transverse sections through the left side of the developing nasal sac.

the nasal cavity. The duct usually becomes completely patent after birth.

Between weeks 7 and 10, the **medial nasal prominences** merge with each other and with the maxillary and lateral nasal prominences (see Fig. 10.23C), resulting in the disintegration of their contacting surface epithelia. This causes the intermingling of the underlying mesenchyme. Fusion of the medial nasal and maxillary prominences results in continuity of the upper jaw and lip and separation of the nasal pits from the stomodeum. As the medial nasal prominences merge, they form an **intermaxillary segment** (see Fig. 10.26C to F). The segment gives rise to the

- Median part (philtrum) of the upper lip
- Premaxillary part of the maxilla and its associated gingiva (gum)
- Primary palate

The lateral parts of the upper lip, most of the maxilla, and the secondary palate form from the **maxillary prominences** (see Fig. 10.23D). These prominences merge laterally with the mandibular prominences. Recent studies indicate that the lower part of the medial nasal prominences appears to become deeply positioned and covered by medial extensions of the maxillary prominences to form the **philtrum**.

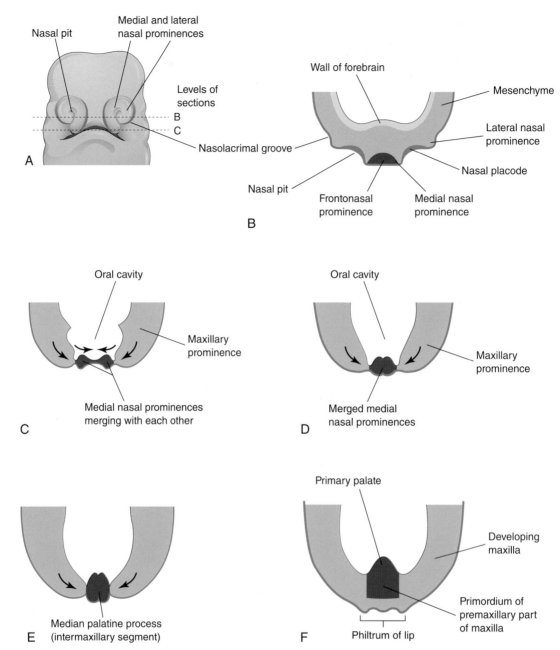

Fig. 10.26   Illustrations of the early development of the maxilla, palate, and upper lip. (A) Facial view of a 5-week embryo. (B and C) Sketches of horizontal sections at the levels shown in (A). The *arrows* in (C) indicate subsequent growth of the maxillary and medial nasal prominences toward the median plane and merging of the prominences with each other. (D–F) Similar sections of older embryos illustrating the merging of the medial nasal prominences with each other and the maxillary prominences to form the upper lip. Recent studies suggest that the upper lip is formed entirely from the maxillary prominences.

The primordial lips and cheeks are invaded by myoblasts from the second pair of pharyngeal arches, which differentiate into the **facial muscles** (see Fig. 10.5 and Table 10.1). The myoblasts from the first pair of arches differentiate into the muscles of mastication. The smallness of the face prenatally results from the following:

- Rudimentary upper and lower jaws
- No erupted deciduous teeth
- Small size of nasal cavities and maxillary sinuses

DEVELOPMENT OF NASAL CAVITIES

As the face develops, the **nasal placodes** become depressed, forming **nasal pits** (see Figs. 10.24 and 10.25). The proliferation of the surrounding mesenchyme forms the medial and lateral **nasal prominences** and results in the deepening of the nasal pits and the formation of primordial **nasal sacs**. Each sac grows dorsally, ventral to the developing forebrain (Fig. 10.27A). At first, the nasal sacs are separated from the oral cavity by the **oronasal membrane**. This membrane

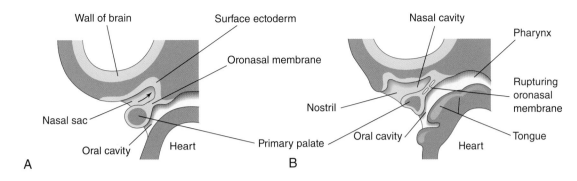

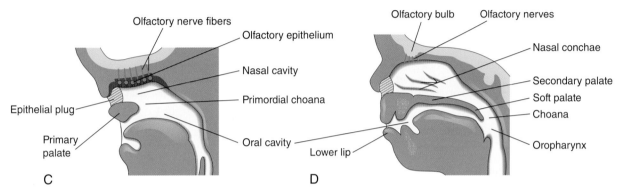

Fig. 10.27 Sagittal sections of the head showing development of the nasal cavities. The nasal septum has been removed. (A) At 5 weeks. (B)) At 6 weeks, showing breakdown of the oronasal membrane. (C) At 7 weeks, showing the nasal cavity communicating with the oral cavity and development of the olfactory epithelium. (D) At 12 weeks, showing that the palate and lateral wall of the nasal cavity are evident.

ruptures by the end of the sixth week, bringing the nasal and oral cavities into communication (see Fig. 10.27B and C). Proliferating epithelial cells (epithelial plug) fill the anterior lumen of the nasal cavity by 7 to 8 weeks. This epithelial plug undergoes apoptosis, and by the 17th week, the nasal passages are reopened, becoming the nasal vestibule.

The regions of continuity between the nasal and oral cavities are the **primordial choanae** (right or left openings from the nasal cavity into the nasal pharynx), which lie posterior to the primary palate. After the **secondary palate** develops, the choanae are located at the junction of the nasal cavity and pharynx (see Fig. 10.27D). While these changes are occurring, the superior, middle, and inferior **nasal conchae** develop as elevations of the lateral walls of the nasal cavities (see Fig. 10.29E and G). Concurrently, the ectodermal epithelium in the roof of each nasal cavity becomes specialized to form the **olfactory epithelium**. Some epithelial cells differentiate into olfactory receptor cells. The axons of these cells constitute the **olfactory nerves**, which grow into the olfactory bulbs of the brain (see Fig. 10.27C and D).

PARANASAL SINUSES

The ethmoid sinuses begin to develop during late fetal life; the remainder of them develop after birth. They form from outgrowths (diverticula) of the walls of the nasal cavities, becoming pneumatic (air-filled) extensions of the nasal cavities in the adjacent bones. The original openings of the diverticula persist as the orifices of the adult sinuses.

Postnatal Development of Paranasal Sinuses

The **maxillary sinuses** are small at birth but pneumatize rapidly from ages 1 to 4 years. They grow slowly until puberty and are not fully developed until all of the permanent teeth have erupted in early adulthood.

No **frontal** or **sphenoid sinuses** are present at birth. The **ethmoid cells** (sinuses) are small before 2 years, and they do not begin to grow rapidly until 6 to 8 years. At approximately 2 years, the two most anterior ethmoid cells grow into the frontal bone, forming a frontal sinus on each side which slowly pneumatizes. Usually, the frontal sinuses are visible on radiographs by 7 years and have an adult appearance by the age of 12 years. The two most anterior ethmoid cells grow into the frontal bone at approximately 2 years, forming a frontal sinus on each side. The two most posterior ethmoid cells grow into the sphenoid bone at approximately 2 years of age, forming two sphenoidal sinuses. Growth of the paranasal sinuses is important in altering the size and shape of the face during infancy and childhood and in adding resonance to the voice during adolescence.

DEVELOPMENT OF PALATE

8

The palate develops from two primordia: the primary palate and the secondary palate. **Palatogenesis** (a regulated morphogenetic process) begins in the sixth week but is not completed until the 12th week. *Multiple molecular pathways, including* Wnt *and* PRICKLE1, *are involved. The critical*

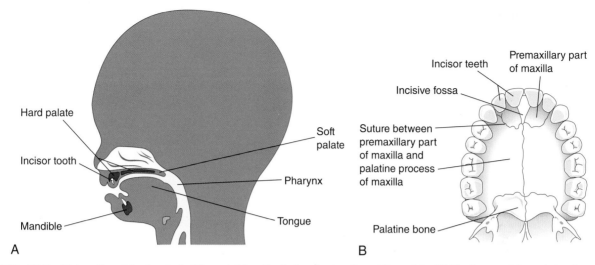

Fig. 10.28   (A) Sagittal section of the head of a 20-week fetus, illustrating the location of the palate. (B) The bony palate and alveolar arch of a young adult. The suture between the premaxillary part of the maxilla and the fused palatal processes of the maxillae is usually visible in the crania (skulls) of young people. The suture is not visible in the hard palates of most dried crania because they are usually from old adults.

period of palatogenesis is from the end of the sixth week until the beginning of the ninth week.

PRIMARY PALATE

Early in the sixth week, the primary palate (**median palatine process**) begins to develop from the deep part of the intermaxillary segment of the maxilla (see Figs. 10.26F and 10.27). Initially, this segment is a wedge-shaped mass of mesenchyme between the internal surfaces of the maxillary prominences of the developing maxillae. The primary palate forms the **premaxillary part of the maxilla** (Fig. 10.28B). It represents only a small part of the adult hard palate (the part anterior to the incisive fossa).

SECONDARY PALATE

The secondary palate (definitive palate) is the primordium of the hard and soft parts of the palate (see Figs. 10.27D and 10.28A and B). It begins to develop early in the sixth week from two mesenchymal projections that extend from the internal aspects of the maxillary prominences. Initially, these structures—**lateral palatine processes** (palatal shelves)—project inferomedially on each side of the tongue (Fig. 10.29A–C). As the jaws develop, they pull the tongue away from its root, and, as a result, the palate is brought lower in the mouth.

During the seventh and eighth weeks, the lateral palatine processes elongate and ascend to a horizontal position superior to the tongue. The release of hyaluronic acid in the palatine process by mesenchyme helps with this elevation. Gradually, the processes approach each other and fuse in the median plane (see Fig. 10.29D–H). They also fuse

with the nasal septum and the posterior part of the primary palate. Elevation of the palatine processes to the horizontal position is believed to be caused by an intrinsic force that is generated by the hydration of hyaluronic acid in the mesenchymal cells within the palatine processes. The medial epithelial seam at the edges of the palatine shelves breaks down, allowing for the fusion of the palatine shelves.

The **nasal septum** develops in a downward growth pattern from internal parts of the merged medial nasal prominences (see Fig. 10.29C, E, and G). The fusion between the nasal septum and the palatine processes begins anteriorly during the ninth week and is completed posteriorly by the 12th week, superior to the primordium of the hard palate (see Fig. 10.29D and F). Bone gradually develops by intramembranous ossification (see Chapter 15) in the primary palate, forming the premaxillary part of the maxilla, which lodges the incisor teeth (see Fig. 10.28B). Concurrently, bone extends from the maxillae and palatine bones into the lateral palatine processes to form the **hard palate** (see Fig. 10.29E and G). The posterior parts of these processes do not become ossified; they extend posteriorly beyond the nasal septum and fuse to form the **soft palate**, including its conical projection, the **uvula** (see Fig. 10.29D, F, and H). The **median palatine raphe** indicates the line of fusion of the lateral palatine processes. A small **nasopalatine canal** persists in the median plane of the palate, between the premaxillary part of the maxilla and the palatine processes of the maxillae. This canal is represented in the adult hard palate by the **incisive fossa** (see Fig. 10.28B). An irregular suture runs from the incisive fossa to the alveolar process of the maxilla, between the lateral incisor and the canine teeth on each side, indicating where the embryonic primary and secondary palates fused.

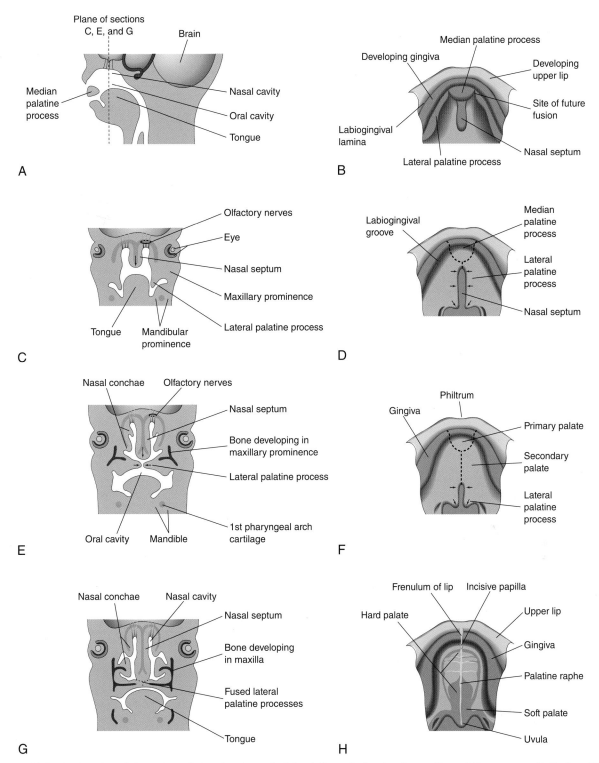

Fig. 10.29 (A) Sagittal section of the embryonic head at the end of the sixth week showing the median palatine process. (B, D, F, and H) Roof of the mouth from the sixth to 12th weeks, illustrating the development of the palate. The *broken lines* in (D and F) indicate the sites of fusion of the palatine processes. The *arrows* indicate medial and posterior growth of the lateral palatine processes. (C, E, and G) Frontal sections of the head, illustrating fusion of the lateral palatine processes with each other and with the nasal septum and separation of the nasal and oral cavities.

Cleft Lip and Cleft Palate

Clefts of the upper lip and palate are common. The defects are usually classified according to developmental criteria, with the incisive fossa and papilla used as reference landmarks (see Figs. 10.28B and 10.33A). Cleft lip and cleft palate are especially conspicuous because they result in an abnormal facial appearance and defective speech (Fig. 10.30). Two major groups of cleft lip and cleft palate are recognized (Figs. 10.31, 10.32, and 10.33):

- **Anterior cleft** defects include cleft lip, with or without cleft of the alveolar part of the maxilla. A complete cleft anomaly is one in which the cleft extends through the lip and the alveolar part of the maxilla to the incisive fossa, separating the anterior and posterior parts of the palate (see Fig. 10.33E and F). Anterior cleft anomalies result from a deficiency of mesenchyme in the maxillary prominences and the median palatine process (see Fig. 10.26D and E).
- **Posterior cleft** defects include clefts of the secondary, or posterior, palate that extend through the soft and hard regions of the palate to the incisive fossa, separating the anterior and posterior parts of the palate (see Fig. 10.33G and H). Posterior cleft defects are caused by defective development of the secondary palate and result from growth distortions in the lateral palatine processes that, in turn, prevent the medial migration and fusion of these processes.

Clefts involving the upper lip, with or without cleft palate, occur in approximately 1 in 1000 births; however, their frequency varies widely, and 60% to 80% of those affected are males. The clefts vary in severity from small notches in the vermilion border of the lip (see Fig. 10.32G) to larger clefts that extend into the floor of the nostril and through the alveolar part of the maxilla (see Figs. 10.31A and 10.33E). Cleft lip can be unilateral or bilateral.

Unilateral cleft lip (see Fig. 10.31A) results from failure of the maxillary prominence on the affected side to unite with the merged medial nasal prominences (see Fig. 10.32A–H), in turn causing a persistent labial groove. The tissues in the floor of the persistent groove break down. As a result, the lip is divided into medial and lateral parts. Sometimes, a bridge of tissue, a *Simonart band*, joins the parts of the incomplete cleft lip.

Bilateral cleft lip (see Figs. 10.31B and 10.33F) results from the failure of the mesenchymal masses in the maxillary prominences to meet and unite with the merged medial nasal prominences. When there is a complete bilateral cleft of the lip and the alveolar part of the maxilla, the intermaxillary segment hangs free and projects anteriorly. These defects are especially deforming

because of the loss of continuity of the **orbicularis oris muscle**, which closes the mouth and purses the lips.

Median cleft lip is an extremely rare defect. It results from partial or complete failure of the medial nasal prominences to merge and form the intermaxillary segment. The median cleft of the lower lip is also very rare and is caused by the failure of the mandibular prominences to merge completely (see Fig. 10.23). The landmark for distinguishing anterior from posterior cleft anomalies is the **incisive fossa** (see Fig. 10.28B). Anterior and posterior cleft defects are embryologically distinct.

Cleft palate, with or without cleft lip, occurs in approximately 1 in 2500 births and is more common in females. It is thought that for isolated cleft palate the difference in incidence is related to a 1-week delay in palate shelf fusion in females versus males. The cleft may involve only the uvula—cleft uvula—giving it a fish-tail appearance (see Fig. 10.33B), or it may extend through the soft and hard regions of the palate (see Fig. 10.33C and D). In severe cases associated with cleft lip, the cleft in the palate extends through the alveolar part of the maxilla and lips on both sides (see Fig. 10.33G and H).

Unilateral and bilateral clefts in the palate are classified into three groups:

- *Clefts of the anterior palate* result from failure of the lateral palatine processes to meet and fuse with the primary palate (see Fig. 10.33F).
- *Clefts of the posterior palate* result from failure of the lateral palatine processes to meet and fuse with each other and with the nasal septum (see Fig. 10.29E).
- *Clefts of the anterior and posterior parts of the palate* result from failure of the lateral palatine processes to meet and fuse with the primary palate, with each other, and with the nasal septum.

Most clefts of the lip and palate result from multiple factors (*multifactorial inheritance*; see Chapter 19). Some clefts of the lip, palate, or both appear as part of syndromes determined by pathogenic variants (mutants) in genes. Other clefts are features of chromosomal syndromes, especially **trisomy 13** (see Fig. 19.6). A few cases of cleft lip or cleft palate appear to be caused by teratogenic agents (e.g., anticonvulsant drugs). A sibling of a child with a cleft palate has an elevated risk of having a cleft palate but no increased risk of cleft lip. A cleft of the lip and the alveolar process of the maxilla that continues through the palate is usually transmitted through a male sex-linked gene.

Facial Clefts

Various types of facial clefts occur, but they are extremely rare. Severe clefts are usually associated with gross anomalies of the head. **Oblique facial clefts** (orbitofacial fissures) are often bilateral and extend from the upper lip to the medial margin of the orbit. When this occurs, the nasolacrimal ducts are open grooves (persistent nasolacrimal grooves). Oblique facial clefts

associated with cleft lip result from the failure of the maxillary prominences to merge with the lateral and medial nasal prominences. Lateral, or transverse, facial clefts run from the mouth toward the ear. Bilateral clefts result in a very large mouth—**macrostomia**. In severe cases, the clefts in the cheeks extend almost to the ears.

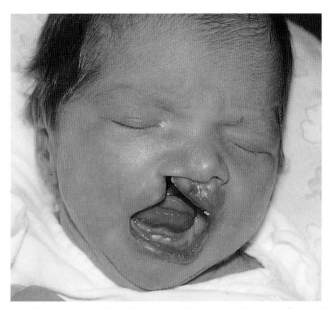

Fig. 10.30   Infant with unilateral cleft lip and cleft palate. Clefts of the lip, with or without a cleft palate, occur in approximately 1 in 1000 births; most affected individuals are males. (Courtesy A.E. Chudley, MD, Professor of Paediatrics and Child Health, Children's Hospital and University of Manitoba, Winnipeg, Manitoba, Canada.)

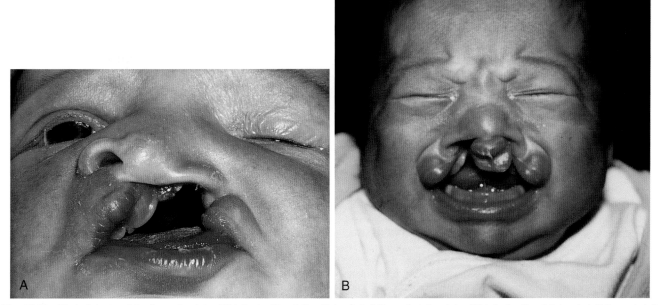

Fig. 10.31   Birth defects of the lip and palate. (A) Infant with a left unilateral cleft lip and cleft palate. (B) Infant with a bilateral cleft lip and cleft palate. (Courtesy Dr. Barry H. Grayson and Dr. Bruno L. Vendittelli, Institute of Reconstructive Plastic Surgery, New York University Medical Center, New York, New York.)

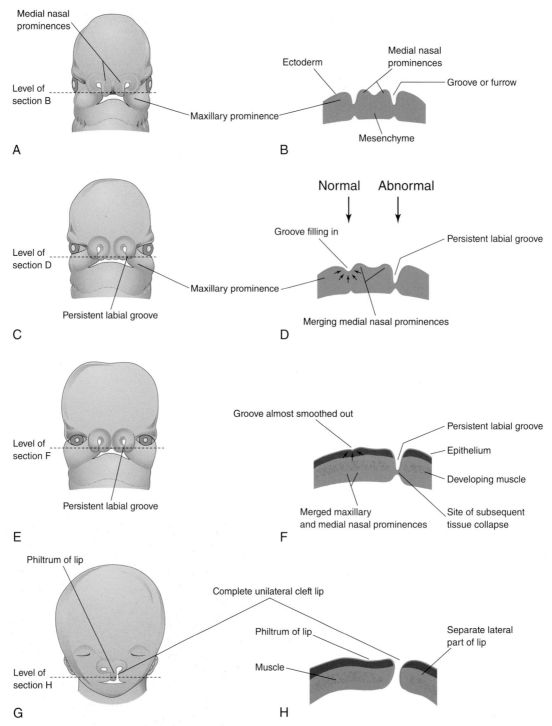

Fig. 10.32 Drawings illustrating the embryologic basis for a complete unilateral cleft lip. (A) A 5-week embryo. (B) Horizontal section through the head illustrating the grooves between the maxillary prominences and the merging medial nasal prominences. (C) 6-week embryo showing a persistent labial groove on the left side. (D) Horizontal section through the head showing the groove gradually filling in on the right side after proliferation of the mesenchyme (*arrows*). (E) A 7-week embryo. (F) Horizontal section through the head showing that the epithelium on the right has almost been pushed out of the groove between the maxillary and medial nasal prominences. (G) A 10-week fetus with a complete unilateral cleft lip. (H) Horizontal section through the head after stretching of the epithelium and breakdown of the tissues in the floor of the persistent labial groove on the left side, forming complete unilateral cleft lip.

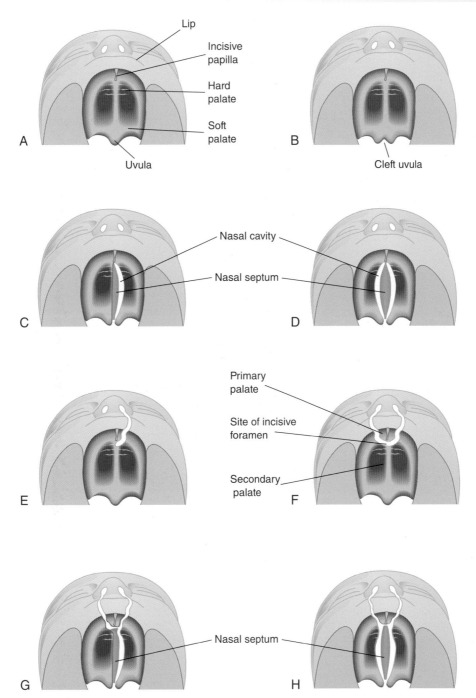

Fig. 10.33 Various types of cleft lip and cleft palate. (A) Normal lip and palate. (B) Cleft uvula. (C) Unilateral cleft of the posterior (secondary) palate. (D) Bilateral cleft of the posterior palate. (E) Complete unilateral cleft of the lip and alveolar process of the maxilla with a unilateral cleft of the anterior (primary) palate. (F) Complete bilateral cleft of the lip and the alveolar processes of the maxillae with bilateral cleft of the anterior palate. (G) Complete bilateral cleft of the lip and the alveolar processes of the maxillae with bilateral cleft of the anterior palate and unilateral cleft of the posterior palate. (H) Complete bilateral cleft of the lip and the alveolar processes of the maxillae with complete bilateral cleft of the anterior and posterior palate.

CLINICALLY ORIENTED QUESTIONS

1. Do embryos have cleft lips? Does this common facial defect represent a persistence of such an embryonic condition?

2. Neither Clare nor her husband Jack has a cleft lip or a cleft palate, and no one in either one of their families is known to have or to have had these anomalies. What are their chances of having a child with a cleft lip, with or without a cleft palate?

3. Mary's son has a cleft lip and a cleft palate. Her brother has a similar defect involving his lip and palate. A friend says that Mary's family genetics are entirely to blame for their son's birth defects. Was the defect likely inherited only from Mary's side of the family?

4. A patient's son has minor anomalies involving his external ears, but he does not have hearing problems or a facial malformation. Would his ear abnormalities be considered pharyngeal (branchial) arch defects?

The answers to these questions are at the back of this book.

Respiratory System 11

The **lower respiratory organs** begin to form during the fourth week. The respiratory system starts as a median outgrowth—the **laryngotracheal groove**—that appears in the floor of the caudal end of the anterior foregut (primordial pharynx) (Fig. 11.1A and B). This primordium of the **tracheobronchial tree** develops caudal to the fourth pair of the pharyngeal pouches. The endodermal lining of the **laryngotracheal groove** gives rise to the pulmonary epithelium and glands of the larynx, trachea, and bronchi. The connective tissue, cartilage, and smooth muscle in these structures develop from the splanchnic mesoderm surrounding the foregut (see Fig. 11.4A). *Signaling pathways of BMP, Wnt, and FGF control patterning of the expression of Sox2 and Nkx2.1 in the early foregut for the differentiation of the trachea from the esophagus. In the ventral areas, Nkx2.1 is activated, whereas Sox2 is suppressed.*

By the end of the fourth week, the laryngotracheal groove has evaginated to form **laryngotracheal diverticulum** (lung bud), located ventral to the caudal part of the foregut (Fig. 11.2A; see also Fig. 11.1A).

As the diverticulum elongates, its distal end enlarges to form a globular **respiratory bud** (see Fig. 11.2B). The laryngotracheal diverticulum soon separates from the **primordial pharynx**, but it maintains communication with it through the **primordial laryngeal inlet** (see Fig. 11.2A and C). As the diverticulum elongates, it is invested with splanchnic mesoderm (see Fig. 11.2B). Longitudinal **tracheoesophageal folds** develop in the laryngotracheal diverticulum, approach each other, and fuse to form a partition—the **tracheoesophageal septum** (see Fig. 11.2D and E).

This septum divides the cranial part of the foregut into a ventral part, the **laryngotracheal tube** (primordium of the larynx, trachea, bronchi, and lungs), and a dorsal part (primordium of the oropharynx and esophagus) (see Fig. 11.2F).

The laryngeal epithelium proliferates rapidly, resulting in temporary occlusion of the laryngeal lumen. Recanalization of the larynx occurs by the 10th week. The laryngeal ventricles form during this recanalization process. These recesses are bound by folds of mucous membrane that evolve into the **vocal folds** (cords) and the **vestibular folds**.

The **epiglottis** develops from the caudal part of the **hypopharyngeal eminence**, a prominence produced by the proliferation of the mesenchyme in the ventral ends of the third and fourth pharyngeal arches (see Fig. 10.21; Fig. 11.3B–D). The rostral part of this eminence forms the posterior third or pharyngeal part of the tongue (see Fig. 10.21). The **laryngeal muscles** develop from myoblasts in the fourth and sixth pairs of pharyngeal arches and are innervated by the laryngeal branches of the vagus nerves (CN X) that supply these arches (see Table 10.1). Growth of the larynx and epiglottis is rapid during the first 3 years after birth, by which time the epiglottis has reached its adult form and position.

Laryngeal Atresia

Laryngeal atresia is a very rare (1:50,000) birth defect that results in obstruction of the upper fetal airway—**congenital high airway obstruction syndrome** (CHAOS syndrome). Distal to the atresia or stenosis (narrowing), the airways become dilated, the lungs are hyperplastic (causing compression of the heart and great vessels), the diaphragm is either flattened or inverted, and **fetal hydrops** (accumulation of fluid in two or more compartments) and/or **ascites** (abdominal fluid) are present. Prenatal ultrasonography permits the diagnosis of this anomaly. Laryngeal atresia is typically a fatal condition but, in some instances, tracheotomy at birth has led to survival.

DEVELOPMENT OF LARYNX

The epithelial lining of the larynx develops from the endoderm of the cranial end of the laryngotracheal tube. The laryngeal cartilages may develop from the fourth and sixth pairs of pharyngeal arches and neural crest mesenchyme (see Chapter 10). The mesenchyme at the cranial end of the laryngotracheal tube proliferates rapidly, producing paired **arytenoid swellings** (Fig. 11.3B). These swellings grow toward the tongue, converting the **primordial glottis** into a T-shaped **laryngeal inlet** (see Fig. 11.3C and D). The opening of the laryngotracheal tube into the pharynx becomes the **primordial laryngeal outlet** (see Figs. 11.2F and 11.3C).

DEVELOPMENT OF TRACHEA

The endodermal lining of the laryngotracheal tube distal to the larynx differentiates into the epithelium and glands of the trachea and the pulmonary epithelium. The cartilage, connective tissue, and muscles of the trachea are derived from the splanchnic mesoderm surrounding the laryngotracheal tube (Fig. 11.4). *The cargo receptor Evi/Wls is involved in the dorsal–ventral patterning of the endodermal lining of the laryngotracheal tube. Proliferation of the surrounding mesenchyme and formation of cartilage and smooth muscles are regulated by Wnt/β-catenin, Bmp, Shh, fgf, and retinoic acid signaling pathways.*

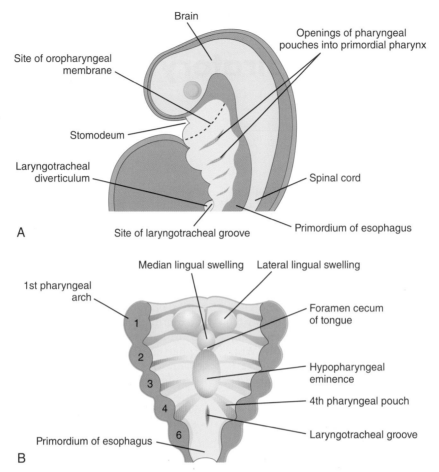

Fig. 11.1   (A) Sagittal section of the cranial half of a 4-week embryo. (B) Horizontal section of the embryo, illustrating the floor of the primordial pharynx and the location of the laryngotracheal groove.

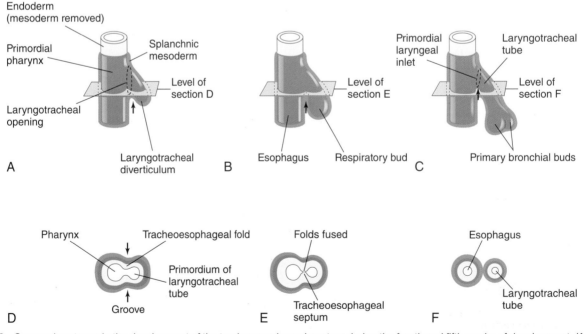

Fig. 11.2   Successive stages in the development of the tracheoesophageal septum during the fourth and fifth weeks of development. (A–C) Lateral views of the caudal part of the primordial pharynx, showing the laryngotracheal diverticulum and partitioning of the foregut into the esophagus and the laryngotracheal tube. (D–F) Transverse sections, illustrating the formation of the tracheoesophageal septum and how it separates the foregut into the laryngotracheal tube and esophagus. The *arrows* represent cellular changes resulting from growth.

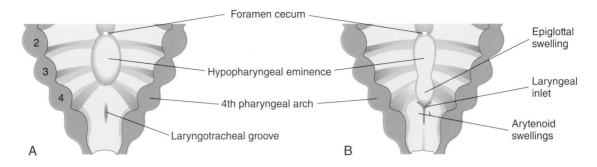

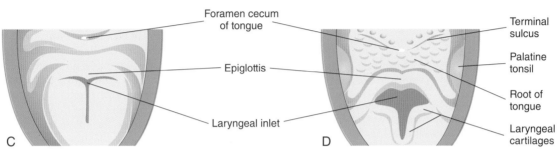

Fig. 11.3 Successive stages in the development of the larynx. (A) Four weeks. (B) Five weeks. (C) Six weeks. (D) Ten weeks. The epithelium lining the larynx is of endodermal origin. The cartilages and muscles of the larynx arise from the mesenchyme in the fourth and sixth pairs of pharyngeal arches. Note that the laryngeal inlet changes in shape from a slit-like opening to a T-shaped inlet as the mesenchyme surrounding the developing larynx proliferates.

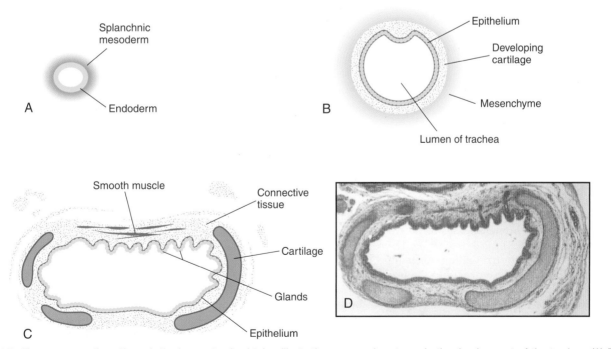

Fig. 11.4 Transverse sections through the laryngotracheal tube, illustrating progressive stages in the development of the trachea. (A) Four weeks. (B) Ten weeks. (C) Eleven weeks (drawing of micrograph in [D]). Note that the endoderm of the tube gives rise to the epithelium and the glands of the trachea and that the mesenchyme surrounding the tube forms the connective tissue, muscle, and cartilage. (D) Photomicrograph of a transverse section of the developing trachea at 12 weeks. From Moore KL, Persaud TVN, Shiota K: *Color atlas of clinical embryology*, ed 2, Philadelphia, 2000, Saunders.

Tracheoesophageal Fistula

A **tracheoesophageal fistula (TEF)** is an abnormal passage between the trachea and esophagus (Figs. 11.5 and 11.6A). This birth defect occurs at a rate of approximately 1 in 3000 to 1 in 4500 live births and more commonly affects males (3:2). In most cases, the fistula is associated with **esophageal atresia**. TEF results from incomplete division of the cranial part of the foregut into respiratory and esophageal parts during the fourth week. Incomplete fusion of the tracheoesophageal folds results in a **defective tracheoesophageal septum** and communication between the trachea and esophagus.

TEF is the most common anomaly of the lower respiratory tract. Four main varieties of TEF may develop (see Fig. 11.5). The usual anomaly is a blind ending of the superior part of the esophagus **(esophageal atresia)** and a joining of the inferior part to the trachea near its bifurcation (see Figs. 11.5A and 11.6B). Infants with this type of TEF and esophageal atresia cough and choke when swallowing because of the accumulation of excessive amounts of liquid in the mouth and upper respiratory tract. When the infant attempts to swallow milk, it rapidly fills the esophageal pouch and is regurgitated. Gastric contents may also reflux from the stomach through the fistula into the trachea and lungs, which may result in **pneumonia** or **pneumonitis**. Other varieties of TEF are shown in Fig. 11.5B–D. **Polyhydramnios** (see Chapter 8) is often associated with esophageal atresia. Excess amniotic fluid accumulates because the fluid cannot pass to the stomach and intestines for absorption and subsequent transfer through the placenta to the maternal blood for disposal.

Tracheal Stenosis and Atresia

Stenosis and atresia of the trachea are uncommon birth defects that are usually associated with one of the varieties of TEF. Stenoses and atresias probably result from unequal partitioning of the foregut into the esophagus and trachea (see Fig. 11.5). In some cases, a web of tissue obstructs airflow (incomplete tracheal atresia).

DEVELOPMENT OF BRONCHI AND LUNGS

The **respiratory bud** (lung bud) develops at the caudal end of the laryngotracheal diverticulum during the fourth week (see Fig. 11.2B). The bud soon divides into two outpouchings—**primary bronchial buds** (see Fig. 11.2C). Later, **secondary and tertiary bronchial buds** form and grow laterally into the pericardioperitoneal canals (Fig. 11.7A).

Together with the surrounding splanchnic mesoderm, the bronchial buds differentiate into the **bronchi** and their ramifications in the lungs (see Fig. 11.7B). Early in the fourth week, the connection of each bronchial bud with the trachea enlarges to form the primordia of **main bronchi** (Fig. 11.8).

The embryonic right main bronchus is slightly larger than the left one and is oriented more vertically. This embryonic relationship persists in adults; consequently, a foreign body is more liable to enter the right main bronchus than the left one.

The main bronchi subdivide into **secondary bronchi that form lobar, segmental, and intrasegmental branches** (see Fig. 11.8). On the right, the superior secondary bronchus supplies the upper (superior) lobe of the lung, whereas the inferior secondary bronchus subdivides into two bronchi, one connecting to the middle lobe of the right lung and the other connecting to the lower (inferior) lobe. On the left, the two secondary bronchi supply the upper and lower lobes of the lung. Each secondary bronchus undergoes progressive branching.

The **segmental bronchi**, 10 in the right lung and 8 or 9 in the left lung, begin to form by the seventh week. As this occurs, the surrounding mesenchyme also divides. Each segmental bronchus, with its surrounding mass of mesenchyme, is the primordium of a **bronchopulmonary segment**. By 24 weeks, approximately 17 orders of branching have occurred, and **respiratory bronchioles** have developed (Fig. 11.9B). An additional seven orders of airways develop after birth.

As the bronchi develop, cartilaginous plates are formed from the surrounding splanchnic mesenchyme. The bronchial smooth muscle and connective tissue and the pulmonary connective tissue and capillaries are also derived from this mesenchyme. As the lungs develop, they acquire a layer of **visceral pleura** from the splanchnic mesoderm (see Fig. 11.7). With expansion, the lungs and pleural cavities grow caudally into the mesenchyme of the body wall and soon lie close to the heart. The thoracic body wall becomes lined by a layer of **parietal pleura** derived from the somatic mesoderm (see Fig. 11.7B). The space between the visceral and parietal pleura is the **pleural cavity**.

MATURATION OF LUNGS

Maturation of the lungs is divided into four overlapping histological stages: pseudoglandular, canalicular, terminal sac (saccular), and alveolar.

PSEUDOGLANDULAR PERIOD (5–17 WEEKS)

The developing lungs resemble, on a histological basis, an exocrine gland during the early part of this period (see Fig. 11.9A). By 16 weeks, all of the major elements of the lung have formed, except those involved with gas exchange. Respiration is not possible; hence, *fetuses born during this period are unable to survive.*

CANALICULAR PERIOD (16–25 WEEKS)

This period overlaps the pseudoglandular period because cranial segments of the lungs mature faster than caudal segments. During the canalicular period, the lumina of the bronchi and the **terminal bronchioles** become larger, and the lung tissue becomes highly vascular (see Fig. 11.9B). By 24 weeks, each terminal bronchiole has given rise to two or more **respiratory bronchioles**, each of which then divides into three to six tubular passages—**primordial alveolar ducts**.

Respiration is possible toward the end of the canalicular stage because some thin-walled **terminal sacs** (primordial alveoli) have developed at the ends of the respiratory bronchioles and the lung tissue is well vascularized (rendered vascular by the formation of new vessels). Although a fetus born at 24 to 26 weeks may survive if given intensive care, it often dies because its respiratory and other systems are relatively immature.

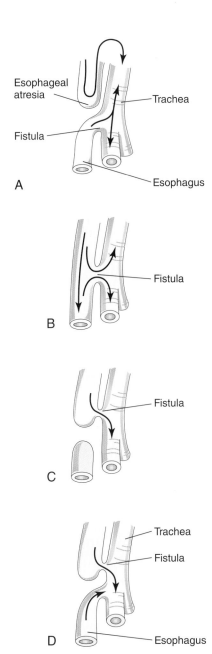

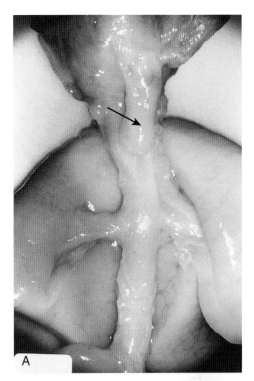

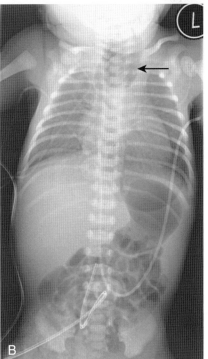

Fig. 11.5 The four main varieties of tracheoesophageal fistula (TEF) are shown in order of frequency. Possible directions of the flow of the contents are indicated by *arrows*. (A) Esophageal atresia is associated with TEF in more than 85% of cases. (B) Fistula between the trachea and esophagus; this type of birth defect accounts for approximately 4% of cases. (C) Atresia of the proximal esophagus ending in a tracheoesophageal fistula with the distal esophagus having a blind pouch. Air cannot enter the distal esophagus and stomach. (D) Atresia of the proximal segment of the esophagus with fistulas between the trachea and both the proximal and distal segments of the esophagus. Air can enter the distal esophagus and stomach. All neonates born with TEF have esophageal dysmotility disorders, and most have reflux (regurgitation of the contents of the stomach).

Fig. 11.6 (A) Tracheoesophageal fistula in a 17-week fetus. The upper esophageal segment ends blindly *(arrow)*. (B) Radiograph of an infant with esophageal atresia. Air in the distal gastrointestinal tract indicates the presence of a tracheoesophageal fistula *(arrow,* blind proximal esophageal sac). A, From Kalousek DK, Fitch N, Paradice BA: *Pathology of the human embryo and previable fetus*, New York, 1990, Springer Verlag; **B**, Courtesy Dr. J. Been, Dr. M. Shuurman, Dr. S. Robben, Maastricht University Medical Centre, Maastricht, Netherlands.

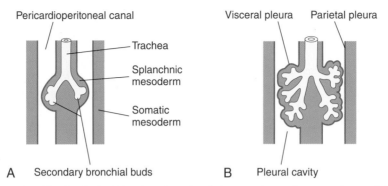

Fig. 11.7 Illustrations of the growth of the developing lungs into the splanchnic mesoderm adjacent to the medial walls of the pericardioperitoneal canals (primordial pleural cavities). Development of the layers of the pleura is also shown. (A) Five weeks. (B) Six weeks.

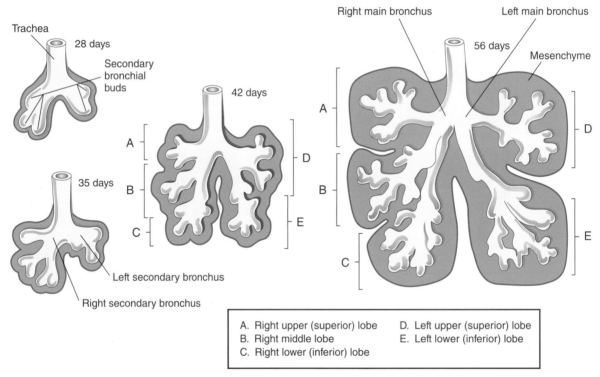

A. Right upper (superior) lobe   D. Left upper (superior) lobe
B. Right middle lobe   E. Left lower (inferior) lobe
C. Right lower (inferior) lobe

Fig. 11.8 Successive stages in the development of the bronchial buds, the bronchi, and the lungs.

TERMINAL SAC (SACCULAR) PERIOD (24 WEEKS TO LATE FETAL PERIOD)

During this period, many more terminal sacs develop and their epithelium becomes very thin. Capillaries begin to bulge into these sacs (see Fig. 11.9C). The intimate contact between epithelial and endothelial cells establishes the **blood–air barrier**, which permits adequate gas exchange for survival.

By 26 weeks, the terminal sacs are lined mainly by squamous epithelial cells of endodermal origin—**type I pneumocytes**—across which gas exchange occurs. The capillary network proliferates rapidly in the mesenchyme around the developing alveoli, and there is concurrent active development of lymphatic capillaries. Scattered among the squamous epithelial cells are rounded secretory epithelial cells—**type II pneumocytes**, which secrete **pulmonary surfactant**, a complex mixture of phospholipids and proteins.

Surfactant forms as a monomolecular film over the interior walls of the alveolar sacs and counteracts surface tension forces at the air–alveolar interface. This facilitates the expansion of the terminal sacs.

The maturation of alveolar type II cells and the production of surfactant vary widely in fetuses of different ages. Surfactant production begins by 20 to 22 weeks, but surfactant is present in only small amounts in premature infants. It does not reach adequate levels until the late fetal period. Both increased surfactant production, induced by antenatal corticosteroids, and **postnatal artificial surfactant replacement therapy** have increased the rates of survival of these infants.

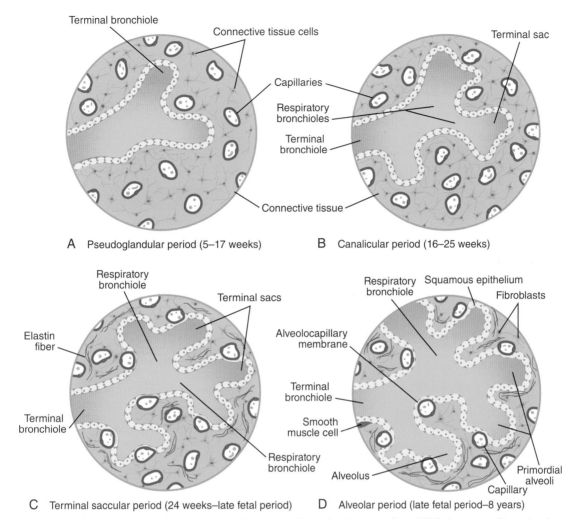

Fig. 11.9 Diagram of histological sections showing progressive stages of lung development. (A and B) Early stages of lung development. (C and D) Note that the alveolocapillary membrane is thin and that some capillaries bulge into the terminal saccules.

ALVEOLAR PERIOD (LATE FETAL PERIOD TO 8 YEARS)

Exactly when the terminal saccular period ends and the alveolar period begins depends on the definition of the term **alveolus** (see Fig. 11.9D). At the beginning of the alveolar period, each respiratory bronchiole terminates in a cluster of thin-walled terminal sacs that are separated from one another by loose connective tissue. These terminal sacs represent future **alveolar ducts**. The **alveolocapillary membrane** (pulmonary diffusion barrier, or respiratory membrane) is sufficiently thin to allow gas exchange. The transition from dependence on the placenta for gas exchange to autonomous gas exchange after birth requires the following adaptive changes in the lungs:

• Production of surfactant in the alveolar sacs
• Transformation of the lungs into gas-exchanging organs
• Establishment of parallel pulmonary and systemic circulations.

*Approximately 95% of **mature alveoli** develop in the postnatal period.* Before birth, the primordial alveoli appear as small bulges on the walls of the respiratory bronchioles and alveolar sacs (see Fig. 11.9D). After birth, the primordial alveoli enlarge as the lungs expand; however, most of the increase in the size of the lungs results from a continued increase in the number of respiratory bronchioles and primordial alveoli rather than from an increase in the size of the alveoli. Alveolar development is largely complete by 3 years of age, but new alveoli may be added until approximately 8 years of age. Unlike mature alveoli, immature alveoli have the potential to form additional primordial alveoli.

Approximately 150 million primordial alveoli, one-half the number in adults, are present in the lungs of full-term neonates. On chest radiographs, therefore, the lungs of neonates appear denser than adult lungs. Between the third and eighth years, the adult complement of 300 million alveoli is achieved.

Three factors that are essential for normal lung development are as follows:

• Adequate thoracic space for lung growth
• Adequate amniotic fluid volume
• Fetal breathing movements.

The mechanism modulating lung morphogenesis and formation of blood vessels in the lungs involves the transcription factors Sox17, SHH, and Wnt signaling. An autonomic nerve–myofibroblast circuit may regulate alveoli formation and patterning through a protein-coding gene VANGL2.

Fetal breathing movements occur before birth, exerting sufficient force to cause the aspiration of some amniotic fluid into the lungs. These fetal breathing movements occur approximately 50% of the time and only during rapid eye movement sleep. These movements stimulate lung development, possibly by creating a pressure gradient between the lungs and the amniotic fluid. By birth, the fetus has had the advantage of several months of breathing exercise. Fetal breathing movements increase as the time of delivery approaches.

At birth, the lungs are approximately half-filled with fluid derived from the amniotic cavity, the lungs, and the tracheal glands. Aeration of the lungs at birth occurs not so much by the inflation of empty collapsed organs as by the rapid replacement of intra-alveolar fluid by air. The fluid in the lungs is cleared at birth by three routes:

- Through the mouth and nose by applying pressure on the thorax during vaginal delivery
- Into the pulmonary capillaries and pulmonary arteries and veins
- Into the lymphatic vessels

Oligohydramnios and Lung Development

When **oligohydramnios** (insufficient amount of amniotic fluid) is severe and chronic, lung development is retarded. It is thought that reduced hydraulic pressure in the lungs and its consequential effects on lung calcium regulation may result in **pulmonary hypoplasia**, which may cause postnatal respiratory distress.

Neonatal Respiratory Distress Syndrome

Respiratory distress syndrome (RDS) affects approximately 2% of live newborns, and those born prematurely are the most susceptible. RDS is also known as **hyaline membrane disease**. *Surfactant deficiency is a major cause of RDS.* Prolonged intrauterine asphyxia may produce irreversible changes in type II alveolar cells, making them incapable of producing surfactant. **Corticosteroids** are potent stimulators of fetal surfactant production and may be given to the mother if early delivery is a risk. Neonates with RDS have rapid, labored breathing shortly after birth. An estimated 30% of all neonatal disease results from RDS or its complications. The lungs are underinflated and the alveoli contain amorphous materials (hyaline membrane) from substances in the circulation and the injured pulmonary epithelium. Treatment includes supplementary oxygen and artificial surfactant—more than 90% of neonates with RDS survive.

Lungs of Neonates

Fresh healthy lungs always contain some air; consequently, pulmonary tissue samples float in water. By contrast, a diseased lung that is partially filled with fluid may not float. Of medicolegal significance is the fact that the lungs of a *stillborn* neonate are firm and sink when placed in water because they contain fluid, not air.

Lung Hypoplasia

In infants with a **congenital diaphragmatic hernia** (see Chapter 9), the lungs may not develop normally. This hypoplasia may be caused by the changes in the growth factors that existed before the abdominal viscera became abnormally positioned. **Lung hypoplasia** is characterized by markedly reduced lung volume. Many infants with a congenital diaphragmatic hernia die of pulmonary insufficiency, despite optimal postnatal care, because their lungs are too hypoplastic to support extrauterine life.

Primary Ciliary Dyskinesia (PCD)

PCD is a rare disease of motile cilia (ciliopathies) and has an incidence of 1:10,000 to 20,000 births. It is a heterogeneous group of inherited as an autosomal recessive disorders. The most common feature of PCD is neonatal respiratory distress due to reduced mucociliary clearance of the respiratory passages. About 50% of individuals with PCD also show other abnormalities due to motile cilia dysfunction, including situs abnormalities (Kartagener syndrome). In total, 90% of males with PCD are infertile because of the dysmotility of the sperm.

CLINICALLY ORIENTED QUESTIONS

1. What stimulates the infant to start breathing at birth? Is "slapping the buttocks" necessary?

2. A neonate reportedly died approximately 72 hours after birth from the effects of respiratory distress syndrome. What is respiratory distress syndrome? By what other name is this condition known? Is the cause genetic or environmental?

3. Can a neonate born 22 weeks after fertilization survive? What can be done to reduce the severity of respiratory distress syndrome?

The answers to these questions are at the back of this book.

Alimentary System

The **alimentary system** extends from the mouth to the anus with all its associative glands and organs. The **primordial gut** forms during the fourth week as the head, caudal eminence (tail), and lateral folds incorporate the dorsal part of the **umbilical vesicle** (yolk sac) (see Fig. 6.1). The primordial gut is initially closed at its cranial end by the **oropharyngeal membrane** (see Fig. 10.1B) and at its caudal end by the **cloacal membrane** (Fig. 12.1). The endoderm of the primordial gut gives rise to most of the gut, epithelium, and glands. The epithelium at the cranial and caudal ends of the alimentary tract is derived from the ectoderm of the **stomodeum** and **anal pit** (proctodeum), respectively (see Fig. 12.1).

The muscular and connective tissue and other layers of the wall of the alimentary tract are derived from the splanchnic mesenchyme surrounding the primordial gut. For descriptive purposes, the gut is divided into three parts: foregut, midgut, and hindgut. *Molecular studies indicate that the regional differentiation of the primordial gut is regulated by Nodal signals,* expression of *Hox and ParaHox genes, as well as Shh, bone morphogenetic protein (BMP), and Wnt and Indian hedgehog genes* (SHH *and* IHH) *that are expressed in the endoderm and the surrounding mesoderm.* The endodermal signaling provides temporal and positional information for the development of the gut.

FOREGUT

The derivatives of the foregut are as follows:

- Primordial pharynx and its derivatives
- Lower respiratory system
- Esophagus and stomach
- Duodenum, just proximal to, and including the opening of the bile duct
- Liver, biliary apparatus (hepatic ducts, gallbladder, and bile duct), and pancreas.

These foregut derivatives, other than the pharynx, lower respiratory tract, and most of the esophagus, are supplied by the **celiac trunk**, the artery of the foregut (Fig. 12.2A; see also Fig. 12.1).

DEVELOPMENT OF ESOPHAGUS

The esophagus develops from the foregut immediately caudal to the pharynx (see Fig. 12.1). Initially, the esophagus is short, but it elongates rapidly and reaches its final relative length by the seventh week. Its epithelium and glands are derived from the endoderm The striated muscle of the esophagus is

derived from mesenchyme in the fourth and sixth pharyngeal arches (see Figs. 10.1 and 10.5B). The smooth muscle, mainly in the inferior third of the esophagus, develops from the surrounding splanchnic mesenchyme.

Esophageal Atresia

Blockage (atresia) of the esophageal lumen occurs in approximately 1 in 3000 to 1 in 4500 neonates. About one-third of affected infants are born prematurely. **Esophageal atresia** is frequently associated with **tracheoesophageal fistula** (see Figs. 11.5 and 11.6). The atresia results from deviation of the **tracheoesophageal septum** in a posterior direction (see Figs. 11.2 and 11.6); as a result, separation of the esophagus from the laryngotracheal tube is incomplete. Isolated atresia (approximately 5% of cases) appears to result from insufficient vascular perfusion. A fetus with esophageal atresia is unable to swallow amniotic fluid, resulting in **polyhydramnios**, the accumulation of excessive amniotic fluid. *BMP and transforming growth factor β (TGF-β) signaling and other molecular pathways play an important role in foregut development.* Incomplete separation, which causes tracheoesophageal fistula or esophageal atresia, is likely caused by both genetic and environmental factors.

Esophageal Stenosis

Stenosis of the esophagus can occur anywhere along the esophagus, but it usually occurs in the distal one-third, either as a web or as a long segment of the esophagus with a thread-like lumen. The stenosis likely results from the failure of esophageal blood vessels to develop in the affected area.

DEVELOPMENT OF STOMACH

During the fourth week, a slight dilation of the tubular foregut indicates the site of the primordial stomach. It first appears as a fusiform enlargement of the caudal part of the foregut that is oriented in the median plane (see Fig. 12.2B). The primordial stomach enlarges and broadens ventrodorsally. Its dorsal border grows more quickly than its ventral border. This site of rapid growth demarcates the **greater curvature** of the stomach (see Fig. 12.2D).

ROTATION OF STOMACH

As the stomach enlarges, it rotates 90 degrees in a clockwise direction around its longitudinal axis. The effects of

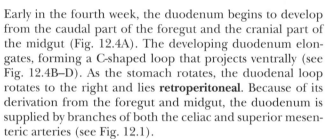

Fig. 12.1 Drawing of the median section of a 4-week embryo, showing the early alimentary system and its blood supply.

rotation on the stomach are as follows (Fig. 12.3; see also Fig. 12.2):

- The ventral border (**lesser curvature**) moves to the right, and the dorsal border (greater curvature) moves to the left (see Fig. 12.2C–F).
- Before rotation, the cranial and caudal ends of the stomach are in the median plane (see Fig. 12.2B).
- During rotation and growth of the stomach, its cranial region moves to the left and slightly inferiorly, and its caudal region moves to the right and superiorly (see Fig. 12.2C–E).
- After rotation, the stomach assumes its final position, with its long axis almost transverse to the long axis of the body (see Fig. 12.2E). This rotation and growth explain why the **left vagus nerve** supplies the anterior wall of the adult stomach and the **right vagus nerve** innervates its posterior wall.

Hypertrophic Pyloric Stenosis

Birth defects of the stomach are uncommon, except for hypertrophic pyloric stenosis, which affects 1 in 150 males and 1 in 750 females. Infants with this birth defect have marked **muscular thickening of the pylorus** of the stomach, the distal **sphincteric region** of the stomach. The muscles in the pyloric region are hypertrophied, which results in severe stenosis of the pyloric canal and obstruction to the passage of food. As a result, the stomach becomes markedly distended and its contents are expelled with considerable force **(projectile vomiting)**. Surgical relief of the obstruction is the usual treatment.

MESENTERIES OF STOMACH

The stomach is suspended from the dorsal wall of the abdominal cavity by the **primordial dorsal mesogastrium** (see Figs. 12.2B and C and 12.3A–E). This mesentery, originally located in the median plane, is carried to the left during the rotation of the stomach and formation of the omental bursa. The **primordial ventral mesogastrium** attaches to the

stomach, duodenum, liver, and ventral abdominal wall (see Figs. 12.2C and 12.3A and B).

OMENTAL BURSA

Isolated clefts develop in the mesenchyme, forming the dorsal mesogastrium (see Fig. 12.3A and B). The clefts soon coalesce to form a single cavity—the **omental bursa** (lesser peritoneal sac)—a large recess of the peritoneal cavity (see Figs. 12.2F and G and 12.3C and D). Rotation of the stomach pulls the dorsal mesogastrium to the left, thereby enlarging the bursa. The pouch-like bursa facilitates movements of the stomach.

The omental bursa lies between the stomach and posterior abdominal wall. As the stomach enlarges, the bursa expands and hangs over the developing intestines (see Fig. 12.3J). This part of the bursa is the **greater omentum** (see Figs. 12.3G–J and 12.13A). The two layers of the greater omentum eventually fuse (see Fig. 12.13F). The omental bursa communicates with the main part of the peritoneal cavity through a small opening—the **omental foramen** (see Figs. 12.2D and F and 12.3C and F).

DEVELOPMENT OF DUODENUM

Early in the fourth week, the duodenum begins to develop from the caudal part of the foregut and the cranial part of the midgut (Fig. 12.4A). The developing duodenum elongates, forming a C-shaped loop that projects ventrally (see Fig. 12.4B–D). As the stomach rotates, the duodenal loop rotates to the right and lies **retroperitoneal**. Because of its derivation from the foregut and midgut, the duodenum is supplied by branches of both the celiac and superior mesenteric arteries (see Fig. 12.1).

During the fifth and sixth weeks, the lumen of the duodenum becomes progressively smaller and is temporarily obliterated because of the proliferation of its epithelial cells. By this time, most of the ventral mesentery of the duodenum has disappeared.

Duodenal Stenosis and Atresia

Duodenal stenosis and **atresia** appear to result from reduced vascular perfusion, leading to luminal narrowing or complete obliteration of the lumen. Most stenoses involve the horizontal (third) and/or ascending (fourth) parts of the duodenum. Because of the stenosis, the stomach's contents (usually containing bile) are often vomited. Duodenal stenosis is often associated with chromosomal and other anomalies, such as trisomy 21. **Duodenal atresia** is not common, with a frequency of 1:5000 to 10,000 births. Most atresias involve the descending and horizontal parts of the duodenum and are located distal to the opening of the bile duct. In neonates with duodenal atresia, vomiting begins within a few hours of birth. The vomitus almost always contains bile. For the survival of the infant, surgery is usually carried out during the first week of life. **Polyhydramnios** also occurs because duodenal atresia prevents the normal absorption of amniotic fluid by the intestines. A diagnosis of duodenal atresia is suggested by the presence of a "double-bubble sign" on plain radiographs or ultrasound scans (Fig. 12.5B). This sign is caused by a distended, gas-filled stomach and the proximal duodenum. Between 20% and 30% of affected infants have Down syndrome and an additional 20% are premature neonates.

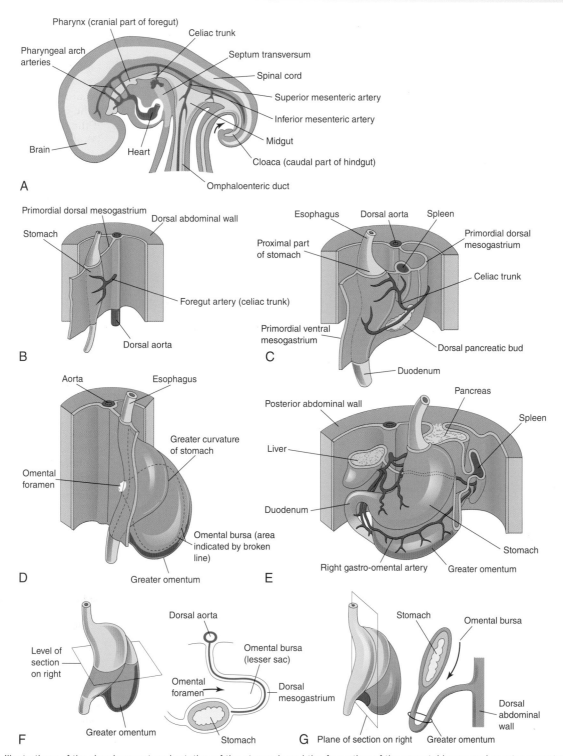

Fig. 12.2 Illustrations of the development and rotation of the stomach and the formation of the omental bursa and greater omentum. (A) Median section of the abdomen of a 28-day embryo. (B) Anterolateral view of the embryo shown in (A). (C) Embryo of approximately 35 days. (D) Embryo at approximately 40 days. (E) Embryo of approximately 48 days. (F) Lateral view of the stomach and greater omentum of an embryo of approximately 52 days. (G) Sagittal section, showing the omental bursa and greater omentum. The *arrows* in (F) and (G) indicate the site of the omental foramen.

▶ DEVELOPMENT OF LIVER AND BILIARY APPARATUS

The liver, gallbladder, and biliary duct system arise as a ventral endodermal outgrowth—**hepatic diverticulum**—from the caudal part of the foregut early in the fourth week (Fig. 12.6A;

see also Fig. 12.4A). *Wnt/β-catenin signaling is involved in the induction of the hepatic diverticulum.*

The diverticulum extends into the **septum transversum** (see Fig. 12.6B), a mass of splanchnic mesoderm between the developing heart and midgut. The diverticulum enlarges

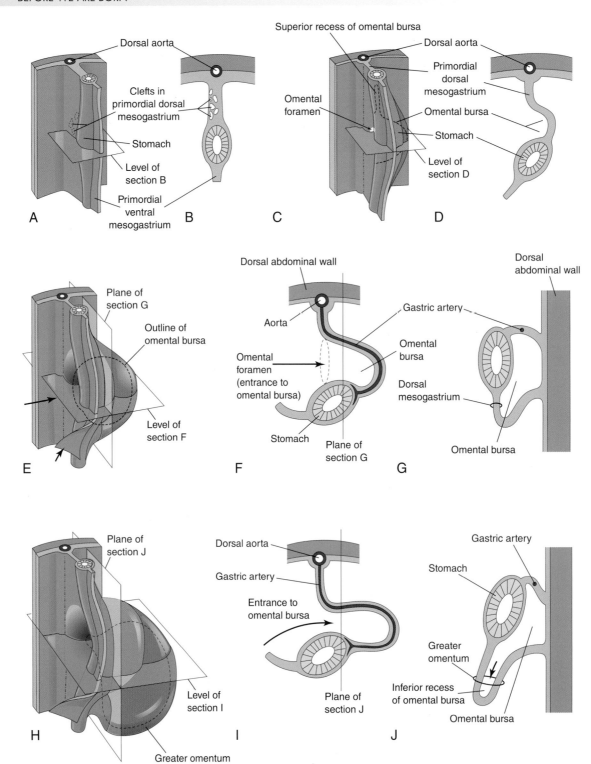

Fig. 12.3 Development of the stomach and mesenteries and formation of the omental bursa. (A) Embryo of 5 weeks. (B) Transverse section showing clefts in the dorsal mesogastrium. (C) Later stage after coalescence of the clefts to form the omental bursa. (D) Transverse section showing the initial appearance of the omental bursa. (E) The dorsal mesentery has elongated and the omental bursa has enlarged. (F and G) Transverse and sagittal sections, respectively, showing elongation of the dorsal mesogastrium and expansion of the omental bursa. (A) Embryo of 6 weeks, showing the greater omentum and expansion of the omental bursa. (I) and (J) Transverse and sagittal sections, respectively, showing the inferior recess of the omental bursa and omental foramen. The *arrows* in (E, F, and I) indicate the site of the omental foramen. (J) The *arrow* indicates the recess of the omental bursa.

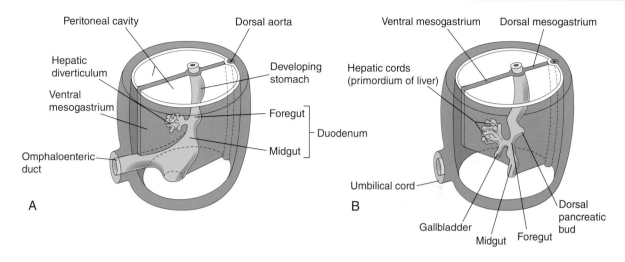

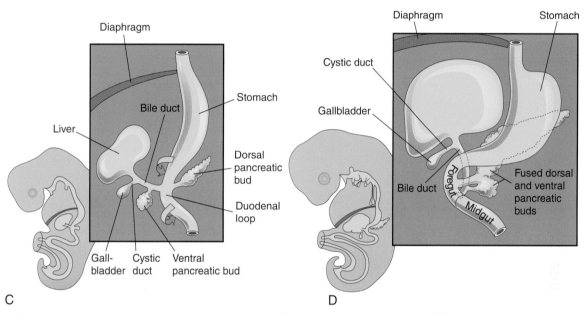

Fig. 12.4 Progressive stages in the development of the duodenum, liver, pancreas, and extrahepatic biliary apparatus. (A) Embryo of 4 weeks. (B) Embryo of early week 5. (C) Embryo of late week 5. (D) Embryo of 6 weeks. The pancreas develops from the dorsal and ventral pancreatic buds that fuse to form the pancreas. Note that the entrance of the bile duct into the duodenum gradually shifts from its initial position to a posterior one. This explains why the bile duct in adults passes posterior to the duodenum and the head of the pancreas.

and divides into two parts as it grows between the layers of the ventral mesogastrium (see Fig. 12.4A). The larger cranial part of the diverticulum is the **primordium of the liver**; the smaller caudal portion becomes the **gallbladder**. The proliferating endodermal cells give rise to interlacing cords of **hepatocytes** (parenchymal liver cells) and to the cholangiocytes, which form the epithelial lining of the intrahepatic part of the biliary apparatus. The **hepatic cords** anastomose around endothelium-lined spaces, the primordia of the hepatic sinusoids. The fibrous and hematopoietic tissue of the liver are derived from mesenchyme in the septum transversum, whereas Kupffer cells originate from precursors in the umbilical vesicle. The liver grows rapidly from the 5th to 10th weeks and fills a large part of the upper abdominal cavity (see Figs. 12.4 and 12.6C and D). By the ninth week, the liver accounts for approximately 10% of the total weight

of the fetus. **Bile formation** by the hepatic cells begins during the 12th week. *Molecular studies reported diverse interacting signaling pathways (Sox4, Sox9, Hnf1b and Notch, TGF-β, Wnt, fibroblast growth factor [FGF], Hippo-Yap, and MAPK) and multiple transcription factors that are involved in the development of the liver.* **Hematopoiesis** (formation and development of various types of blood cells) begins in the liver during the sixth week when hematopoietic stem cells migrate into the liver from the dorsal aorta.

The small caudal part of the hepatic diverticulum becomes the **gallbladder**, and the stalk forms the **cystic duct** (see Fig. 12.4B and C). Initially, the extrahepatic biliary apparatus is occluded with epithelial cells. The extrahepatic cholangiocytes are also derived from the endoderm. The stalk connecting the hepatic and cystic ducts to the duodenum becomes the **bile duct**; this duct attaches to the ventral

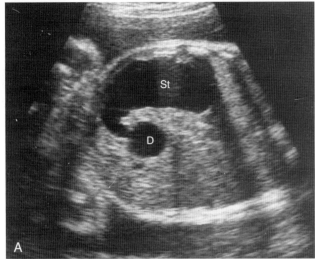

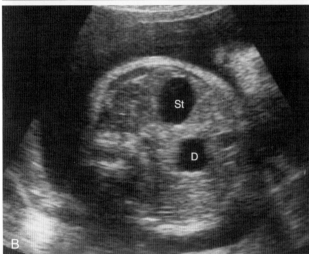

Fig. 12.5 Ultrasound scans of a fetus at 33 weeks' gestation (31 weeks after fertilization), showing duodenal atresia. (A) An oblique scan shows the dilated, fluid-filled stomach *(St)* entering the proximal duodenum *(D)*, which is also enlarged because of the atresia (blockage) distal to it. (B) Transverse ultrasound scan, showing the characteristic "double-bubble" appearance of the stomach and duodenum when there is duodenal atresia. Courtesy Dr. Lyndon M. Hill, Magee-Women's Hospital, Pittsburgh, Pennsylvania.

aspect of the duodenal loop. As the duodenum grows and rotates, the entrance of the bile duct is carried to the dorsal aspect of the duodenum (see Fig. 12.4C and D). The bile entering the duodenum through the bile duct after the 13th week gives the meconium (first intestinal discharges of neonates) a dark green color.

Birth Defects of Liver

Minor variations of liver lobulation are common; however, birth defects are rare. Variations of hepatic ducts, bile duct, and cystic duct are common and clinically significant. **Accessory hepatic ducts** are present in approximately 5% of the population, and awareness of their possible presence is of importance in some surgical situations (e.g., liver transplantation).

Extrahepatic Biliary Atresia

This is the most serious birth defect involving the **extrahepatic biliary system**, and it occurs in 1 in 5000 to 20,000 live births. These neonates have the loss or absence of all or a significant portion of the extrahepatic biliary system. The cause is unclear but may include a viral infection or defects in circulation. **Jaundice** typically occurs between 2 and 6 weeks postpartum, and surgical correction to enhance bile flow, although not curative, can provide temporary palliation. Definitive therapy requires liver transplantation.

VENTRAL MESENTERY

The thin, double-layered ventral membrane (Fig. 12.7; see also Fig. 12.6C and D) gives rise to:

- The **lesser omentum**, passing from the liver to the lesser curvature of the stomach (**hepatogastric ligament**) and from the liver to the duodenum (**hepatoduodenal ligament**)
- The **falciform ligament**, extending from the liver to the ventral abdominal wall.

The **umbilical vein** passes through the free border of the falciform ligament on its way from the umbilical cord to the liver. The ventral mesentery, derived from the mesogastrium, also forms the **visceral peritoneum of the liver**.

DEVELOPMENT OF PANCREAS

The pancreas develops between the layers of the mesenteries from dorsal and ventral **pancreatic buds**, which arise from the caudal part of the foregut (Fig. 12.8A). Most of the pancreas is derived from the larger **dorsal pancreatic bud**, which appears first.

Formation of the dorsal pancreatic bud depends on signals from the notochord (activin and FGF2) that block the expression of SHH in the endoderm. Expression of pancreatic and duodenal homeobox factors (PDX-1 and MafA) is critical for the development of the pancreas.

The smaller **ventral pancreatic bud** develops near the entry of the bile duct into the duodenum (see Fig. 12.8A and B). As the duodenum rotates to the right and becomes C-shaped, the bud is carried dorsally with the bile duct (see Fig. 12.8C–F). It soon lies posterior to the dorsal pancreatic bud and later fuses with it (see Fig. 12.8G). As the pancreatic buds fuse, their ducts anastomose. The ventral pancreatic bud forms the **uncinate process** and is part of the **head of the pancreas**. As the stomach, duodenum, and ventral mesentery rotate, the pancreas comes to lie along the dorsal abdominal wall (retroperitoneal) (see Fig. 12.8D and G).

The **pancreatic duct** forms from the duct of the ventral bud and the distal part of the duct of the dorsal bud (see Fig. 12.8G). In approximately 9% of people, the proximal part of the duct of the dorsal bud persists as an **accessory pancreatic duct** that opens into the minor duodenal papilla.

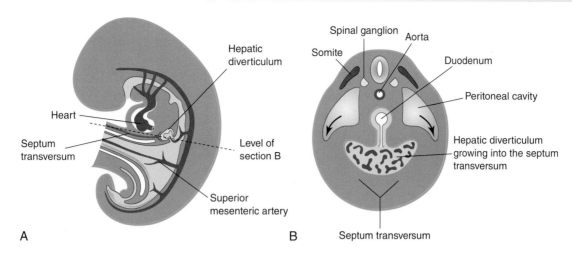

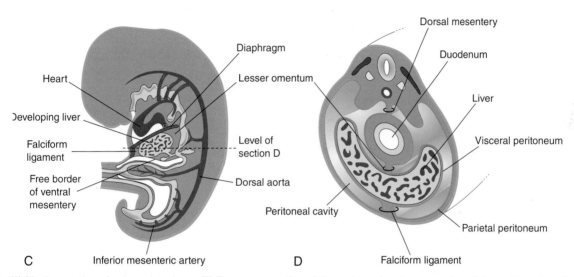

Fig. 12.6 (A) Median section of a 4-week embryo. (B) Transverse section of the embryo showing expansion of the peritoneal cavity *(arrows)*. (C) Sagittal section of a 5-week embryo. (D) Transverse section of the embryo after formation of the dorsal and ventral mesenteries.

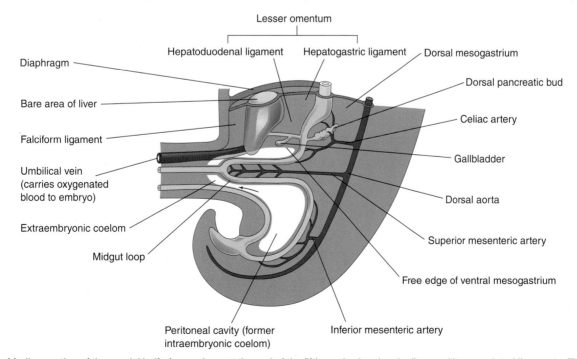

Fig. 12.7 Median section of the caudal half of an embryo at the end of the fifth week, showing the liver and its associated ligaments. The *arrow* indicates the communication of the peritoneal cavity with the extraembryonic coelom.

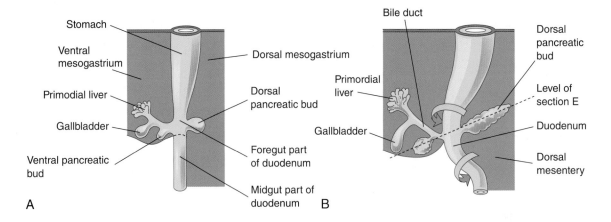

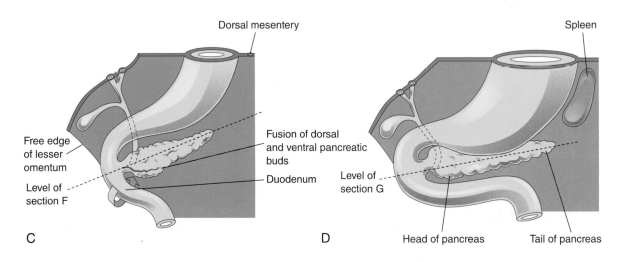

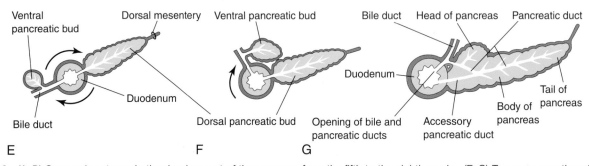

Fig. 12.8   (A–D) Successive stages in the development of the pancreas from the fifth to the eighth weeks. (E–G) Transverse sections through the duodenum and developing pancreas. Growth and rotation *(arrows)* of the duodenum bring the ventral pancreatic bud toward the dorsal bud, where the two buds subsequently fuse.

The connective tissue sheath and interlobular septa of the pancreas develop from the surrounding splanchnic mesenchyme. **Insulin secretion** begins at approximately 10 weeks. The glucagon- and somatostatin-containing cells develop before differentiation of the insulin-secreting cells occurs. With increasing fetal age, total pancreatic insulin and glucagon content also increase.

Annular Pancreas

Annular pancreas is an uncommon birth defect, but it warrants attention because it may cause duodenal obstruction (Fig. 12.9C). This defect probably results from the growth of a bifid ventral pancreatic bud around the duodenum (see Fig. 12.9A–C). The parts of the bifid ventral bud then fuse with

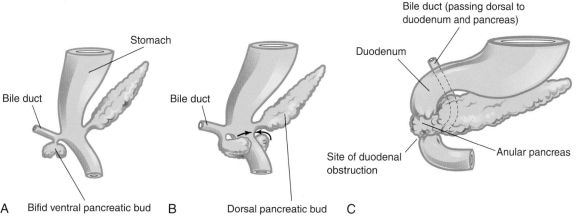

Fig. 12.9 (A and B) The probable basis of an annular pancreas. (C) An annular pancreas encircling the duodenum. This birth defect produces complete obstruction (atresia) or partial obstruction (stenosis) of the duodenum.

the dorsal bud, forming a pancreatic ring. The ring-like, annular part of the pancreas consists of a thin, flat band of pancreatic tissue surrounding the descending or second part of the duodenum. An annular pancreas may cause obstruction of the duodenum shortly after birth, but many cases are not diagnosed until adulthood. Females are affected more frequently.

DEVELOPMENT OF SPLEEN

The spleen is derived from a mass of mesenchymal cells located between the layers of the dorsal mesogastrium (Fig. 12.10A and B). The spleen, a vascular lymphatic organ, begins to develop during the fifth week but does not acquire its characteristic shape until early in the fetal period. The spleen in a fetus is lobulated, but the lobules normally disappear before birth. The notches in the superior border of the adult spleen are remnants of the grooves that separate the fetal lobules.

Accessory Spleens

One or more small splenic masses (about 1 cm in diameter) of fully functional splenic tissue may exist in one of the peritoneal folds, usually near the hilum of the spleen or the tail of the pancreas. These accessory spleens **(polysplenia)** occur in approximately 10% of people.

MIDGUT

The derivatives of the midgut are as follows:

- The small intestine, including the duodenum distal to the opening of the bile duct
- The cecum, appendix, ascending colon, and right half to two-thirds of the transverse colon.

Each of these derivatives is supplied by the **superior mesenteric artery** (see Figs. 12.1 and 12.7). The **midgut loop** is suspended from the dorsal abdominal wall by an elongated **mesentery**. The midgut elongates and forms a ventral, U-shaped loop that projects into the proximal part of the **umbilical cord** (Fig. 12.11A). The loop of the intestine, a **physiological umbilical herniation**, occurs at the beginning of the sixth week (Fig. 12.12; see also Fig. 12.11C). The loop communicates with the **umbilical vesicle** through the narrow **omphaloenteric duct** until the 10th week (see Fig. 12.11A and C). The herniation occurs because there is not enough room in the abdominal cavity for the rapidly growing midgut. The shortage of space is caused mainly by the relatively massive liver and kidneys. The cranial limb grows rapidly and forms small **intestinal loops** (see Fig. 12.11C). The caudal limb undergoes very little change except for the development of the **cecal swelling**, the primordium of the cecum, and appendix (see Fig. 12.11C–E).

ROTATION OF MIDGUT LOOP

While it is in the umbilical cord, the midgut loop rotates 90 degrees counterclockwise around the axis of the **superior mesenteric artery** (see Fig. 12.11B). This rotation brings the cranial limb (small intestine) of the midgut loop to the right and the caudal limb (large intestine) to the left. During rotation, the cranial limb elongates and forms **intestinal loops** (e.g., primordia of the jejunum and ileum). It appears that rotation is a result of differential growth of portions of the gut.

RETRACTION OF INTESTINAL LOOPS

During the 10th week, the intestines return to the abdomen (reduction of midgut hernia) (see Fig. 12.11C and D). The small intestine returns first, passing posterior to the superior mesenteric artery, and occupies the central part of the abdomen. As the large intestine returns, it undergoes a further 180-degree counterclockwise rotation (see Fig. 12.11C$_1$ and D$_1$). Later, it comes to occupy the right side of the abdomen. The

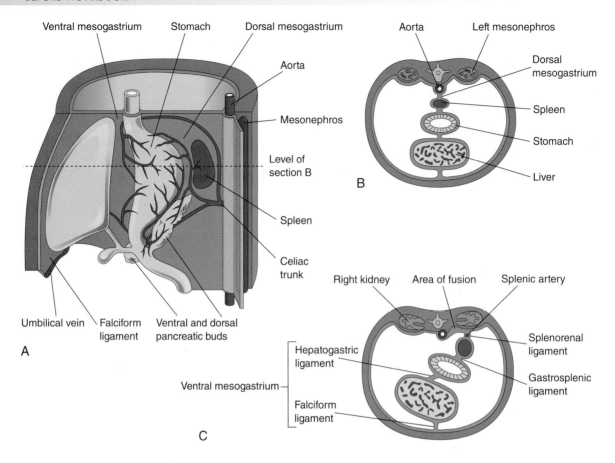

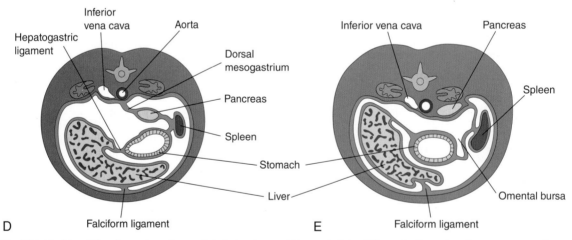

Fig. 12.10 (A) Left side of the stomach and associated structures at the end of the fifth week. Note that the pancreas, spleen, and celiac trunk are between the layers of the dorsal mesogastrium. (B) Transverse section of the liver, stomach, and spleen at the level shown in (A) illustrating their relationship to the dorsal and ventral mesenteries. (C) Transverse section of a fetus showing fusion of the dorsal mesogastrium with the peritoneum on the posterior abdominal wall. (D and E) Similar sections show the movement of the liver to the right and the rotation of the stomach. Observe the fusion of the dorsal mesogastrium to the dorsal abdominal wall. As a result, the pancreas becomes retroperitoneal.

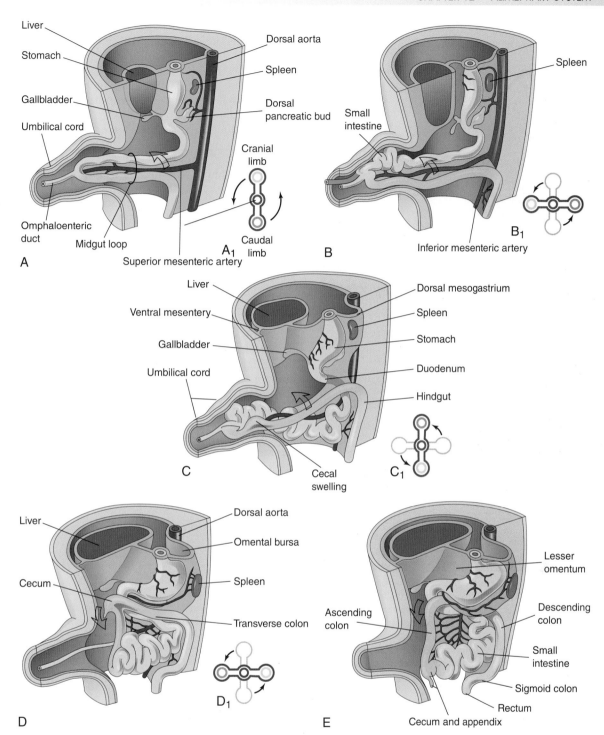

Fig. 12.11 Drawings illustrating herniation and rotation of the midgut loop. (A) At the beginning of the sixth week. (A₁) Transverse section through the midgut loop, illustrating the initial relationship of the limbs of the midgut loop to the superior mesenteric artery. Note that the midgut loop is in the proximal part of the umbilical cord. (B) Later stage showing the beginning of midgut rotation. (B₁) Illustration of the 90-degree counterclockwise rotation that carries the cranial limb of the midgut to the right. (C) At approximately 10 weeks, showing the intestines returning to the abdomen. (C₁) Illustration of a further rotation of 90 degrees. (D) At approximately 11 weeks, showing the location of the viscera (internal organs) after contraction of the intestines. (D₁) Illustrations of a further 90-degree rotation of the viscera, for a total of 270 degrees. (E) Later in the fetal period, showing the cecum rotating to its normal position in the lower right quadrant of the abdomen.

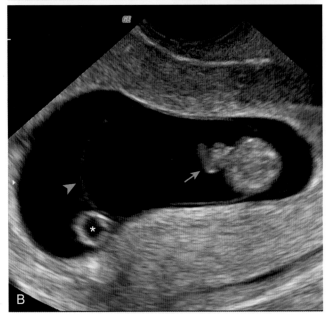

Fig. 12.12 (A) Physiological hernia in a fetus of approximately 58 days attached to its placenta. Note the herniated intestine in the proximal part of the umbilical cord *(arrow)*. (B) Transverse section through the abdomen of a 9-week and 5-day-old fetus demonstrates irregular intestinal (bowel) loops just outside the anterior abdominal wall *(thin arrow)*. At this gestational age, this is the normal appearance of physiological midgut herniation. Conversely, herniation of abdominal contents beyond 12 weeks of gestation would suggest the presence of a pathological anterior wall defect such as gastroschisis or an omphalocele. Note also the normal location of the umbilical vesicle (yolk sac) *(asterisk)* at this gestational age, just outside the thin-walled amniotic sac *(arrowhead)*. A, Courtesy Dr. D.K. Kalousek, Department of Pathology, University of British Columbia, Children's Hospital, Vancouver, British Columbia, Canada; B, Courtesy Dr. Alexandra Stanislavsky, Radiopaedia.org.

ascending colon becomes recognizable with the elongation of the posterior abdominal wall (see Fig. 12.11E).

FIXATION OF INTESTINES

Rotation of the stomach and duodenum causes the duodenum and pancreas to fall to the right. The enlarged colon presses the duodenum and pancreas against the posterior abdominal wall. The adjacent layers of peritoneum fuse and subsequently disappear (Fig. 12.13C and F); consequently, most of the duodenum and head of the pancreas become retroperitoneal. The mesentery of the ascending colon fuses with the parietal peritoneum on the posterior abdominal wall. The mesentery of the ascending colon becomes retroperitoneal (see Fig. 12.13B and E). The other derivatives of the midgut loop retain their mesenteries.

FORMATION OF VILLI

Flattened luminal cells undergo morphogenesis to form finger-like epithelial villi. The formation of villi results in an enormous increase in the surface area of the gut, which provides the means of absorption. Villi begin to form in the gut at approximately 51 to 54 days. Proliferation and differentiation of gut epithelial cells continue, resulting in the formation of other specialized cells in the gut, including Paneth cells.

CECUM AND APPENDIX

The primordium of the cecum and appendix—the cecal **diverticulum**— appears in the sixth week as a swelling on the antimesenteric border of the caudal limb of the midgut loop (Fig. 12.14A; see also Fig. 12.11C–E). Initially, the appendix is a small diverticulum (pouch) of the cecum. It subsequently increases rapidly in length so that at birth, it is a relatively long tube arising from the distal end of the **cecum** (see Fig. 12.14D). After birth, the unequal growth of the walls of the cecum results in the appendix entering its medial side (see Fig. 12.14E). *The appendix is subject to considerable variation in position.* As the ascending colon elongates, the appendix may pass posterior to the cecum (retrocecal appendix) or colon (retrocolic appendix).

Congenital Omphalocele

This birth defect results in the persistence of the **herniation of the abdominal contents** into the proximal part of the umbilical cord (Figs. 12.15 and 12.16). It is caused by the failure of the body walls to fuse at the umbilical ring because of defective growth of the mesenchyme. Herniation of the intestines occurs in approximately 1 in 5000 births. Herniation of the liver and intestines occurs less frequently (1 in 10,000 births). The size of the hernia depends on its contents. Because the impetus for the abdominal cavity to grow is reduced, it is proportionately small when an omphalocele is present.

Umbilical Hernia

When the intestines herniate through an imperfectly closed umbilicus, an umbilical hernia forms. This common type of hernia differs from an omphalocele. In umbilical hernias, the protruding mass (usually consisting of part of the greater omentum and small intestine) is covered by subcutaneous tissue and skin. The hernia protrudes during crying, straining, or coughing.

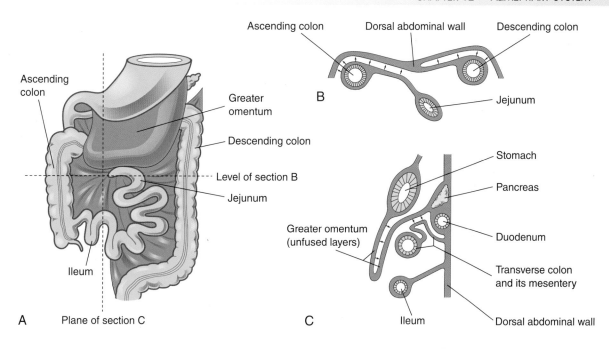

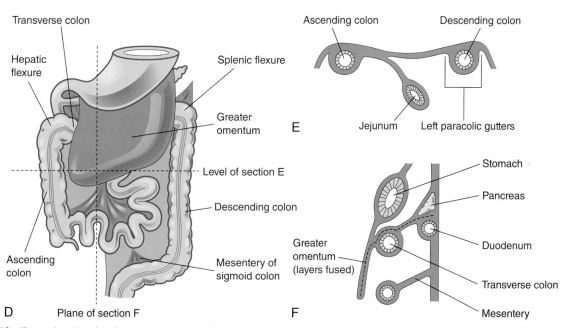

Fig. 12.13 Illustration showing the mesenteries and fixation of the intestines. (A) Ventral view of the intestines before their fixation. (B) Transverse section at the level shown in (A). The *arrows* indicate areas of subsequent fusion. (C) Sagittal section at the plane shown in (A), illustrating the greater omentum overhanging the transverse colon. The *arrows* indicate areas of subsequent fusion. (D) Ventral view of the intestines after their fixation. (E) Transverse section at the level shown in (D) after disappearance of the mesentery of the ascending and descending colon. (F) Sagittal section at the plane shown in (D), illustrating fusion of the greater omentum with the mesentery of the transverse colon and fusion of the layers of the greater omentum.

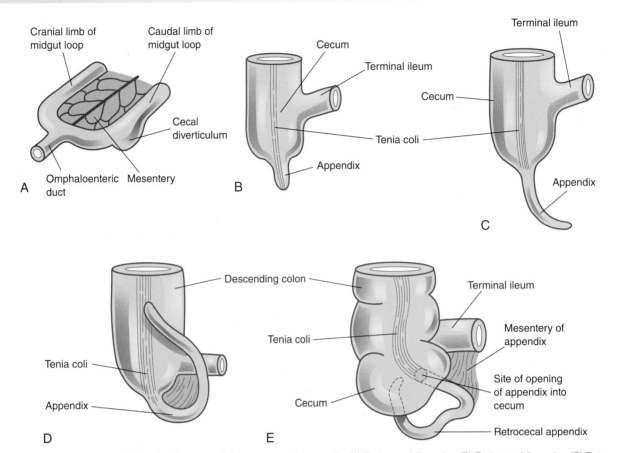

Fig. 12.14 Successive stages in the development of the cecum and appendix. (A) Embryo of 6 weeks. (B) Embryo of 8 weeks. (C) Fetus of 12 weeks. (D) Neonate. Note that the appendix is relatively long and is continuous with the apex of the cecum. (E) Child. Note that the appendix is now relatively short and its opening is located posterior to the cecum. In approximately 64% of people, the appendix is located posterior to the cecum (retrocecal).

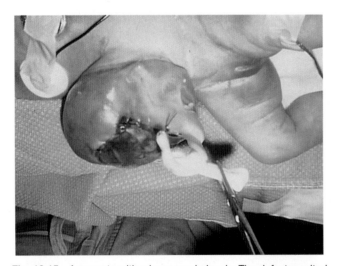

Fig. 12.15 A neonate with a large omphalocele. The defect resulted in the herniation of intraabdominal structures (liver and intestine) into the proximal end of the umbilical cord. The omphalocele is covered by a membrane composed of peritoneum and amnion. *Courtesy Dr. N.E. Wiseman, Department of Surgery, Children's Hospital, Winnipeg, Manitoba, Canada.*

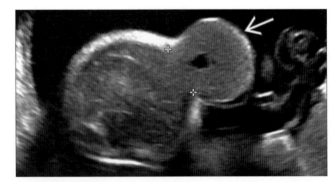

Fig. 12.16 Ultrasonogram (sonogram) of the abdomen. This fetus with an abdominal wall defect (calipers) and eviscerated liver (*arrow*). *From Kamaya A, Wong-You-Cheong J, Woodward PJ, et al: Diagnostic ultrasound for sonographers, Philadelphia, PA, 2019, Elsevier, pp 604–605.*

Gastroschisis

Gastroschisis occurs approximately once in every 2000 live births. It results from a defect near the median plane of the abdominal wall (Fig. 12.17). The viscera protrude into the amniotic cavity and are bathed by amniotic fluid. The term *gastroschisis*, which literally means "split stomach," is a misnomer because it is the anterior abdominal wall, not the stomach, that is split. The defect usually occurs on the right side, lateral to the median plane, and is more common in males. This birth defect results from incomplete closure of the lateral folds during the fourth week of development (see Fig. 6.1). The exact cause of gastroschisis is uncertain but may involve genetic factors and ischemic injury to the developing abdominal wall musculature.

Nonrotation of Midgut

Birth defects of the intestines are common; most of them are defects of gut rotation (e.g., **malrotation of the gut**). Nonrotation of the midgut (left-sided colon) is a relatively common defect (Fig. 12.18A and B), resulting in the caudal limb of the midgut loop returning to the abdomen first. The small intestine then lies on the right side of the abdomen, and the entire large intestine lies on the left. Although patients are generally asymptomatic, if **volvulus** (twisting) occurs, the superior mesenteric artery may be obstructed, resulting in infarction and gangrene of the associated intestine.

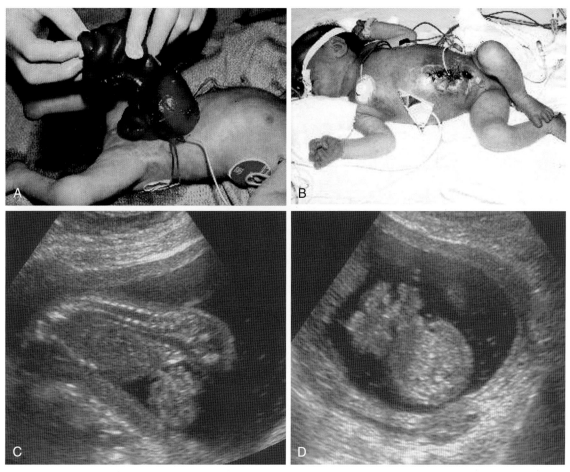

Fig. 12.17 (A) Photograph of a neonate with an anterior abdominal wall birth defect—gastroschisis (congenital fissure with protrusion of viscera). The defect was relatively small (2–4 cm long) and involved all layers of the abdominal wall. The defect was located to the right of the umbilicus. (B) Photograph of the same neonate after the viscera were returned to the abdomen and the defect was surgically closed. (C and D) Sonogram (ultrasonogram) of an 18-week fetus with gastroschisis. Loops of intestine (bowel) can be seen in the amniotic fluid ventral to the fetus on the sagittal scan (C) and the axial scan (D) of the fetal abdomen. A and B, Courtesy A.E. Chudley, MD, Section of Genetics and Metabolism, Department of Pediatrics and Child Health, Children's Hospital, Winnipeg, Manitoba, Canada; C and D, Courtesy Dr. E.A. Lyons, Professor of Radiology, Obstetrics and Gynecology, and Anatomy, Health Sciences Centre, University of Manitoba, Winnipeg, Manitoba, Canada.

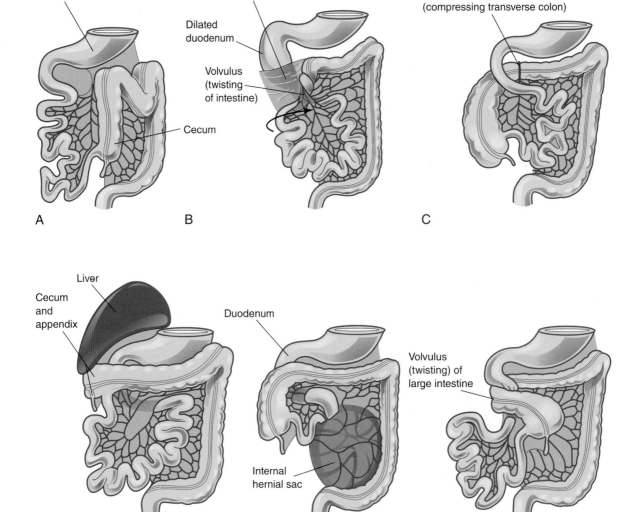

Fig. 12.18 Birth defects of midgut rotation. (A) Nonrotation. (B) Mixed rotation and volvulus (twisting of the intestine). The *arrow* indicates the twisting of the intestine. (C) Reversed rotation. (D) Subhepatic (below the liver) cecum and appendix. (E) Internal hernia. (F) Midgut volvulus with duodenal obstruction.

Mixed Rotation and Volvulus

With mixed rotation and volvulus, the cecum lies just inferior to the pylorus of the stomach and is fixed to the posterior abdominal wall by peritoneal bands that pass over the duodenum (see Fig. 12.18B). These bands and volvulus usually cause **duodenal obstruction**. This type of malrotation results from the failure of the midgut loop to complete the final 90 degrees of rotation (see Fig. 12.11D); consequently, the terminal part of the ileum returns to the abdomen first.

Subhepatic Cecum and Appendix

If the cecum adheres to the inferior surface of the liver when it returns to the abdomen (see Fig. 12.11D), it is drawn superiorly to the liver. As a result, the cecum remains in its fetal position (see Fig. 12.18D). Subhepatic cecum and appendix are more common in males. This birth defect may create problems in diagnostic procedures for and surgical removal of the appendix in adults.

Reversed Rotation

In very unusual cases, the midgut loop rotates in a clockwise rather than a counterclockwise direction (see Fig. 12.18C). As a result, the duodenum lies anterior to the superior mesenteric artery, rather than posterior to it, and the transverse colon lies posterior to the superior mesenteric artery instead of anterior to it. In these infants, the transverse colon may be obstructed by pressure from the superior mesenteric artery.

Internal Hernia

In this rare birth defect, the small intestine passes into the mesentery of the midgut loop during the return of the intestines to the abdomen (see Fig. 12.18E). As a result, a hernia-like sac forms. This very uncommon condition does not usually produce symptoms and is often detected at postmortem examination.

Midgut Volvulus

Midgut volvulus is a birth defect in which the small intestine does not enter the abdominal cavity normally, and the mesenteries do not undergo normal fixation. As a result, **volvulus** of the intestines occurs (see Fig. 12.18F). Only two parts of the intestine—the duodenum and proximal colon—are attached to the posterior abdominal wall. The small intestine hangs by a narrow stalk that contains the superior mesenteric artery and vein. These vessels are usually twisted and may become obstructed at or near the **duodenojejunal junction**. The circulation to the twisted intestine is often restricted; if the vessels are completely obstructed, necrosis develops.

Stenosis and Atresia of Intestine

Stenosis and atresia of the intestinal lumen (see Fig. 12.5) account for approximately one-third of cases of intestinal obstruction in neonates. The obstructive lesion occurs most often in the ileum (50%) and duodenum (25%). Most atresias of the ileum are probably caused by infarction of the fetal intestine as a result of impairment of its blood supply secondary to volvulus. This impairment most likely occurs during the 10th week as the intestines return to the abdomen.

Ileal Diverticulum and Other Omphaloenteric Duct Remnants

A congenital **ileal diverticulum**—Meckel diverticulum (Fig. 12.19)—occurs in 2% to 4% of infants and is three to five times more prevalent in males. It represents a remnant of the proximal portion of the **omphaloenteric duct**. It typically appears as a finger-like pouch approximately 3 to 6 cm long that arises from the antimesenteric border of the ileum, 40 to 50 cm from the ileocecal junction. An ileal diverticulum is of clinical significance because it sometimes becomes inflamed and causes symptoms that mimic appendicitis. The wall of the diverticulum contains all layers of the ileum and may also contain small patches of gastric and pancreatic tissues. The gastric mucosa often secretes acid, producing ulceration and bleeding (Fig. 12.20A–C). An ileal diverticulum may be connected to the umbilicus by a fibrous cord or an **omphaloenteric fistula** (see Fig. 12.20B and C); other possible remnants of the omphaloenteric duct are shown in Fig. 12.20D–F.

HINDGUT

The derivatives of the hindgut are as follows:

- The left third to half of the transverse colon, the descending colon and sigmoid colon, the rectum, and the superior part of the anal canal
- The epithelium of the urinary bladder and most of the urethra.

All hindgut derivatives are supplied by the **inferior mesenteric artery** (see Fig. 12.7). The descending colon becomes

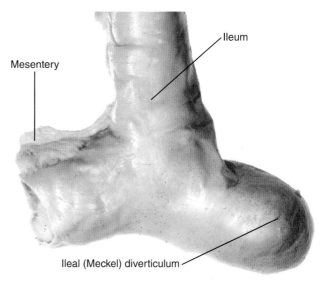

Fig. 12.19 A typical ileal diverticulum—Meckel diverticulum (cadaveric specimen). Only a small percentage of these diverticula produce symptoms. Ileal diverticula are one of the most common birth defects of the alimentary tract. From Moore KL, Persaud TVN, Shiota K: *Color atlas of clinical embryology*, ed 2, Philadelphia, 2000, Saunders.

retroperitoneal as its mesentery fuses with the peritoneum on the left posterior abdominal wall (see Fig. 12.13B and E). The mesentery of the sigmoid colon is retained (see Fig. 12.13D).

CLOACA

The cloaca is the expanded terminal part of the hindgut before division into the rectum, bladder, and genital primordia. The cloaca is an endoderm-lined chamber that is in contact with the surface ectoderm at the cloacal membrane (Fig. 12.21A and B). This membrane is composed of the endoderm of the cloaca and ectoderm of the anal pit (see Fig. 12.21C and D). The cloaca receives the allantois, which is a finger-like diverticulum (see Fig. 12.21A), ventrally.

PARTITIONING OF CLOACA

The cloaca is divided into dorsal and ventral parts by mesenchyme—the **urorectal septum**—that develops in the angle between the allantois and hindgut (see Fig. 12.21C and D). *Endodermal β-catenin signaling is required for the formation of the urorectal septum.* As the septum grows toward the cloacal membrane, it develops fork-like extensions that produce infoldings of the lateral walls of the cloaca (see Fig. 12.21B₁). These folds grow toward each other and fuse, forming a partition that divides the cloaca into three parts (see Fig. 12.21D and E)—the **rectum**, the cranial part of the **anal canal**, and the **urogenital sinus**.

The cloaca plays a crucial role in anorectal development. New information indicates that the urorectal septum does not fuse with the cloacal membrane; therefore an anal membrane does not exist. After the cloacal membrane ruptures by **apoptotic cell death**, the **anorectal lumen** is temporarily closed by an **epithelial plug**, which may have been interpreted as the anal membrane (see Fig. 12.21E).

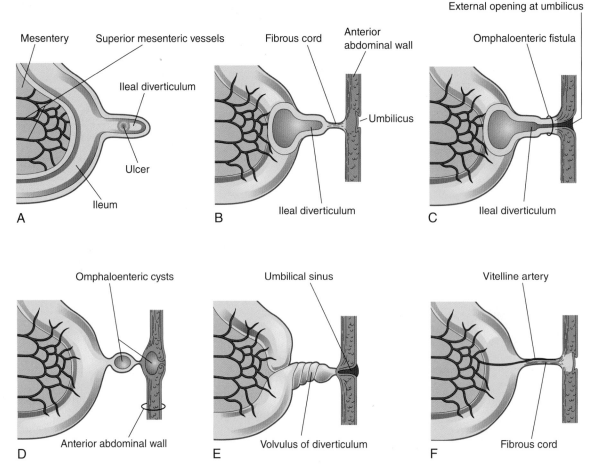

Fig. 12.20 Ileal diverticula and remnants of the omphaloenteric duct. (A) Section of the ileum and a diverticulum with an ulcer. (B) A diverticulum connected to the umbilicus by a fibrous remnant of the omphaloenteric duct. (C) Omphaloenteric fistula resulting from persistence of the intraabdominal part of the omphaloenteric duct. (D) Omphaloenteric cysts at the umbilicus and in a fibrous remnant of the omphaloenteric duct. (E) Volvulus (twisted) ileal diverticulum and an umbilical sinus resulting from the persistence of the omphaloenteric duct in the umbilicus. (F) The omphaloenteric duct has persisted as a fibrous cord connecting the ileum with the umbilicus. A persistent vitelline artery extends along the fibrous cord to the umbilicus. This artery carried blood to the umbilical vesicle from the anterior wall of the embryo.

Mesenchymal proliferations produce elevations of the surface ectoderm around the epithelial anal plug. Recanalization of the anorectal canal occurs by apoptosis of the epithelial anal plug, which forms the **anal pit** (see Fig. 12.21) by the eighth week of development.

ANAL CANAL

10 The superior two-thirds of the anal canal are derived from the **hindgut**; the inferior one-third develops from the anal pit (Fig. 12.22).

Because of its hindgut origin, the superior two-thirds of the anal canal are supplied mainly by the **superior rectal artery**, the continuation of the inferior mesenteric artery. Its nerves are from the autonomic nervous system. Because of its origin from the anal pit, the inferior one-third of the anal canal is supplied mainly by the **inferior rectal arteries**, branches of the internal pudendal artery. The inferior part of the anal canal is innervated by the inferior rectal nerve and is sensitive to pain, temperature, touch, and pressure.

Therefore tumors in the superior part are typically painless, whereas those in the inferior part are painful.

The differences in originating cells (columnar versus squamous epithelium), blood supply, nerve supply, and venous and lymphatic drainage of the anal canal are important clinically, such as when considering the metastasis of cancer cells. The characteristics of **carcinomas** involving the two parts differ.

ENTERIC NERVOUS SYSTEM

The functions of the gastrointestinal system include transportation, secretion, digestion, and protection. These are controlled by the enteric nervous system (ENS), the gut's intrinsic system that can maintain functions autonomously without brain or spinal cord input. The ENS is highly complex and composed of ganglionic plexuses and more than 200 million neurons of 20 subtypes. Neural crest cells migrate to the foregut, along the length of the developing

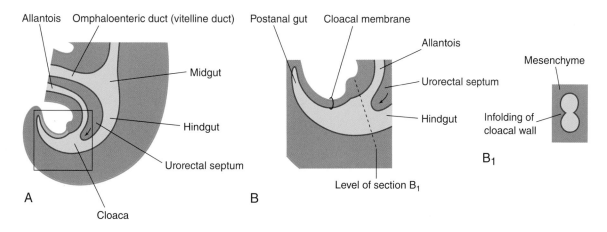

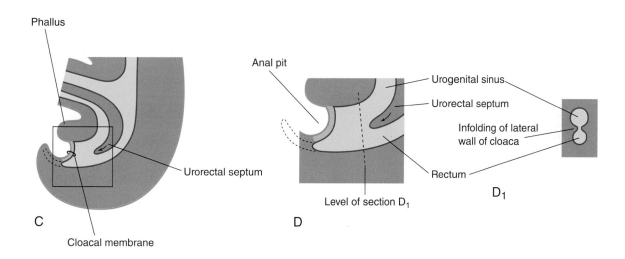

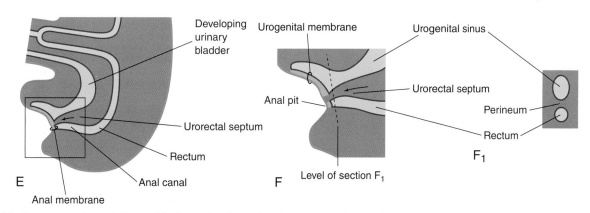

Fig. 12.21 Successive stages in the partitioning of the cloaca into the rectum and urogenital sinus by the urorectal septum. (A, C, and E) Views from the left side at 4, 6, and 7 weeks, respectively. (B, D, and F) Enlargements of the cloacal region. (B₁, D₁, and F₁) Transverse sections of the cloaca at the levels shown in (B, D, and F), respectively. Note that the postanal portion (shown in B) degenerates and disappears as the rectum forms. The *arrows* in (A–E) indicate the growth of the urorectal septum.

gut, populating and differentiating into neurons and other ENS cell types. The population in the gut by these cells occurs approximately between week 3 and week 7. Molecular s*tudies have shown that several interacting genes, including RET, EDNRB, GDNF, SOX10, PHOX2B, EDN3, and* *other signaling pathways are* associated with the development of the ENS. Defects in the migration, proliferation, and differentiation of neural crest cells with failure in the formation of associated ganglia can lead to Hirschsprung disease (Fig. 12.23).

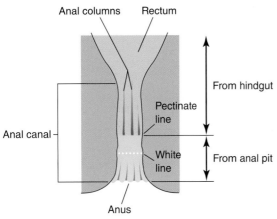

Fig. 12.22 The rectum and anal canal, showing their developmental origins. Note that the superior two-thirds of the anal canal are derived from the hindgut, whereas the inferior one-third of the anal canal is derived from the anal pit. Because of their different embryological origins, the superior and inferior parts of the anal canal are supplied by different arteries and nerves and have different venous and lymphatic drainages.

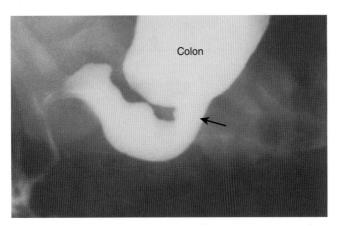

Fig. 12.23 Radiograph of the colon, after a barium enema, in a 1-month-old infant with megacolon (Hirschsprung disease). The distal aganglionic segment is narrow, with a dilated proximal colon full of fecal material. Note the transition zone *(arrow)*. Courtesy Dr. Martin H. Reed, Department of Radiology, University of Manitoba and Children's Hospital, Winnipeg, Manitoba, Canada.

Congenital Megacolon

In infants with **congenital megacolon**, or **Hirschsprung (HSCR) disease** (see Fig. 12.23), a part of the colon is dilated because of the absence of autonomic ganglion cells in the **myenteric plexus** distal to the dilated segment of the colon. The dilation results from failure of peristalsis in the aganglionic segment, which prevents movement of the intestinal contents, resulting in dilation.

Males are affected more than females (4:1). HSCR is a neurocristopathy with the failure of neural crest cells to migrate into the wall of the colon during the fifth to seventh weeks of development. *Of the genes involved in the pathogenesis of HSCR, the RET (oncogene product) proto-oncogene accounts for most cases.* HSCR is the most common cause of neonatal obstruction of the colon and accounts for 33% of all neonatal obstructions; this disease affects 1 in 5000 neonates.

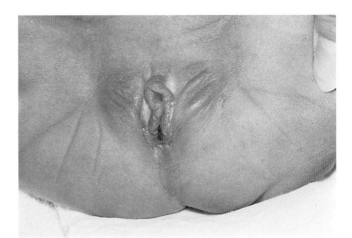

Fig. 12.24 Female neonate with membranous anal atresia (imperforate anus—lacking a normal opening). In most cases of this atresia, a thin layer of tissue separates the anal canal from the exterior. Some form of imperforate anus occurs approximately once in every 5000 neonates; it is more common in males. Courtesy A.E. Chudley, MD, Section of Genetics and Metabolism, Department of Pediatrics and Child Health, Children's Hospital, Winnipeg, Manitoba, Canada.

Anorectal Birth Defects

Imperforate anus occurs in approximately 1 in 5000 neonates, and it is more common in males than females (Figs. 12.24 and 12.25C). Most anorectal defects result from abnormal development of the urorectal septum, resulting in incomplete separation of the cloaca into urogenital and anorectal parts (see Fig. 12.25A). Lesions are classified as low or high, depending on whether the rectum ends superior or inferior to the puborectalis muscle, which maintains fetal continence and relaxes to allow defecation.

Low Anorectal Birth Defects

Anal Agenesis, With or Without a Fistula

The anal canal may end blindly, or there may be an **ectopic anus** or an **anoperineal fistula** that opens into the perineum (see Fig. 12.25D and E). The abnormal canal may, however, open into the vagina in females or the urethra in males (see Fig. 12.25F and G). Most low anorectal defects are associated with an external fistula. **Anal agenesis with a fistula** results from incomplete separation of the cloaca by the urorectal septum. *These anomalies have been associated with disruption of β-catenin signaling.*

Anal Stenosis

In anal stenosis, the anus is in a normal position, but the anus and anal canal are narrow (see Fig. 12.25B). This defect is probably caused by a slight dorsal deviation of the **urorectal septum** as it grows caudally (see Fig. 12.21D).

Membranous Atresia of Anus

The anus is in the normal position, but a thin layer of tissue separates the anal canal from the exterior (see Figs. 12.24 and 12.25C). The thin remnant of the epithelial plug bulges on straining and appears blue from the presence of **meconium** (feces of neonate) above it. This defect results from the failure of the epithelial plug to perforate at the end of the eighth week.

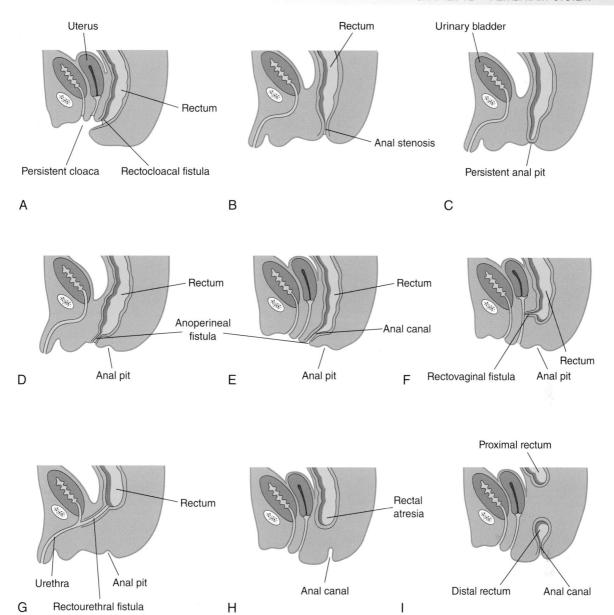

Fig. 12.25   Various types of anorectal birth defects. (a) Persistent cloaca. Note the common outlet of the intestinal, urinary, and reproductive tracts. (B) Anal stenosis. (C) An atresia (imperforate anus). (D and E) Anal agenesis with a perineal fistula. (F) Anorectal agenesis with a rectovaginal fistula. (G) Anorectal agenesis with a rectourethral fistula. (H and I) Rectal atresia.

High Anorectal Birth Defects

Anorectal Agenesis With or Without a Fistula

In **high defects** of the anorectal region, the rectum ends superior to the puborectalis muscle when there is anorectal agenesis. This is the most common type of anorectal defect, and it accounts for approximately two-thirds of anorectal defects. There is usually a fistula to the bladder **(rectovesical fistula)** or urethra **(rectourethral fistula)** in males, or to the vagina **(rectovaginal fistula)** or the vestibule of the vagina **(rectovestibular fistula)** in females (see Fig. 12.25F and G). Anorectal agenesis with a fistula is the result of incomplete separation of the cloaca from the urogenital sinus by the urorectal septum (see Fig. 12.21C–E).

Rectal Atresia

In this atresia, the anal canal and rectum are present but separated (see Fig. 12.25H and I). Sometimes the two segments of the intestine are connected by a fibrous cord, the remnant of the atretic portion of the rectum. The cause of rectal atresia may be abnormal recanalization of the colon or, more likely, a defective blood supply.

CLINICALLY ORIENTED QUESTIONS

1. About 2 weeks after birth, a neonate began to vomit shortly after feeding. Each time, the vomitus was propelled approximately 2 feet. The physician told the mother that her infant has an obstructing benign growth that causes a narrow outlet from the stomach. Is there an embryological basis for this defect?

2. Do infants with Down syndrome have an increased incidence of duodenal atresia? Can the condition be corrected?

3. A man claimed that his appendix was on his left side. Is this possible, and, if so, how could this happen?

4. A patient reported that she had two appendices and had separate operations to remove them. Do people ever have two appendices?

5. What is Hirschsprung disease? Some sources state that it is a congenital condition resulting from large intestine obstruction. Is this correct? If so, what is its embryological basis?

6. A nurse observed what appeared to be feces being expelled from a baby's umbilicus. How could this happen? If so, what conditions would likely be present?

The answers to these questions are at the back of this book.

Urogenital System 13

The **urogenital system** is divided functionally into the **urinary system** and **genital system** and develops from the **intermediate mesenchyme** from the dorsal body wall of the embryo (Fig. 13.1A and B). During folding of the embryo in the horizontal plane (see Chapter 6), the mesenchyme is carried ventrally and loses its connection with the somites (see Fig. 13.1C and D). A longitudinal elevation of the mesenchyme—the **urogenital ridge**—forms on each side of the dorsal aorta (see Fig. 13.1D). The part of the urogenital ridge giving rise to the urinary system is the **nephrogenic cord** (see Fig. 13.1C and D); the part that gives rise to the genital system is the **gonadal ridge** (see Fig 13.2C).

DEVELOPMENT OF URINARY SYSTEM

The urinary system begins to develop before the genital system and consists of the kidneys, ureters, urinary bladder, and urethra.

DEVELOPMENT OF KIDNEYS AND URETERS

Three sets of successive kidneys develop in human embryos. The first set—the **pronephroi**—is rudimentary and nonfunctional. The second set—the **mesonephroi**—is well developed and functions briefly during the early period. The third set—the **metanephroi**—forms the permanent kidneys.

PRONEPHROI

The bilateral, transitory pronephroi appear early in the fourth week. They are represented by a few cell clusters in the neck region (Fig. 13.3A). The pronephric ducts run caudally and open into the cloaca (see Fig. 13.3B). The pronephroi soon degenerate; however, most parts of the **pronephric ducts** persist and are used by the second set of kidneys.

MESONEPHROI

These large, elongated excretory organs appear late in the fourth week, caudal to the pronephroi (see Fig. 13.3). The mesonephric kidneys consist of approximately 40 **glomeruli** with **mesonephric tubules** (Fig. 13.4C–F). The tubules open into the **mesonephric ducts**, originally the pronephric ducts. The mesonephric ducts open into the cloaca (see Fig. 12.21A). The mesonephroi create urine between weeks 6 and 10, until the permanent kidneys begin to function (see Fig. 13.4). The mesonephroi degenerate toward the end of the first trimester (3 months); however, their tubules become the **efferent ductules of the testes**. The mesonephric ducts have several adult derivatives in males (Table 13.1).

METANEPHROI

The metanephroi—**primordia of the permanent kidneys**—begin to develop early in the fifth week (Fig. 13.5) and become functional approximately 4 weeks later. **Urine formation** continues throughout fetal life. The urine is excreted through the urethra into the amniotic cavity and forms a portion of the amniotic fluid.

The permanent kidneys develop from two sources (see Fig. 13.5A):

- The ureteric bud (metanephric diverticulum)
- The metanephrogenic blastema (metanephric mass of mesenchyme)

The **ureteric bud** is a diverticulum (outgrowth) from the mesonephric duct near its entrance into the cloaca. The ureteric bud is the primordium of the ureter, renal pelvis, calices (subdivisions of the renal pelvis), and collecting tubules (see Fig. 13.5B–E). The elongating bud penetrates the **metanephrogenic blastema**—a mass of cells derived from the **nephrogenic cord**—that forms the nephrons (see Fig. 13.5A). The **stalk of the ureteric bud** becomes the **ureter**, and the cranial part of the diverticulum undergoes repetitive branching. The branches differentiate into the **collecting tubules of the metanephros** (Fig. 13.6; see also Fig. 13.5C–E).

The **straight collecting tubules** undergo repeated branching, forming successive generations of collecting tubules. The first four generations of tubules enlarge and coalesce to form the **major calices** (see Fig. 13.5C–E); the second four generations coalesce to form the **minor calices**. The end of each **arched collecting tubule** induces clusters of mesenchymal cells in the metanephrogenic blastema to form small **metanephric vesicles** (see Fig. 13.6A). These vesicles elongate and become the metanephric tubules (see Fig. 13.6B and C). The proximal ends of these tubules are invaginated by **glomeruli**. The renal corpuscle (glomerulus and its capsule) and its proximal convoluted tubule, the **nephron loop** (Henle loop), and the distal convoluted tubule constitute a **nephron** (see Fig. 13.6D). Each distal convoluted tubule contacts an arched collecting tubule. The collecting tubules become confluent, forming a **uriniferous tubule**.

Branching of the metanephric diverticulum depends on an inductive signal from the metanephric mesoderm. Differentiation of the nephrons depends on induction by the collecting tubules. The molecular aspects of the reciprocal interactions between the metanephric mesenchyme and collecting tubules are shown in Fig. 13.7.

The **fetal kidneys are subdivided into lobes**. The lobulation usually disappears during infancy as the nephrons increase in size. Nephron formation is complete at birth,

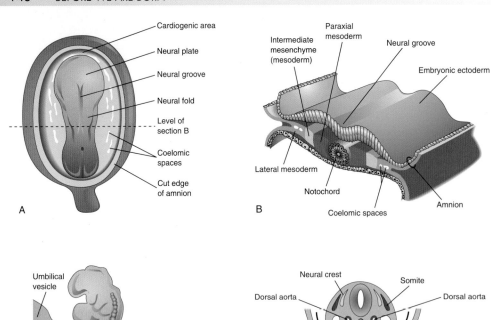

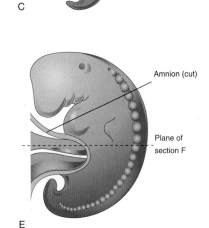

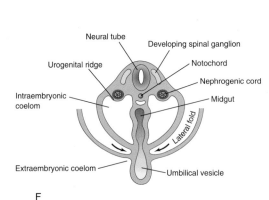

Fig. 13.1 (A) Dorsal view of an embryo during the third week (approximately 18 days). (B) Transverse section of the embryo showing the position of the intermediate mesenchyme before lateral folding occurs. (C) Transverse section of the embryo after the commencement of folding, showing the nephrogenic cords. (D) Transverse section of the embryo, showing the lateral folds meeting each other ventrally. (E) Lateral view of an embryo later in the fourth week (approximately 26 days). (F) Transverse section of the embryo, showing the lateral folds meeting each other ventrally.

except in premature infants. Each kidney contains between 200,000 and 2 million nephrons. Functional maturation of the kidneys occurs between 14 and 16 weeks with increasing rate of filtration until after birth, but no additional nephrons are formed, and limited numbers may result in significant consequences in the child and adult.

POSITIONAL CHANGES OF KIDNEYS

The developing metanephric kidneys lie close to each other in the pelvis (Fig. 13.8A). As the abdomen and pelvis grow, the kidneys gradually become repositioned to the abdomen and move farther apart (see Fig. 13.8B and C). They attain their adult position on either side of the vertebral column by the ninth week (see Fig. 13.8D) resulting mainly from straightening of the vertebral

curvature and the relative growth of the embryo's thorax and abdomen caudal to the kidneys. As the kidneys change their positions, they also rotate medially almost 90 degrees. By the ninth week, the kidneys come in contact with the **suprarenal glands** as the former attain their adult position (see Fig. 13.8D).

CHANGES IN BLOOD SUPPLY OF KIDNEYS

Initially, the **renal arteries** are branches of the **common iliac arteries** (see Fig. 13.8A and B). Later, the kidneys receive their blood supply from the distal end of the aorta (see Fig. 13.8C). The kidneys receive their most cranial arterial branches, which become the renal arteries, from the **abdominal aorta**. Normally, the caudal primordial branches undergo involution and disappear (see Fig. 13.8C and D).

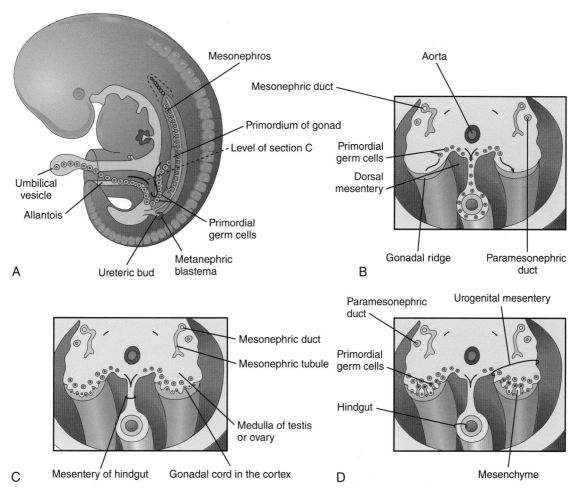

Fig. 13.2 (A) Sketch of a 5-week embryo illustrating the migration of primordial germ cells from the umbilical vesicle into the embryo. (B) Transverse section showing the gonadal ridges and the migration of primordial germ cells into the developing gonads. (C) Transverse section of a 6-week embryo showing the gonadal cords. (D) Similar section at a later stage showing the indifferent gonads and paramesonephric ducts.

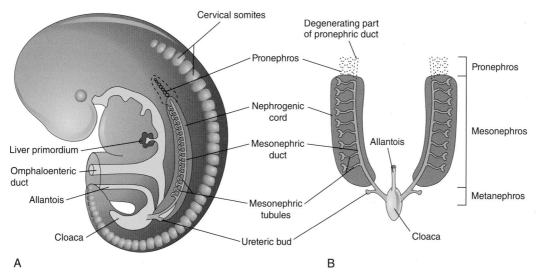

Fig. 13.3 Illustrations of the three sets of nephric systems in an embryo during the fifth week. (A) Lateral view. (B) Ventral view. The mesonephric tubules are pulled laterally; their normal position is shown in (A).

Table 13.1   Adult Derivatives and Vestigial Remains of Embryonic Urogenital Structures[a]

Embryonic Structure	Female	Male
Indifferent gonad	*Ovary*	*Testis*
Cortex	*Ovarian follicles*	*Seminiferous tubules*
Medulla	*Rete ovarii*	*Rete testis*
Gubernaculum	*Ovarian ligament*	Gubernaculum testis
	Round ligament of uterus	
Mesonephric tubules	Epoophoron	*Efferent ductules of testis*
	Paroophoron	Paradidymis
Mesonephric duct	Appendix vesiculosa	Appendix of epididymis
	Duct of epoophoron	*Duct of epididymis*
	Longitudinal duct (Gartner duct)	*Ductus deferens*
		Ejaculatory duct and seminal gland
Stalk of ureteric bud	*Ureter, pelvis, calices, and collecting tubules*	*Ureter, pelvis, calices, and collecting tubules*
Paramesonephric duct	Hydatid (of Morgagni)	Appendix of testis
	Uterine tube	
	Uterus, cervix	
Urogenital sinus	*Urinary bladder*	*Urinary bladder*
	Urethra	*Urethra (except navicular fossa)*
	Vagina	Prostatic utricle
	Urethral and paraurethral glands	*Prostate*
	Greater vestibular glands	*Bulbourethral glands*
Sinus tubercle	Hymen	Seminal colliculus
Primordial phallus	*Clitoris*	*Penis*
	Glans clitoris	*Glans penis*
	Corpora cavernosa of clitoris	*Corpora cavernosa of penis*
	Bulb of vestibule	*Corpus spongiosum of penis*
Urogenital folds	*Labia minora*	*Ventral aspect of penis*
Labioscrotal swellings	*Labia majora*	*Scrotum*

[a]Functional derivatives are in italics.

Accessory Renal Arteries

The common variations in the blood supply to the kidneys reflect the manner in which the blood supply continually changes during embryonic and early fetal life (see Fig. 13.8). Approximately 25% of adult kidneys have two to four renal arteries. **Accessory (supernumerary) renal arteries** usually arise from the aorta, superior or inferior to the main renal artery (Fig. 13.9A and B). An accessory artery to the inferior pole (polar renal artery) may cross anterior to the ureter and obstruct it, causing **hydronephrosis**—distention of the pelvis and calices with urine (see Fig. 13.9B). Accessory renal arteries are end arteries; consequently, if an accessory artery is damaged or ligated, the part of the kidney supplied by it will become ischemic. Accessory arteries are approximately twice as common as accessory veins. Diagnostic computed tomographic imaging and identification of accessory renal arteries are essential for surgical procedures to avoid a fatal outcome.

Congenital Anomalies of Kidneys and Ureters

Unilateral renal agenesis (absence of kidney) occurs in approximately 1 in 1000 neonates (Fig. 13.10A). Males are affected more often than females, and the left kidney is usually the one that is absent. The other kidney usually undergoes **compensatory hypertrophy** and performs the function of the missing kidney.

Bilateral renal agenesis is associated with oligohydramnios because little or no urine is excreted into the amniotic cavity. This condition occurs in approximately 1 in 3000 births and is incompatible with postnatal life. This defect is three times more common in males. These infants also have **pulmonary hypoplasia**. Failure of the ureteric bud to penetrate the metanephric blastema results in the absence of renal development because no nephrons are induced by the collecting tubules to develop from the blastema.

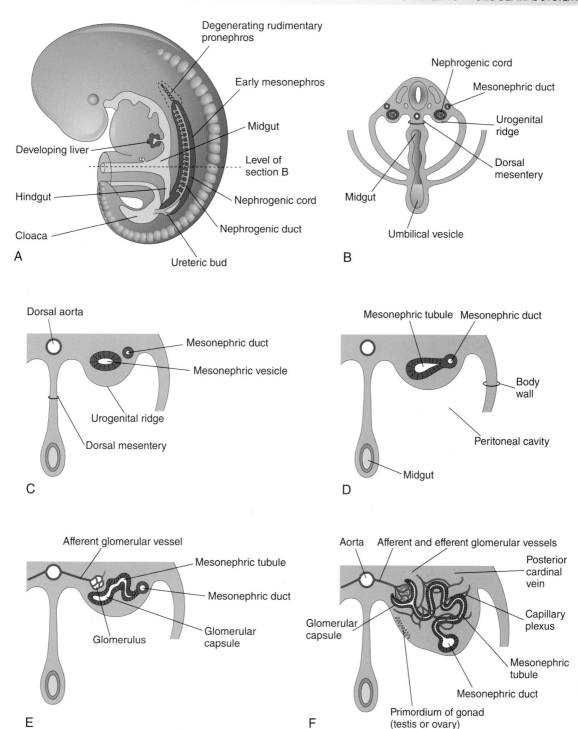

Fig. 13.4   (A) Lateral view of a 5-week embryo showing the extent of the early mesonephros and ureteric bud, the primordium of the metaneph-ros (primordium of the permanent kidney). (B) Transverse section of the embryo showing the nephrogenic cords from which the mesonephric tubules develop. (C–F) Successive stages in the development of mesonephric tubules between the 5th and 11th weeks. The expanded medial end of the mesonephric tubule is invaginated by blood vessels to form a glomerular capsule.

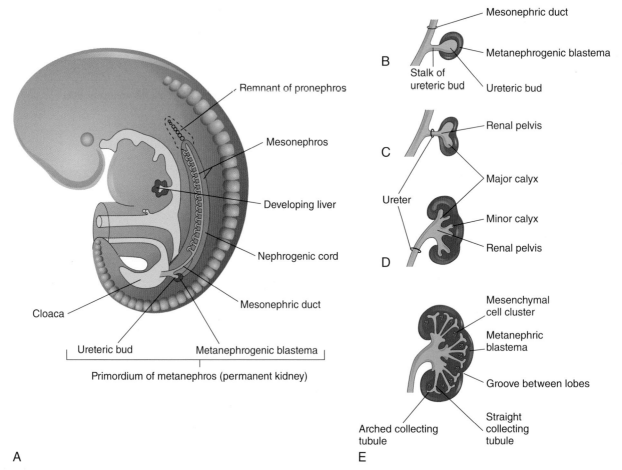

Fig. 13.5 Development of the permanent kidney. (A) Lateral view of a 5-week embryo showing the ureteric bud, the primordium of the meta-nephros. (B–E) Successive stages in the development of the ureteric bud (fifth to eighth weeks). Observe the development of the kidney: ureter, renal pelvis, calices, and collecting tubules.

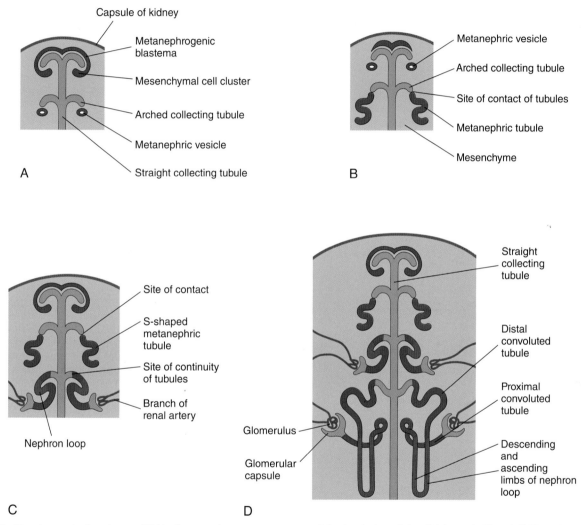

Fig. 13.6 Development of nephrons. (A) Nephrogenesis commences around the beginning of the eighth week. (B and C) Note that the metanephric tubules, the primordia of the nephrons, connect with the collecting tubules to form uriniferous tubules. (D) Observe that nephrons are derived from the metanephric blastema, and the collecting tubules are derived from the ureteric bud.

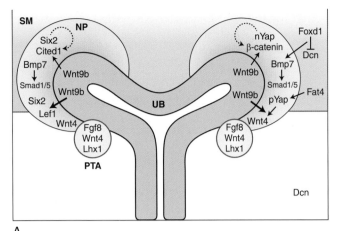

A

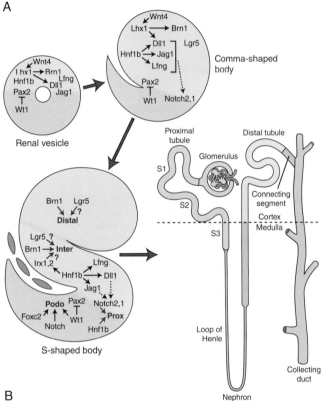

B

Fig. 13.7   Molecular control of kidney development. (A) Regulation of nephron progenitor induction. The self-renewing nephron progenitors are demarcated by the expression of Six2 and Cited1. Six2 promotes self-renewal in addition to Wnt9b signals from the ureteric bud, which directly promote the expression of progenitor genes such as Cited1. nYap signaling may also cooperate with β-catenin induced from canonical Wnt9b signals to promote progenitor self-renewal. Bmp7-SMAD signaling promotes the conversion of nephron progenitors to a Six2+Cited1- state, where they can be induced by Wnt9b and turn on differentiation markers Lef1 and Wnt4. These cells form the pretubular aggregate (PTA) highlighted by the expression of critical differentiation factors Fgf8, Wnt4, and Lhx1. Foxd1+ stromal cells promote Bmp7-SMAD signaling in the nephron progenitors by repressing Dcn, an antagonist of Bmp7 activity. Stromal Fat4 regulates the induction process by inducing nuclear export and phosphorylation of Yap, which allows Wnt9b inductive signals to promote differentiation of the nephron progenitors. *Dotted arrow* represents promotion of self-renewal. (B) Regulation of nephron patterning. Proximal/distal polarity is established in the renal vesicle and demarcated by the expression of several genes, including three Notch ligands: Dll1, Lfng, and Jag1. The Notch pathway establishes a proximal polarity that is carried through the comma- and S-shaped body stages and integral for proximal tubule and podocyte development. Wt1 also promotes proximal fate, specifically that of the podocyte, by antagonizing Pax2, and cooperating with Notch pathway components and Foxc2, to regulate genes necessary for podocyte development. Endothelial cells are recruited by signals from developing podocytes of the S-shaped body. Hnf1b promotes proximal and intermediate/medial fate through the regulation of Notch ligand expression and other factors such as Irx1/2, which may play a role in medial segment differentiation. Intermediate and distal fates are regulated by Brn1, which establishes distal polarity starting at the renal vesicle stage. Lgr5 is expressed in the distal segment of the comma-shaped body and the distal and intermediate segments of the S-shaped body; however, a direct role in establishing or maintaining these segments has not been shown. Proximal polarity establishes the glomerulus and S1–S3 segments of the proximal tubule. Intermediate segments give rise to the loop of Henle. Distal segments establish the distal tubule, which hooks up to the collecting duct through a connecting segment. *?* represents direct role not established; *dashed arrow* represents ligand–receptor engagement. *Inter,* Intermediate; *NP,* nephron progenitors; *Podo,* podocyte; *Prox,* proximal; *SM,* stromal mesenchyme; *UB,* ureteric bud. (From O'Brien LL, McMahon AP: Induction and patterning of the metanephric nephron, *Semin Cell Devel Biol* 36:31–38, 2014.)

Cystic Kidney Disease

Autosomal dominant polycystic kidney disease (ADPKD) is the most common of all heritable cystic kidney diseases (1:500). Most commonly, PKD-1 and PKD-2 pathogenic variants (mutations) are responsible; these encode for polycystin 1 and 2, respectively. These two molecules are mechanoreceptors localized to primary cilia of the kidney—they detect urine flow in the tubules. The main clinical findings in ADPKD are cysts involving <5% of nephrons. These cysts can enlarge and reduce normal kidney function.

Malrotation of Kidneys

If the kidney does not rotate, the hilum faces anteriorly (see Fig. 13.10C). If the hilum faces posteriorly, rotation has progressed too far; if it faces laterally, medial rotation has occurred. Malrotation of the kidneys is often associated with ectopic kidneys.

Ectopic Kidneys

One or both kidneys may be in an abnormal position (see Fig. 13.10B and E). Most ectopic kidneys are located in the pelvis, but some lie in the inferior part of the abdomen. Pelvic kidneys and other forms of ectopia result from the failure of the kidneys to ascend.

Fusion Anomalies

Crossed Fused Ectopia

Sometimes a kidney crosses to the other side, resulting in crossed renal ectopia, with or without fusion. An unusual kidney defect is **unilateral fused kidneys** (see Fig. 13.10D). In such cases, the developing kidneys fuse while they are in the pelvis, and one kidney moves to its normal position, carrying the other one with it.

Horseshoe Kidney

Horseshoe kidney is the most common renal fusion defect. In 0.2% of the population, the poles of the kidneys are fused (usually the inferior poles) (Fig. 13.11). The large U-shaped (horseshoe) kidney is usually located in the pelvic region, anterior to the inferior lumbar vertebrae. In 60% of cases, normal ascent of the fused kidneys does not occur, and it is found below the **inferior mesenteric artery**. The function of these kidneys is preserved, and each has a normal ureter and blood supply. A horseshoe kidney may produce no symptoms but is prone to increased occurrence of renal stones and infection. Approximately 15% of people with Turner syndrome have horseshoe kidneys (see Fig. 19.3).

Duplications of Urinary Tract

Duplications of the abdominal part of the ureter and renal pelvis are common, but a kidney in excess of the normal number **(supernumerary kidney)** is rare (see Fig. 13.10C and F). These duplicates often result from the division of a ureteric bud. Partial division results in a divided kidney with a bifid ureter (see Fig. 13.10B). Complete division results in a double kidney with a bifid ureter or with separate ureters (see Fig. 13.10C). A supernumerary kidney with its own ureter probably results from the formation of two ureteric buds (see Fig. 13.10F).

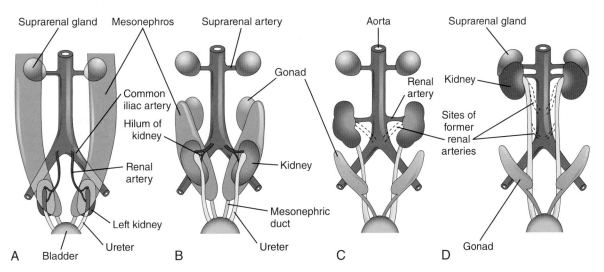

Fig. 13.8 (A–D) Diagrammatic ventral views of the abdominopelvic region of embryos and fetuses (sixth to ninth weeks), showing medial rotation and relocation of the kidneys from the pelvis to the abdomen. (C and D) Note that, as the kidneys relocate (ascend), they are supplied by arteries at successively higher levels and that the hila of the kidneys (where the vessels and nerves enter) are directed anteromedially.

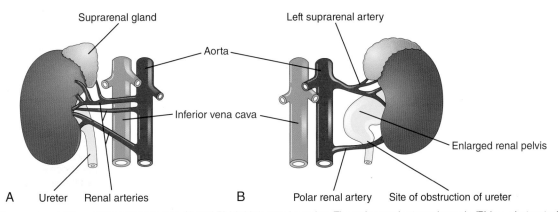

Fig. 13.9 Common variations of the renal arteries. (A and B) Multiple renal arteries. The polar renal artery shown in (B) has obstructed the ureter and produced an enlarged renal pelvis.

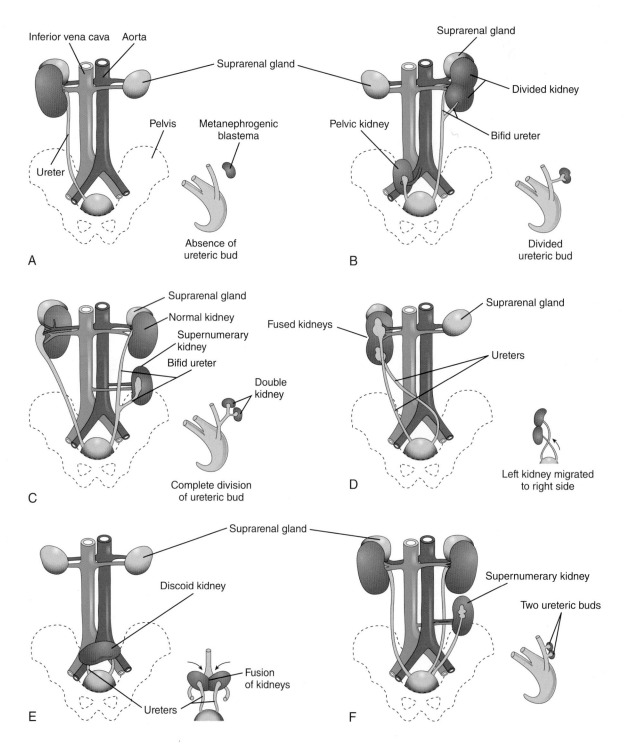

Fig. 13.10   Various birth defects of the urinary system. The small sketch to the lower right of each drawing illustrates the probable embryologic basis of the defect. (A) Unilateral renal agenesis. (B) Right side, pelvic kidney; left side, divided kidney with a bifid ureter. (C) Right side, malrotation of the kidney; the hilum is facing laterally. Left side, bifid ureter and the normal and a supernumerary kidney. (D) Crossed renal ectopia. The left kidney crossed to the right and fused with the right kidney. (E) Pelvic kidney or discoid kidney, resulting from fusion of the kidneys while they were in the pelvis. (F) Supernumerary left kidney resulting from the development of two ureteric buds.

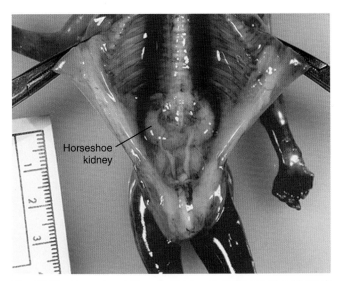

Fig. 13.11 Horseshoe kidney in the lower abdomen of a 13-week female fetus. This anomaly resulted from the fusion of the inferior poles of the kidneys while they were in the pelvis. (Courtesy Dr. D.K. Kalousek, Department of Pathology, University of British Columbia, Children's Hospital, Vancouver, British Columbia, Canada.)

DEVELOPMENT OF URINARY BLADDER

The urogenital sinus is divided into three parts (Fig. 13.12C):

- A **vesical part** that forms most of the bladder and is continuous with the allantois
- A **pelvic part** that becomes the urethra in the neck of the bladder, the prostatic part of the urethra in males, and the entire urethra in females
- A **phallic part** that grows toward the genital tubercle—the primordium of the penis or the clitoris

The bladder develops mainly from the vesical part of the urogenital sinus (see Fig. 13.12C), but the **trigone** of the bladder is derived from the caudal ends of the mesonephric ducts (see Fig. 13.12A and B). Initially, the bladder is continuous with the **allantois** (see Fig. 13.12C). The allantois constricts and becomes a thick, fibrous cord, the **urachus** (see Fig. 13.12G and H). In adults, the urachus is represented by the **median umbilical ligament**. As the bladder enlarges, distal parts of the mesonephric ducts are incorporated into its dorsal wall (see Fig. 13.12B–H). The epithelium of the entire bladder is derived from the endoderm of the urogenital sinus. The other layers of the bladder wall develop from the adjacent splanchnic mesenchyme. As the mesonephric ducts are absorbed, the ureters open separately into the urinary bladder (see Fig. 13.12C–H). In males, the orifices of the mesonephric ducts move close together and enter the prostatic part of the urethra (see Fig. 13.13C) as the caudal ends of these ducts become the ejaculatory ducts (see Fig. 13.13A). In females, the distal ends of the mesonephric ducts degenerate.

DEVELOPMENT OF URETHRA

The epithelium of most of the male urethra and the entire female urethra is derived from the endoderm of the **urogenital sinus** (Fig. 13.17; see also Fig. 13.12A and B). The

Ectopic Ureter

In males, an ectopic ureter may open into the neck of the bladder or the prostatic part of the urethra. It may also enter the ductus deferens, prostatic utricle, or seminal gland (see Fig. 13.13). In females, an ectopic ureter may enter the neck of the bladder, urethra, vagina, or vestibule of the vagina. An ectopic ureter results when the ureter is carried caudally with the mesonephric duct and is incorporated into the caudal portion of the vesical part of the urogenital sinus. **Incontinence** may result and urine may leak from the urethra in males and the urethra and/or vagina in females.

Urachal Anomalies

A remnant of the urachal lumen may persist, typically in the inferior part of the **urachus**. In approximately 50% of cases, the lumen is continuous with the cavity of the bladder. Remnants of the epithelial lining of the urachus may give rise to **urachal cysts** (Fig. 13.14A). The patent inferior end of the urachus may dilate to form a **urachal sinus** that opens into the bladder. The lumen in the superior part of the urachus may also remain patent and form a urachal sinus that opens at the umbilicus (see Fig. 13.14B). Very rarely, the entire urachus remains patent and forms a **urachal fistula** that allows urine to escape from its umbilical orifice (see Fig. 13.14C).

Exstrophy of Bladder

Exstrophy of the bladder is a severe birth defect that occurs in approximately 1 in every 30,000 to 50,000 births, predominantly affecting females (Fig. 13.15). Exposure and protrusion of the mucosal surface of the posterior wall of the bladder characterize this birth defect. The trigone of the bladder and ureteric orifices are exposed, and urine dribbles intermittently from the everted bladder. In some cases, the penis is divided into two parts, and the scrotum is bifid (split). Exstrophy of the bladder is believed to be caused by the failure of the mesenchymal cells to migrate between the ectoderm and endoderm of the abdominal wall **(cloacal membrane)** during the fourth week (Fig. 13.16B and C). As a result, no muscle or connective tissue forms in the abdominal wall over the urinary bladder. **Rupture of the cloacal membrane** results in wide communication between the exterior and the mucous membrane of the bladder. Rupture of the cloacal membrane before division of the cloaca by the urorectal septum leads to **exstrophy of the cloaca**, resulting in exposure of both the bladder and hindgut.

distal part of the urethra in the **glans penis** is derived from a solid cord of ectodermal cells that grows from the tip of the glans and joins the rest of the spongy urethra (see Fig. 2.1B; Fig. 13.17A–C). Consequently, the epithelium of the terminal part of the urethra is derived from the surface ectoderm. The connective tissue and smooth muscle of the urethra in both sexes are derived from splanchnic mesenchyme.

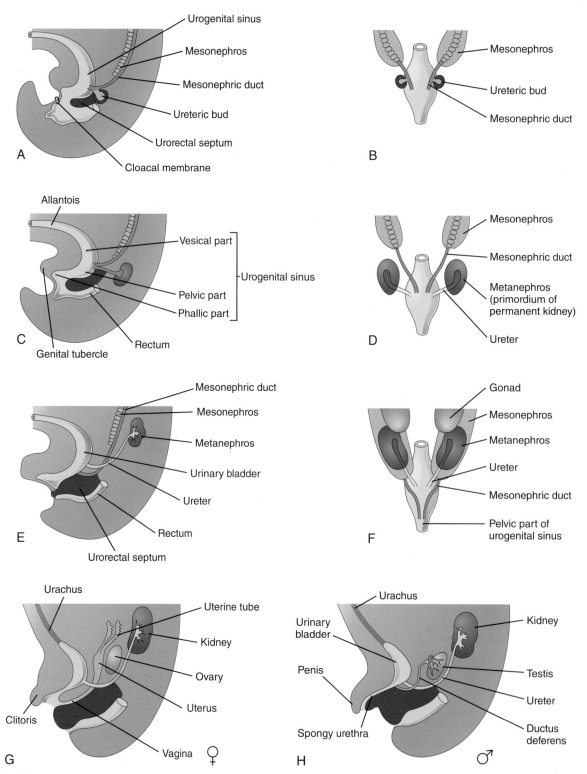

Fig. 13.12 (A) Lateral view of a 5-week embryo showing division of the cloaca by the urorectal septum into the urogenital sinus and rectum. (B, D, and F) Dorsal views showing the development of the kidneys and bladder and changes in the location of kidneys. (C, E, G, and H) Lateral views. The stages shown in (G) and (H) are reached by the 12th week.

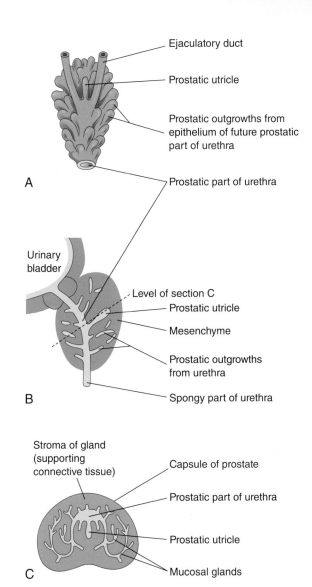

Fig. 13.13 (A) Dorsal view of the developing prostate in an 11-week fetus. (B) Sketch of a median section of the developing urethra and prostate showing numerous endodermal outgrowths from the prostatic urethra. The vestigial prostatic utricle is also shown. (C) Section of the prostate (16 weeks) at the level shown in (B).

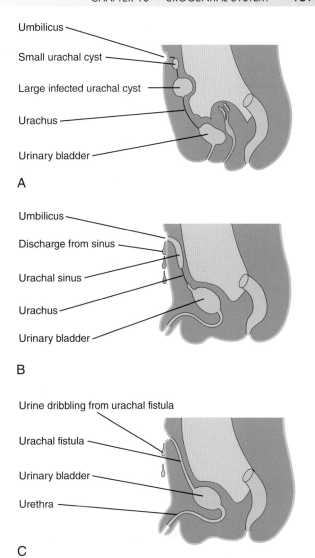

Fig. 13.14 Urachal anomalies. (A) Urachal cysts; the common site for them is in the superior end of the urachus, just inferior to the umbilicus. (B) Two types of urachal sinus are shown: one that opens into the bladder and another that opens at the umbilicus. (C) A urachal fistula connects the bladder and umbilicus.

DEVELOPMENT OF SUPRARENAL GLANDS

The **cortex and medulla** of the suprarenal glands have different origins (Fig. 13.18). The **cortex** develops from mesenchyme of the urogenital ridge and the **medulla** from **neural crest cells** (see Fig. 13.12A and B). During the sixth week, the cortex begins an aggregation of mesenchymal cells on each side of the embryo between the root of the dorsal mesentery and the developing gonad (see Fig. 13.18C). *DAX1, Sf1, and Pbx1 have been shown to be critical for cortex development.* Differentiation of the characteristic suprarenal cortical zones begins during the late fetal period (see Fig. 13.18C–E). The **zona glomerulosa** and the **zona fasciculata** are present at birth, but the **zona reticularis** is not recognizable until the end of the third year (see Fig. 13.18H).

Relative to body weight, the suprarenal glands of the fetus are 10 to 20 times larger than the adult glands and are large compared with the kidneys because of the extensive size of

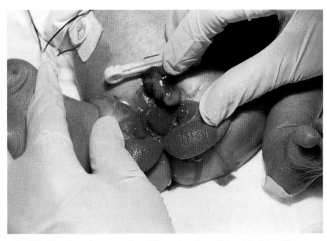

Fig. 13.15 A male neonate with exstrophy of the bladder. Because of defective closure of the inferior part of the anterior abdominal wall and anterior wall of the bladder, the urinary bladder appears as an everted, bulging mass inferior to the umbilicus. (Courtesy Dr. A.E. Chudley, Department of Pediatrics and Child Health, University of Manitoba, Children's Hospital, Winnipeg, Manitoba, Canada.)

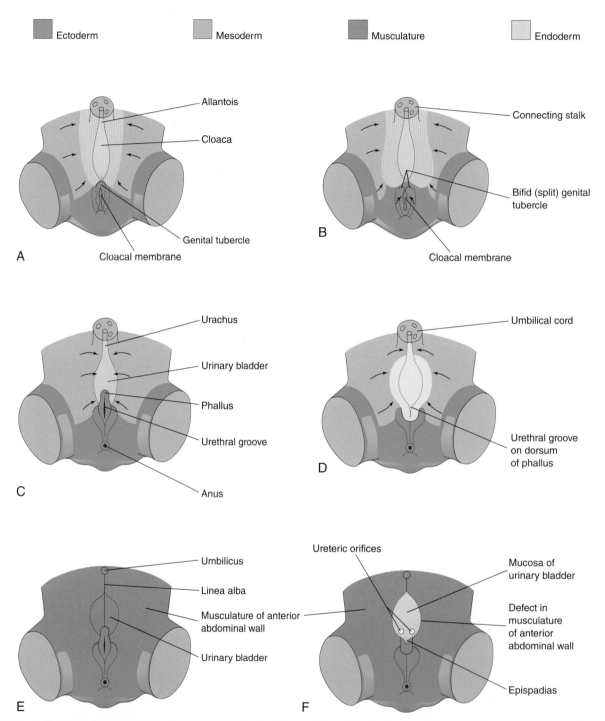

Ectoderm   Mesoderm   Musculature   Endoderm

A
Allantois
Cloaca
Genital tubercle
Cloacal membrane

B
Connecting stalk
Bifid (split) genital tubercle
Cloacal membrane

C
Urachus
Urinary bladder
Phallus
Urethral groove
Anus

D
Umbilical cord
Urethral groove on dorsum of phallus

E
Umbilicus
Linea alba
Musculature of anterior abdominal wall
Urinary bladder

F
Ureteric orifices
Mucosa of urinary bladder
Defect in musculature of anterior abdominal wall
Epispadias

Fig. 13.16 (A, C, and E) Normal stages in the development of the infraumbilical abdominal wall and the penis during the fourth to eighth weeks. (B, D, and F) Probable stages in the development of epispadias and exstrophy of the bladder with epispadias. (B and D) Note that the mesoderm fails to extend into the anterior abdominal wall anterior to the urinary bladder. Also note that the genital tubercle is located in a more caudal position than usual and that the urethral groove has formed on the dorsal surface of the penis. (F) The surface ectoderm and anterior wall of the bladder have ruptured, resulting in exposure of the posterior wall of the bladder. Note that the musculature of the anterior abdominal wall is present on each side of the defect. (Modified from Patten BM, Barry A: The genesis of exstrophy of the bladder and epispadias, *Am J Anat* 90:35, 1952.)

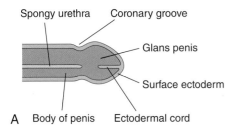

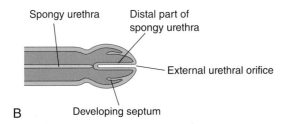

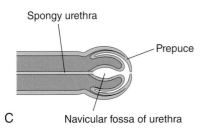

Fig. 13.17 Schematic longitudinal sections of the developing penis, illustrating development of the prepuce (foreskin) and the distal part of the spongy urethra. (A) At 11 weeks. (B) At 12 weeks. (C) At 14 weeks. The epithelium of the spongy urethra has a dual origin; most of it is derived from endoderm of the phallic part of the urogenital sinus; the distal part of the urethra lining the navicular fossa is derived from surface ectoderm.

the fetal suprarenal cortex. The medulla remains small until after birth (see Fig. 13.18F). The suprarenal glands rapidly become smaller as the cortex regresses during the first year of infancy (see Fig. 13.18G).

DEVELOPMENT OF GENITAL SYSTEM

The early genital systems in the two sexes are similar, and the initial period of genital development is referred to as the *indifferent stage of sexual development.*

DEVELOPMENT OF GONADS

The gonads, testes, and ovaries are the organs that produce sperms and oocytes, respectively. The gonads are derived from three sources (Fig. 13.12):

- Mesothelium (mesodermal epithelium) lining the posterior abdominal wall
- Underlying mesenchyme
- Primordial germ cells (earliest undifferentiated sex cells)

INDIFFERENT (BIPOTENTIAL) GONADS

Gonadal development begins during the fifth week when a thickened area of mesothelium develops on the medial side of the **mesonephros** (see Fig. 13.2A–C). Proliferation of this epithelium and underlying mesenchyme produces a bulge on the medial side of the mesonephros—the **gonadal ridge** (see Fig. 13.2A and C). Finger-like epithelial cords—**gonadal cords**—soon grow into the underlying mesenchyme (see Fig. 13.2D). The indifferent gonads now consist of an external cortex and an internal medulla (Fig. 13.19). *It appears that FOG2, WT1, and NR5A1 are required to form the bipotential gonad.*

In embryos with an **XX sex chromosome complex**, the cortex of the indifferent gonad differentiates into an ovary and the medulla regresses. In embryos with an **XY sex chromosome complex**, the medulla differentiates into a testis and the cortex regresses (see Fig. 13.2D).

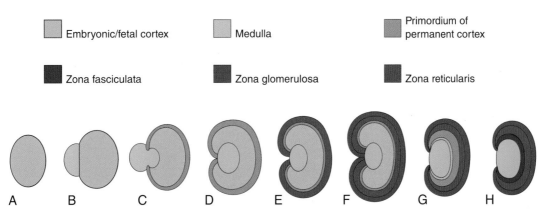

Fig. 13.18 Schematic drawings illustrating the development of the suprarenal glands. (A) At 6 weeks, showing the mesodermal primordium of the embryonic cortex. (B) At 7 weeks, showing the addition of neural crest cells. (C) At 8 weeks, showing the fetal cortex and early permanent cortex beginning to encapsulate the medulla. (D and E) Later stages of encapsulation of the medulla by the cortex. (F) Gland of a neonate showing the fetal cortex and two zones of the permanent cortex. (G) At 1 year the fetal cortex has almost disappeared. (H) At 4 years, showing the adult pattern of cortical zones. Observe that the fetal cortex has disappeared and that the gland is smaller than it was at birth (F).

PRIMORDIAL GERM CELLS

The **primordial germ cells** originate in the wall of the umbilical vesicle (from the epiblast) and migrate along the dorsal mesentery of the hindgut to the gonadal ridges (see Fig. 13.2D). *Early chemotactic signaling by stem cell factor and later nerve tract guidance appears to help the cells migrate to the gonadal ridges.* During the sixth week, the primordial germ cells enter the underlying mesenchyme and are incorporated into the **gonadal cords** (see Fig. 13.2D). They eventually differentiate into oocytes or sperms.

SEX DETERMINATION

Chromosomal and genetic sex, established at fertilization, depends on whether an X-bearing or a Y-bearing sperm fertilizes the X-bearing oocyte. The type of gonads that develop is normally determined by the **sex chromosome complex** of the embryo (XX or XY). Before the seventh week, the gonads of the two sexes are identical in appearance (see Fig. 13.19). Development of a male phenotype requires a functional Y chromosome. Two X chromosomes are required for the development of the female phenotype.

DEVELOPMENT OF TESTES

A coordinated sequence of genes induces the development of testes. The *SRY* gene (sex-determining region on the Y) for a **testis-determining factor (TDF)** acts as the switch that directs the development of the indifferent gonad into a testis. TDF induces the gonadal cords to condense and extend into the medulla of the indifferent gonad, where they branch and anastomose to form the **rete testis** (see Fig. 13.19). The connection of the prominent gonadal cords—the **seminiferous cords**—with the surface epithelium is lost when the **tunica albuginea** develops. This dense tunica, a thick fibrous capsule, is a characteristic feature of testicular development. Gradually, the testis separates from the degenerating mesonephros and becomes suspended by its own mesentery, the **mesorchium**. The seminiferous cords develop into the seminiferous tubules, tubuli recti, and rete testis.

The **seminiferous tubules** are separated by mesenchyme, giving rise to the **interstitial cells** (Leydig cells). By the eighth week, these cells secrete the androgenic hormone **testosterone**, which induces masculine differentiation of the mesonephric ducts and external genitalia. Testosterone production is stimulated by human chorionic gonadotropin, which reaches peak amounts during the 8th to 12th week. The fetal testes also produce a glycoprotein, **antimüllerian hormone (AMH)** or müllerian-inhibiting substance, beginning in week 8. AMH is produced by the **sustentacular cells (Sertoli cells)**, which continues until puberty, after which the levels of the hormone decrease. *Expression of the transcription factor SOX9 is essential in the differentiation of Sertoli cells in the testes.* AMH suppresses the development of the paramesonephric ducts, which form the uterus and uterine tubes. The seminiferous tubules remain until puberty, when lumina begin to develop. In addition to sustentacular cells, the walls of the seminiferous tubules are composed of (see Fig. 13.19):

- **Spermatogonia**, the primordial sperm cells derived from the primordial germ cells
- **Sertoli cells**, which constitute most of the seminiferous epithelium in the fetal testis (see Fig. 13.19)

The **rete testis** becomes continuous with 15 to 20 mesonephric tubules, which become **efferent ductules**. These ductules are connected with the mesonephric duct, which becomes the **ductus epididymis** (Fig. 13.20A; see also Figs. 13.19).

DEVELOPMENT OF OVARIES

Ovarian development occurs approximately 3 weeks later (by week 10) than testicular development. *The X chromosomes have genes that contribute to ovarian development (e.g., DAX1); autosomal genes also appear to play a role in ovarian organogenesis with factors including FOXL2, WNT, and Iroquois-1 involved.* The ovary is not identifiable by histologic examination until approximately the 10th week. **Gonadal cords** extend into the medulla of the ovary and form a rudimentary **rete ovarii** (see Figs. 13.2D and 13.19). This network of canals and gonadal cords normally degenerates and disappears. **Cortical cords** extend from the surface epithelium of the developing ovary into the underlying mesenchyme during the early fetal period. As the cortical cords increase in size, **primordial germ cells** are incorporated into them. At approximately 16 weeks, these cords begin to break up into isolated cell clusters—**primordial follicles**—each of which consists of an **oogonium** (derived from a primordial germ cell). The follicles are surrounded by a layer of follicular cells derived from the surface epithelium (see Fig. 13.19). Active mitosis produces many oogonia during fetal life.

No oogonia form postnatally. Although many oogonia degenerate before birth, 2 million or so enlarge to become **primary oocytes** (see Fig. 2.5) before birth. After birth, the surface epithelium of the ovary flattens to a single layer of cells that is continuous with the mesothelium of the peritoneum. The surface epithelium becomes separated from the follicles in the cortex by a thin fibrous capsule, the **tunica albuginea**. As the ovary separates from the regressing mesonephros, it is suspended by its mesentery, the **mesovarium** (see Fig. 13.19).

DEVELOPMENT OF GENITAL DUCTS

12

Both male and female embryos have two pairs of genital ducts: **mesonephric ducts** (wolffian ducts) and **paramesonephric ducts** (müllerian ducts) (Fig. 13.21A). The mesonephric ducts play an essential role in the development of the male reproductive system (see Fig. 13.20A), and the paramesonephric ducts play an essential role in the development of the female reproductive system (see Table 13.1 and Fig. 13.20B and C). During conversion of the mesonephric and paramesonephric ducts into adult structures, some parts of the ducts remain as **vestigial structures** (see Fig. 13.20A–C). These vestiges are rarely seen unless pathologic changes develop in them (e.g., Gartner duct cysts; see Fig. 13.20C).

DEVELOPMENT OF MALE GENITAL DUCTS AND GLANDS

Testosterone stimulates the mesonephric ducts to form male genital ducts, whereas AMH causes the paramesonephric ducts to regress by epithelial–mesenchymal transformation. As the mesonephros degenerates, some mesonephric tubules persist and are transformed into **efferent ductules** (see Fig. 13.20A). These ductules open into the mesonephric

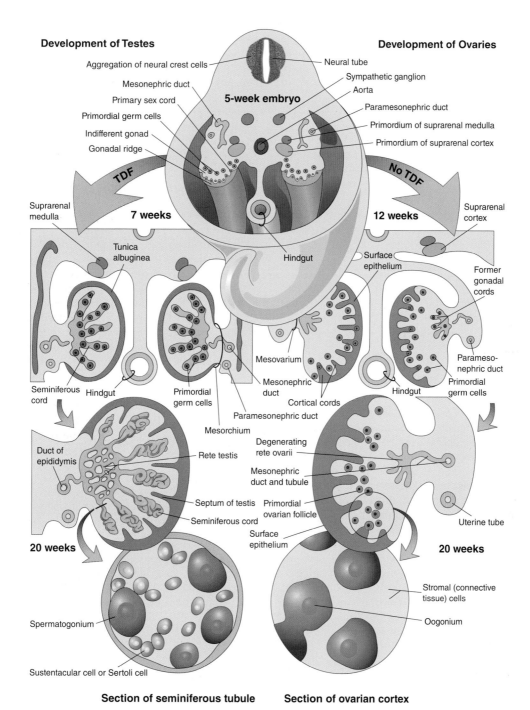

Development of Testes

Development of Ovaries

Aggregation of neural crest cells — Neural tube
— Sympathetic ganglion
Mesonephric duct — Aorta
Primary sex cord — Paramesonephric duct
Primordial germ cells — Primordium of suprarenal medulla
Indifferent gonad — Primordium of suprarenal cortex
Gonadal ridge

5-week embryo

TDF   No TDF

Suprarenal medulla   **7 weeks**   **12 weeks**   Suprarenal cortex

Tunica albuginea   Surface epithelium   Former gonadal cords

Hindgut   Mesovarium   Paramesonephric duct
Seminiferous cord   Hindgut   Mesonephric duct   Hindgut   Primordial germ cells
Primordial germ cells   Cortical cords
Paramesonephric duct
Mesorchium

Duct of epididymis   Rete testis   Degenerating rete ovarii
Mesonephric duct and tubule
Septum of testis   Primordial ovarian follicle   Uterine tube
Seminiferous cord
Surface epithelium
20 weeks   **20 weeks**

Stromal (connective tissue) cells
Spermatogonium   Oogonium

Sustentacular cell or Sertoli cell

Section of seminiferous tubule   **Section of ovarian cortex**

Fig. 13.19 Schematic illustrations showing differentiation of the indifferent gonads in a 5-week embryo (*top*) into ovaries or testes. The **left side** of the drawing shows the development of testes resulting from the effects of the testis-determining factor (TDF) located on the Y chromosome. Note that the gonadal cords become seminiferous cords, the primordia of the seminiferous tubules. The parts of the gonadal cords that enter the medulla of the testis form the rete testis. In the section of the testis at the *bottom left*, observe that there are two kinds of cells: spermatogonia, derived from the primordial germ cells; and sustentacular or Sertoli cells, derived from mesenchyme. The **right side** shows the development of ovaries in the absence of TDF. Cortical cords have extended from the surface epithelium of the gonad, and primordial germ cells have entered them. They are the primordia of the oogonia. Follicular cells are derived from the surface epithelium of the gonad, and primordial germ cells have entered them. They are the primordia of the oogonia. Follicular cells are derived from the surface epithelium of the ovaries. The *arrows* indicate the changes that occur as the gonads (testes and ovaries) develop.

duct, which has been transformed into the **duct of epididymis** in this region. Distal to the epididymis, the mesonephric duct acquires a thick investment of smooth muscle and becomes the **ductus deferens** (see Fig. 13.20A).

Seminal Glands. Lateral outgrowths from the caudal end of each mesonephric duct become **seminal glands** (vesicles). The secretions of this pair of glands nourish the sperms. The part of the mesonephric duct between the duct of this gland and the urethra becomes the **ejaculatory duct** (see Fig. 13.20A).

Prostate. Multiple endodermal outgrowths arise from the prostatic part of the urethra and grow into the surrounding urogenital sinus mesenchyme (Fig. 13.13). The glandular epithelium of the prostate differentiates from these endodermal cells, and the associated mesenchyme differentiates into the dense stroma and smooth muscle of the prostate. Secretions from the prostate contribute to the semen.

Bulbourethral Glands. The bulbourethral glands are pea-sized structures that develop from paired outgrowths derived from the spongy part of the urethra (see Fig. 13.20A). The smooth muscle fibers and the stroma differentiate from the adjacent mesenchyme. Secretions from these glands also contribute to the semen.

DEVELOPMENT OF FEMALE GENITAL DUCTS AND GLANDS

The mesonephric ducts of female embryos regress because of the absence of testosterone. The paramesonephric ducts develop because of the absence of AMH. Female sexual development does not depend on the presence of ovaries or hormones until puberty. The **paramesonephric ducts** form most of the female genital tract. The **uterine tubes** develop from the unfused cranial parts of the paramesonephric ducts (see Fig. 13.20B and C). The caudal, fused portions of these ducts form the **uterovaginal primordium**, which gives rise to the **uterus** and the superior portion of the **vagina** (see Fig. 13.21). *Expression of Hox genes in the paramesonephric ducts regulates the development of the female genital ducts.* The endometrial stroma and myometrium are derived from splanchnic mesenchyme. Fusion of the paramesonephric ducts also forms a peritoneal fold that becomes the **broad ligament** and forms two peritoneal compartments—the **rectouterine pouch** and **vesicouterine pouch** (Fig. 13.22B–D).

Development of the Vagina. The vaginal epithelium is derived from the endoderm of the **urogenital sinus**. The fibromuscular wall of the vagina develops from the surrounding mesenchyme. Contact of the **uterovaginal primordium** with the urogenital sinus, forming the **sinus tubercle** (see Fig. 13.21B), induces the formation of paired endodermal outgrowths—**sinovaginal bulbs** (see Fig. 13.22A). They extend from the urogenital sinus to the caudal end of the uterovaginal primordium. The sinovaginal bulbs fuse to form a **vaginal plate** (see Fig. 13.20B). The central cells of this plate break down, forming the **lumen of the vagina**. The peripheral cells of the plate form the vaginal epithelium or lining (see Fig. 13.20C). Until late in fetal life, the lumen of the vagina is separated from the cavity of the urogenital sinus by a membrane—the **hymen** (Fig. 13.23H; see

also Fig. 13.20C). The hymen is formed by invagination of the posterior wall of the urogenital sinus. The hymen usually ruptures during the perinatal period and remains as a thin mucous membrane just within the vaginal orifice.

Female Auxiliary Genital Glands. Outgrowths from the urethra into the surrounding mesenchyme form the bilateral mucus-secreting urethral glands and **paraurethral glands** (see Fig. 13.20B). Outgrowths from the urogenital sinus form the **greater vestibular glands** in the lower one-third of the **labia majora** (see Fig. 13.23F). These tubuloalveolar glands also secrete mucus and are homologous to the bulbourethral glands in males (see Table 13.1).

DEVELOPMENT OF EXTERNAL GENITALIA

Up to the seventh week, the external genitalia are sexually undifferentiated (see Fig. 13.23A and B). Distinguishing sexual characteristics begin to appear during the 9th week, but the external genitalia are not fully differentiated until the 12th week. Early in the fourth week, the proliferating mesenchyme produces a **genital tubercle** (see Fig. 13.23A)—**primordium of penis or clitoris**—in both sexes at the cranial end of the cloacal membrane. *FGF8 is involved in the signaling pathways in the early development of the external genitalia.*

Labioscrotal swellings and **urogenital folds** soon develop on each side of the cloacal membrane. The genital tubercle soon elongates to form a **primordial phallus—penis or clitoris** (see Fig. 13.23B). In female fetuses, the urethra and vagina open into a common cavity, the **vestibule of the vagina** (see Fig. 13.23B and H).

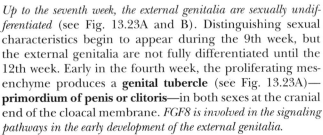

Determination of Fetal Sex

Several studies indicate that sex assignment before birth by transabdominal ultrasound imaging is highly accurate in most cases (99%–100%) after 13 weeks of gestation, provided the external genitalia are not malformed. The accuracy of diagnosis increases with gestational age, and it depends on the experience of the sonographer, the equipment, the position of the fetus, and the amount of amniotic fluid.

DEVELOPMENT OF MALE EXTERNAL GENITALIA

Masculinization of the indifferent external genitalia is induced by dihydrotestosterone produced peripherally by 5α-reductase conversion of testosterone from the testicular Leydig cells (see Fig. 13.23C, E, and G). The **primordial phallus** enlarges and elongates to become the penis. A **urethral plate** forms in the ventral portion of the phallus. The urethral plate canalizes and opens to form the **urethral groove**. This groove is bounded by the **urethral folds**, which form the lateral walls. This groove is lined by a proliferation of endodermal cells from the **urethral plate** (see Fig. 13.23C), which extends from the phallic portion of the urogenital sinus. Under the influence of androgens, the **urethral folds** fuse with each other along the ventral surface of the penis to form the **spongy urethra** (see Fig. 13.24D$_1$ to D$_3$). The surface ectoderm fuses

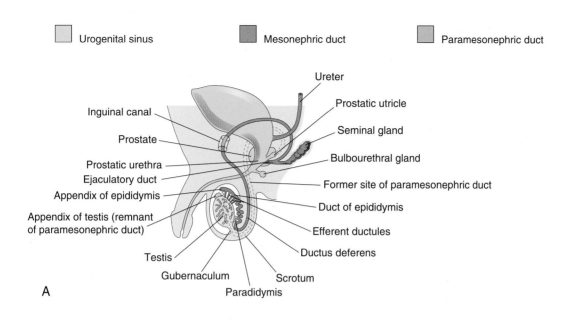

Urogenital sinus   Mesonephric duct   Paramesonephric duct

A

Ureter
Prostatic utricle
Inguinal canal
Seminal gland
Prostate
Bulbourethral gland
Prostatic urethra
Ejaculatory duct
Former site of paramesonephric duct
Appendix of epididymis
Duct of epididymis
Appendix of testis (remnant
of paramesonephric duct)
Efferent ductules
Testis
Ductus deferens
Gubernaculum
Scrotum
Paradidymis

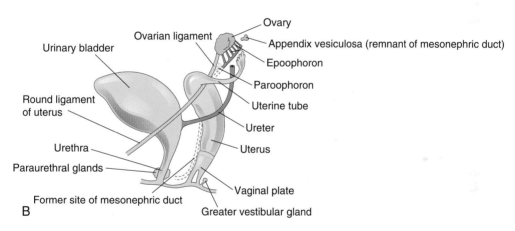

B

Ovary
Ovarian ligament
Appendix vesiculosa (remnant of mesonephric duct)
Urinary bladder
Epoophoron
Paroophoron
Round ligament
of uterus
Uterine tube
Ureter
Urethra
Uterus
Paraurethral glands
Vaginal plate
Former site of mesonephric duct
Greater vestibular gland

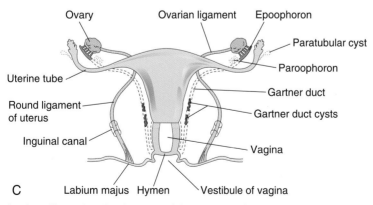

C

Ovary   Ovarian ligament   Epoophoron
Paratubular cyst
Paroophoron
Uterine tube
Gartner duct
Round ligament
of uterus
Gartner duct cysts
Inguinal canal
Vagina
Labium majus   Hymen   Vestibule of vagina

Fig. 13.20 Schematic drawings illustrating development of the male and female reproductive systems from the genital ducts and urogenital sinus. Vestigial structures are also shown. (A) Reproductive system in a male neonate. (B) Female reproductive system in a 12-week fetus. (C) Reproductive system in a female neonate.

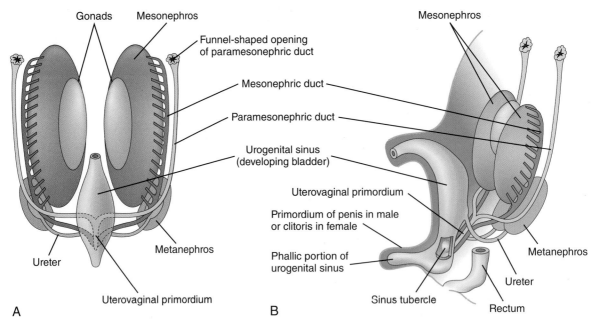

Fig. 13.21 (A) Sketch of a ventral view of the posterior abdominal wall of a 7-week embryo, showing the two pairs of genital ducts present during the indifferent stage of sexual development. (B) Lateral view of a 9-week fetus showing the sinus tubercle on the posterior wall of the urogenital sinus. It becomes the hymen in females (see Fig. 13.20C) and the seminal colliculus in males.

in the median plane of the penis, forming the **penile raphe** and enclosing the spongy urethra within the penis. At the tip of the **glans penis**, an ectodermal ingrowth forms a cellular ectodermal cord, which extends toward the root of the penis to meet the spongy urethra (see Fig. 13.17A). This cord canalizes and joins the previously formed spongy urethra (see Fig. 13.17B). This juncture completes the terminal part of the urethra and moves the **external urethral orifice** to the tip of the glans penis (see Figs. 13.17C and 13.23G). During the 12th week, a circular ingrowth of ectoderm occurs at the periphery of the glans penis (see Fig. 13.17B). When this ingrowth breaks down, it forms the **prepuce** (foreskin) (see Fig. 13.23G). The **corpora cavernosa** and **corpus spongiosum** develop from mesenchyme in the phallus. The **labioscrotal swellings** grow toward each other and fuse to form the **scrotum** (see Fig. 13.23E). The line of fusion of these folds is clearly visible as the **scrotal raphe** (see Fig. 13.23G).

DEVELOPMENT OF FEMALE EXTERNAL GENITALIA

Growth of the primordial phallus in the female fetus gradually decreases as it becomes the **clitoris** (see Fig. 13.15D, F, and H). The clitoris is still relatively large at 18 weeks (see Fig. 13.23D). The clitoris develops in a similar way to the penis, except that the urogenital folds do not fuse, except posteriorly, where they join to form the **frenulum of labia minora**. The unfused parts of the urogenital folds form the **labia minora**. The labioscrotal folds fuse posteriorly to form the **posterior labial commissure** and anteriorly to form the **anterior labial commissure** and the **mons pubis**. Most parts of the **labioscrotal folds** remain unfused and form two large folds of skin, the **labia majora** (see Fig. 13.23H).

Disorders of Sexual Development

Careful fetal ultrasound examination of the perineum may detect **ambiguous genitalia**. Errors in sex determination and differentiation result in various degrees of intermediate sex. Advances in molecular genetics have led to a better understanding of abnormal sexual development and **ambiguous genitalia**.

Disorders of sexual development (DSD) implies a discrepancy between the morphology of the gonads (testes or ovaries) and the appearance of the external genitalia. A DSD can be classified as:

- **Sex chromosome DSD,** including Turner syndrome and Klinefelter syndrome
- **Gonadal dysgenesis,** including ovotesticular DSD, XX testicular DSD, and XY gonadal dysgenesis
- **Virilizing congenital adrenal hyperplasia (CAH)**
- **Disorders of androgen action**

Sex Chromosome DSD

In embryos with **abnormal sex chromosome complexes**, such as XXX or XXY (see Fig. 19.7), the number of X chromosomes appears to be unimportant in sex determination. If a normal Y chromosome is present, the embryo develops as a male. If no Y chromosome is present or the testis-determining region of the Y chromosome is absent, female development occurs. The loss of an X chromosome does not appear to interfere with the migration of primordial germ cells to the gonadal ridges, because some germ cells have been observed in the fetal gonads of 45,XO females with **Turner syndrome** (see Fig. 19.3). Two X chromosomes are needed, however, to bring about normal ovarian development.

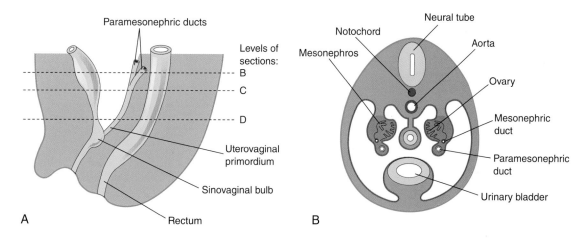

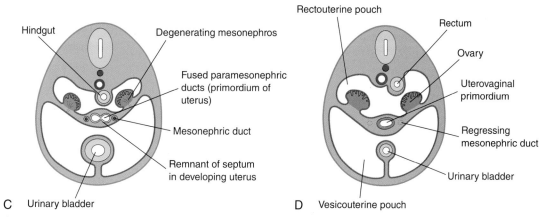

Fig. 13.22 Early development of the ovaries and uterus. (A) Schematic drawing of a sagittal section of the caudal region of an 8-week female embryo. (B) Transverse section showing the paramesonephric ducts approaching each other. (C) Similar section at a more caudal level illustrating fusion of the paramesonephric ducts. A remnant of the septum that separates the paramesonephric ducts is shown. (D) Similar section showing the uterovaginal primordium, broad ligament, and pouches in the pelvic cavity. Note that the mesonephric ducts have regressed.

Gonadal Dysgenesis

Ovotesticular DSD

Persons with **ovotesticular DSD**, a very rare (1:100,000) intersexual condition, usually have **chromatin-positive nuclei**. Approximately 70% of these persons have a 46,XX chromosome constitution; 20% have 46,XX/46,XY **mosaicism** (the presence of two or more cell lines), and 10% have a 46,XY chromosome constitution. The causes of ovotesticular DSD are still poorly understood.

Persons with this condition can have **an ovotestis**, with combined testicular and ovarian tissue within one gonad, or a testicle and ovary each on opposite sides. These tissues are not usually functional. The phenotype may be male or female, but the external genitalia are always ambiguous.

XX Testicular DSD

Persons with XX Testicular **DSD** have chromatin-positive nuclei and a 46,XX chromosome constitution. This anomaly occurs when the *SRY* gene is translocated to an X chromosome, resulting in a male appearance of the external genitalia, although some individuals may have ambiguous-appearing genitalia.

XY Gonadal Dysgenesis

Persons with this intersexual condition have **chromatin-negative nuclei** (no sex chromatin) and a 46,XY chromosome constitution. The external genitalia are developmentally variable, as is the development of the internal genitalia, due to the varying degrees of development of the paramesonephric ducts. *These anomalies are caused by inadequate production of testosterone and AMH by the fetal testes.*

Virilizing Congenital Adrenal Hyperplasia

CAH represents a group of *autosomal-recessive disorders* in which an abnormal increase in the cells of the suprarenal cortex results in **excessive androgen production** during the fetal period. In females, this usually causes masculinization of the external genitalia (Fig. 13.24). Affected male infants have normal external genitalia, and the disorder may go undetected in early infancy. Later in childhood in both sexes, androgen excess leads to rapid growth and accelerated skeletal maturation.

CAH is most often caused by a steroid 21-hydroxylase deficiency due to pathogenic variants (mutations) of *CYP21A2* gene. This results in a deficiency of suprarenal cortical enzymes, which are necessary for the biosynthesis of various steroid hormones. The reduced hormone output results in increased release of adrenocorticotropic hormone by the anterior pituitary, which causes hyperplasia of the suprarenal glands and overproduction of androgens. In some cases of CAH, aldosterone may also be affected, resulting in salt wasting.

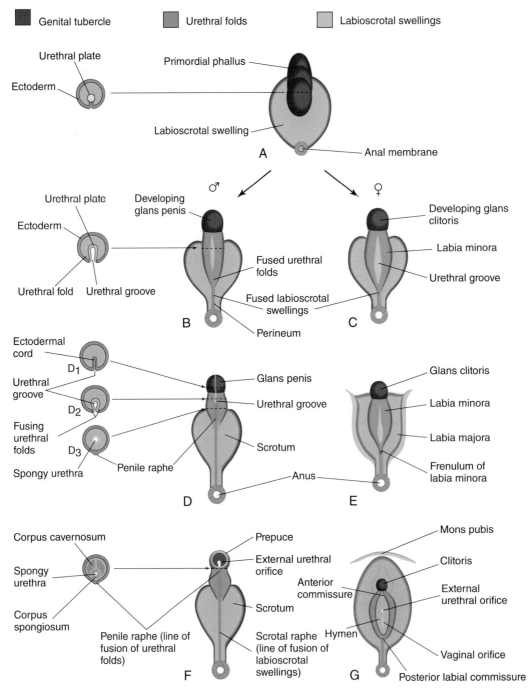

Fig. 13.23 Development of the external genitalia. (A) Diagram illustrating appearance of the genitalia during the indifferent stage (fourth to seventh weeks). (B, D, and F) Stages in the development of the male external genitalia at 9, 11, and 12 weeks, respectively. To the *left* are schematic transverse sections of the developing penis illustrating formation of the spongy urethra and scrotum. (C, E, and G) Stages in the development of the female external genitalia at 9, 11, and 12 weeks, respectively. The mons pubis is a pad of fatty tissue over the symphysis pubis.

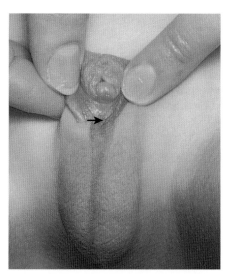

Fig. 13.24 External genitalia of a 6-year-old girl showing an enlarged clitoris and a scrotum-like structure formed by fusion of the labia majora. The *arrow* indicates the opening into the urogenital sinus (see Fig. 13.12C). This extreme masculinization is the result of congenital adrenal hyperplasia. (Courtesy Dr. Heather Dean, Department of Pediatrics and Child Health, University of Manitoba, Winnipeg, Manitoba, Canada.)

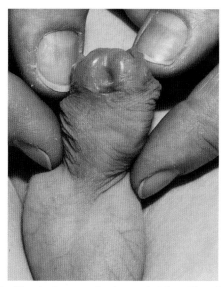

Fig. 13.25 Glanular hypospadias in a male infant. There is a shallow pit in the glans penis at the usual site of the urethral orifice. (Courtesy Dr. A.E. Chudley, Department of Pediatrics and Child Health, University of Manitoba, Children's Hospital, Winnipeg, Manitoba, Canada.)

Disorders of Androgen Action

Androgen Insensitivity Syndrome

Persons with androgen insensitivity syndrome, which occurs in 1 in 20,000 live births, are normal-appearing females, despite the presence of testes and a 46,XY chromosome constitution. The external genitalia are female; however, the vagina usually ends in a blind pouch, and the uterus and uterine tubes are absent or rudimentary. At puberty, there is normal development of breasts and female characteristics; however, menstruation does not occur.

The testes are usually in the abdomen or inguinal canals, but they may be within the labia majora. The failure of masculinization to occur in these individuals results from a **resistance to the action of testosterone** at the cellular level in the genital tubercle and labioscrotal and urethral folds.

Persons with **partial androgen insensitivity syndrome** exhibit some masculinization at birth, such as ambiguous external genitalia, and they may have an enlarged clitoris. Androgen insensitivity syndrome follows X-linked recessive inheritance, and hundreds of gene variations encoding the androgen receptor have been described.

Hypospadias

There are four types of hypospadias: glanular (most common type), penile, penoscrotal, and perineal hypospadias. **Hypospadias is the most frequent anomaly** involving the penis and is found in 1 in 125 male infants. In **glanular hypospadias**, the external urethral orifice is on the ventral surface of the glans penis. In **penile hypospadias**, the external urethral orifice is on the ventral surface of the body of the penis. The glanular and penile types of hypospadias are the common types (Fig. 13.25). In **penoscrotal hypospadias**, the urethral orifice is at the junction of the penis and scrotum. In **perineal hypospadias**, the external urethral orifice is located between the unfused halves of the scrotum. Hypospadias results from inadequate production of androgens by the fetal testes. It is believed that environmental factors may disrupt testosterone-related gene expression.

Epispadias

In 1 of every 30,000 male neonates, the urethra opens on the dorsal surface of the penis. Although epispadias may occur as a separate entity, it is often associated with exstrophy of the bladder (see Fig. 13.15). Epispadias may result from inadequate ectodermal–mesenchymal interactions during the development of the genital tubercle. As a consequence, the genital tubercle develops more dorsally than in normal embryos. Consequently, when the urogenital membrane ruptures, the urogenital sinus opens on the dorsal surface of the penis. Urine is expelled at the root of the malformed penis.

Birth Defects of Female Genital Tract

Various types of uterine duplication and vaginal defects result from developmental arrest of the uterovaginal primordium during the eighth week of development (Fig. 13.26B–G). The main developmental defects are as follows:

- Incomplete fusion of the paramesonephric ducts
- Incomplete development of one or both paramesonephric ducts
- Failure of parts of one or both paramesonephric ducts to develop
- Incomplete canalization of the vaginal plate that forms the vagina

In some cases, the uterus is divided internally by a septum (see Fig. 13.26F). If the duplication involves only the superior part of the body of the uterus, the condition is a **bicornuate uterus** (see Fig. 13.26D and E). If growth of one paramesonephric duct is retarded and the duct does not fuse with the other one, a **bicornuate uterus with a rudimentary horn** develops (see Fig. 13.26E). The horn may not communicate with the cavity of the uterus. A **unicornuate uterus** develops when one paramesonephric duct does not develop; this results in a uterus with one uterine tube (see Fig. 13.26G).

Continued

In many of these cases, the individuals are fertile but may have an increased incidence of premature delivery. A **double uterus** (uterus didelphys) results from the failure of fusion of the inferior parts of the paramesonephric ducts. It may be associated with a double or a single vagina (see Fig. 13.26B and C).

Agenesis of the vagina results from the **failure of the sinovaginal bulbs to develop** and form the vaginal plate (see Fig. 13.20B). When the vagina is absent, the uterus is usually also absent because the developing uterus (uterovaginal primordium) induces the formation of sinovaginal bulbs, which fuse to form the **vaginal plate** (see Fig. 13.23C). Failure of canalization of the vaginal plate results in blockage of the vagina. Failure of the inferior end of the vaginal plate to perforate results in an **imperforate hymen** (see Fig. 13.20C).

DEVELOPMENT OF INGUINAL CANALS

The inguinal canals form pathways for the testes to descend from the dorsal abdominal wall through the anterior abdominal wall into the scrotum. Inguinal canals develop in both sexes because of the morphologically indifferent stage of sexual development. Through a series of condensations of mesenchyme, a connective tissue structure—the **gubernaculum** develops on each side of the abdomen from the inferior pole of the gonad (Fig. 13.27A). The gubernaculum passes obliquely through the developing anterior abdominal wall at the site of the future inguinal canal (see Fig. 13.27B–D). The gubernaculum is associated cranially with the mesenchyme of the mesonephros.

The **processus vaginalis**, an evagination of peritoneum, develops ventral to the gubernaculum and herniates through the abdominal wall along the path formed by the gubernaculum (see Fig. 13.27B–E). The processus vaginalis carries along extensions of the layers of the abdominal wall before it, which form the walls of the inguinal canal. These layers also form the coverings of the spermatic cord and testis (see Fig. 13.27E and F). The opening in the transversalis fascia produced by the vaginal process becomes the **deep inguinal ring**, and the opening created in the external oblique aponeurosis forms the **superficial inguinal ring**.

RELOCATION OF TESTES AND OVARIES

12

DESCENT OF TESTES

By 26 weeks, the testes have descended retroperitoneally from the posterior abdominal wall to the deep inguinal rings (see Fig. 13.27B and C). This change in position occurs as the fetal pelvis enlarges and the trunk of the embryo elongates. Transabdominal relocation of the testes is largely a relative movement that results from the growth of the cranial part of the abdomen away from the future pelvic region. Increased abdominal pressure may also play a role.

Testicular descent through the **inguinal canals** and into the scrotum is controlled by androgens (e.g., testosterone) produced by the fetal testes. The gubernaculum guides the path of the process vaginalis. The relocation of the testes through the inguinal canals and into the scrotum usually begins during the 26th week, and it may take 2 to 3 days.

By 32 weeks, both testes are in the scrotum in most cases. More than 97% of full-term neonates have both testes in the scrotum. During the first 3 months after birth, most undescended testes descend into the scrotum. When the testes descend, they carry the ductus deferens and vessels with them. As the testis and ductus deferens descend, they are ensheathed by the fascial extensions of the abdominal wall (see Fig. 13.27F):

- The extension of the transversalis fascia becomes the **internal spermatic fascia**.
- The extensions of the internal oblique muscle and fascia become the **cremasteric muscle** and **fascia**.
- The extension of the external oblique muscle and aponeurosis become the external spermatic fascia.

Within the scrotum, the testis projects into the distal end of the processus vaginalis. During the perinatal period, the connecting stalk of the process normally obliterates, forming a serous membrane—the **tunica vaginalis**—that covers the front and sides of the testis (see Fig. 13.27F).

Cryptorchidism

Cryptorchidism (undescended testes) is the most common birth defect in neonates and occurs in about 30% of premature males and in approximately 3% to 4% of full-term males. Cryptorchidism may be unilateral or bilateral. In most cases, the testes descend into the scrotum by the end of the first year. If both testes remain within or just outside the abdominal cavity, they do not mature and sterility is common. If uncorrected, there is a significantly higher risk for the development of **germ cell tumors**, especially in cases of abdominal cryptorchidism. **Cryptorchid testes** may be in the abdominal cavity or anywhere along the usual path of descent of the testis, but they are usually in the inguinal canal (Fig. 13.28A). The cause of most cases of cryptorchidism is unknown, but a deficiency of androgen production by the fetal testes is an important factor.

Ectopic Testes

After traversing the inguinal canal, the testis may deviate from its usual path of descent and lodge in various abnormal locations (see Fig. 13.28B):

- Interstitial (external to the aponeurosis of the external oblique muscle)
- In the proximal part of the medial thigh
- Dorsal to the penis
- On the opposite side **(crossed ectopia)**

All types of ectopic testis are rare, but **interstitial ectopia** occurs most frequently. Ectopic testis occurs when a part of the gubernaculum passes to an abnormal location and the testis follows it.

DESCENT OF OVARIES

The ovaries also descend from the lumbar region of the posterior abdominal wall and relocate to the pelvis; however, they do not pass from the pelvis and enter the inguinal canals. The gubernaculum is attached to the uterus near the attachment

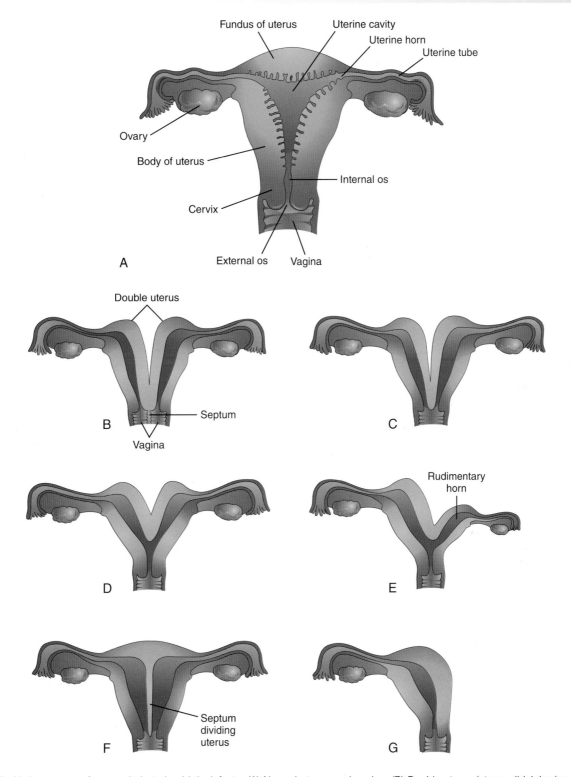

Fig. 13.26 Various types of congenital uterine birth defects. (A) Normal uterus and vagina. (B) Double uterus (uterus didelphys) and double vagina. Note the septum dividing the vagina. (C) Double uterus with a single vagina. (D) Bicornuate uterus (two uterine horns). (E) Bicornuate uterus with a rudimentary left horn. (F) Septate uterus. Note the septum dividing the uterus. (G) Unicornuate uterus. Note that only half of the uterus exists.

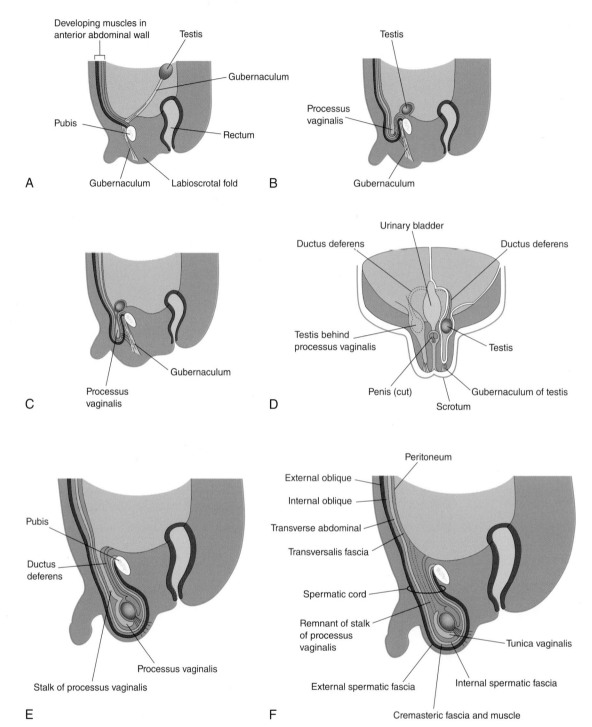

Fig. 13.27 Formation of the inguinal canals and descent of the testes. (A) Sagittal section of a 7-week embryo showing the testis before its descent from the dorsal abdominal wall. (B and C) Similar sections at approximately 28 weeks showing the processus vaginalis and testis beginning to pass through the inguinal canal. Note that the processus vaginalis carries fascial layers of the abdominal wall before it. (D) Frontal section of a fetus approximately 3 days later illustrating descent of the testis posterior to the processus vaginalis. The processus has been cut away on the *left side* to show the testis and ductus deferens. (E) Sagittal section of a male infant neonate showing the processus vaginalis communicating with the peritoneal cavity by a narrow stalk. (F) Similar section of a 1-month-old neonate after obliteration of the stalk of the processus vaginalis. Note that the extended fascial layers of the abdominal wall now form the coverings of the spermatic cord.

of the uterine tube. The cranial part of the gubernaculum becomes the **ovarian ligament** and the caudal part forms the **round ligament** of the uterus (see Fig. 13.20C). The round ligaments pass through the inguinal canals and terminate in the labia majora. The relatively small processus vaginalis in the female is usually obliterated, and it disappears long before birth. A patent processus in a fetus is known as **a vaginal process of peritoneum** (canal of Nuck).

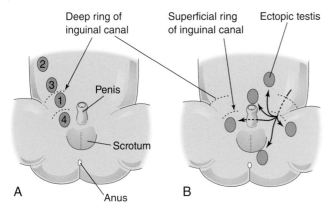

Fig. 13.28 Possible sites of cryptorchid and ectopic testes. (A) Positions of cryptorchid testes, numbered 1 to 4 in order of increasing frequency. (B) Usual locations of ectopic testes.

Congenital Inguinal Hernia

If the communication between the tunica vaginalis and peritoneal cavity does not close, a **persistent processus vaginalis** occurs. A loop of intestine may herniate through it into the scrotum or labia majora (Fig. 13.29A and B). Embryonic remnants resembling the ductus deferens or epididymis are often found in inguinal hernial sacs. Congenital inguinal hernia is much more common in males, especially when there are undescended testes. The hernias are also common with ectopic testes and in **androgen insensitivity syndrome** (see Fig. 13.24).

Hydrocele

Occasionally the abdominal end of the processus vaginalis remains open but is too small to permit herniation of intestine (see Fig. 13.29D). Peritoneal fluid passes into the patent processus vaginalis and forms a **scrotal hydrocele**. If only the middle part of the processus vaginalis remains open, fluid may accumulate and give rise to a **hydrocele of the spermatic cord** (see Fig. 13.29C).

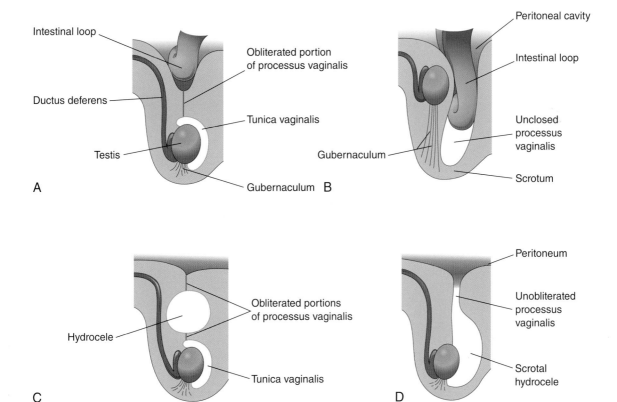

Fig. 13.29 Diagrams of sagittal sections illustrating conditions resulting from failure of closure of the processus vaginalis. (A) Incomplete congenital inguinal hernia into the scrotum resulting from persistence of the proximal part of the processus vaginalis. (B) Complete congenital inguinal hernia entering the unobliterated processus in the scrotum. Cryptorchidism, a commonly associated birth defect, is also shown. (C) Large hydrocele that arose from an unobliterated portion of the processus vaginalis. (D) Hydrocele of the testis and spermatic cord resulting from peritoneal fluid passing into an unclosed processus vaginalis.

CLINICALLY ORIENTED QUESTIONS

1. Does a horseshoe kidney usually function normally? What problems may occur with this anomaly, and how can they be corrected?

2. A man was told by a doctor that he has two kidneys on one side and none on the other. How did this birth defect probably happen? Are there likely to be any problems associated with this condition?

3. Are individuals with ovotesticular DSD ever fertile?

4. When a baby is born with ambiguous external genitalia, how long does it take to assign the appropriate sex?

What does the physician tell the parents? How is the appropriate sex determined?

5. What is a common type of disorder that produces ambiguous external genitalia? Will masculinizing, or androgenic, hormones given during the fetal period of development cause ambiguity of the external genitalia in female fetuses?

The answers to these questions are at the back of this book.

Cardiovascular System 14

The cardiovascular system is the first major system to function in the embryo. The primordial heart and vascular system appear in the middle of the third week (Fig. 14.1). *The heart begins to beat at 22 to 23 days* (Fig. 14.2). This precocious development is necessary because diffusion alone cannot satisfy the nutritional and oxygen requirements of the rapidly growing embryo. The cardiovascular system is derived from:

- Splanchnic mesoderm, which forms the primordium of the heart (see Fig. 14.1A and B)
- Paraxial and lateral mesoderm near the otic placodes (see Fig. 17.9A and B).

EARLY DEVELOPMENT OF HEART AND BLOOD VESSELS

Multipotential cardiac progenitor cells contribute to the formation of the heart. These include distinct mesodermal populations—a primary, or first heart field (FHF) and a secondary heart field (SHF)—and neural crest cells. Mesodermal cells from the primitive streak migrate to form bilateral paired strands (FHF), and those from the pharyngeal mesoderm form the SHF, located medial to the FHF. These strands canalize to form two thin **heart tubes** that soon fuse into a single heart tube late in the third week as a result of embryo folding (see Fig. 14.5). An inductive influence from the anterior endoderm stimulates early formation of the heart. Specified cardiac progenitor cells express *Nkx2-5* and can already be identified during gastrulation. *Morphogenesis of the heart is controlled by a cascade of regulatory genes and transcription factors. The role of the canonical Wnt pathway, β-catenin, in cardiogenesis is well established.*

DEVELOPMENT OF VEINS ASSOCIATED WITH EMBRYONIC HEART

Three paired veins drain into the tubular heart of a 4-week embryo (see Fig. 14.2):

- **Vitelline veins** return poorly oxygenated blood from the umbilical vesicle.
- **Umbilical veins** carry well-oxygenated blood from the chorionic sac.
- **Common cardinal veins** return poorly oxygenated blood from the body of the embryo to the heart.

The vitelline veins enter the venous end of the primordial heart—the **sinus venosus** (Figs. 14.3 and 14.4; see also Fig. 4.2). As the liver primordium grows into the septum transversum, the **hepatic cords** anastomose around preexisting endothelium-lined spaces. These spaces, the primordia of the hepatic sinusoids, later become linked to the vitelline veins. The **hepatic veins** form from the remains of the right vitelline vein in the region of the developing liver. The **portal vein** develops from a network of vitelline veins around the duodenum (see Fig. 14.4B).

The transformation of the umbilical veins may be summarized as follows (see Fig. 14.4B):

- The right umbilical vein and the cranial part of the left umbilical vein between the liver and the sinus venosus degenerate.
- The persistent caudal part of the left umbilical vein becomes the umbilical vein, which carries well-oxygenated blood from the placenta to the embryo.
- A large venous shunt—the ductus venosus—develops within the liver and connects the umbilical vein with the inferior vena cava (IVC).

The cardinal veins (see Figs. 14.2 and 14.3A) constitute the main venous drainage system of the embryo. The anterior and posterior cardinal veins drain the cranial and caudal parts of the embryo, respectively (see Fig. 14.3A). These join the **common cardinal veins**, which enter the sinus venosus (see Fig. 14.4A). During the eighth week, the **anterior cardinal veins** are connected by an oblique anastomosis (see Fig. 14.4B) that shunts blood from the left to the right anterior cardinal vein. This anastomotic shunt becomes the **left brachiocephalic vein** when the caudal part of the left anterior cardinal vein degenerates (see Figs. 14.3D and 14.4C). The **superior vena cava** (SVC) forms from the right anterior cardinal vein and the right common cardinal vein. The only adult derivatives of the **posterior cardinal veins** are the root of the **azygos vein** and the **common iliac veins** (see Figs. 14.3D and 14.4C). The subcardinal and supracardinal veins gradually replace and supplement the posterior cardinal veins.

The **subcardinal veins** appear first (see Fig. 14.3A) and form the stem of the left renal vein, the suprarenal veins, the gonadal veins (testicular and ovarian), and a segment of the IVC (see Fig. 14.3D). The supracardinal veins become disrupted in the region of the kidneys (see Fig. 14.3C). Cranial to this, they anastomose and form the **azygos** and the **hemiazygos veins** (see Figs. 14.3D and 14.4C). Caudal to the kidneys, the left supracardinal vein degenerates, but the right supracardinal vein becomes the inferior part of the IVC (see Fig. 14.3D). The **IVC** forms as blood returning from the caudal part of the embryo is shunted from the left to the right side of the body.

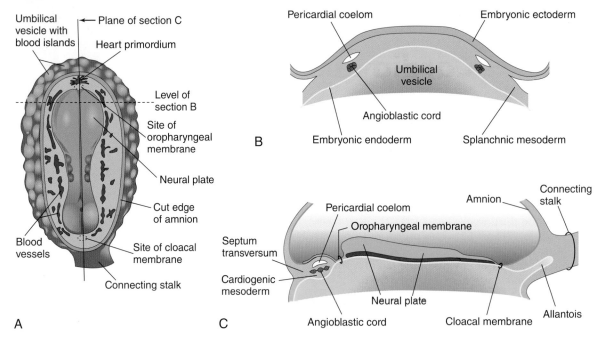

Fig. 14.1   Early development of the heart. (A) Drawing of a dorsal view of an embryo (approximately 18 days). (B) Transverse section of the embryo showing angioblastic cords in the cardiogenic mesoderm and their relationship to the pericardial coelom. (C) Longitudinal section through the embryo illustrating the relationship of the angioblastic cords to the oropharyngeal membrane, pericardial coelom, and septum transversum.

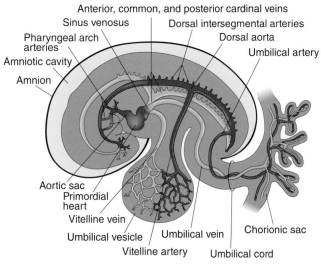

Fig. 14.2   Drawing of the embryonic cardiovascular system (at approximately 26 days) showing vessels on the left side only. The umbilical vein carries well-oxygenated blood and nutrients from the chorionic sac to the embryo. The umbilical arteries carry poorly oxygenated blood and waste products from the embryo to the chorionic sac (outermost embryonic membrane; see Fig. 8.1A and B).

Anomalies of Venae Cavae

The most common (3–5:1000) anomaly of the venae cavae is a persistent left SVC. The most common (6:1000) IVC anomaly is interrupted IVC with azygous circulation; as a result, blood drains from the lower limbs, abdomen, and pelvis to the heart through the azygos system of veins (see Fig. 14.3).

PHARYNGEAL ARCH ARTERIES AND OTHER BRANCHES OF THE DORSAL AORTA

As the pharyngeal arches form during the fourth and fifth weeks, they are supplied by **pharyngeal arch arteries** arising from the **aortic sac** and terminating in the **dorsal aortae** (see Fig. 14.2). Neural crest cells delaminate from the neural tube and contribute to the formation of the outflow tract of the heart and pharyngeal arches. Initially, the paired dorsal aortae run through the entire length of the embryo. Later, the caudal portions of the paired dorsal aortae fuse to form a single lower thoracic/abdominal aorta. Of the remaining paired dorsal aortae, the right regresses and the left becomes the primordial aorta.

INTERSEGMENTAL ARTERIES

Thirty or so branches of the dorsal aorta, the **intersegmental arteries**, pass between and carry blood to the somites and their derivatives (see Fig. 14.2). The intersegmental arteries in the neck join to form the **vertebral arteries**. Most of the original connections of the intersegmental arteries to the dorsal aorta disappear.

In the thorax, the intersegmental arteries persist as **intercostal arteries**. Most of the intersegmental arteries in the abdomen become **lumbar arteries**; however, the fifth pair of lumbar intersegmental arteries remains as the **common iliac arteries**. In the sacral region, the intersegmental arteries form the **lateral sacral arteries**.

FATE OF VITELLINE AND UMBILICAL ARTERIES

The unpaired ventral branches of the dorsal aorta supply the umbilical vesicle, allantois, and chorion (see Fig. 14.2). The vitelline arteries supply the umbilical vesicle and, later, the primordial gut, which forms from the incorporated part of the

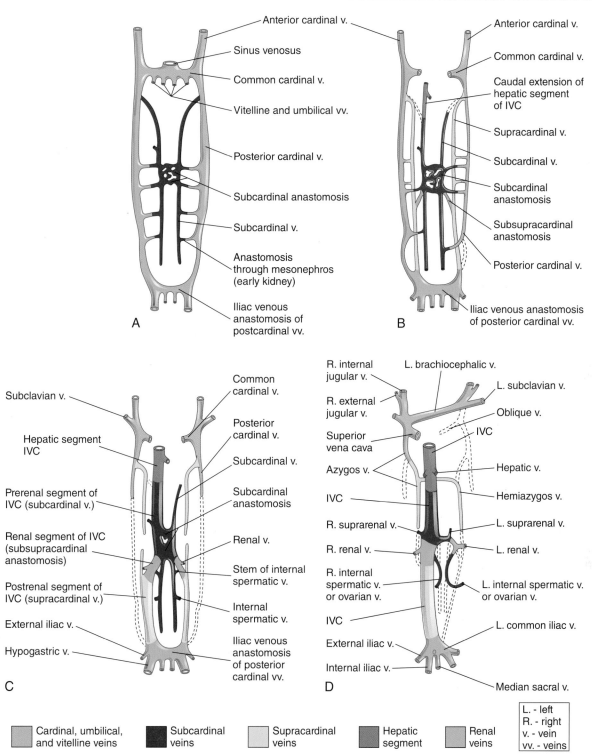

Fig. 14.3   Illustrations of the primordial veins of the trunk of an embryo (ventral views). Initially, three systems of veins are present: the umbilical veins from the chorionic sac, the vitelline veins from the umbilical vesicle, and the cardinal veins from the body of the embryo. Next, the subcardinal veins appear, and finally the supracardinal veins develop. (A) At 6 weeks. (B) At 7 weeks. (C) At 8 weeks. (D) Drawing illustrating the transformations that produce the adult venous pattern. *IVC*, Inferior vena cava. Modified from Arey LB: *Developmental anatomy*, ed 7, Philadelphia, 1974, Saunders.

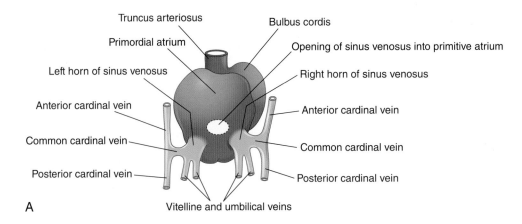

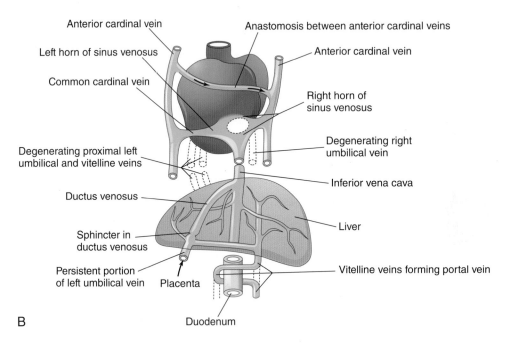

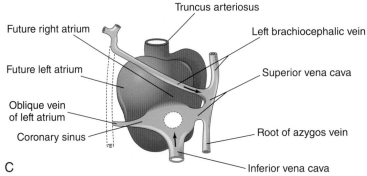

Fig. 14.4 Dorsal views of the developing heart. (A) During the fourth week (approximately 24 days), showing the primordial atrium, sinus venosus, and veins draining into them. (B) At 7 weeks, showing the enlarged right sinus horn and venous circulation through the liver. The organs are not drawn to scale. (C) At 8 weeks, indicating the adult derivatives of the cardinal veins shown in A and B. *Arrows* indicate the flow of blood.

umbilical vesicle. Only three vitelline arteries remain: the **celiac arterial trunk** to the foregut, the **superior mesenteric artery** to the midgut, and the **inferior mesenteric artery** to the hindgut.

The paired umbilical arteries pass through the connecting stalk and join the vessels in the chorion. The umbilical arteries carry poorly oxygenated fetal blood to the placenta (see Fig. 14.2). The proximal parts of these arteries become the **internal iliac arteries** and **superior vesical arteries**, whereas the distal parts are obliterated after birth and become **medial umbilical ligaments**.

LATER DEVELOPMENT OF HEART

The external layer of the embryonic heart tube—the **primordial myocardium** (cardiac precursor of the primary heart field)—is formed from the splanchnic mesoderm surrounding the **pericardial cavity** (Figs. 14.5 and 14.6B and C). At this stage, the developing heart is composed of a thin endothelial tube, separated from a thick primordial myocardium by a gelatinous extracellular matrix—**cardiac jelly** (see Fig. 14.6C and D).

The endothelial tube becomes the internal endothelial lining of the heart—**endocardium**—and the primordial myocardium becomes the muscular wall of the heart, the **myocardium**. The **epicardium** is derived from the SHF and from mesothelial cells that arise from the external surface of the sinus venosus and spread over the myocardium (see Fig. 14.6F).

As folding of the head region occurs, the heart and pericardial cavity appear ventral to the foregut and caudal to the **oropharyngeal membrane** (Fig. 14.7A–C). Concurrently, the tubular heart elongates and develops alternate dilations and constrictions (see Fig. 14.5C–E): the **bulbus cordis** (composed of the **truncus arteriosus**, **conus arteriosus**, and **conus cordis**), ventricle, atrium, and sinus venosus. The growth of the heart tube results from the addition of cells (cardiomyocytes) that differentiate from the mesoderm at the dorsal wall of the pericardium.

The tubular **truncus arteriosus** is continuous cranially with the aortic sac (Fig. 14.8A), from which the pharyngeal arch arteries arise. Progenitor cells from the SHF contribute to the formation of the arterial and venous ends of the developing heart. The **sinus venosus** receives the umbilical, vitelline, and common cardinal veins from the chorion, umbilical vesicle, and embryo, respectively (see Fig. 14.4A). The arterial and venous ends of the heart are fixed in place

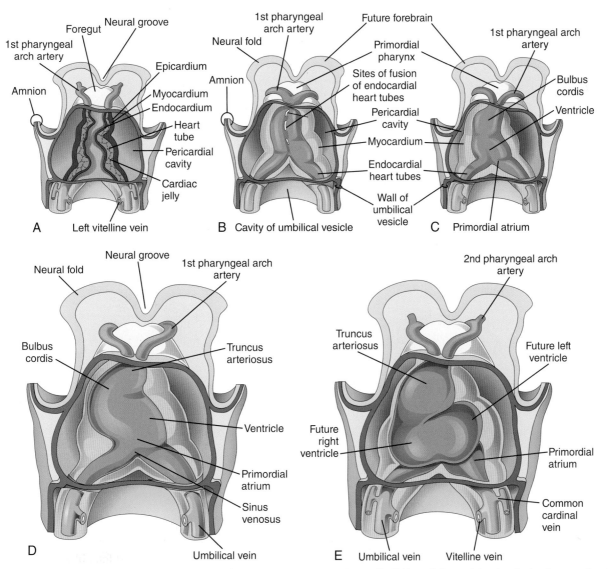

Fig. 14.5 Drawings showing fusion of the heart tubes and looping of the tubular heart. (A–C) Ventral views of the developing heart and pericardial region (22–35 days). The ventral pericardial wall has been removed to show the developing myocardium and fusion of the two heart tubes to form a tubular heart. The endothelium of the heart tube forms the endocardium of the heart. (D and E) As the straight tubular heart elongates, it bends and undergoes looping, which forms a D-loop that produces an S-shaped heart.

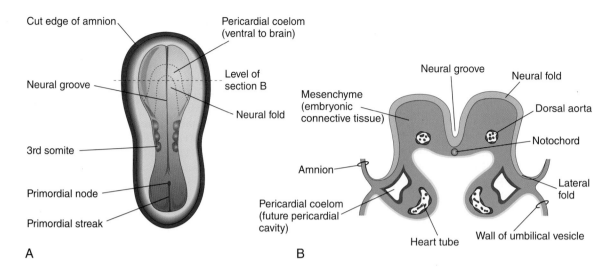

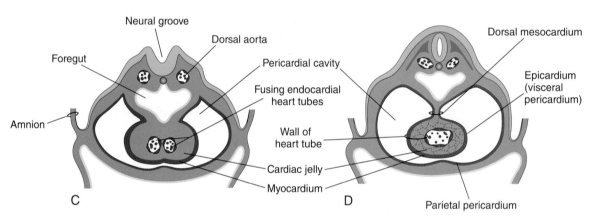

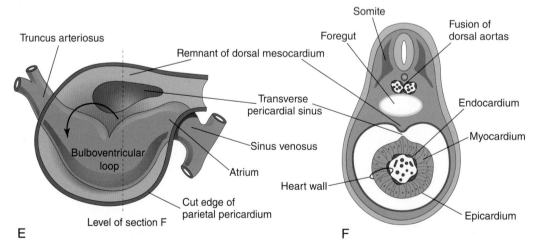

Fig. 14.6 (A) Dorsal view of an embryo (approximately 20 days). (B) Schematic transverse section of the heart region of the embryo illustrated in (A) showing the two endocardial heart tubes and lateral folds of the body. (C) Transverse section of a slightly older embryo, showing the formation of the pericardial cavity and fusion of the heart tubes. (D) Similar section (approximately 22 days) showing the tubular heart suspended by the dorsal mesocardium. (E) Schematic drawing of the heart (approximately 28 days) showing degeneration of the central part of the dorsal mesocardium and formation of the transverse pericardial sinus. The *arrow* shows bending of the primordial heart. The tubular heart now has a D-loop. (F) Transverse section of the embryo at the level seen in (E) showing the layers of the heart wall.

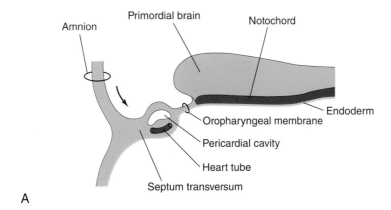

A

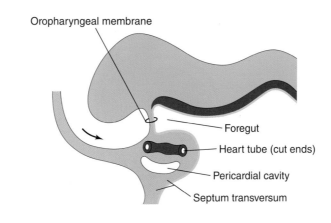

B

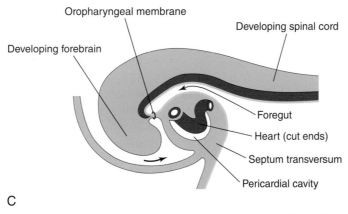

C

Fig. 14.7 Illustrations of longitudinal sections through the cranial half of embryos during the fifth week, showing the effect of the head fold *(arrows)* on the position of the heart and other structures. (A and B) As the head fold develops, the heart tube and pericardial cavity move ventral to the foregut and caudal to the oropharyngeal membrane. (C) Note that the positions of the pericardial cavity and septum transversum have reversed with respect to each other. The septum transversum now lies posterior to the pericardial cavity, where it will form the central tendon of the diaphragm.

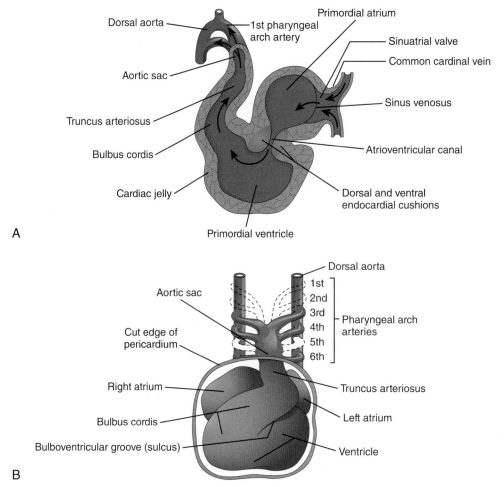

Fig. 14.8   (A) Sagittal section of the primordial heart at approximately 24 days, showing blood flowing through it *(arrows)*. (B) Ventral view of the heart and pharyngeal arch arteries at approximately 35 days. The ventral wall of the pericardial sac has been removed to show the heart in the pericardial cavity.

by the pharyngeal arches and septum transversum, respectively. Because the **bulbus cordis** and ventricle grow faster than the other regions, the heart bends on itself, forming a U-shaped **bulboventricular loop** (see Fig. 14.6E). *Complex signaling pathways involving BMP, Notch, Wnt, and SHH are essential regulators in the remodeling of the heart tube. Nodal (belonging to the transforming growth factor-β superfamily) is involved in the looping of the heart tube.*

As the primordial heart bends, the atrium and sinus venosus appear dorsal to the truncus arteriosus, bulbus cordis, and ventricle (see Fig. 14.8A and B). By this stage, the sinus venosus has developed lateral expansions, the **right and left horns of the sinus venosus**.

As the heart develops, it gradually invaginates the **pericardial cavity** (see Figs. 14.6C and D and 14.7C). The heart is initially suspended from the dorsal wall by a mesentery, the **dorsal mesocardium**. However, the central part of this mesentery degenerates, forming a communication—the **transverse pericardial sinus**—between the right and left sides of the pericardial cavity (see Fig. 14.6E and F). At this stage, the heart is attached only at its cranial and caudal ends.

CIRCULATION THROUGH PRIMORDIAL HEART

Blood enters the sinus venosus (see Figs. 14.8A and 14.4A) from the:

- Embryo through the common cardinal veins
- Developing placenta through the umbilical veins
- Umbilical vesicle through the vitelline veins.

Blood from the **sinus venosus** enters the **primordial atrium**; its flow is controlled by **sinuatrial (SA) valves** (see Fig. 14.8A). The blood then passes through the **atrioventricular (AV) canal** into the **primordial ventricle**. When the ventricle contracts, blood is pumped through the bulbus cordis and truncus arteriosus into the **aortic sac**, from which it is distributed to the pharyngeal arch arteries (see Fig. 14.8B). The blood then passes into the dorsal aortae for distribution to the embryo, umbilical vesicle, and placenta (see Fig. 14.2).

PARTITIONING OF PRIMORDIAL HEART

Partitioning of the AV canal, primordial atrium, ventricle, and outflow tract begins at the middle of the fifth week and is essentially completed by the end of the eighth week.

13

Toward the end of the fifth week, **atrioventricular endocardial cushions** form on the dorsal and ventral walls of the AV canal (see Fig. 14.8A). These cushions approach each other and fuse, dividing the AV canal into right and left AV canals (Fig. 14.9B). These canals partially separate the primordial atrium from the ventricle, and the cushions function as AV valves. The endocardial cushions develop initially from cardiac jelly.

Transforming growth factor-β (TGF-β₁ and TGF-β₂), bone morphogenetic proteins (BMP-2A and BMP-4) expression in the endocardial lineage, the zinc finger protein Slug, and an activin receptor–like kinase (ChALK2) have been reported to be involved in the epithelial–mesenchymal transformation and formation of the endocardial cushions.

PARTITIONING OF PRIMORDIAL ATRIUM

The primordial atrium is divided into right and left atria by the formation and fusion of two septa, the septum primum and septum secundum (Fig. 14.10; see also Fig. 14.9A–E). The **septum primum** grows toward the fusing endocardial cushions from the roof of the primordial atrium, partially dividing the atrium into right and left halves. As this muscular septum develops, a large opening—the **foramen primum**—forms between its free edge and the endocardial cushions (see Figs. 14.9C and 14.10A to C). This foramen allows the shunting of oxygenated blood from the right to the left atrium. The foramen becomes progressively smaller and disappears as the mesenchymal cap of the septum primum fuses with the fused endocardial cushions to form the **primordial AV septum** (see Fig. 14.10D and D₁). *Molecular studies have revealed that a distinct population of extracardiac progenitor cells, from the SHF, migrate through the dorsal mesocardium to complete the atrial septum. SHH signaling plays a critical role in this process.*

Before the foramen primum disappears, perforations produced by **apoptosis** appear in the central part of the septum primum. As the septum fuses with the endocardial cushions, obliterating the foramen primum (see Figs. 14.9D and 14.10D), the perforations coalesce to form another opening in the septum primum—the **foramen secundum** (see Fig. 14.10C). This foramen ensures continued shunting of oxygenated blood from the right to the left atrium.

The **septum secundum** grows from the muscular ventrocranial wall of the atrium, immediately to the right of the septum primum (see Fig. 14.10D₁). As this thick septum grows during the fourth and sixth weeks, it gradually overlaps the foramen secundum in the septum primum (see Fig. 14.10E and F). The septum secundum forms an incomplete partition between the atria: the **oval foramen** (foramen ovale) results. The cranial part of the septum primum gradually disappears (see Fig. 14.10G₁). The remaining part of the septum, attached to the endocardial cushions, forms the **valve of the oval foramen**.

Before birth, the oval foramen allows most of the oxygenated blood entering the right atrium from the IVC to pass into the left atrium (see Fig. 14.10H₁). It also prevents the passage of blood in the opposite direction because the septum primum closes against the relatively rigid septum secundum (see Fig. 14.10G₁).

After birth, the oval foramen functionally closes because of higher pressure in the left atrium than in the right atrium.

At approximately 3 months, the valve of the oval foramen fuses with the septum secundum, forming the **oval fossa** (fossa ovalis). As a result, the interatrial septum becomes a complete partition between the atria (see Fig. 14.10G).

CHANGES IN SINUS VENOSUS

Initially, the sinus venosus opens into the center of the posterior wall of the primordial atrium. By the end of the fourth week, the right sinual horn becomes larger than the left sinual horn (Fig. 14.11A and B). As this occurs, the **sinoatrial orifice** moves to the right and opens in the part of the primordial atrium that will become the adult right atrium (see Fig. 14.11C). As the right sinual horn enlarges, it receives all the blood from the head and neck through the SVC and from the placenta and caudal regions of the body through the IVC.

The left horn of the sinus venosus becomes the **coronary sinus**, and the right horn is incorporated into the wall of the right atrium (see Fig. 14.11B and C) and becomes the smooth part of the internal wall of the right atrium—the **sinus venarum** (see Fig. 14.11B and C). The remainder of the anterior internal surface of the wall of the right atrium and that of the **right auricle** have a rough, trabeculated appearance (see Fig. 14.11C). These latter two parts are derived from the primordial atrium. The smooth part and rough part are demarcated internally in the right atrium by a vertical ridge—**crista terminalis**, or terminal crest (see Fig. 14.11C)—and externally by a shallow groove—the **sulcus terminalis**, or terminal groove (see Fig. 14.11B).

The crista terminalis represents the cranial part of the **right sinoatrial valve** (see Fig. 14.11C); the caudal part of this valve forms the valves of the IVC and coronary sinus. The **left sinoatrial valve** fuses with the septum secundum and is incorporated with it into the interatrial septum.

PRIMORDIAL PULMONARY VEIN AND FORMATION OF LEFT ATRIUM

Most of the wall of the left atrium is smooth because it is formed by the incorporation of the **primordial pulmonary vein** (Fig. 14.12A). This vein develops as an outgrowth of the dorsal atrial wall, just to the left of the septum primum. As the atrium expands, the primordial pulmonary vein and its main branches are gradually incorporated into the wall of the left atrium (see Fig. 14.12B). As a result, four pulmonary veins are formed (see Fig. 14.12C and D). The small left auricle is derived from the primordial atrium; its internal surface has a rough, trabeculated appearance (see Fig. 14.12D).

PARTITIONING OF PRIMORDIAL VENTRICLE

Division of the primordial ventricle into two ventricles is first indicated by a median ridge—the **muscular interventricular (IV) septum**—in the floor of the ventricle near its apex (see Fig. 14.9B). This fold has a concave superior free edge (Fig. 14.13A). Initially, most of its increase in height results from dilation of the ventricles on each side of the muscular IV septum (see Fig. 14.13B). Myocytes from both the right and left primordial ventricles contribute to the formation of the **muscular part of the IV septum**.

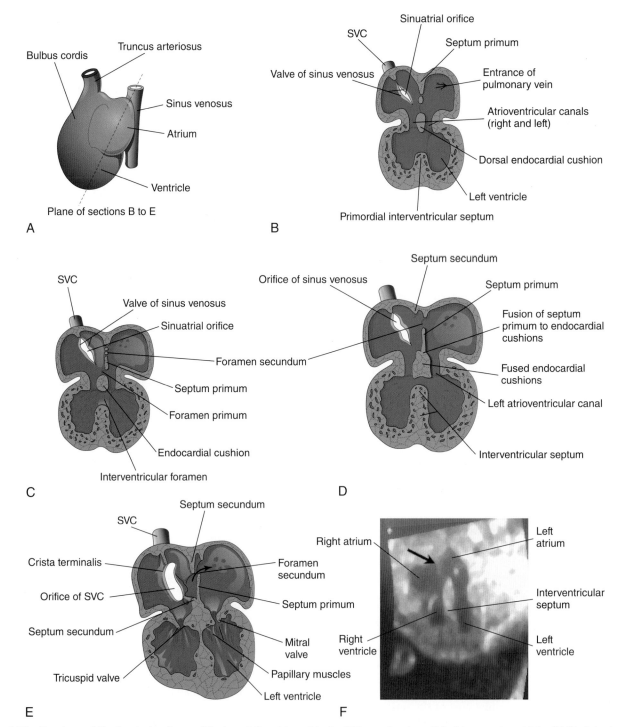

Fig. 14.9 Drawings of the heart showing partitioning of the atrioventricular (AV) canal, primordial atrium, and ventricle. (A) Sketch showing the plane of sections (B–E). (B) Frontal section of the heart during the fourth week (approximately 28 days) showing the early appearance of the septum primum, interventricular septum, and dorsal endocardial cushion. (C) Frontal section of the heart (approximately 32 days) showing perforations in the dorsal part of the septum primum. (D) Frontal section of the heart (approximately 35 days), showing the foramen secundum. (E) At approximately 8 weeks, the heart is partitioned into four chambers. The *arrow* indicates the flow of well-oxygenated blood from the right to the left atrium. (F) Sonogram of a second-trimester fetus showing the four chambers of the heart. Note the septum secundum *(arrow)*. *SVC*, Superior vena cava. Courtesy Dr. G.J. Reid, Department of Obstetrics, Gynecology and Reproductive Sciences, University of Manitoba, Women's Hospital, Winnipeg, Manitoba, Canada.

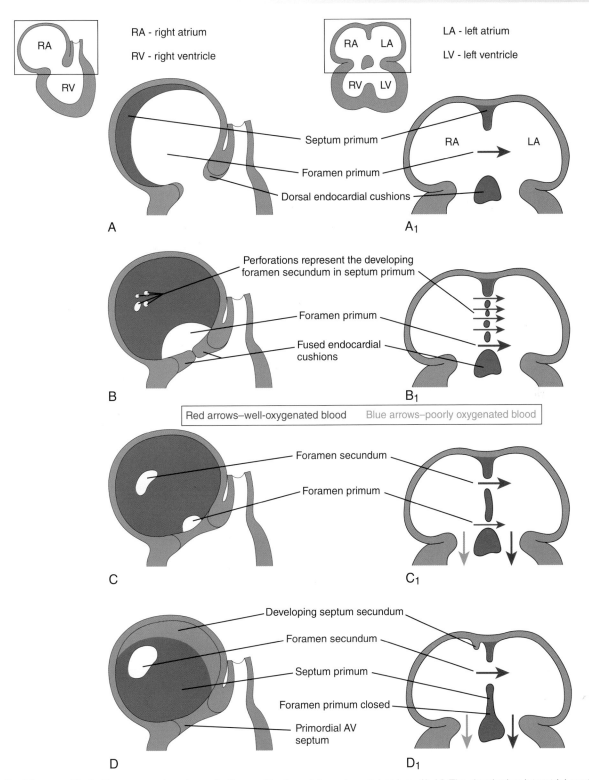

RA - right atrium

RV - right ventricle

LA - left atrium

LV - left ventricle

Septum primum

Foramen primum

Dorsal endocardial cushions

A

A₁

Perforations represent the developing foramen secundum in septum primum

Foramen primum

Fused endocardial cushions

B

B₁

Red arrows—well-oxygenated blood   Blue arrows—poorly oxygenated blood

Foramen secundum

Foramen primum

C

C₁

Developing septum secundum

Foramen secundum

Septum primum

Foramen primum closed

Primordial AV septum

D

D₁

Fig. 14.10 Diagrams illustrating progressive stages in the partitioning of the primordial atrium. (A–H) The developing interatrial septum, as viewed from the right side. (A₁–H₁) Coronal sections of the developing interatrial septum. As the septum secundum grows, note that it overlaps the opening in the septum primum, the foramen secundum. Observe the valve of the oval foramen in (G₁ and H₁). When the pressures are equal or higher in the left atrium, the valve closes the oval foramen (G₁).

Continued

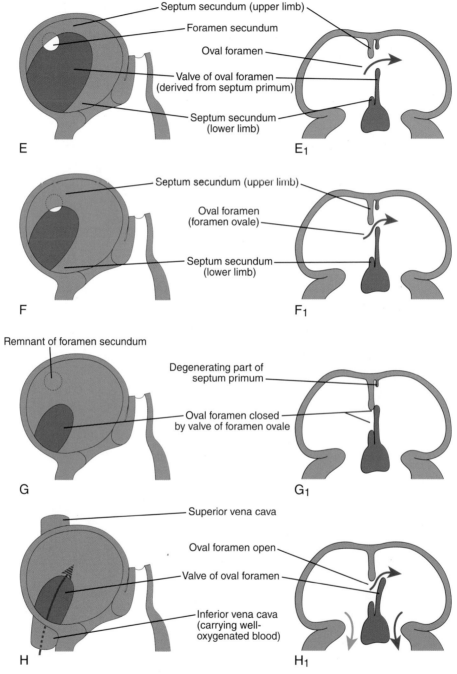

Fig. 14.10   Cont'd

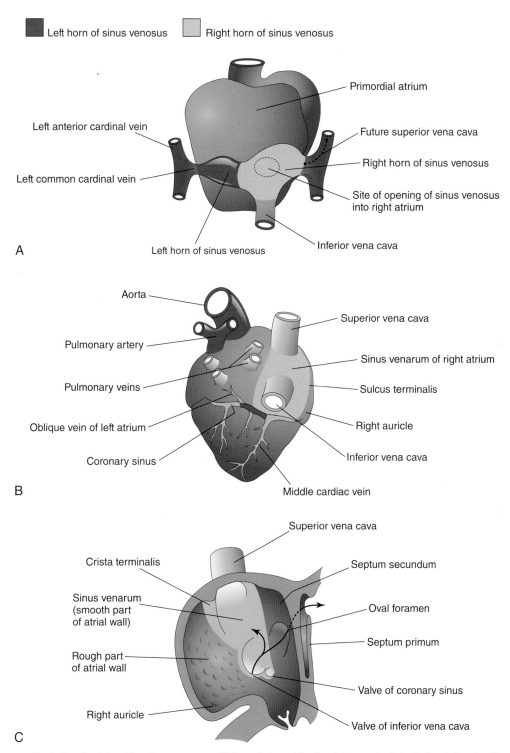

Fig. 14.11 Diagrams illustrating the fate of the sinus venosus. (A) Dorsal view of the heart (approximately 26 days) showing the primordial atrium and sinus venosus. (B) Dorsal view at 8 weeks after incorporation of the right horn of the sinus venosus into the right atrium. The left horn has become the coronary sinus. (C) Internal view of the fetal right atrium showing: (1) the smooth part of the wall of the right atrium (sinus venarum), derived from the right horn of the sinus venosus; and (2) the crista terminalis and valves of the inferior vena cava and coronary sinus, derived from the right sinuatrial valve. The primordial right atrium becomes the right auricle, a conical muscular pouch. *Arrows* indicate the flow of blood.

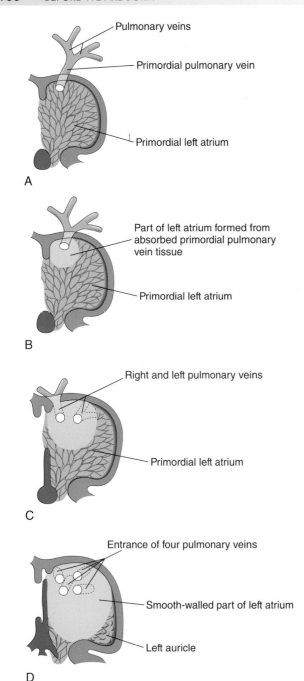

Fig. 14.12 Diagrammatic sketches illustrating absorption of the pulmonary vein into the left atrium. (A) At 5 weeks, showing the primordial pulmonary vein opening into the primordial left atrium. (B) Later stage showing partial absorption of the primordial pulmonary vein. (C) At 6 weeks, showing the openings of two pulmonary veins into the left atrium resulting from absorption of the primordial pulmonary vein. (D) At 8 weeks, showing four pulmonary veins with separate atrial orifices. The primordial left atrium becomes the left auricle, a tubular pouch of the atrium. Most of the left atrium is formed by the absorption of the primordial pulmonary vein and its branches.

Until the seventh week, there is a crescent-shaped opening **(IV foramen)** between the free edge of the IV septum and the fused endocardial cushions. The IV foramen permits communication between the right and left ventricles (Fig. 14.4B; see also Fig. 14.13B). The IV foramen usually closes by the end of the seventh week as the **bulbar ridges** fuse with the endocardial cushion (see Fig. 14.14C–E).

Closure of the IV foramen and formation of the membranous part of the IV septum result from the fusion of tissues from three sources: the right bulbar ridge, the left bulbar ridge, and the endocardial cushion. The **membranous part of the IV septum** is derived from an extension of tissue from the right side of the endocardial cushion to the muscular part of the IV septum. This tissue merges with the **aortico-pulmonary septum** and the muscular part of the IV septum (Fig. 14.15A and B). Closure of the IV foramen and formation of the membranous part of the IV septum result in communication of the pulmonary trunk with the right ventricle (and the aorta communicates with the left ventricle) (see Fig. 14.14E). Cavitation of the ventricular walls forms a sponge-like mass of muscular bundles—**trabeculae carneae**. Other bundles become the **papillary muscles** and **tendinous cords** (chordae tendineae). The tendinous cords run from the papillary muscles to the AV valves (see Fig. 14.15B).

PARTITIONING OF BULBUS CORDIS AND TRUNCUS ARTERIOSUS

During the fifth week, active proliferation of mesenchymal cells in the walls of the **bulbus cordis** results in the formation of **bulbar ridges** (Fig. 14.16B and C; see also Figs. 14.14C and D). Similar ridges form in the truncus arteriosus; these ridges are continuous with the bulbar ridges. The **bulbar** and **truncal ridges** are derived mainly from the neural crest mesenchyme. *Bone morphogenetic protein and other signaling systems in the SHF, such as Wnt and fibroblast growth factor, have been implicated in the induction and migration of neural crest cells through the primordial pharynx and the pharyngeal arches.*

Concurrently, the bulbar and truncal ridges undergo 180-degree spiraling. The spiral orientation of the bulbar and truncal ridges, possibly caused in part by the streaming of blood from the ventricles, results in the formation of a spiral **aorticopulmonary septum** when the ridges fuse (see Fig. 14.16D–G). This septum divides the bulbus cordis and the truncus arteriosus into two arterial channels, the **aorta** and the **pulmonary trunk**. Because of the spiraling of the aorticopulmonary septum, the pulmonary trunk twists around the ascending aorta (see Fig. 14.16H).

The **bulbus cordis** is incorporated into the walls of the definitive ventricles in several ways (see Fig. 14.14A and B):

- In the right ventricle, the bulbus cordis is represented by the **conus arteriosus** (infundibulum), which gives origin to the pulmonary trunk.
- In the left ventricle, the bulbus cordis forms the walls of the **aortic vestibule**, the part of the ventricular cavity just inferior to the aortic valve.

Fetal Cardiac Ultrasonography

Echocardiography and Doppler ultrasonography have made it possible for sonographers to recognize normal and abnormal fetal cardiac anatomy. Most studies are first performed at 18 to 22 weeks' gestation, when the heart is large enough to be examined easily; however, real-time ultrasound images of the fetal heart can be obtained at 16 weeks.

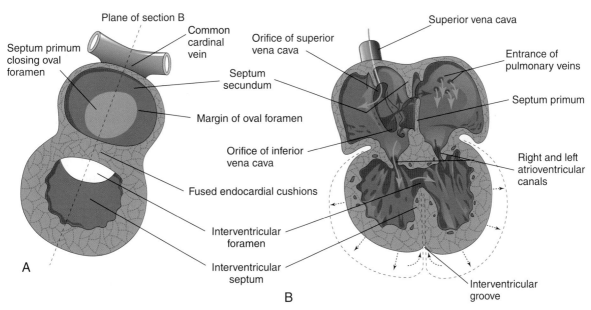

Fig. 14.13 Illustrations of partitioning of the primordial heart. (A) Sagittal section late in the fifth week, showing the cardiac septa and foramina. (B) Frontal section at a slightly later stage, showing the directions of blood flow through the heart *(blue arrows)* and the expansion of the ventricles *(black arrows)*.

DEVELOPMENT OF CARDIAC VALVES

The semilunar valves develop from three swellings of subendocardial tissue around the orifices of the aorta and pulmonary trunk (Fig. 14.17B–F). Cardiac precursors, from neural crest cells, also contribute to this formation. These swellings are hollowed out and reshaped to form three thin-walled cusps. The **atrioventricular valves** (tricuspid and mitral valves) develop similarly from localized proliferations of tissue around the AV canals.

CONDUCTING SYSTEM OF HEART

- Initially, the muscle layers of the atrium and ventricle are continuous. As the chambers form, their myocardium conducts the wave of depolarization faster than the rest of the myocardium. Throughout development, the impulse moves from the venous to the arterial pole of the heart. The atrium acts as the interim pacemaker of the heart, but the sinus venosus soon takes over this function. The **sinuatrial node** develops during the fifth week. This node is located in the right atrium, near the entrance of the SVC (see Fig. 14.15B). After incorporation of the sinus venosus, cells from its left wall are found at the base of the interatrial septum, near the opening of the coronary sinus. Together with cells from the AV region, they form the **AV node and bundle**, located just superior to the endocardial cushions (see Fig. 14.15B). The atrial and ventricular chambers become electrically isolated from each other by fibrous tissue, resulting in only the AV node and bundle being able to conduct the impulses. The fibers arising from the AV bundle pass from the atrium into the ventricle 23/73 and split into right and left **bundle branches**, which are distributed throughout the ventricular myocardium (see Fig. 14.15B). The SA node, AV node, and AV bundle are richly supplied by nerves; however, the conducting system is well developed before these nerves enter the heart. Parasympathetic innervation of the heart occurs through contributions from the neural crest cells.

Congenital Long QT Syndrome (LQTS)

LQTS results in an imbalance between depolarization and repolarization and a prolonged action potential duration. CLQT has a prevalence of 1:2000 and is the cause of approximately 10% of sudden cardiac deaths in young people. The defective genes include KCNQ1/2 and SCN5A.

BIRTH DEFECTS OF HEART AND GREAT VESSELS

Congenital heart defects (CHDs) occur with a frequency of 6 to 8 cases in 1000 live births and are a leading cause of neonatal morbidity. Some CHDs are caused by single-gene or chromosomal mechanisms; others result from exposure to teratogens such as the rubella virus (see Chapter 19). Most CHDs appear to be caused by multiple factors, both genetic and environmental (i.e., multifactorial inheritance). Real-time, three-dimensional echocardiography has permitted the detection of fetal CHDs as early as the 16th week.

Dextrocardia

If the embryonic heart tube bends to the left instead of to the right, the heart is displaced to the right (Fig. 14.18), and there is transposition whereby the heart and its vessels are reversed, left to right, as in a mirror image. **Dextrocardia** is rare (1:12,000) but it is the most frequent positional defect of the heart. In **dextrocardia with situs inversus** (transposition of abdominal viscera), such as in primary ciliary dyskinesia (see Chapters 11 and 20), the incidence of accompanying cardiac defects is low. In **isolated dextrocardia**, the abnormal position of the heart is not accompanied by displacement of other viscera, and it is usually complicated by severe cardiac defects (e.g., single ventricle and transposition of the great vessels).

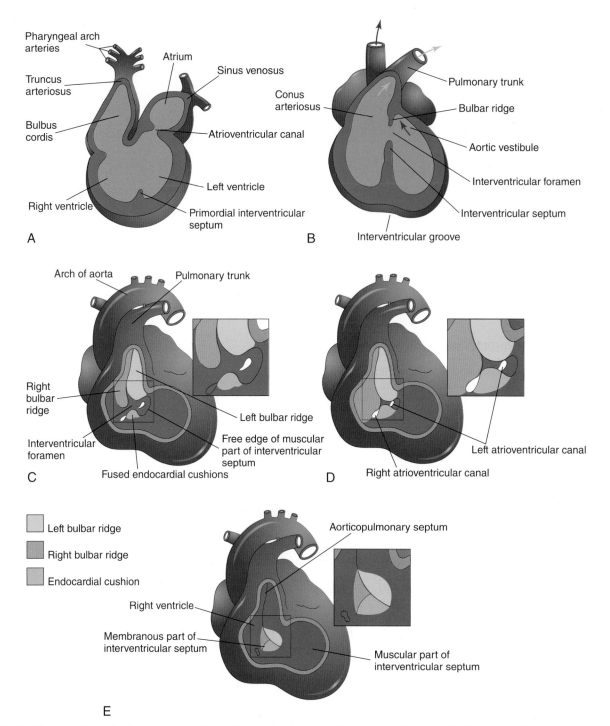

Fig. 14.14 Sketches illustrating incorporation of the bulbus cordis into the ventricles and partitioning of the bulbus cordis and truncus arteriosus into the aorta and pulmonary trunk. (A) Sagittal section at 5 weeks showing the bulbus cordis as one of the chambers of the primordial heart. (B) Schematic coronal section at 6 weeks, after the bulbus cordis has been incorporated into the ventricles to become the conus arteriosus of the right ventricle, which gives origin to the pulmonary trunk and aortic vestibule of the left ventricle. The *arrows* indicate blood flow. (C–E) Schematic drawings illustrating closure of the interventricular (IV) foramen and formation of the membranous part of the IV septum. The walls of the truncus arteriosus, bulbus cordis, and right ventricle have been removed. (C) At 5 weeks, showing the bulbar ridges and fused endocardial cushions. (D) At 6 weeks, showing how the proliferation of subendocardial tissue diminishes the IV foramen. (E) At 7 weeks, showing the fused bulbar ridges, the membranous part of the IV septum formed by extensions of tissue from the right side of the endocardial cushions, and closure of the IV foramen.

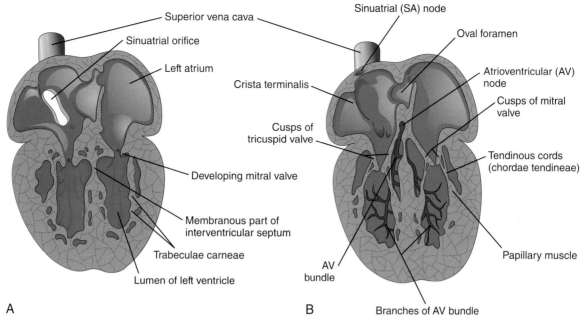

Fig. 14.15 Schematic sections of the heart illustrating successive stages in the development of the atrioventricular valves, tendinous cords *(chordae tendineae)*, and papillary muscles. (A) At 7 weeks. (B) At 20 weeks, showing the conducting system of the heart.

Ectopia Cordis

In ectopia cordis (Fig. 14.19), an extremely rare (5:1,000,000) condition, the heart is in an abnormal location. In the **thoracic form of ectopia cordis**, the heart is partly or completely exposed on the surface of the thorax. It results from faulty development of the sternum and pericardium secondary to incomplete fusion of the lateral folds in the formation of the thoracic wall during the fourth week. Death occurs in most cases during the early neonatal period, usually from infection, cardiac failure, or **hypoxemia**.

Patent Foramen Ovale (PFO)

A **patent foramen ovale (PFO)**, a variant seen in approximately 25% of people, usually results from abnormal resorption of the septum primum during the formation of the foramen secundum. If excessive resorption of the septum primum occurs, the resulting short septum primum will not close the foramen ovale (see Fig. 14.21B). If an abnormally large foramen ovale occurs because of defective development of the septum secundum, a normal septum primum will not close the abnormal foramen ovale at birth. The size of a PFO ranges from approximately 1 to 20 mm with the size increasing with age. A small isolated PFO is of no hemodynamic significance (Fig. 14.20B); however, if there are other defects (e.g., pulmonary stenosis or atresia), blood is shunted through the foramen ovale into the left atrium, resulting in **cyanosis** (deficient oxygenation of blood). A larger PFO in adults may also be associated with migraine, cryptogenic stroke, and places individuals at higher risk of decompression sickness when scuba diving.

Atrial Septal Defects (ASDs)

There are four clinically significant types of ASD (Fig. 14.21), of which the first two are relatively common:

- Ostium secundum defect
- Endocardial cushion defect with a foramen primum defect
- Sinus venosus defect
- Common atrium.

Ostium secundum ASDs (see Fig. 14.21A–D) occur in the area of the oval fossa and include defects of the septum primum and septum secundum. Females with ASDs outnumber males three to one. This ASD is one of the most common, yet least severe, types of CHD, and usually results from abnormal resorption of the septum primum during the formation of the foramen secundum. If resorption occurs in abnormal locations, the septum primum is fenestrated or net-like (see Fig. 14.21A). If excessive resorption of the septum primum occurs, the resulting short septum primum does not close the oval foramen (see Fig. 14.21B). If an abnormally large oval foramen develops as a result of defective development of the septum secundum, a normal septum primum does not close the abnormal oval foramen at birth (see Fig. 14.21D). Large ostium secundum ASDs may also occur because of a combination of excessive resorption of the septum primum and a large oval foramen.

Endocardial cushion defects with a foramen primum (see Fig. 14.21E) results when the septum primum does not fuse with the endocardial cushions, resulting in a patent foramen primum. Usually, there is also a cleft in the anterior cusp of the mitral valve.

Sinus venosus ASDs are located in the superior part of the interatrial septum, close to the entry of the SVC (see Fig. 14.21F). These defects result from incomplete absorption of the sinus venosus into the right atrium, abnormal development of the septum secundum, or both.

Common atrium occurs in patients with all three types of defects simultaneously: ostium secundum, ostium primum, and sinus venosus.

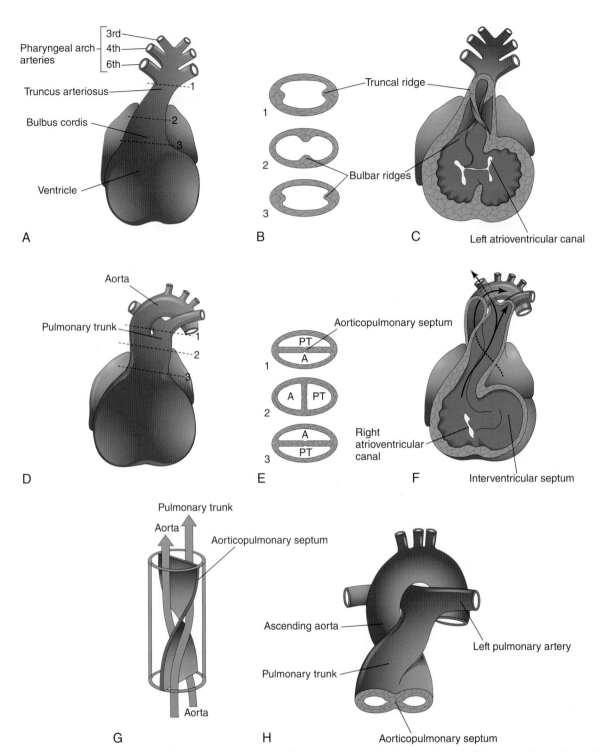

Fig. 14.16 Partitioning of the bulbus cordis and truncus arteriosus. (A) Ventral aspect of the heart at 5 weeks. The *broken lines* indicate the levels of the sections shown in (B). (B) Transverse sections of the truncus arteriosus and bulbus cordis, illustrating the truncal and bulbar ridges. (C) The ventral wall of the heart and truncus arteriosus has been removed to demonstrate these ridges. (D) Ventral aspect of the heart after partitioning of the truncus arteriosus. The *broken lines* indicate the levels of the sections shown in (E). (E) Sections through the newly formed aorta *(A)* and pulmonary trunk *(PT)* showing the aorticopulmonary septum. (F) Ventral aspect of the heart at 6 weeks. The ventral wall of the heart and pulmonary trunk have been removed to show the aorticopulmonary septum. (G) Diagram illustrating the spiral form of the aorticopulmonary septum. (H) Drawing showing the great arteries (ascending aorta and pulmonary trunk) twisting around each other as they leave the heart.

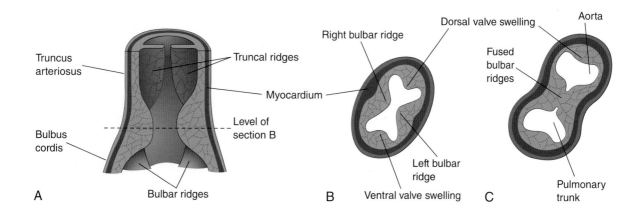

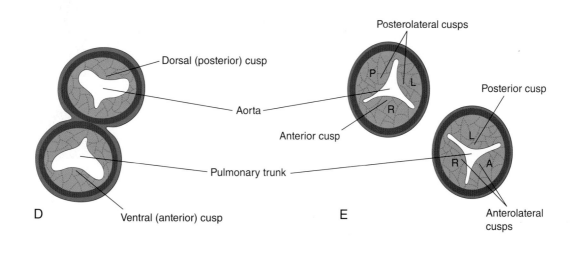

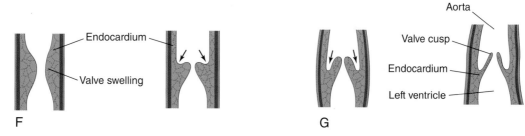

Fig. 14.17 Development of the semilunar valves of the aorta and pulmonary trunk. (A) Sketch of a section of the truncus arteriosus and bulbus cordis showing the valve swellings. (B) Transverse section of the bulbus cordis. (C) Similar section after fusion of the bulbar ridges. (D) Formation of the walls and valves of the aorta and pulmonary trunk. (E) Rotation of the vessels has established the adult positions of the valves in relation to each other. (F and G) Longitudinal sections of the aorticoventricular junction illustrating successive stages in the hollowing *(arrows)* and thinning of the valve swellings to form the valve cusps. *A,* Anterior; *L,* left; *P,* posterior; *R,* right.

NORMAL

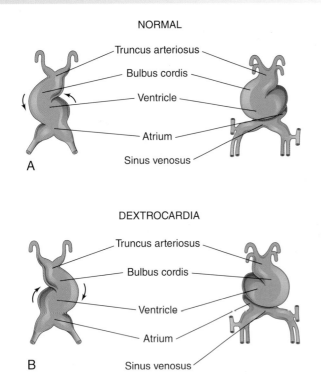

DEXTROCARDIA

Fig. 14.18   The embryonic heart tube during the fourth week. (A) Normal looping of the tubular heart to the right *(arrows)*. (B) Abnormal looping to the left.

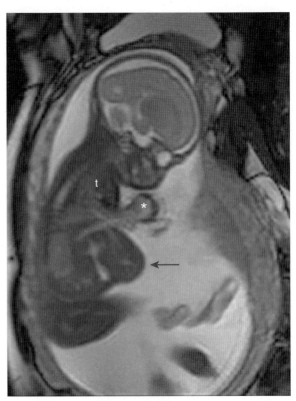

Fig. 14.19   Magnetic resonance image of a fetus demonstrating exteriorization of the heart *(*)* from its normal position within the thorax *(t)*. An omphalocele (see Chapter 12) can also be seen *(arrow)*. From Leyder M, van Berkel K, Done E, Cannie M, Van Hecke W, Voeselmans A: Ultrasound meets magnetic resonance imaging in the diagnosis of pentalogy of Cantrell with complete ectopy of the heart, *Gynecol Obstet [Sunnyvale]* 4:200, 2014.

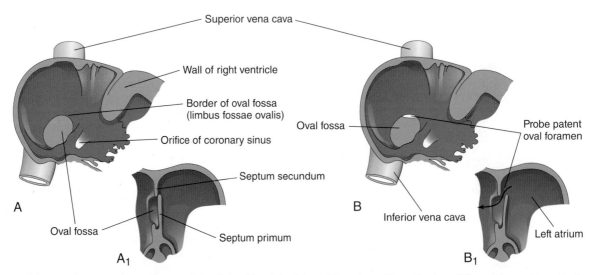

Fig. 14.20   (A) Normal postnatal appearance of the right side of the interatrial septum after adhesion of the septum primum to the septum secundum. (A$_1$) Sketch of a section of the interatrial septum illustrating formation of the oval fossa in the right atrium. Note that the floor of the fossa is formed by the septum primum. (B and B$_1$) Similar views of a probe-patent oval foramen result from incomplete adhesion of the septum primum to the septum secundum. Some well-oxygenated blood can enter the right atrium via a patent oval foramen; however, if the opening is small, it is usually of no hemodynamic significance.

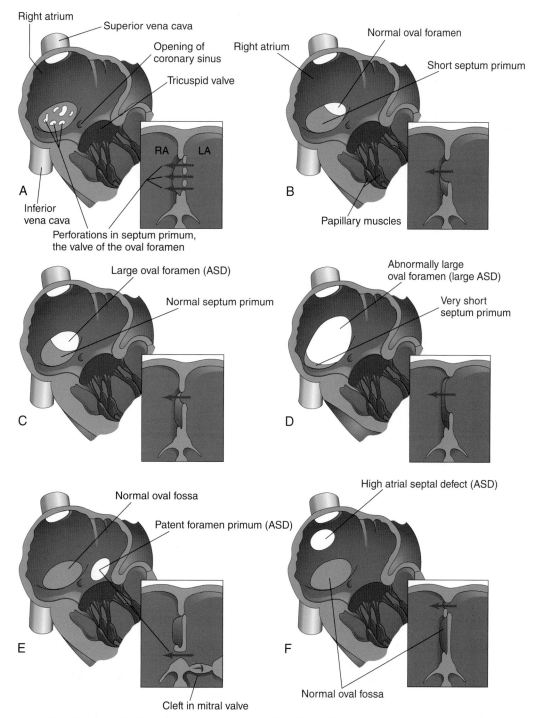

Fig. 14.21 Drawings of the right aspect of the interatrial septum. The adjacent sketches of sections of the septa illustrate various types of atrial septal defect *(ASD)*. (A) Patent oval foramen resulting from resorption of the septum primum in abnormal locations. (B) Patent oval foramen caused by excessive resorption of the septum primum (short flap defect). (C) Patent oval foramen resulting from an abnormally large oval foramen. (D) Patent oval foramen resulting from an abnormally large oval foramen and excessive resorption of the septum primum. (E) Endocardial cushion defect with a primum-type ASD. The adjacent section shows the cleft in the anterior cusp of the mitral valve. (F) Sinus venosus ASD. The high septal defect resulted from abnormal absorption of the sinus venosus into the right atrium. (E and F) Note that the oval fossa has formed normally. *Arrows* indicate the direction of flow of blood. *LA,* Left atrium; *RA,* right atrium.

Ventricular Septal Defects

Ventricular septal defects (VSDs) are the most common (isolated VSD 3:1000) type of CHD, accounting for approximately 35% of cases. VSDs occur more frequently in males. septum-Most VSDs involve the membranous part of the IV septum (Fig. 14.22B). Many small VSDs close spontaneously, usually during the first year. Most individuals with a large VSD have massive left-to-right shunting of blood. **Muscular VSD** is a less common type of defect that may appear anywhere in the muscular part of the IV septum. **Transposition of great arteries** (Fig. 14.23) and a rudimentary outlet chamber are present in most infants with this severe type of CHD.

Persistent Truncus Arteriosus

Persistent truncus arteriosus (TA) (7:100,000 live births) results from failure of the truncal ridges and aorticopulmonary septum to develop normally and to divide the TA into the aorta and pulmonary trunk (see Fig. 14.22). The most common type of persistent TA is a **single arterial trunk** that branches to form the pulmonary trunk and ascending aorta (see Fig. 14.22A and B), supplying the systemic, pulmonary, and coronary circulations. A VSD is always present with a TA defect; the TA straddles the VSD (see Fig. 14.22B).

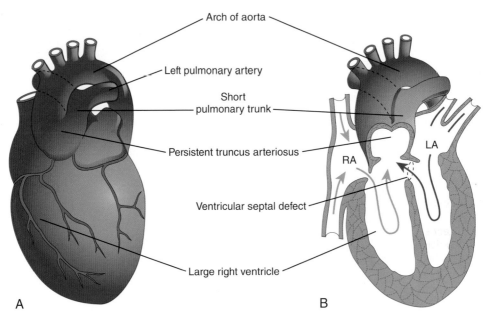

Fig. 14.22   Illustrations of the main type of persistent truncus arteriosus. (A) The common trunk divides into the aorta and a short pulmonary trunk. (B) Coronal section of the heart is shown in (A). Observe the circulation of blood in this heart *(arrows)* and the ventricular septal defect. *LA*, Left atrium; *RA*, right atrium.

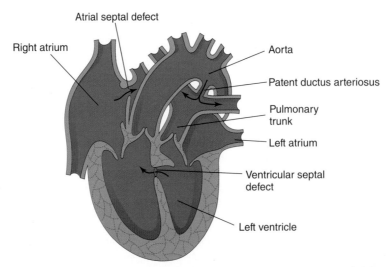

Fig. 14.23   Drawing of a heart illustrating transposition of the great arteries (TGA). The ventricular septal defect (VSD) and atrial septal defect (ASD) allow mixing of the arterial and venous blood. TGA is the most common single cause of **cyanotic heart disease** in neonates. This birth defect is often associated with other cardiac defects, as shown (VSD and ASD). The *arrows* indicate the flow of blood. In TGA, when there is an ASD, blood flows from the right atrium to the left atrium.

Transposition of Great Arteries

Transposition of the great arteries (TGA) is a severe congenital heart defect with an incidence of approximately 1:4000 live births. It is the most common cause of **cyanotic heart disease** in neonates (see Fig. 14.23). In typical cases, the aorta lies anterior and to the right of the pulmonary trunk and arises anteriorly from the morphological right ventricle, whereas the pulmonary trunk arises from the morphological left ventricle. There is also an ASD, with or without an associated patent ductus arteriosus (PDA) and VSD. This defect is believed to result from *failure of the conus arteriosus to develop normally* during incorporation of the bulbus cordis into the ventricles. Defective neural crest cell migration may also be involved.

Unequal Division of Truncus Arteriosus

Unequal division of the truncus arteriosus (Fig. 14.24A and B; also see Fig. 14.22) results when partitioning of the TA superior to the valves is unequal, producing one large great artery and one small one. As a result, the aorticopulmonary septum is not aligned with the IV septum, and a VSD results. The larger vessel (aorta or pulmonary trunk) usually straddles the VSD (see Fig. 14.24A and B).

Pulmonary Valve Stenosis

In **pulmonary valve stenosis**, the cusps of the pulmonary valve are fused to form a dome with a narrow central opening. In **infundibular stenosis**, the conus arteriosus of the right ventricle is underdeveloped. The two types of pulmonary stenosis may be concurrent. Depending on the degree of obstruction to blood flow, there is a variable degree of hypertrophy of the right ventricle (see Fig. 14.24B).

Tetralogy of Fallot

The classic group of four cardiac defects—**tetralogy of Fallot** consists of the following (see Fig. 14.24A and B):

- Pulmonary stenosis (obstructed right ventricular outflow)
- Ventricular septal defect
- Dextroposition of the aorta (straddling or overriding both ventricles)
- Right ventricular hypertrophy.

In these cardiac defects, the pulmonary trunk is usually small and there may be varying degrees of **pulmonary artery stenosis** as well.

Aortic Stenosis and Aortic Atresia

In **aortic valve stenosis**, the edges of the valve are usually fused with a narrow opening. This defect may be present at birth or it may develop after birth (acquired). The valvular stenosis causes extra work for the heart and results in **hypertrophy** of the left ventricle and abnormal heart sounds (**heart murmurs**).

In *subaortic stenosis*, there is often a band of fibrous tissue just inferior to the aortic valve. The narrowing of the aorta results from the persistence of tissue that normally degenerates as the valve forms. **Aortic atresia** is present when obstruction of the aorta or its valve is complete.

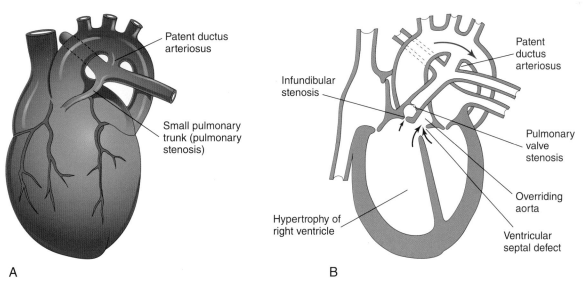

Fig. 14.24 Drawings illustrating tetralogy of Fallot. (A) Drawing of an infant's heart showing a small **(pulmonary stenosis)** and a large aorta resulting from unequal partitioning of the truncus arteriosus. There is also hypertrophy of the right ventricle and a patent ductus arteriosus. (B) Frontal section of this heart, illustrating the tetralogy of Fallot. Observe the four cardiac defects of this tetralogy: pulmonary valve stenosis, ventricular septal defect, overriding aorta, and hypertrophy of the right ventricle. In this case infundibular stenosis is also shown. The *arrows* indicate the flow of blood into the great vessels (aorta and pulmonary trunk).

DERIVATIVES OF PHARYNGEAL ARCH ARTERIES

13

14

As the pharyngeal arches develop during the fourth week, they are supplied by **pharyngeal arch arteries** arising from the aortic sac (Fig. 14.25B). These arteries terminate in the dorsal aorta on the ipsilateral (same) side. Although six pairs of arch arteries usually develop, they are not present at the same time (see Fig. 14.25B and C).

DERIVATIVES OF FIRST PAIR OF PHARYNGEAL ARCH ARTERIES

The first pair of arteries largely disappears but remnants of them form part of the **maxillary arteries**, which supply the ears, teeth, and muscles of the eyes and face. They may also contribute to the formation of the external carotid arteries (see Fig. 14.25B).

DERIVATIVES OF SECOND PAIR OF PHARYNGEAL ARCH ARTERIES

Dorsal parts of these arteries persist and form the stems of the small **stapedial arteries**; these small vessels run through the ring of the **stapes**, a small bone in the middle ear (see Fig. 17.11C).

DERIVATIVES OF THIRD PAIR OF PHARYNGEAL ARCH ARTERIES

Proximal parts of these arteries form the **common carotid arteries**, which supply structures in the head (Fig. 14.26D). Distal parts of these arteries join with the dorsal aortae to form the **internal carotid arteries**, which supply the middle ears, orbits, brain and its meninges, and pituitary gland.

DERIVATIVES OF FOURTH PAIR OF PHARYNGEAL ARCH ARTERIES

The left fourth artery forms part of the **arch of the aorta** (see Fig. 14.26C and D). The proximal part of the arch artery develops from the **aortic sac**, and the distal part is derived from the **left dorsal aorta**. The right fourth artery becomes the proximal part of the **right subclavian artery**. The distal part of the right subclavian artery forms from the **right dorsal aorta** and **right seventh intersegmental artery**. The left subclavian artery is not derived from a pharyngeal arch artery; it forms from the **left seventh intersegmental artery** (see Fig. 14.26A). As development proceeds, differential growth shifts the origin of the left subclavian artery cranially. Consequently, it lies close to the origin of the left common carotid artery (see Fig. 14.26D).

FATE OF FIFTH PAIR OF PHARYNGEAL ARCH ARTERIES

Approximately 50% of the time, the fifth pair of arteries consists of rudimentary vessels that soon degenerate, leaving no vascular derivatives. In other embryos, these arches do not develop.

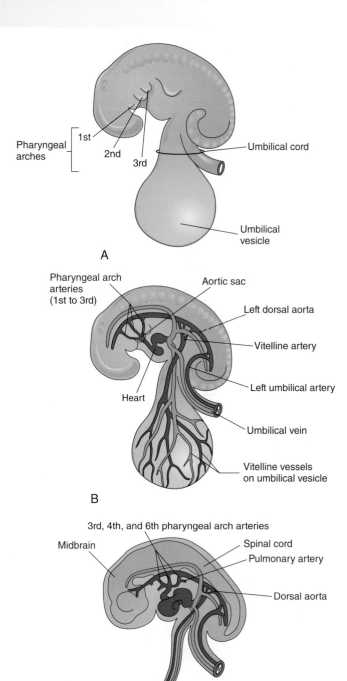

Fig. 14.25 Pharyngeal arches and pharyngeal arch arteries. (A) Left side of an embryo (approximately 26 days). (B) Schematic drawing of this embryo showing the left pharyngeal arch arteries arising from the aortic sac, running through the pharyngeal arches, and terminating in the left dorsal aorta. (C) An embryo (approximately 37 days) showing the single dorsal aorta and that most of the first two pairs of pharyngeal arch arteries have degenerated.

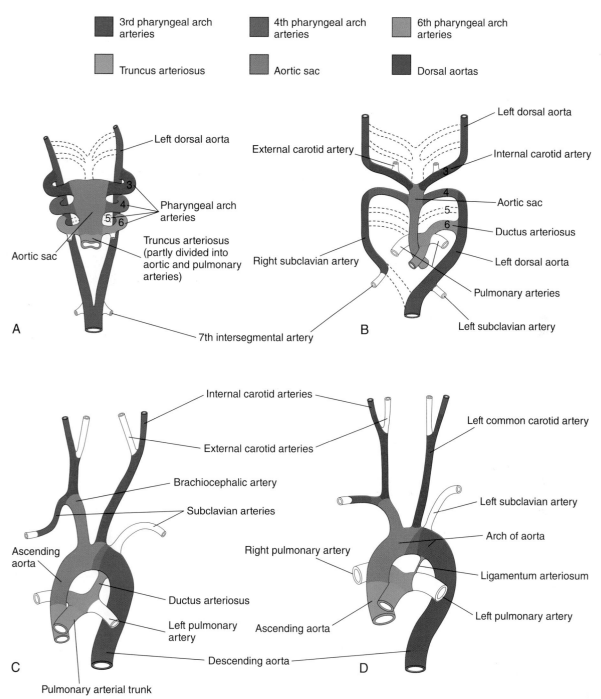

3rd pharyngeal arch arteries

4th pharyngeal arch arteries

6th pharyngeal arch arteries

Truncus arteriosus

Aortic sac

Dorsal aortas

Left dorsal aorta

Pharyngeal arch arteries

Truncus arteriosus (partly divided into aortic and pulmonary arteries)

Aortic sac

A

7th intersegmental artery

External carotid artery

Left dorsal aorta

Internal carotid artery

Aortic sac

Ductus arteriosus

Left dorsal aorta

Right subclavian artery

Pulmonary arteries

Left subclavian artery

B

Internal carotid arteries

External carotid arteries

Brachiocephalic artery

Subclavian arteries

Ascending aorta

Ductus arteriosus

Left pulmonary artery

C

Pulmonary arterial trunk

Descending aorta

Left common carotid artery

Left subclavian artery

Arch of aorta

Right pulmonary artery

Ligamentum arteriosum

Ascending aorta

Left pulmonary artery

D

Fig. 14.26 Schematic drawings illustrating the arterial changes that result during the transformation of the truncus arteriosus, aortic sac, pharyngeal arch arteries, and dorsal aortae into the adult arterial pattern. The vessels that are not colored are not derived from these structures. (A) Pharyngeal arch arteries at 6 weeks; by this stage, the first two pairs of arteries have largely disappeared. (B) Pharyngeal arch arteries at 7 weeks; the parts of the dorsal aortae and pharyngeal arch arteries that normally disappear are indicated with *broken lines*. (C) Arterial arrangement at 8 weeks. (D) Sketch of the arterial vessels of a 6-month-old neonate. Note that the ascending aorta and pulmonary arteries are considerably smaller in (C) than in (D). This represents the relative flow through these vessels at the different stages of development. Observe the large size of the ductus arteriosus (DA) in (C) and that it is essentially a direct continuation of the pulmonary trunk. The DA normally becomes closed within the first few days after birth. Eventually the DA becomes the ligamentum arteriosum, as shown in (D).

DERIVATIVES OF SIXTH PAIR OF PHARYNGEAL ARCH ARTERIES

The **left sixth artery** develops as follows (see Fig. 14.26B and C):

- The proximal part of the artery persists as the proximal part of the left pulmonary artery.
- The distal part of the artery passes from the left pulmonary artery to the dorsal aorta and forms a prenatal shunt, the ductus arteriosus.

The **right sixth artery** develops as follows:

- The proximal part of the artery persists as the proximal part of the right pulmonary artery.
- The distal part of the artery degenerates.

The transformation of the sixth pair of arteries explains why the course of the **recurrent laryngeal nerves** differs on the two sides. These nerves supply the sixth pair of arches and hook around the sixth pair of arteries on their way to the developing larynx (Fig. 14.27A). On the right, because the distal part of the right sixth artery degenerates, the right recurrent laryngeal nerve moves superiorly and hooks around the proximal part of the right subclavian artery, the derivative of the fourth artery (see Fig. 14.27B). On the left, the left recurrent laryngeal nerve hooks around the **ductus arteriosus (DA)** formed by the distal part of the sixth artery. When this arterial shunt involutes after birth, the nerve remains around the **ligamentum arteriosum** (remnant of DA) and the arch of the aorta (see Fig. 14.27C).

Coarctation of Aorta

Aortic coarctation occurs in approximately 10% of children with CHDs and is characterized by an **aortic constriction** of varying length (Fig. 14.28). Most constrictions occur distal to the origin of the left subclavian artery, at the entrance of the DA (**juxtaductal coarctation**).

A classification system of preductal and postductal coarctations is commonly used; however, in 90% of cases, the coarctation is directly opposite the DA. **Coarctation** occurs two times as often in males as in females and is associated with a **bicuspid aortic valve** in 70% of cases (see Fig. 14.15B).

Double Aortic Arch

This rare (5–7:100,000) anomaly is characterized by a vascular ring around the trachea and esophagus (Fig. 14.29). The ring results from failure of the distal part of the right dorsal aorta to disappear (see Fig. 14.29A); as a result, right and left arches form. Usually, the right arch of the aorta is the larger one and it passes posterior to the trachea and esophagus (see Fig. 14.29B). If the compression is significant, it causes wheezing respirations that are aggravated by crying, feeding, and flexion of the neck; rarely it can cause life-threatening tracheal obstruction in infants.

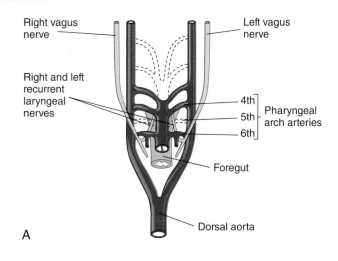

A

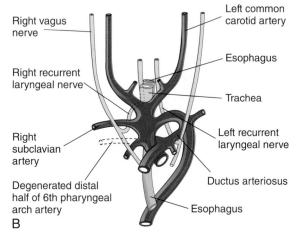

B

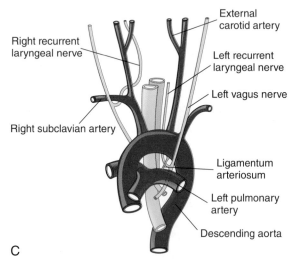

C

Fig. 14.27 The relation of the recurrent laryngeal nerves to the pharyngeal arch arteries. (A) At 6 weeks, showing that the recurrent laryngeal nerves are hooked around the sixth pair of pharyngeal arch arteries. (B) At 8 weeks, showing that the right recurrent laryngeal nerve is hooked around the right subclavian artery, and the left recurrent laryngeal nerve is hooked around the ductus arteriosus and arch of the aorta. (C) After birth, showing that the left recurrent laryngeal nerve is hooked around the ligamentum arteriosum and the arch of the aorta.

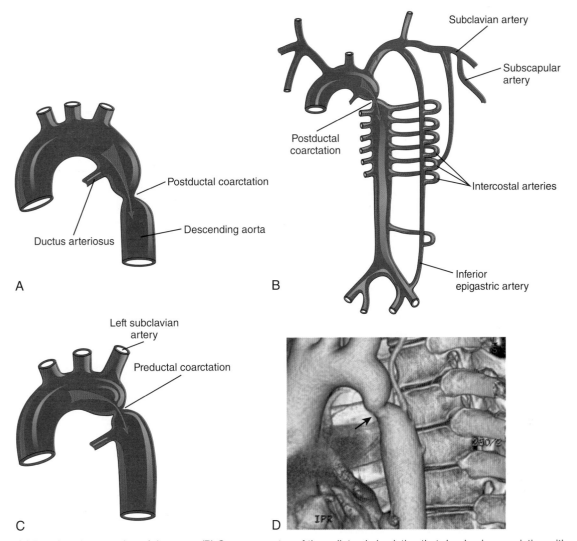

Fig. 14.28 (A) Postductal coarctation of the aorta. (B) Common routes of the collateral circulation that develop in association with postductal coarctation of the aorta. (C) Preductal coarctation. *Arrows* indicate flow of blood. (D) Three-dimensional computed tomography reconstruction image of preductal coarctation *(arrow)* in the aorta in an adult. D, Courtesy Dr. James Koenig, Department of Radiology, Health Sciences Centre, Winnipeg, Manitoba, Canada.

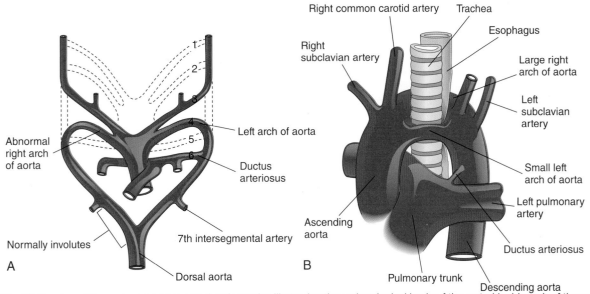

Fig. 14.29 (A) Drawing of the embryonic pharyngeal arch arteries illustrating the embryological basis of the aorta (double arch of the aorta). (B) A large right arch of the aorta and a small left arch of the aorta arise from the ascending aorta and form a vascular ring around the trachea and esophagus. Observe that there is compression of the esophagus and trachea. The right common carotid and subclavian arteries arise separately from the large right arch of the aorta.

Right Arch of Aorta

When the entire right dorsal aorta persists (Fig. 14.30A) and the distal part of the left dorsal aorta involutes, a right arch of the aorta results (0.1–1:1000). There are two main types:

- **Right arch of the aorta without a retroesophageal component** (see Fig. 14.30B). The ductus arteriosus (ligamentum arteriosum) passes from the right pulmonary artery to the right arch of the aorta.
- **Right arch of the aorta with a retroesophageal component** (see Fig. 14.30C). Originally, a small left arch of the aorta probably involuted, leaving the right arch of the aorta posterior to the esophagus. The DA attaches to the distal part of the arch of the aorta and forms a ring that may constrict the esophagus and trachea.

Anomalous Right Subclavian Artery

The right subclavian artery normally arises from the distal part of the arch of the aorta and passes posterior to the trachea and esophagus to supply the right upper limb (Fig. 14.31). A **retroesophageal right subclavian artery** occurs when the right fourth pharyngeal arch artery and the right dorsal aorta disappear cranial to the seventh intersegmental artery. As a result, the right subclavian artery forms from the right seventh intersegmental artery and the distal part of the right dorsal aorta. As development proceeds, differential growth shifts the origin of the right subclavian artery cranially, until it comes to lie close to the origin of the left subclavian artery.

Although an anomalous right subclavian artery is fairly common and always forms a vascular ring (see Fig. 14.31C), it is rarely clinically significant because the ring is usually not tight enough to constrict the esophagus and trachea very much.

PHARYNGEAL ARCH ARTERIAL BIRTH DEFECTS

Because of the many changes involved in the transformation of the embryonic pharyngeal arch system of arteries into the adult arterial pattern, it is understandable why defects may occur. Most defects result from the persistence of parts of the pharyngeal arch arteries that usually disappear or from the disappearance of parts that normally persist.

FETAL AND NEONATAL CIRCULATION

The fetal cardiovascular system is designed to serve prenatal needs (Fig. 14.32). Modifications at birth establish the neonatal pattern (Fig. 14.33). Good respiration in the neonatal period is dependent on normal circulatory changes occurring at birth, which results in oxygenation of the blood occurring in the lungs when fetal blood flow through the placenta ceases. Before birth, the lungs do not provide gas exchange and the pulmonary vessels are vasoconstricted. The three vascular structures most important in the transitional circulation are the ductus venosus, oval foramen, and ductus arteriosus (see Fig. 14.33).

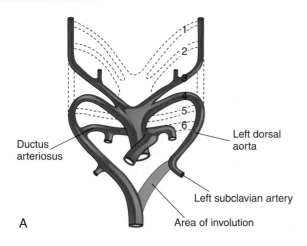

A

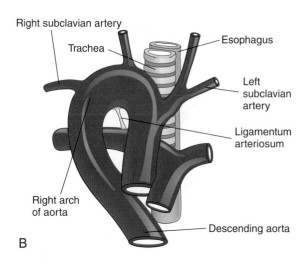

B

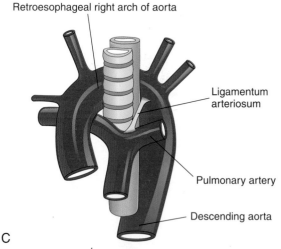

C

Fig. 14.30 (A) Sketch of the pharyngeal arch arteries showing normal involution of the distal portion of the left dorsal aorta. There is also persistence of the entire right dorsal aorta and the distal part of the right sixth pharyngeal arch artery. (B) Right pharyngeal arch artery without a retroesophageal component. (C) Right arch of the aorta with a retroesophageal component. The abnormal right arch of the aorta and ligamentum arteriosum (postnatal remnant of the ductus arteriosus) form a vascular ring that compresses the esophagus and trachea.

FETAL CIRCULATION

Highly oxygenated (80% O₂ saturation) (Note: all O₂ saturation values noted are approximate), nutrient-rich blood returns under high pressure from the placenta in the **umbilical vein** (see Fig. 14.32). On approaching the liver, approximately one-half of the blood passes directly into the **ductus venosus**, a fetal vessel connecting the umbilical vein to the IVC; consequently, this blood bypasses the liver. The other half of the blood in the umbilical vein flows into the sinusoids of the liver and enters the IVC through the **hepatic veins**. Blood flow through the ductus venosus is regulated by a sphincter mechanism close to the umbilical vein. After a short course in the IVC, all of the blood enters the right atrium of the heart. Most blood from the IVC is directed by the **crista dividens**, through the oval foramen into the left atrium (65% O₂ saturation). There, it mixes with the relatively small amount of poorly oxygenated blood returning from the lungs through the pulmonary veins. Fetal lungs use the oxygen from the blood instead of replenishing it. From the left atrium, the blood then passes to the left ventricle and leaves through the ascending aorta. The arteries to the heart, neck, head, and upper limbs receive well-oxygenated blood from the ascending aorta (60% O₂ saturation). The liver also receives well-oxygenated blood from the umbilical vein.

The small amount of well-oxygenated blood from the IVC in the right atrium mixes with poorly oxygenated blood from the SVC and coronary sinus and passes into the right ventricle. This blood, with medium oxygen content (55% O₂ saturation), leaves the heart through the pulmonary trunk. Because of the high pulmonary vascular resistance in fetal life, pulmonary blood flow is low. Approximately 10% of this blood flow goes to the lungs; most blood passes through the DA (80% O₂ saturation) into the aorta to the fetal body. It then returns to the placenta through the umbilical arteries (see Fig. 14.32). Approximately 10% of blood from the ascending aorta enters the descending aorta to supply the viscera and the inferior part of the body. Most of the blood in the descending aorta passes into the umbilical arteries (40% O₂ saturation) and is returned to the placenta for reoxygenation.

TRANSITIONAL NEONATAL CIRCULATION

Important circulatory adjustments occur at birth, when the circulation of fetal blood through the placenta ceases and the infant's lungs expand and begin to function (see Fig. 14.33). *As soon as the fetus is born, the oval foramen, DA, ductus venosus, and umbilical vessels are no longer needed.* The sphincter in the ductus venosus constricts and all blood entering the liver passes through the hepatic sinusoids. This, combined with occlusion of the placental circulation, causes an immediate decrease in blood pressure in the IVC and right atrium.

Because of increased pulmonary blood flow, the pressure in the left atrium is higher than in the right atrium. The *increased left atrial pressure closes the oval foramen* by pressing the valve of the foramen against the septum secundum (see Fig. 14.33). The output from the right ventricle then flows entirely into the pulmonary circulation. Because pulmonary vascular resistance is lower than systemic vascular resistance, blood flow in the DA reverses, passing from the aorta to the pulmonary trunk.

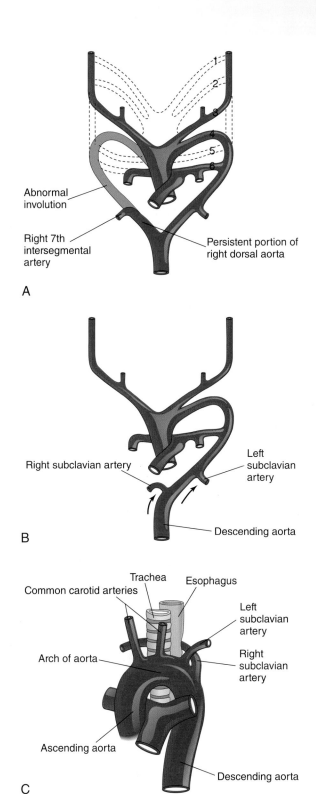

Fig. 14.31 Sketches illustrating the possible embryological basis for an abnormal origin of the right subclavian artery. (A) The right fourth pharyngeal arch artery and the cranial part of the right dorsal aorta have involuted. As a result, the right subclavian artery forms from the right seventh intersegmental artery and the distal segment of the right dorsal aorta. (B) As the arch of the aorta forms, the right subclavian artery is carried cranially *(arrows)* with the left subclavian artery. (C) The abnormal right subclavian artery arises from the aorta and passes posterior to the trachea and esophagus.

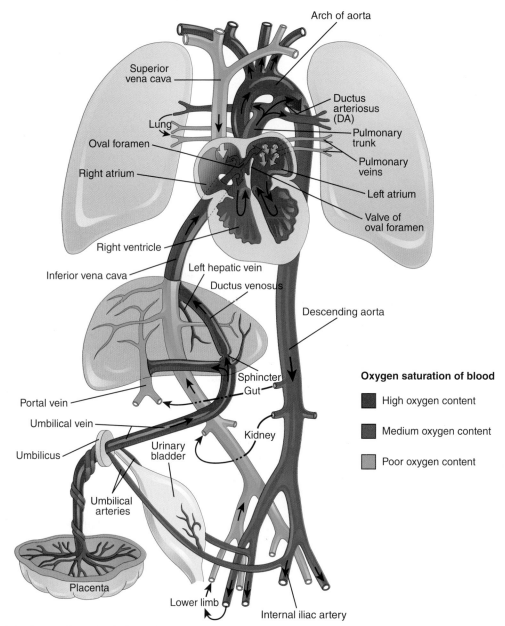

Fig. 14.32 Fetal circulation. The colors indicate the oxygen saturation of the blood, and the *arrows* show the course of the blood from the placenta to the heart. The organs are not drawn to scale. A small amount of highly oxygenated blood from the inferior vena cava remains in the right atrium and mixes with poorly oxygenated blood from the superior vena cava. The medium-oxygenated blood then passes into the right ventricle. Observe that three shunts permit most of the blood to bypass the liver and lungs: (1) ductus venosus, (2) oval foramen, and (3) ductus arteriosus. The poorly oxygenated blood returns to the placenta for oxygen and nutrients through the umbilical arteries.

The *DA begins to constrict at birth*, but for a few days there is often a small shunt of blood from the aorta to the pulmonary trunk in healthy, full-term neonates. In premature neonates and those with persistent hypoxia (decreased oxygen), the DA may remain open much longer. In full-term neonates, oxygen is the most important factor in controlling closure of the DA, and it appears to be mediated by **bradykinin** (a substance released from the lungs) and **prostaglandins** that act on the smooth muscle in the wall of the DA.

The *umbilical arteries constrict at birth*, preventing the loss of neonatal blood. The umbilical cord is not tied for a minute or so; consequently, blood flow through the umbilical vein continues, transferring fetal blood from the placenta to the neonate.

The change from the fetal to the adult pattern of blood circulation is not a sudden occurrence. Some changes occur with the first breath; others take place over hours and days. The closure of fetal vessels and the oval foramen is initially a functional change. Later, anatomic closure results from the proliferation of endothelial and fibrous tissues.

DERIVATIVES OF FETAL VESSELS AND STRUCTURES

Because of the changes in the cardiovascular system at birth, some vessels and structures are no longer required. Over

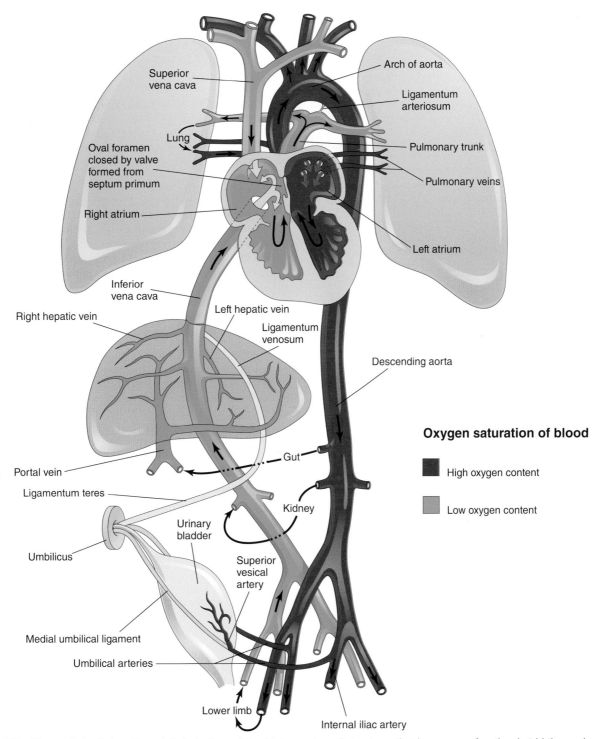

Fig. 14.33 Neonatal circulation. The adult derivatives of the fetal vessels and structures that become nonfunctional at birth are shown. The *arrows* indicate the course of the blood in the infant. The organs are not drawn to scale. After birth, the three fetal shunts cease to function, and the pulmonary and systemic circulations become separated.

a period of months, these fetal vessels form nonfunctional ligaments.

UMBILICAL VEIN AND ROUND LIGAMENT OF LIVER

The intraabdominal part of the umbilical vein eventually becomes the round ligament of the liver (ligamentum teres) (see Fig. 14.33). The umbilical vein remains patent for a considerable period and may be used for blood transfusions

or administration of medications during the early neonatal period. These transfusions are often performed to prevent brain damage and death in neonates with anemia as a result of erythroblastosis fetalis (hemolytic disease of the newborn).

DUCTUS VENOSUS AND LIGAMENTUM VENOSUM

The ductus venosus becomes the ligamentum venosum; however, its closure is more prolonged than that of the DA.

The ligamentum venosum passes through the liver from the left branch of the portal vein to the IVC, to which it is attached (see Fig. 14.33).

Patent Ductus Arteriosus

Patent ductus arteriosus (PDA) is uncommon in full-term live births (3–8:1000) and occurs two to three times more frequently in females than in males (Fig. 14.34B). Functional closure of the PDA usually occurs soon after birth; however, if the ductus arteriosus remains patent, aortic blood is shunted into the pulmonary artery. PDA is the most common birth defect associated with **maternal rubella infection** during early pregnancy. Preterm neonates and those born at high altitude may have PDA; this patency is the result of **hypoxia** and immaturity. The embryological basis of PDA is the failure of the DA to involute after birth and form the ligamentum arteriosum.

UMBILICAL ARTERIES AND ABDOMINAL LIGAMENTS

Most of the intraabdominal parts of the umbilical arteries become the **medial umbilical ligaments** (see Fig. 14.33); the proximal parts of these vessels persist as the **superior vesical arteries**, which supply the urinary bladder.

OVAL FORAMEN AND OVAL FOSSA

The oval foramen normally closes functionally at birth (see Fig. 14.33). Anatomic closure occurs by the third month and results from tissue proliferation and adhesion of the septum primum to the left margin of the septum secundum. The septum primum forms the floor of the oval fossa. The inferior edge of the septum secundum forms a rounded fold, the border of the oval fossa, which marks the former boundary of the oval foramen (see Fig. 14.20).

DUCTUS ARTERIOSUS AND LIGAMENTUM ARTERIOSUM

Functional closure of the DA is usually completed 10 to 15 hours after birth. Anatomic closure of the DA and formation of the ligamentum arteriosum usually occurs by the 12th postnatal week.

DEVELOPMENT OF THE LYMPHATIC SYSTEM

The lymphatic system begins to develop at the end of the sixth week. The precursor lymphatic endothelial cells are derived from the cardinal veins. Lymphatic vessels develop in a manner similar to that described for blood vessels, and they make connections with the venous system. The early lymphatic capillaries join each other to form a network of lymphatics. There are **six primary lymph sacs** present at the end of the embryonic period (Fig. 14.35A):

- Two **jugular lymph sacs** near the junction of the subclavian veins with the anterior cardinal veins (future internal jugular veins)
- Two **iliac lymph sacs** near the junction of the iliac veins with the posterior cardinal veins
- One **retroperitoneal lymph sac** in the root of the mesentery on the posterior abdominal wall
- One **cisterna chyli (chyle cistern)** located dorsal to the retroperitoneal lymph sac.

Lymphatic vessels soon connect to the lymph sacs and pass along main veins: to the head, neck, and upper limbs from the jugular lymph sacs; to the lower trunk and lower limbs from the iliac lymph sacs; and to the primordial gut from the retroperitoneal lymph sac and the cisterna chyli. Two large channels (right and left thoracic ducts) connect the jugular lymph sacs with this cistern. Soon, a large anastomosis forms between these channels (see Fig. 14.35B).

The **thoracic duct** develops from:

- Caudal part of the right thoracic duct
- Anastomosis between the thoracic ducts and the cranial part of the left thoracic duct.

The **right lymphatic duct** is derived from the cranial part of the right thoracic duct (see Fig. 14.35C). The thoracic duct and right lymphatic duct connect with the venous system at the **venous angle** between the internal jugular and subclavian veins (see Fig. 14.35B).

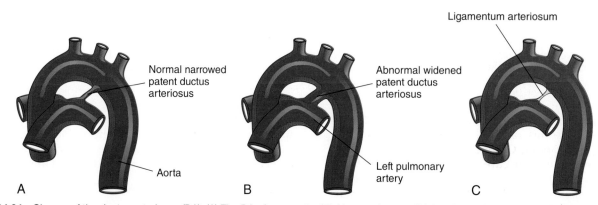

Fig. 14.34   Closure of the ductus arteriosus (DA). (A) The DA of a neonate. (B) Abnormal patent DA in a 6-month-old infant. (C) The ligamentum arteriosum in a 6-month-old infant.

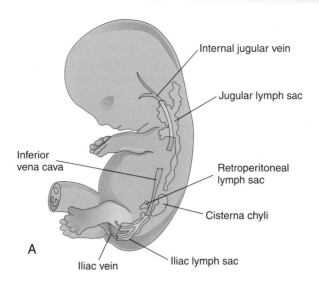

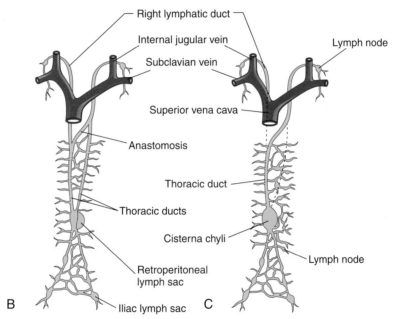

Fig. 14.35 Development of the lymphatic system. (A) Left side of a 7½ week embryo, showing the primary lymph sacs. (B) Ventral view of the lymphatic system at 9 weeks, showing the paired thoracic ducts. (C) Later in the fetal period, showing formation of the thoracic duct and right lymphatic duct.

DEVELOPMENT OF LYMPH NODES

Except for the superior part of the cisterna chyli, the lymph sacs are transformed into groups of lymph nodes during the early fetal period. Mesenchymal cells invade each lymph sac and form a network of lymphatic channels, the primordia of the **lymph sinuses**. Other mesenchymal cells give rise to the capsules and connective tissue framework of the lymph nodes.

The **lymphocytes** are derived originally from **primordial stem cells** in the umbilical vesicle mesenchyme and later from the **liver and spleen**. The early lymphocytes eventually enter the **bone marrow**, where they divide to form **lymphoblasts**. The lymphocytes that appear in the lymph nodes before birth are derived from the thymus, a derivative of the third pair of pharyngeal pouches (see Chapter 10). Small lymphocytes leave the **thymus** and circulate to other lymphoid organs. Later, some mesenchymal cells in the lymph nodes also differentiate into lymphocytes.

Payers patches begin to develop by week 19. These aggregations of lymphoid tissue with immune function are found in the small intestine, mostly in the ileum.

Birth Defects of Lymphatic System

Birth defects of the lymphatic system are uncommon. There may be diffuse swelling of a part of the body, termed **congenital lymphedema**. This condition may result from dilation of the primordial lymphatic channels or from **congenital hypoplasia** of the lymphatic vessels. In **cystic hygroma**, large swellings usually appear in the inferolateral part of the neck and consist of large, single, or multilocular, fluid-filled cavities. **Hygromas** may be present at birth, but they often enlarge and become evident during later infancy. Hygromas are believed to arise from parts of a jugular lymph sac that are pinched off or from lymphatic spaces that do not establish connections with the main lymphatic channels.

DEVELOPMENT OF SPLEEN AND TONSILS

The **spleen** develops from an aggregation of mesenchymal cells in the dorsal mesogastrium (see Chapter 12). The **palatine tonsils** develop from the endoderm of the second pair of pharyngeal pouches and nearby mesenchyme (see Fig. 10.7). The **tubal tonsils** develop from aggregations of lymph nodules around the pharyngeal openings of the pharyngotympanic tubes. The **pharyngeal tonsils** (adenoids) develop from an aggregation of lymph nodules in the wall of the nasopharynx. The **lingual tonsil** develops from an aggregation of lymph nodules in the root of the tongue. Lymph nodules also develop in the mucosa of the respiratory and alimentary systems.

CLINICALLY ORIENTED QUESTIONS

1. A pediatrician diagnosed a heart murmur in a neonate. What does this mean? What causes this condition, and what does it indicate?

2. Are birth defects of the heart common? What is the most common congenital heart defect in neonates?

3. What are the causes of birth defects of the cardiovascular system? Can drugs taken by the mother during pregnancy cause cardiac defects? Could maternal alcohol abuse cause the neonate's heart defect?

4. Can viral infections cause heart disease? If a mother had measles during pregnancy, could the neonate have a defect of the cardiovascular system? Can a pregnant woman be vaccinated to protect the unborn fetus against certain viruses?

5. In a neonate, the aorta arose from the right ventricle and the pulmonary artery arose from the left ventricle. The neonate died during the early neonatal period. What is this defect called, and how common is this disorder? Can the condition be corrected surgically? If so, how is this done?

6. During a routine examination of 40-year-old identical twin sisters, it was found that one had a reversed heart. Is this a serious heart defect? How common is this among identical twins, and what causes this condition to develop?

The answers to these questions are at the back of this book.

Musculoskeletal System

SKELETAL SYSTEM

As the notochord and neural tube form in the third week, the **intraembryonic mesoderm** lateral to these structures thickens to form two longitudinal columns of **paraxial mesoderm** (Fig. 15.1A and B). By the end of the third week, these columns become compacted and segmented into blocks of mesoderm—**somites** (see Fig. 15.1C). The somites appear as bead-like elevations along the dorsolateral surface of the embryo. Each somite differentiates into two parts (see Fig. 15.1D and E):

- The ventromedial part is the **sclerotome**; its cells form the vertebrae and ribs.
- The dorsolateral part is the **dermomyotome**; cells from its myotome region form **myoblasts** (primordial muscle cells), and those from its dermatome region form the **dermis** (fibroblasts).

The bones and connective tissue of the craniofacial structures are formed from mesenchyme in the head region that is derived from cranial **neural crest cells**.

DEVELOPMENT OF CARTILAGE AND BONE

HISTOGENESIS OF CARTILAGE

Cartilage develops from mesenchyme during the fifth week as the mesenchyme condenses to form **chondrification centers**. The mesenchymal cells differentiate into **chondroblasts**, which secrete collagenous fibrils and extracellular matrix. Subsequently, collagenous and/or elastic fibers are deposited in the intercellular substance or **matrix**.

Three types of cartilage are distinguished according to the type of matrix that is formed:

- **Hyaline cartilage**, the most widely distributed type (e.g., in synovial joints)
- **Fibrocartilage** (e.g., in intervertebral discs)
- **Elastic cartilage** (e.g., in auricles of the external ears).

HISTOGENESIS OF BONE

Bone develops primarily in two types of connective tissue, mesenchyme, and cartilage, but it can also develop in muscle and tendons (e.g., patella). Most **flat bones** develop in mesenchyme within preexisting membranous sheaths; this type of osteogenesis is **intramembranous bone formation**. Mesenchymal models of most limb bones are transformed into cartilaginous bone models, which later become ossified by **endochondral bone formation**. Like cartilage, bone consists of cells and an organic intercellular substance, **bone matrix**, which comprises collagen fibrils embedded in an amorphous component.

Osteogenesis and chondrogenesis are programmed early in development and are independent processes under the influence of molecular and vascular events. *The Hox genes, bone morphogenetic proteins (BMPs) 5 and 7, growth and differentiation factor 5—members of the transforming growth factor-β (TGF-β) superfamily—and vascular endothelial growth factor, and other signaling molecules, have been implicated as endogenous regulators of chondrogenesis and skeletal development. Lineage commitment of skeletal precursor cells to chondrocytes and osteoblasts is determined by β-catenin levels.*

INTRAMEMBRANOUS OSSIFICATION

During intramembranous ossification, precursor mesenchymal stem cells differentiate into **osteoblasts** (bone-forming cells) and begin to deposit unmineralized matrix rich in type I collagen **(osteoid)** (Fig. 15.2) with a high concentration of type I collagen. **Calcium phosphate** is then deposited in **osteoid tissue** as it is organized into bone. Osteoblasts are trapped in the matrix and become **osteocytes**. Spicules of bone soon become organized and coalesce into **lamellae** (layers). *Tyrosine phosphatase (SHP2), transcription factors Foxf2, RUNX2, and Wnt signaling are key regulating factors in osteoblast differentiation.*

Concentric lamellae develop around blood vessels, forming **osteons** (Haversian systems). Some osteoblasts remain at the periphery of the bone and continue to lay down lamellae, forming plates of compact bone on the surfaces. Between the **surface plates**, the intervening bone remains spiculated or spongy. This spongy environment is accentuated by the action of **osteoclasts** that reabsorb bone. In the interstices of the spongy bone, the mesenchyme differentiates into **bone marrow**. During fetal and postnatal life, continuous remodeling of bone occurs by the coordinated action of osteoclasts and osteoblasts.

ENDOCHONDRAL OSSIFICATION

Endochondral ossification is a type of bone formation that occurs in preexisting cartilaginous models (Fig. 15.3A–E). In a long bone, the **primary center of ossification** appears in the **diaphysis**, which forms the **shaft of a bone**. Here the cartilage cells undergo hypertrophy, they synthesize an extracellular matrix rich in type X collagen, the matrix then becomes calcified, and the cells die (see Fig. 15.3B). Concurrently, a thin layer of bone is deposited under the **perichondrium** surrounding the diaphysis; thus the perichondrium becomes the **periosteum** (see Fig. 15.3A and B).

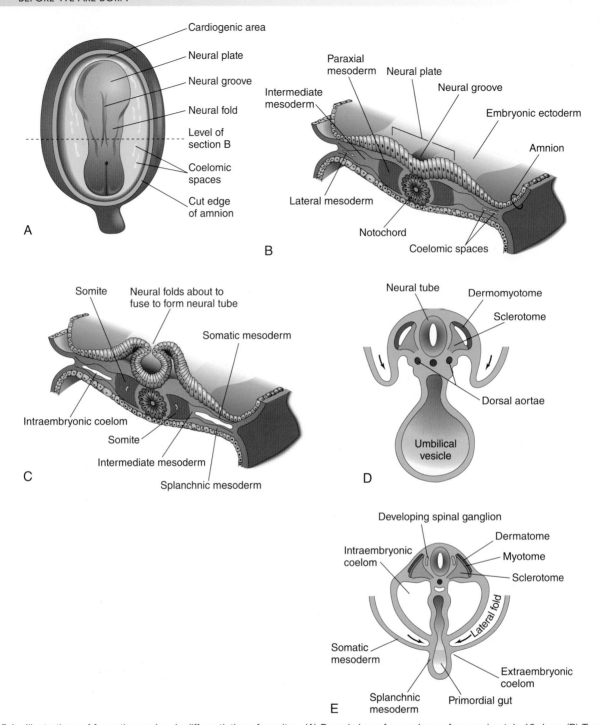

Fig. 15.1 Illustrations of formation and early differentiation of somites. (A) Dorsal view of an embryo of approximately 18 days. (B) Transverse section of the embryo shown in (A) illustrating the paraxial mesoderm from which the somites are derived. (C) Transverse section of an embryo of approximately 22 days showing the appearance of the early somites. Note that the neural folds are about to fuse to form the neural tube. (D) Transverse section of an embryo of approximately 24 days showing folding of the embryo in the horizontal plane *(arrows)*. The dermomyotome region of the somite gives rise to the dermatome and myotome. (E) Transverse section of an embryo of approximately 26 days showing the dermatome, myotome, and sclerotome regions of the somite. The *arrows* in (D) and (E) indicate movement of the lateral body folds.

Invasion of the vascular connective tissue by the blood vessels surrounding the periosteum breaks up the cartilage. Some invading progenitor cells differentiate into **hematopoietic cells** (blood cells of the bone marrow). This process continues toward the **epiphyses**. The spicules of bone are remodeled by the action of osteoclasts and osteoblasts.

Lengthening of the long bones occurs at the diaphyseal–epiphyseal junction. The lengthening of bone depends on the **epiphyseal cartilage plates** (growth plates), whose chondrocytes proliferate and participate in endochondral bone formation (see Fig. 15.3D and E). Toward the **diaphysis**, the cartilage cells increase in size and the matrix becomes

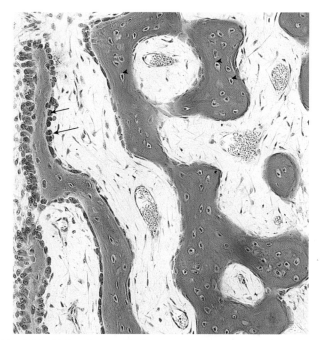

Fig. 15.2 Light micrograph of intramembranous ossification (×132). The trabeculae of the bone are being formed by osteoblasts lining their surface *(arrows)*. Observe that osteocytes are trapped in the lacunae *(arrowheads)* and that primordial osteons are beginning to form. The osteons (canals) contain blood capillaries. From Gartner LP, Hiatt JL: *Color textbook of histology*, ed 2, Philadelphia, 2001, Saunders.

calcified. The spicules are isolated from each other by vascular invasion from the **medullary cavity** (marrow) of long bone (see Fig. 15.3E). Bone is deposited on these spicules by osteoblasts; resorption of this bone keeps the spongy bone masses relatively constant in length and enlarges the medullary cavity.

Rickets

Rickets (hereditary or acquired) is a disease in children attributable to deficiency of the active form of **vitamin D**. This vitamin is required for calcium and phosphorus absorption by the intestine. The resulting calcium and phosphorus deficiency causes disturbances in the formation of chondrocytes and ossification of the epiphyseal cartilage plates There is disorientation of cells at the **metaphysis**—the flared part of the diaphysis nearest the epiphysis (see Fig. 15.3D). The limbs are shortened and deformed, with severe bowing of the limb bones. Rickets may also delay closure of the **fontanelles** of the cranial bones in infants (see Fig. 15.8).

Ossification of limb bones begins at the end of the embryonic period. Thereafter, it makes demands on the maternal supply of calcium and phosphorus beginning at approximately 8 weeks. At birth, the diaphysis is largely ossified, but most of the epiphyses are still cartilaginous. **Secondary ossification centers** appear in the epiphyses during the first few years after birth. The epiphyseal cartilage cells become hypertrophied, and there is invasion

by vascular connective tissue. Ossification spreads radially, and only the articular cartilage and **epiphyseal cartilage plate** remain cartilaginous (see Fig. 15.3E). On completion of growth, the cartilage plate is replaced by spongy bone; the epiphyses and diaphysis are united, and no further elongation of the bone occurs.

In most bones, the epiphyses have fused with the diaphysis by the age of 20 years. Growth in the diameter of a bone results from the deposition of bone at the **periosteum** (see Fig. 15.3B) and from resorption on the internal medullary surface. The rate of deposition and resorption is balanced to regulate the thickness of the compact bone and the size of the medullary cavity (see Fig. 15.3E).

DEVELOPMENT OF JOINTS

Joints begin to develop with the appearance of the **interzone** within the continuous cartilaginous bone model. The cells in the interzone begin to flatten and form a separation at the joint location. *Factors involved in the interzone formation appear to be Wnt-14 and Noggin.* During the sixth week (Fig. 15.4A), and by the end of the eighth week, they resemble adult joints (see Fig. 15.4B).

FIBROUS JOINTS

During the development of fibrous joints, the interzonal mesenchyme between the developing bones differentiates into dense fibrous tissue (see Fig. 15.4D). The sutures of the cranium are an example of fibrous joints (see Fig. 15.8).

CARTILAGINOUS JOINTS

During the development of cartilaginous joints, the interzonal mesenchyme between the developing bones differentiates into **hyaline cartilage** (e.g., costochondral joints) or **fibrocartilage** (e.g., pubic symphysis) (see Fig. 15.4C).

SYNOVIAL JOINTS

During development of synovial joints (e.g., knee joint), the interzonal mesenchyme between the developing bones differentiates as follows (see Fig. 15.4B):

- Peripherally, the interzonal mesenchyme forms the **joint capsular ligament** and other ligaments.
- Centrally, the mesenchyme undergoes cavitation late in development and postnatal life. The resulting space becomes the **synovial cavity** (joint cavity).
- Where the mesenchyme lines the joint capsule and articular surfaces, it forms the **synovial membrane**, which secretes synovial fluid.

DEVELOPMENT OF AXIAL SKELETON

The axial skeleton is composed of the cranium, vertebral column, ribs, and sternum. During the fourth week, cells in the sclerotomes surround the neural tube and notochord, the structure around which the **primordia**

Cartilage Model of Bone

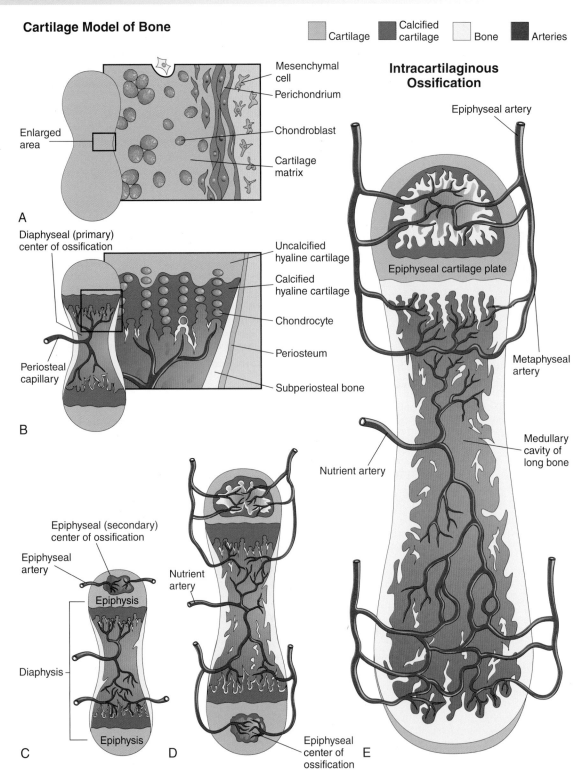

Cartilage   Calcified cartilage   Bone   Arteries

A

- Mesenchymal cell
- Perichondrium
- Chondroblast
- Cartilage matrix

Enlarged area

B

- Diaphyseal (primary) center of ossification
- Periosteal capillary
- Uncalcified hyaline cartilage
- Calcified hyaline cartilage
- Chondrocyte
- Periosteum
- Subperiosteal bone

Intracartilaginous Ossification

- Epiphyseal artery
- Epiphyseal cartilage plate
- Metaphyseal artery
- Nutrient artery
- Medullary cavity of long bone

C

- Epiphyseal (secondary) center of ossification
- Epiphyseal artery
- Epiphysis
- Diaphysis
- Epiphysis

D

- Nutrient artery
- Epiphyseal center of ossification

E

Fig. 15.3   (A–E) Schematic longitudinal sections of a 5-week embryo, illustrating endochondral ossification in a developing long bone.

of the vertebrae develop. This positional change of the sclerotomal cells is affected by differential growth of the surrounding structures and not by the migration of sclerotomal cells. *TBX6, Hox, and Pax genes regulate the patterning and regional development of the vertebrae along the anterior–posterior axis.*

DEVELOPMENT OF VERTEBRAL COLUMN

During the precartilaginous or mesenchymal stage, mesenchymal cells from the **sclerotomes** are found in three main areas (Fig. 15.5A): around the notochord, surrounding the neural tube, and in the body wall. In a frontal section of a

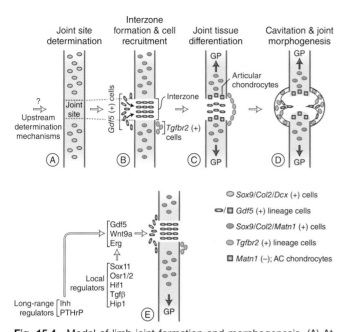

Fig. 15.4 Model of limb joint formation and morphogenesis. (A) At early developmental stages, as yet unknown upstream determination mechanisms would identify and prescribe the location of the joints along *Sox9/Col2/Dcx*-expressing anlagen. (B) Soon after, *Gdf5* expression would be activated along with other interzone-specific genes (E) that would define the initial interzone mesenchymal population within the *Sox9/Col2/Matn1*-positive cartilaginous anlagen. This would be accompanied by cell immigration from the flank, and cells located dorsally and ventrally would activate *Tgfbr2* expression. (C) *Gdf5*-positive cells adjacent their respective cartilaginous anlagen — with a *Sox9/Col2* history but negative for *matrilin-1* expression — would differentiate into articular chondrocytes. (D) Additional differentiation processes and mechanisms such as muscle movement would bring about cavitation and genesis of other joint tissues, such as ligaments and other meniscus, involving *Gdf5*- and *Tgfbr2*-positive and -negative cell progenies. Note that the above distinct spatiotemporal steps — presented here as distinct for illustration purposes — may actually occur more closely and involve overlapping events. Also, the model may not entirely apply to other joints, including intervertebral and temporomandibular joints, that involve additional and/or diverse mechanisms. (E) Schematic summarizing local and long-range regulators that converge to regulate interzone gene expression at the early stages of joint formation. Note that this list is not exhaustive. *AC*, Articular cartilage; *GP*, growth plate. From Decker RS, Koyama E, Pacifici M: Genesis and morphogenesis of limb synovial joints and articular cartilage, *Matrix Biol* 39:5, 2014.

4-week embryo, the **sclerotomes** appear as paired condensations of mesenchymal cells around the notochord (see Fig. 15.5B). Each sclerotome consists of loosely arranged cells cranially and densely packed cells caudally.

Some densely packed cells migrate cranially, opposite the center of the myotome, where they form the **intervertebral disc** (see Fig. 15.5C and D). The remaining densely packed cells fuse with the loosely arranged cells of the immediately caudal sclerotome to form the mesenchymal **centrum**, the primordium of the body of a vertebra. Thus each centrum develops from two adjacent sclerotomes and becomes an intersegmental structure.

The spinal nerves now lie in close relationship to the intervertebral discs, and the intersegmental arteries lie on each side of the vertebral bodies. In the thorax, the dorsal

intersegmental arteries become the **intercostal arteries**. *Studies indicate that the regional development of the vertebral column is regulated along the anterior–posterior axis by homeobox (HOX) and paired box (PAX) genes.*

Where it is surrounded by the developing vertebral bodies, the notochord degenerates and disappears. Between the vertebrae, the notochord expands to form the gelatinous center of the IV disc—the **nucleus pulposus** (see Fig. 15.5D), which becomes surrounded by circularly arranged fibers that form the **anulus fibrosus**. The nucleus pulposus and anulus fibrosus together constitute the **intervertebral disc**. The mesenchymal cells that surround the neural tube form the **neural arch**, the primordium of the **vertebral arch** (Fig. 15.6D; see also Fig. 15.5C). The mesenchymal cells in the body wall form the **costal processes**, which form the ribs in the thoracic region.

Chordoma

Remnants of the notochord may persist and form a **chordoma**, an extremely rare (1:1,000,000) form of sarcoma. Approximately one-third of these slowly growing, malignant tumors occur at the base of the cranium and extend to the nasopharynx (the part of the pharynx that lies above the soft palate).

Chordomas infiltrate bone and are difficult to remove. They also develop in the lumbosacral region. Surgical resection, when feasible, has provided long-term disease-free survival for many people.

CARTILAGINOUS STAGE OF VERTEBRAL DEVELOPMENT

During the sixth week, **chondrification centers** appear in each mesenchymal vertebra (see Fig. 15.6A and B). At the end of the embryonic period, the two centers in each **centrum** fuse to form a cartilaginous centrum. Concomitantly, the centers in the neural arches fuse with each other and the centrum. The spinous and transverse processes develop from extensions of chondrification centers in the neural arch. Chondrification spreads until a cartilaginous vertebral column is formed.

BONY STAGE OF VERTEBRAL DEVELOPMENT

Ossification of typical vertebrae begins during the embryonic period and usually ends by the 25th year. There are two **primary ossification centers** in the centrum—ventral and dorsal (see Fig. 15.6C), which soon fuse to form one center. Three primary centers are present by the eighth week: one in the centrum and one in each half of the neural arch.

Ossification becomes evident in the **neural arches** during the eighth week. At birth, each vertebra consists of three bony parts connected by cartilage (see Fig. 15.6D). The bony halves of the **vertebral arch** usually fuse during the first 3 to 5 years. The arches first unite in the lumbar region and union progresses cranially. The vertebral arch articulates with the **centrum** at cartilaginous **neurocentral joints**, which permit the vertebral arches to grow as the spinal cord enlarges. These joints disappear when the vertebral arch fuses with the centrum during the third to sixth years.

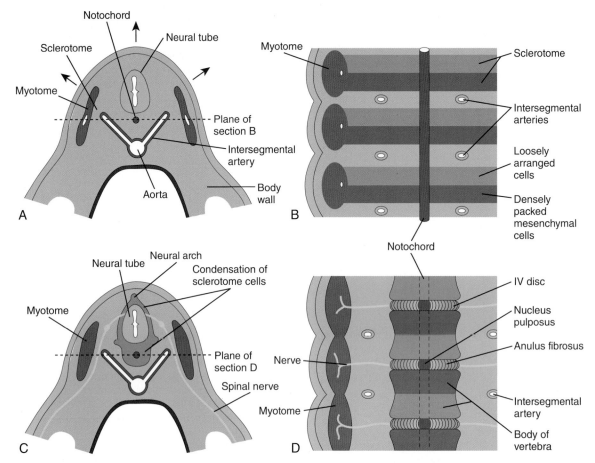

Fig. 15.5 (A) Transverse section through a 4-week embryo. The *arrows* indicate the dorsal growth of the neural tube and the simultaneous dorsolateral movement of the somite remnant, leaving behind a trail of sclerotomal cells. (B) Diagrammatic frontal section of the same embryo showing that the condensation of sclerotomal cells around the notochord consists of a cranial area of loosely packed cells and a caudal area of densely packed cells. (C) Transverse section through a 5-week embryo showing the condensation of sclerotomal cells around the notochord and neural tube, which forms a mesenchymal vertebra. (D) Diagrammatic frontal section illustrating that the vertebral body forms from the cranial and caudal halves of two successive sclerotomal masses. The intersegmental arteries now cross the bodies of the vertebrae and the spinal nerves lie between the vertebrae. The notochord is degenerating, except in the region of the intervertebral disc, where it forms the nucleus pulposus.

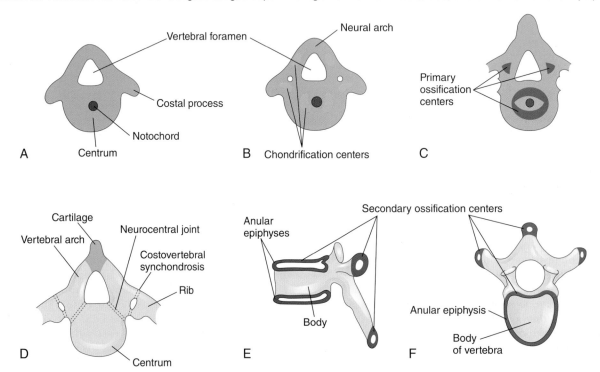

Fig. 15.6 Stages of vertebral development. (A) Mesenchymal vertebra at 5 weeks. (B) Chondrification centers in a mesenchymal vertebra at 6 weeks. The neural arch is the primordium of the vertebral arch of the vertebra. (C) Primary ossification centers in a cartilaginous vertebra at 7 weeks. (D) Thoracic vertebra at birth consisting of three bony parts: vertebral arch, body of vertebra, and transverse processes. Note the cartilage between the halves of the vertebral arch and between the arch and the centrum (neurocentral joint). (E and F) Two views of a typical thoracic vertebra at puberty showing the location of the secondary centers of ossification.

Five **secondary ossification centers** appear in the vertebrae after puberty (see Fig. 15.6E and F):

- One for the tip of the spinous process
- One for the tip of each transverse process
- Two anular epiphyses, one on the superior rim and one on the inferior rim of the vertebral body.

The **vertebral body** is a composite of the anular epiphyses and the mass of bone between them. All secondary centers unite with the rest of the vertebrae at approximately 25 years of age. Variations in the ossification of vertebrae occur in C1 (atlas), C2 (axis), and C7 vertebrae, as well as in the lumbar vertebrae, sacrum, and coccyx.

Variations in the Number of Vertebrae

Most people have 7 cervical, 12 thoracic, 5 lumbar, and 5 sacral vertebrae. A few have one or two additional vertebrae or one fewer. An apparent extra (or absent) vertebra in one segment of the column may be compensated for by an absent (or extra) vertebra in an adjacent segment.

Klippel–Feil Sequence

The main features of this sequence are shortness of the neck, low hairline, restricted neck movements, fusion of cervical vertebral bodies, and abnormalities of the brainstem and cerebellum. Persons with this syndrome may have other birth defects, including **scoliosis**, deafness, and urinary tract disorders. Klippel–Feil sequence is associated with pathogenic variants in genes including MYO18B and RIPPLY2.

DEVELOPMENT OF RIBS

The ribs develop from the mesenchymal **costal processes** of the thoracic vertebrae (see Fig. 15.6A). They become cartilaginous during the embryonic period and ossify during the fetal period. The original site of union of the costal processes with the vertebrae is replaced by **costovertebral synovial joints** (see Fig. 15.6D). Seven pairs of ribs (1–7)—**true ribs**—attach by their own cartilages to the sternum. Five pairs of ribs (8–12)—**false ribs**—attach to the sternum through the cartilage of another rib or ribs. The last two pairs of ribs (11 and 12)—**floating ribs**—do not attach to the sternum.

DEVELOPMENT OF STERNUM

A pair of vertical mesenchymal bands—**sternal bars**—develops ventrolaterally in the body wall. Chondrification occurs in these bars as they move medially. They fuse craniocaudally in the median plane to form cartilaginous models of the **manubrium, sternebrae** (segments of sternal body), and **xiphoid process**. Centers of ossification appear craniocaudally in the sternum before birth, except the ossification center for the xiphoid process, which appears during childhood. The xiphoid may never completely ossify.

DEVELOPMENT OF CRANIUM

The cranium develops from mesenchyme and neural crest cells around the developing brain. The cranium consists of:

- **Neurocranium**, the bones of the cranium enclosing the brain
- **Viscerocranium**, the bones of the facial skeleton derived from the pharyngeal arches.

CARTILAGINOUS NEUROCRANIUM

Endochondral ossification of the neurocranium forms the bones of the base of the cranium. The ossification pattern of these bones has a definite sequence, beginning with the **occipital bone, body of the sphenoid**, and **ethmoid bone**. The **parachordal cartilage**, or basal plate, forms around the cranial end of the notochord (Fig. 15.7A) and fuses with the cartilages derived from the sclerotome regions of the occipital somites. This cartilaginous mass contributes to the **base of the occipital bone**; later, extensions grow around the cranial end of the spinal cord and form the boundaries of the **foramen magnum**—a large opening in the basal part of the occipital bone—(see Fig. 15.7C).

The **hypophyseal cartilage** forms around the developing pituitary gland and fuses to form the body of the sphenoid bone (see Fig. 15.7B). The **trabeculae cranii** fuse to form the body of the **ethmoid bone**, and the **ala orbitalis** forms the lesser wing of the sphenoid bone. Otic capsules develop around the otic vesicles, the primordia of the internal ears (see Chapter 17), and form the **petrous** and **mastoid parts** of the **temporal bone**. Nasal capsules develop around the nasal sacs (see Chapter 10) and contribute to the formation of the ethmoid bone.

MEMBRANOUS NEUROCRANIUM

Membranous ossification occurs in the head mesenchyme at the sides and top of the brain, forming the **calvaria** During fetal life, the flat bones of the calvaria are separated by dense connective tissue membranes that form fibrous joints—the **sutures** of the calvaria (Fig. 15.8). Six large fibrous areas—**fontanelles**—are present where several sutures meet. The softness of the bones and their loose connections at the sutures enable the calvaria to undergo changes of shape during birth (**molding of fetal cranium**) made possible by flexion of the coronal and lambdoid sutures. Within a few days after birth, the shape of the calvaria returns to normal.

CARTILAGINOUS VISCEROCRANIUM

The cartilaginous viscerocranium is derived from the cartilaginous skeleton of the first two pairs of **pharyngeal arches** (see Chapter 10). Most of the craniofacial skeleton is derived from neural crest cells. The neural crest cells migrate into the pharyngeal arches with positional and patterning information.

- The dorsal end of the first pharyngeal arch cartilage forms the **malleus** and **incus** of the middle ear.
- The dorsal end of the second pharyngeal arch cartilage forms a portion of the **stapes** of the middle ear and styloid process of the temporal bone. Its ventral end ossifies to form the **lesser horn** of the **hyoid bone**.

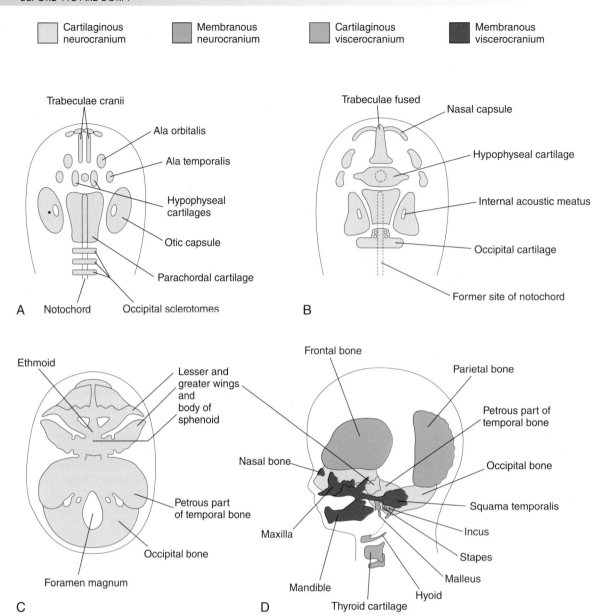

Fig. 15.7 Stages in the development of the cranium. The base of the developing cranium is viewed superiorly (A–C) and laterally (D). (A) At 6 weeks, showing the various cartilages that will fuse to form the chondrocranium. (B) At 7 weeks, after fusion of some of the paired cartilages. (C) At 12 weeks, showing the cartilaginous base of the cranium formed by the fusion of various cartilages. (D) At 20 weeks, indicating the derivation of the bones of the fetal cranium.

• The third, fourth, and sixth pharyngeal arch cartilages form only in the ventral parts of the arches. The third arch cartilages form the greater horns of the hyoid bone and the superior cornu of the **thyroid cartilage**.

• The fourth pharyngeal arch cartilages appear to fuse to form the **laryngeal cartilages**, except for the **epiglottis** (see Chapter 10).

MEMBRANOUS VISCEROCRANIUM

Membranous ossification occurs in the maxillary prominence of the first pharyngeal arch (see Chapter 10) and subsequently forms the **squamous temporal**, **maxillary**, and **zygomatic bones**. The **squamous temporal bones** become part of the neurocranium. The **mandibular prominence** forms the

mandible. Some endochondral ossification occurs in the median plane of the chin and in the mandibular condyle.

POSTNATAL GROWTH OF CRANIUM

The cranium of a neonate is large in proportion to the rest of the skeleton, and the face is relatively small compared with the calvaria (roof of cranium). The small facial region of the cranium results from the small size of the jaws, the virtual absence of paranasal sinuses, and underdevelopment of the facial bones.

After molding, the neonate's cranium is rather round and its bones are thin. The fibrous sutures permit the brain and calvaria to enlarge during infancy and childhood. The increase in size is greatest during the first 2 years, the

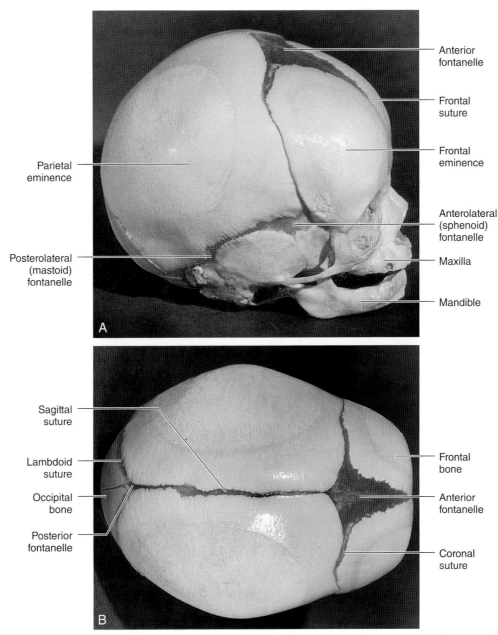

Fig. 15.8 Fetal cranium (skull) showing the bones, fontanelles, and sutures. (A) Lateral view. (B) Superior view. The posterior and anterolateral fontanelles disappear within 2 or 3 months after birth because of the growth of the surrounding bones, but they remain as sutures for several years. The posterolateral fontanelles disappear in a similar manner by the end of the first year and the anterior fontanelle disappears by the end of the second year. The halves of the frontal bone normally begin to fuse during the second year, and the frontal suture is usually obliterated by the eighth year.

period of most rapid postnatal growth of the brain. The calvaria continues to expand to conform to brain growth until approximately 16 years, after which its size usually increases slightly for 3 to 4 years because of the thickening of its bones.

There is also rapid growth of the face and jaws, coinciding with the eruption of the primary (deciduous) teeth. These facial changes are more marked after the secondary (permanent) teeth erupt (see Chapter 18). There is concurrent enlargement of the frontal and facial regions, associated with the increase in the size of the paranasal sinuses (e.g., the maxillary sinuses). The growth of these sinuses is important in adding resonance to the voice.

Accessory Ribs

Costal processes usually form only in the thoracic region. The ectopic development of costal processes from the cervical or lumbar vertebrae results in **accessory ribs** (see Fig. 15.6A). The most common accessory rib is a **lumbar rib** (1%), but it is usually clinically insignificant. A **cervical rib** occurs in 0.5% to 1% of people (Fig. 15.9A) and is often fused with the first rib; it is usually attached to the manubrium of the sternum or the seventh cervical vertebra. Accessory ribs may be unilateral or bilateral. Pressure of a cervical rib on the brachial plexus of nerves, partly in the neck and axilla, or on the subclavian artery often produces neurovascular symptoms (e.g., paralysis and anesthesia of the upper limb).

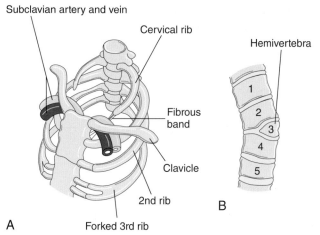

A

Forked 3rd rib

B

Fig. 15.9 Vertebral and rib abnormalities. (A) Cervical and forked ribs. Observe that the left cervical rib has a fibrous band that passes posterior to the subclavian vessels and attaches to the sternum. (B) Anterior view of the vertebral column showing a hemivertebra. The right half of the third thoracic vertebra is absent. Note the associated lateral curvature (scoliosis) of the vertebral column.

Hemivertebra

Developing vertebral bodies usually have two chondrification centers that soon unite. A hemivertebra (1:1000) results from the failure of one of the chondrification centers to appear and the subsequent failure of half of the vertebra to form. Hemivertebra is the most common cause of **congenital scoliosis** of the vertebral column (see Fig. 15.9B).

Spinal Dysraphism

Spinal dysrapthism is a broad category of defects that result from the faulty closure of the neural tube. Spinal dysraphia includes a number of conditions: spinal bifida, tethered spinal cord, split cord, spinal cord lipoma, and dermal sinus tract. Symptoms vary from mild to debilitating, depending on the nature and severity of the defect (Fig. 15.10).

Acrania

In acrania, the neurocranium is absent, and there are major birth defects of the vertebral column that are incompatible with life (see Fig. 15.10). Acrania associated with **meroencephaly** (partial absence of the brain) occurs in approximately 1 in 10,000 births and is not compatible with life. It occurs when the cranial end of the neural tube does not close during the fourth week of development, resulting in the subsequent failure of the calvaria to form.

Craniosynostosis

Several birth defects result from prenatal fusion of the cranial sutures (Fig. 15.11). The cause of craniosynostosis is unclear, but genetic factors appear to be important. *Homeobox gene (MSX2 and ALX4) pathogenic variants (mutations) have been implicated in cases of craniosynostosis and other cranial defects.* These

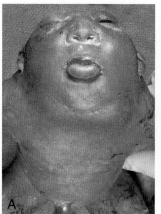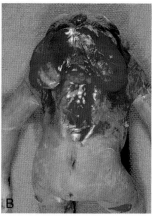

Fig. 15.10 Anterior (A) and posterior (B) views of a 20-week fetus with severe defects, including acrania (absence of calvaria), cervical rachischisis (extensive clefts in vertebral arches), cerebral regression (meroencephaly), and iniencephaly (defect in occiput—back of cranium). Courtesy Dr. Marc Del Bigio, Department of Pathology [Neuropathology], University of Manitoba, Winnipeg, Manitoba, Canada.

defects are much more common in males than in females, and they are often associated with other skeletal defects.

The type of cranial deformation produced depends on which sutures close prematurely. The closed suture prevents perpendicular bone growth, resulting in parallel bone growth in the region of the suture. For instance, if the sagittal suture closes early, the cranium becomes elongated and wedge-shaped—**scaphocephaly** (see Fig. 15.11A and C). This type of cranial deformity constitutes approximately half of the cases of craniosynostosis. Other types of craniosynostosis include **brachycephaly** (see Fig. 15.11B), **plagiocephaly**, and **trigonocephaly** (see Fig. 15.8).

DEVELOPMENT OF APPENDICULAR SKELETON

The appendicular skeleton consists of the pectoral and pelvic girdles and limb bones. During the sixth week, the mesenchymal bone models in the limbs undergo chondrification to form hyaline cartilage bone models (Fig. 15.12). The **clavicle** initially develops by intramembranous ossification, and it later forms growth cartilages at both ends. The models of the pectoral girdle and upper limb bones appear slightly before those of the pelvic girdle and lower limb bones. The bone models appear in a proximodistal sequence. *The molecular mechanism of limb morphogenesis is regulated by specialized signaling centers along three axes of development (proximal/distal, ventral/dorsal, and anterior/posterior). Patterning in the developing limbs is controlled by Hox and other complex signaling pathways* (see Chapter 20).

Ossification begins in the long bones by the eighth week (Fig. 15.3B and C). By 12 weeks, primary ossification centers have appeared in nearly all limb bones (see Fig. 15.13). The clavicles begin to ossify before any other bones in the body, followed by the femurs. Virtually all primary (diaphyseal) centers of ossification are present at birth.

The secondary ossification centers for the distal end of the femur and the proximal end of the tibia usually appear during the last month of intrauterine life (34–38 weeks). The centers of the other bones appear after birth. The part of the bone ossified from the secondary center is the epiphysis. The bone

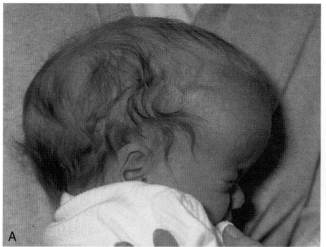
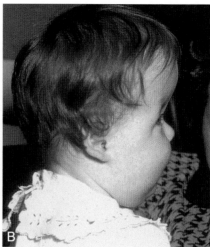
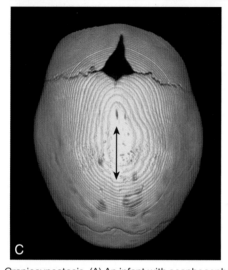

Fig. 15.11   Craniosynostosis. (A) An infant with scaphocephaly (long narrow head) resulting from premature closure of the sagittal suture. (B) An infant with bilateral premature closure of the coronal suture—brachycephaly—resulting in a high, tower-like forehead. (C) Cranium of a 9-month-old infant with scaphocephaly resulting from premature closure of the sagittal suture (sagittal synostosis; *double arrow*). Computed tomography reconstructed image. A and B, Courtesy Dr. John A. Jane, Sr., Department of Neurological Surgery, University of Virginia Health System, Charlottesville, Virginia; C, Courtesy Dr. Gerald S. Smyser, Altru Health System, Grand Forks, North Dakota.

formed from the primary center in the diaphysis does not fuse at the epiphyseal cartilage plate with that formed from the secondary centers in the epiphyses until the bone grows to its adult length (see Fig. 15.3E). This delay enables lengthening of the bone to continue until the final size is reached.

Bone Age

Bone age is a good index of general maturation. Using a radiograph of the left wrist, hand, and fingers, a radiologist can determine bone age by assessing the ossification centers using two criteria:

- The time of appearance of calcified material in the diaphysis, epiphysis, or both is specific for each diaphysis and epiphysis and for each bone and sex.
- The disappearance of the dark line on the X-ray representing the epiphyseal cartilage plate indicates that the epiphysis has fused with the diaphysis.

Fusion of the diaphyseal–epiphyseal centers, which occurs at specific times for each epiphysis, happens 1 to 2 years earlier in females.

Generalized Skeletal Malformations

Achondroplasia is the most common cause of **dwarfism—short stature** (see Fig. 19.9). It occurs in approximately 1 in 15,000 births. The limbs become bowed and short because of a disturbance of endochondral ossification at the epiphyseal cartilage plates, particularly of the long bones, during fetal life (Fig. 15.14). The trunk is usually short, and the head is enlarged with a bulging forehead and a flatened nasal bone.

Achondroplasia is an **autosomal dominant disorder**, and approximately 80% of cases arise from new pathogenic variants; the rate increases with paternal age. *The majority of cases are due to a point mutation in the fibroblast growth factor receptor 3 (FGFR3) gene*, which results in magnification of the normal inhibiting effect of endochondral ossification, specifically in the zone of chondrocyte proliferation. This results in shortened bones but does not affect growth of bone width (periosteal growth). **Thanatophoric dysplasia**, a short-limb dwarfism syndrome, is associated with pathogenic variants of the *FGFR3* gene. Most infants with this condition typically die in the perinatal period because of respiratory failure resulting from a small thoracic cage.

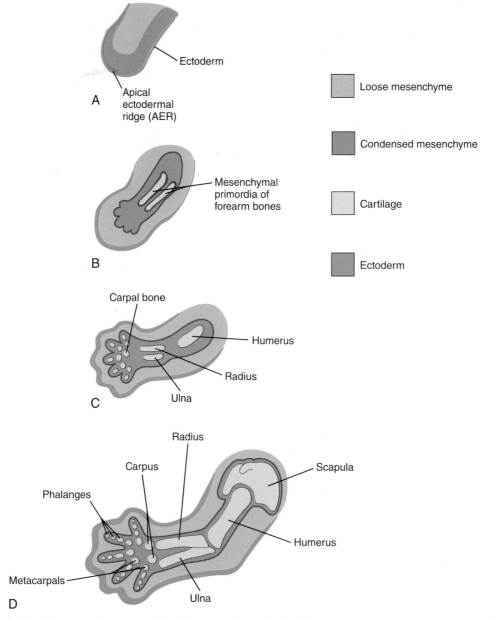

Loose mesenchyme

Condensed mesenchyme

Cartilage

Ectoderm

Fig. 15.12 Longitudinal sections through an upper limb bud of an embryo showing development of the cartilaginous bones. (A) At 28 days. (B) At 44 days. (C) At 48 days. (D) At 56 days.

MUSCULAR SYSTEM

The muscular system develops from the **mesoderm**, except for the muscles of the iris, which develop from the **neuroectoderm**. Myoblasts—embryonic muscle cells—are derived from mesenchyme.

DEVELOPMENT OF SKELETAL MUSCLE

The myoblasts that form the skeletal muscles of the trunk are derived from the mesenchyme in the myotome regions of the somites. The limb muscles develop from **myogenic precursor cells** in the limb buds. These cells originate from the ventral **dermomyotome of somites** in response to molecular signals from nearby tissues (Fig. 15.15). The myogenic precursor cells migrate into the limb buds, where they undergo epithelial–mesenchymal transformation. The first indication of **myogenesis** is the elongation of the nuclei and cell bodies of mesenchymal cells as they differentiate into myoblasts.

The myoblasts soon fuse to form elongated, multinucleated, cylindrical structures—**myotubes**. *At the molecular level, these events are preceded by gene activation and expression of the MyoD family of muscle-specific basic helix-loop-helix transcription factors (MyoD, myogenin, Myf-5, and MRF4) in the precursor myogenic cells. It has been suggested that signaling molecules from the ventral neural tube (SHH), the notochord (SHH), the dorsal neural tube (Wnt, BMP-4), and the overlying ectoderm (Wnt, BMP-4) regulate the beginning of myogenesis and the induction of the myotome.*

Muscle growth results from the ongoing fusion of myoblasts and myotubes. **Myofilaments** develop in the cytoplasm of the myotubes during or after fusion of the myoblasts.

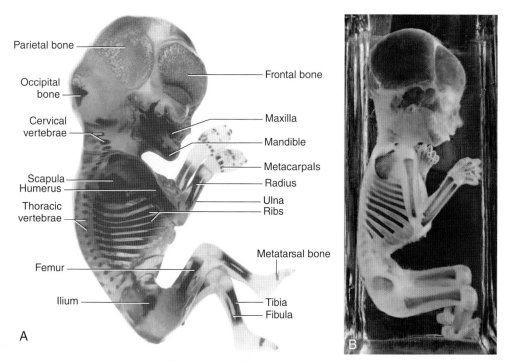

Parietal bone

Occipital bone

Cervical vertebrae

Scapula
Humerus

Thoracic vertebrae

Femur

Ilium

Frontal bone

Maxilla

Mandible

Metacarpals

Radius

Ulna
Ribs

Metatarsal bone

Tibia
Fibula

A

B

Fig. 15.13 (A) Alizarin-stained, 12-week fetus. (B) Alizarin-stained, 20-week fetus. Observe the degree of progression of ossification from the primary centers of ossification, which are endochondral in the appendicular and axial parts of the skeleton, except for most of the cranial bones. Note that the carpus and tarsus are wholly cartilaginous at this stage, as are the epiphyses of all long bones. A, Courtesy Dr. David Bolender, Department of Cell Biology, Neurobiology, and Anatomy, Medical College of Wisconsin, Milwaukee, Wisconsin; B, Courtesy Dr. Gary Geddes, Lake Oswego, Oregon.

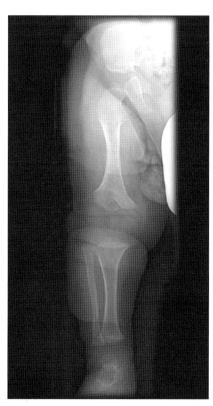

Fig. 15.14 Radiograph of the skeletal system of a 2-year-old child with achondroplasia, showing proximal shortening of the femur with metaphyseal flaring. Courtesy Dr. Prem M Sahni, formerly of the Department of Radiology, Children's Hospital, Winnipeg, Manitoba, Canada.

Soon after that, **myofibrils** and other organelles characteristic of striated muscle cells develop. Because muscle cells are long and narrow, they are called **muscle fibers**. As the myotubes differentiate, they become invested with external laminae, which segregate them from the surrounding connective tissue. **Fibroblasts** produce the perimysium and epimysium layers of the fibrous sheath; the endomysium is formed by the external lamina, which is derived from the muscle fiber, and by reticular fibers.

Most skeletal muscle develops before birth, and almost all remaining muscles are formed by age one. The increase in the size of a muscle after the first year results from an increase in the diameter of the fibers because of the formation of more myofilaments. Muscles increase in length and width to grow with the skeleton.

MYOTOMES

Each myotome part of a somite divides into a dorsal **epaxial division** and a ventral **hypaxial division** (Fig. 15.16). Each developing **spinal nerve** also divides and sends a branch to each division, with the **dorsal primary ramus** supplying the epaxial division and the **ventral primary ramus** supplying the hypaxial division. Some muscles, such as the intercostal muscles, remain segmentally arranged like the somites, but most myoblasts migrate away from the myotome and form nonsegmented muscles.

DERIVATIVES OF EPAXIAL DIVISIONS OF MYOTOMES

Myoblasts from the epaxial divisions of the myotomes form the segmental muscles of the main body axis, the extensor muscles of the neck, and vertebral column (Fig. 15.17). The embryonic extensor muscles that are derived from the sacral

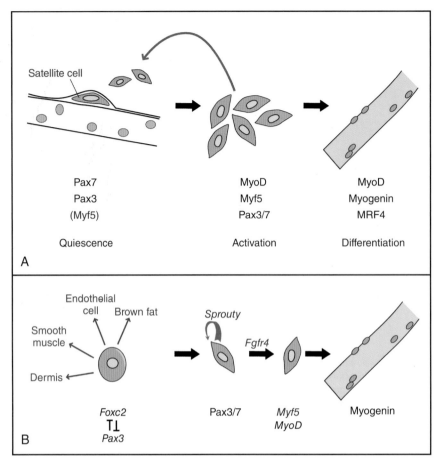

Fig. 15.15 Progression of muscle progenitor cells toward formation of differentiated skeletal muscle. (A) The progression of adult muscle satellite cells toward new muscle fiber formation. Myf-5 is shown in *red* in the quiescent state to indicate that transcripts are present but not the protein. (B) The progression of somitic cells toward myogenesis, showing how Pax3 activates target genes that regulate different stages of this process. Pax3 target genes are shown in *red*. From Buckingham M, Rigby PWJ: Gene regulatory networks and transcriptional mechanisms that control myogenesis, *Dev Cell* 28:225, 2014.

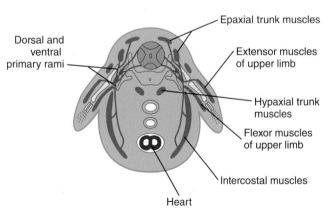

Fig. 15.16 Transverse section of the embryo showing the epaxial and hypaxial derivatives of a myotome.

and coccygeal myotomes degenerate; their adult derivatives are the dorsal sacrococcygeal ligaments.

DERIVATIVES OF HYPAXIAL DIVISIONS OF MYOTOMES

Myoblasts from the hypaxial divisions of the cervical myotomes form the scalene, prevertebral, geniohyoid, and infrahyoid muscles (see Fig. 15.17A). Those from the thoracic myotomes form the lateral and ventral flexor muscles of the vertebral column, whereas the lumbar myotomes form the quadratus lumborum muscle. The muscles of the limbs, the intercostal muscles, and the abdominal muscles are also derived from the hypaxial division of the myotomes. The sacrococcygeal myotomes form the muscles of the pelvic diaphragm and probably the striated muscles of the anus and sex organs.

PHARYNGEAL ARCH MUSCLES

Myoblasts from the pharyngeal arches form the muscles of mastication and facial expression and those of the pharynx and larynx (see Chapter 10). These muscles are innervated by the pharyngeal arch nerves.

OCULAR MUSCLES

Paraxial head mesoderm and mesoderm in the prechordal plate area are believed to give rise to three **preotic myotomes** from which myoblasts differentiate (see Fig. 15.17B). Groups of myoblasts, each supplied by its own cranial nerve (CN III, CN IV, or CN VI), form the extrinsic muscles of the eye.

TONGUE MUSCLES

Myoblasts from the **occipital (postotic) myotomes** form the tongue muscles, which are innervated by the hypoglossal nerve (CN XII).

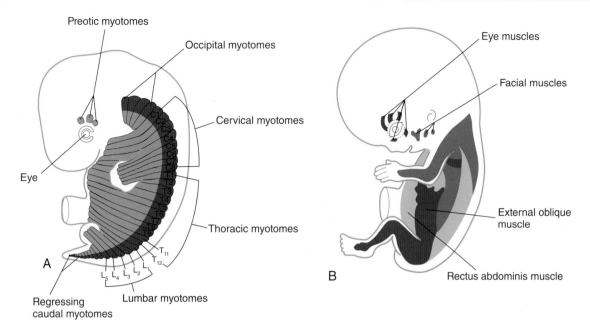

Fig. 15.17   Illustrations of the developing muscular system. (A) A 6-week embryo showing the myotome regions of the somites that give rise to most skeletal muscles. (B) An 8-week embryo showing the developing trunk and limb musculature.

LIMB MUSCLES

The musculature of the limbs develops from myoblasts surrounding the developing bones (see Fig. 15.16). The **precursor myogenic cells** in the limb buds originate from the somites. These cells are first located in the ventral part of the dermomyotome, and they are epithelial (see Fig. 15.1D). After **epitheliomesenchymal transformation**, the cells migrate into the primordium of the limb.

DEVELOPMENT OF SMOOTH MUSCLE

Some smooth muscle fibers differentiate from the **splanchnic mesenchyme** surrounding the endoderm of the primordial gut and its derivatives (see Fig. 15.1E). The smooth muscle in the walls of many blood and lymphatic vessels arises from the somatic mesoderm. The muscles of the iris (sphincter and dilator pupillae) and the **myoepithelial** cells in the mammary and sweat glands are believed to be derived from mesenchymal cells that originate from the ectoderm.

The first sign of differentiation in smooth muscle is the development of elongated nuclei in spindle-shaped myoblasts. During early development, new myoblasts continue to differentiate from mesenchymal cells but do not fuse; they remain mononucleated. During later development, the division of existing myoblasts gradually replaces the differentiation of new myoblasts in the production of new smooth muscle tissue. Filamentous, but non-sarcomeric, contractile elements develop in their cytoplasm, and the external surface of each differential cell acquires a surrounding external lamina. As smooth muscle fibers develop into sheets or bundles, they receive autonomic innervation; fibroblasts and muscle cells synthesize and lay down collagenous, elastic, and reticular fibers.

DEVELOPMENT OF CARDIAC MUSCLE

The lateral splanchnic mesoderm gives rise to the mesenchyme surrounding the developing heart tube (see Chapter 14). **Cardiac myoblasts** are derived from this mesenchyme by the differentiation and growth of single cells, unlike striated skeletal muscle fibers, which develop by the fusion of cells. The myoblasts adhere to each other as in developing skeletal muscle, but the intervening cell membranes do not disintegrate; these areas of adhesion give rise to **intercalated discs**. Growth of cardiac muscle fibers results from the formation of new **myofilaments**. Late in the embryonic period, special bundles of muscle cells develop that have relatively few myofibrils and relatively larger diameters than typical cardiac muscle fibers. The cells develop from original trabeculated myocardium, have fast-conducting gap junctions, and form the conducting system of the heart (Purkinje fibers) (see Chapter 14).

Anomalies of Muscles

Any muscle in the body may occasionally be absent; common examples are the sternocostal head of the pectoralis major, the palmaris longus, the trapezius, the serratus anterior, and the quadratus femoris. Absence of the pectoralis major, often its sternal part, is usually associated with *syndactyly* (fusion of digits). This defect is part of the **Poland syndrome** (1:20,000), which also includes breast and nipple aplasia or hypoplasia, deficiencies of axillary hair and subcutaneous fat, and shortened arms and fingers.

The sternocleidomastoid muscle (SCM) is sometimes injured at birth, resulting in **congenital torticollis**. There is fixed rotation and tilting of the head because of concomitant muscle fibrosis and shortening of the SCM on one side (Fig. 15.18). Although birth trauma is commonly considered a cause of congenital torticollis, this may also result from malpositioning in utero and primary SCM myopathy.

Accessory Muscles

Accessory muscles occasionally develop. For example, an **accessory soleus muscle** is present in approximately 3% of the population. It has been suggested that the primordium of the soleus muscle may undergo early splitting to form an accessory soleus.

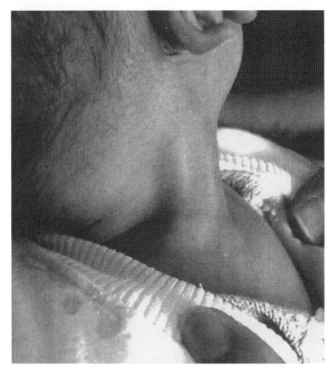

Fig. 15.18 Congenital muscular torticollis (wry neck) showing extensive involvement of the left sternocleidomastoid muscle in an infant at 2 months. Courtesy Professor Jack C.Y. Cheng, Department of Orthopaedics & Traumatology, The Chinese University of Hong Kong, Hong Kong, China.

DEVELOPMENT OF LIMBS

▶ EARLY STAGES OF LIMB DEVELOPMENT

15

The **limb buds** first appear toward the end of the fourth week as small elevations of the ventrolateral body wall (Fig. 15.19, week 5). Limb development begins with the activation of a group of mesenchymal cells in the lateral mesoderm. The upper limb buds are visible by day 26 or 27, whereas the lower limb buds appear 1 to 2 days later. Each limb bud consists of a mass of mesenchyme covered by ectoderm (see Fig. 15.12A and B). The mesenchyme is derived from the somatic layer of the lateral mesoderm.

The limb buds elongate with the proliferation of the mesenchyme. Although the early stages of limb development are alike for the upper and lower limbs (see Fig. 6.11), there are distinct differences because of their form and function. The **upper limb buds** develop opposite the caudal cervical segments, whereas the **lower limb buds** form opposite the lumbar and upper sacral segments.

At the apex of each limb bud, the ectoderm thickens to form an **apical ectodermal ridge** (AER) (Fig. 15.12A). The AER, a specialized multilayered epithelial structure, interacts with the mesenchyme in the limb bud, promoting outgrowth of the bud *for which BMP is essential. Retinoic acid promotes the formation of the limb bud by inhibiting fibroblast growth factor 8 (FGF8) signaling.* The AER exerts an inductive influence on the limb mesenchyme that initiates growth and development of the limbs along a proximodistal axis. Mesenchymal cells aggregate at the posterior margin of the limb bud to form a **zone of polarizing activity**. *FGFs from the AER activate the zone of polarizing activity, causing expression of sonic hedgehog (SHH), which controls the patterning of the limb along the anteroposterior axis.*

Expression of Wnt7 from the dorsal epidermis of the limb bud and engrailed-1 (En-1) from the ventral aspect is involved in specifying the dorsoventral axis. Curiously, the AER itself is maintained by inductive signals from SHH and Wnt7. The mesenchyme adjacent to the AER consists of undifferentiated, rapidly proliferating cells, whereas the mesenchymal cells proximal to it differentiate into blood vessels and cartilage bone models. *For cartilage formation, TGF-β signaling plays a key role.* The distal ends of the limb buds eventually flatten into hand and foot plates (see Fig. 15.19).

By the end of the sixth week of development, mesenchymal tissue in the **hand plates** has condensed to form **finger buds—digital rays** (Fig. 15.20A–C; see also Fig. 15.19), which outline the pattern of the digits. During the seventh week, similar condensations of mesenchyme in foot plates form **toe buds**—digital rays (see Fig. 15.20G–I). At the tip of each digital ray, a part of the AER induces development of the mesenchyme into the mesenchymal primordia of the phalanges. The intervals between the digital rays are occupied by loose mesenchyme. Soon the intervening regions of mesenchyme undergo **apoptosis**, forming notches between the digital rays (see Figs. 15.19 and 15.20D and J). As this tissue breakdown progresses, separate digits are produced by the end of the eighth week of development (see Fig. 15.19). *Molecular studies show that antagonism between retinoic acid and TGF-β control the interdigital cell apoptosis.* Blocking of cellular and molecular events during this process may account for webbing, or fusion, of the fingers or toes, a condition known as **syndactyly** (see Fig. 15.25C and D).

FINAL STAGES OF LIMB DEVELOPMENT

The mesenchyme in a limb bud gives rise to bones, ligaments, and blood vessels (see Fig. 15.12). As the limb buds elongate during the early part of the fifth week, mesenchymal models of the bones are formed by cellular aggregations (see Fig. 15.12A and B). **Chondrification centers** appear later in the fifth week. By the end of the sixth week, the entire limb skeleton is cartilaginous (see Fig. 15.12C and D).

Osteogenesis of the long bones begins in the seventh week from primary ossification centers in the diaphysis of the long bones. **Ossification centers** are present in all long bones by the 12th week. Primary ossification of the carpal (wrist) bones begins during the first year after birth.

From the **dermomyotome regions of the somites**, myogenic precursor cells also migrate into the limb bud and later differentiate into myoblasts, the precursors of muscle cells. As the long bones form, myoblasts aggregate and form a large muscle mass in each limb bud (see Fig. 15.16). In general, this muscle mass separates into dorsal (extensor) and ventral (flexor) components.

Early in the seventh week, the limbs extend ventrally, and the preaxial and postaxial borders are cranial and caudal, respectively (see Fig. 15.22A and D). The upper limbs rotate laterally through 90 degrees on their longitudinal axes; thus the future elbows point dorsally, and the extensor muscles lie on the lateral and posterior aspects of the limb. The lower limbs rotate medially through almost 90 degrees; thus the future knees face ventrally, and the extensor muscles lie on the anterior aspect of the lower limb (Fig. 15.21A–D).

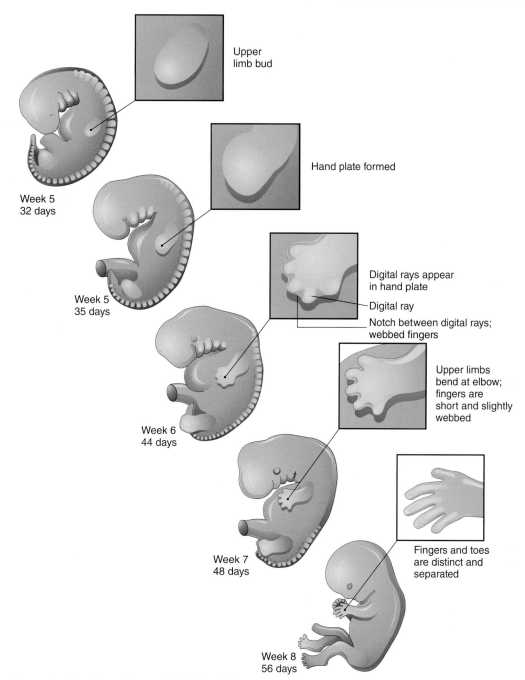

Upper
limb bud

Hand plate formed

Digital rays appear
in hand plate

Digital ray

Notch between digital rays;
webbed fingers

Upper limbs
bend at elbow;
fingers are
short and slightly
webbed

Fingers and toes
are distinct and
separated

Week 5
32 days

Week 5
35 days

Week 6
44 days

Week 7
48 days

Week 8
56 days

Fig. 15.19 Development of the limbs of fetuses (32–56 days). Note that development of the upper limbs precedes that of the lower limbs.

The radius and tibia are homologous bones, as are the ulna and fibula, just as the thumb and great toe are homologous digits. **Synovial joints** appear at the beginning of the fetal period, coinciding with functional differentiation of the limb muscles and their innervation.

CUTANEOUS INNERVATION OF LIMBS

Motor axons arising from the spinal cord enter the limb buds during the fifth week and grow into the dorsal and ventral muscle masses. **Sensory axons** enter the limb buds after the motor axons and use them for guidance. **Neural crest cells**, the precursors of Schwann cells, surround the motor and sensory nerve fibers in the limbs and form the neurolemmal and myelin sheaths (see Chapter 16).

A **dermatome** is the area of skin supplied by a single spinal nerve and its spinal ganglion. During the fifth week, the peripheral nerves grow from the developing **limb** (brachial and lumbosacral) **plexuses** into the mesenchyme of the limb buds (Fig. 15.22A and B). The spinal nerves are distributed in segmental bands, supplying both the dorsal and ventral surfaces of the limb buds. As the limbs elongate, the cutaneous distribution of the spinal nerves migrates along the limbs and no longer reaches the surface in the distal part of the limbs. Although the original **dermatomal pattern** changes during growth of the limbs, an orderly sequence of distribution can still be recognized in the adult (see Fig. 15.22C and F). In the upper limb, the areas supplied by C5 and C6 adjoin the areas supplied by T2, T1, and C8, but the overlap between them is minimal at the ventral axial line.

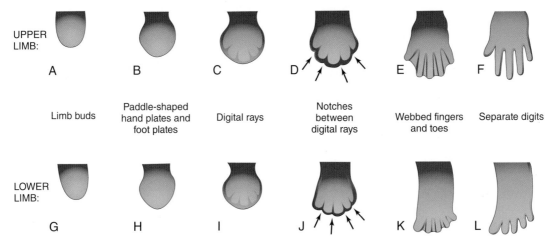

Fig. 15.20 Development of the hands and feet between the fourth and eighth weeks. The early stages of limb development are similar, except that the development of the hands precedes that of the feet by approximately 1 day. (A) At 27 days. (B) At 32 days. (C) At 41 days. (D) At 46 days. (E) At 50 days. (F) At 52 days. (G) At 28 days. (H) At 36 days. (I) At 46 days. (J) At 49 days. (K) At 52 days. (L) At 56 days. The *arrows* in (D) and (J) indicate the tissue breakdown processes that separate the fingers and toes.

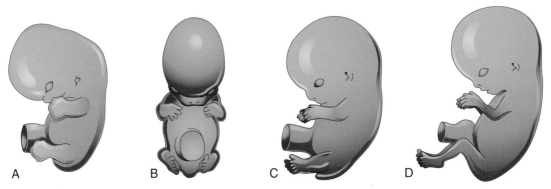

Fig. 15.21 Positional changes of the developing limbs of embryos. (A) At approximately 48 days showing the limbs extending ventrally and the hand plates and foot plates facing each other. (B) At approximately 51 days showing the upper limbs bent at the elbows and the hands curved over the thorax. (C) At approximately 54 days showing the soles of the feet facing medially. (D) At approximately 56 days. Note that the elbows now point caudally and the knees, cranially.

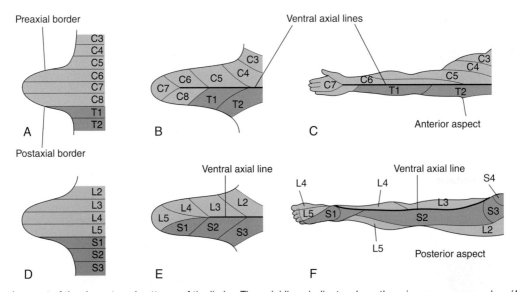

Fig. 15.22 Development of the dermatomal patterns of the limbs. The axial lines indicate where there is no sensory overlap. (A and D) Ventral aspect of the limb buds early in the fifth week. At this stage, the dermatomal patterns show the primordial segmental arrangement. (B and E) Similar views later in the fifth week showing the modified arrangement of dermatomes. (C and F) The dermatomal patterns in the adult upper and lower limbs. The primordial dermatomal pattern has disappeared, but an orderly sequence of dermatomes can still be recognized. (F) Note that most of the original ventral surface of the lower limb lies on the back of the adult limb. This results from the medial rotation of the lower limb that occurs toward the end of the embryonic period. In the upper limb, the ventral axial line extends along the anterior surface of the arm and forearm. In the lower limb, the ventral axial line extends along the medial side of the thigh and knee to the posteromedial aspect of the leg to the heel.

Because there is an overlap of dermatomes, a particular area of skin is not exclusively innervated by a single segmental nerve. The limb dermatomes may be traced progressively down the lateral aspect of the upper limb and back up its medial aspect. A comparable distribution of dermatomes occurs in the lower limbs and may be traced down the ventral aspect and then up the dorsal aspect of the lower limb. When the limbs extend and rotate, they carry their nerves with them; this explains the oblique course of the nerves arising from the brachial and lumbosacral plexuses.

BLOOD SUPPLY OF LIMBS

The limb buds are supplied by branches of the **intersegmental arteries** (Fig. 15.23A), which arise from the dorsal aorta and form a fine capillary network throughout the

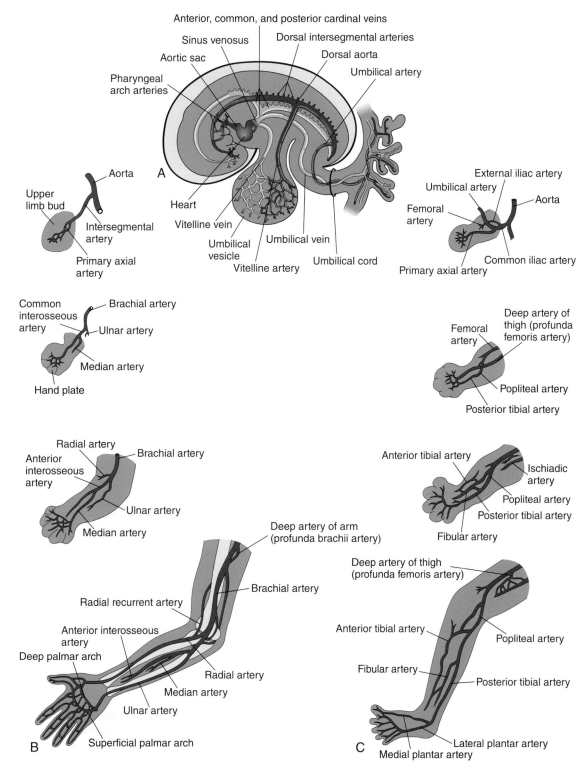

Fig. 15.23 Development of the limb arteries. (A and B) Development of the arteries in the upper limb. (C) Development of the arteries in the lower limb.

mesenchyme. The primordial vascular pattern consists of a **primary axial artery** and its branches (see Fig. 15.23B and C), which drain into a peripheral marginal sinus. Blood in the sinus drains into a peripheral vein.

The vascular pattern changes as the limbs develop, chiefly as a result of new vessels sprouting from existing vessels **(angiogenesis)**. The new vessels coalesce with other sprouts to form larger vessels. The primary axial artery forms the **brachial artery** in the arm and the **ulnar and radial arteries** in the forearm, arise from the terminal branches of the brachial artery (see Fig. 15.23B). As the digits form, the marginal sinus breaks up and the final venous pattern, represented by the basilic and cephalic veins and their tributaries, develops. In the thigh, the primary axial artery is represented by the **deep artery of the thigh** (profunda femoris artery). In the leg, the primary axial artery is represented by the anterior and posterior **tibial arteries** (see Fig. 15.23C).

Split-Hand/Foot Malformations

In the rare **cleft hand** or **cleft foot** defects, one or more central digits are absent—**ectrodactyly**—resulting from the failure of one or more digital rays to develop (Fig. 15.24A and B). The hand or foot is divided into two parts that oppose each other. The remaining digits are partially or completely fused **(syndactyly)**. This autosomal dominant (incomplete penetrance) defect affects 1:20,000 live births.

Radial Aplasia

In rare cases (1:30,000), the radius is partially or completely absent. The hand deviates laterally (radially), and the ulna bows with the concavity on the lateral side of the forearm. This defect results from the failure of the mesenchymal primordium of the radius to form during the fifth week. Absence of the radius is usually caused by genetic factors.

Polydactyly

Supernumerary digits are common (1:500 to 1:1000 infants) (Fig. 15.25A and B). Often, the extra digit is incompletely formed and lacks proper muscular development, rendering it useless. If the hand is affected, the extra digit is most commonly medial or lateral rather than central. In the foot, the extra toe is usually on the lateral side. Polydactyly is inherited as a dominant trait.

Syndactyly

This birth defect occurs approximately 1 in 2200 births. **Cutaneous syndactyly** (simple webbing of digits) is the most common limb defect (see Fig. 15.25C). It occurs more frequently in the foot than in the hand (see Fig. 15.25C and D). Syndactyly is most frequently observed between the third and fourth fingers and between the second and third toes (see Fig. 15.25D). It is inherited as a simple dominant or simple recessive trait. Cutaneous syndactyly results from the failure of the webs to degenerate between two or more digits. In some cases, there is **synostosis** (fusion of bones). **Osseous syndactyly** occurs when the notches between the digital rays do not develop during the seventh week; as a result, separation of the digits does not occur.

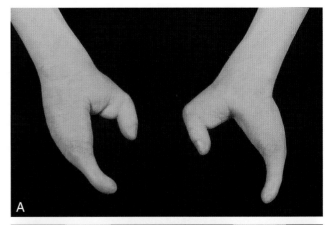
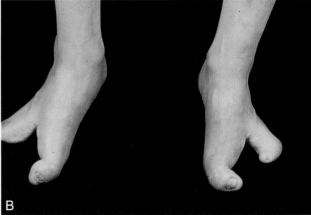

Fig. 15.24   Birth defects of the hands and feet. (A) Ectrodactyly in a child. Note the absence of the central digits of the hands, resulting in split hands. (B) A similar type of defect involving the feet. These limb defects can be inherited in an autosomal dominant pattern. *Courtesy A.E. Chudley, MD, Section of Genetics and Metabolism, Department of Pediatrics and Child Health, University of Manitoba, Children's Hospital, Winnipeg, Manitoba, Canada.*

Arthrogryposis

Arthrogryposis multiplex congenita refers to a heterogeneous group of musculoskeletal disorders characterized by multiple contractures and immobility of two or more joints from birth. The incidence of this birth defect is 1 in 3000 live births; males are more affected in sex-linked cases. The causes may be both neurological (central and peripheral nervous system defects) and nonneurological (cartilaginous defects and restricted movement in utero).

Congenital Talipes

Talipes occurs at a rate of approximately 1 in 1000 births. **Talipes equinovarus**, the most common type, occurs approximately twice as frequently in males as in females. The sole of the foot is turned medially, and the foot is inverted (Fig. 15.26). There is much uncertainty about the cause of talipes. Hereditary factors are involved in some cases, and it appears that environmental factors are involved in most cases. Talipes appears to follow a **multifactorial pattern of inheritance**. It may be caused by radial and longitudinal uneven growth and muscular imbalance.

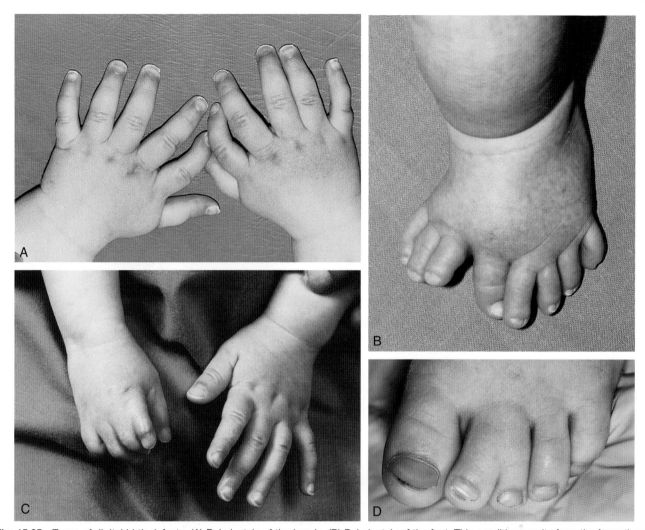

Fig. 15.25 Types of digital birth defects. (A) Polydactyly of the hands. (B) Polydactyly of the foot. This condition results from the formation of one or more extra digital rays during the embryonic period. (C) and (D) Various forms of syndactyly involving the fingers and toes. Cutaneous syndactyly (C) is probably caused by incomplete apoptosis (programmed cell death) in the tissues between the digital rays during embryonic life. (D) Syndactyly of the second and third toes. In osseous syndactyly, the digital rays merge as a result of lack of apoptosis, causing fusion of the bones. Courtesy A.E. Chudley, MD, Section of Genetics and Metabolism, Department of Pediatrics and Child Health, University of Manitoba, Children's Hospital, Winnipeg, Manitoba, Canada.

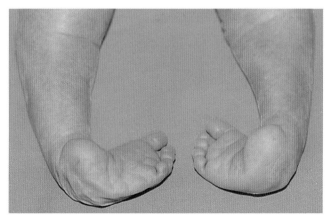

Fig. 15.26 Neonate with bilateral talipes equinovarus deformities (club feet) illustrating the classic type of this birth defect, characterized by inversion and medial rotation of the soles of the feet. Courtesy A.E. Chudley, MD, Section of Genetics and Metabolism, Department of Pediatrics and Child Health, University of Manitoba, Children's Hospital, Winnipeg, Manitoba, Canada.

Limb Anomalies

There are two main types of limb defects:

- **Amelia**—complete absence of a limb
- **Meromelia**—such as **hemimelia**, partial absence of a limb (e.g., absence of the fibula in the leg), and **phocomelia**, hands and feet are attached close to the body

Anomalies of the limbs originate at different stages of development. Suppression of limb bud development during the early part of the fifth week results in **amelia** (Fig. 15.27A). Arrest or disturbance of the differentiation or growth of the limbs during the fifth week results in **meromelia** (see Fig. 15.27B and C). Some limb defects are caused by the following:

- **Genetic factors**, such as chromosomal abnormalities associated with trisomy 18 (see Chapter 19)

- **Pathogenic Variant (Mutant) in genes**, as in skeletal dysplasias (achondroplasia), brachydactyly (shortness of digits), or osteogenesis imperfecta (connective tissue disorders). *Molecular studies have implicated pathogenic variants (mutation) in genes (HOX, BMP, SHH, WNT7, EN1, FGFR3, and others) in some cases of limb anomalies*
- **Environmental factors**, such as teratogens (e.g., thalidomide)
- **Combination of genetic and environmental factors** (multifactorial inheritance), as in congenital dislocation of the hip
- **Vascular disruption and ischemia (diminished blood supply)**, as in limb reduction defects

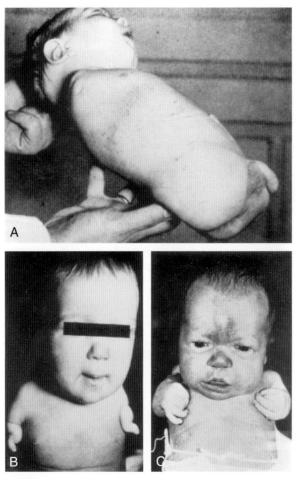

Fig. 15.27 Birth defects caused by maternal ingestion of thalidomide. (A) Quadruple amelia (absence of the upper and lower limbs). (B) Meromelia (partial absence) of the upper limbs; the limbs are represented by rudimentary stumps. (C) Meromelia with rudimentary upper limbs attached directly to the trunk. From Lenz W, Knapp K: Foetal malformations due to thalidomide, *Ger Med Mon* 7:253, 1962.

CLINICALLY ORIENTED QUESTIONS

1. Occasionally, accessory ribs are associated with the seventh cervical vertebra and the first lumbar vertebra. Are these accessory ribs of clinical importance?

2. What vertebral defect can produce scoliosis? Define this condition. What is the embryological basis of a vertebral defect?

3. What is meant by the term craniosynostosis? What results from this developmental abnormality? Give a common example and describe it.

4. A child presented with characteristics of Klippel–Feil syndrome. What are the main features of this condition? What vertebral defects are usually present?

5. A neonate was born with the prune-belly syndrome. What do you think would cause this birth defect? What urinary defect results from the abnormal development of the anterior abdominal wall?

6. A boy presents with one nipple much lower than the other one. How would you explain the abnormally low position of the nipple to the parents?

7. An 8-year-old girl asked her doctor why the muscle on one side of her neck was so prominent. What would you tell her? What would happen if this is not treated?

8. After strenuous exercise, a young athlete complained of pain on the posteromedial aspect of his ankle. He was told that he had an accessory calf muscle. Is this possible? If so, what is the embryological basis of this defect?

9. An infant had short limbs. His trunk was normally proportioned, but his head was slightly larger than normal. Both parents had normal limbs and these problems had never occurred in either of their families. Could the mother's ingestion of drugs during pregnancy have caused these abnormalities? If not, what would be the probable cause of these skeletal disorders? Could they occur again if the couple had more children?

10. A man has very short fingers (brachydactyly). He says that two of his relatives have short fingers, but none of his brothers or sisters have them. What are the chances that his children would have brachydactyly if his wife has normal digits?

11. A female gave birth to a child with no right hand. She had taken a drug that contained doxylamine and dicyclomine to alleviate nausea during the 10th week of her pregnancy (8 weeks after fertilization). The woman is instituting legal proceedings against the company that makes the drug. Does this drug cause limb defects? If it does, could it have caused the child's hand to fail to develop?

12. An infant had syndactyly of the left hand and the absence of the left sternal head of the pectoralis major muscle. The infant was otherwise normal, except that the nipple on the left side was approximately 2 inches lower than the other one. What is the cause of these defects? Can they be corrected?

13. What is the most common type of talipes? How common is it? What is the appearance of the feet of neonates born with this defect?

The answers to these questions are at the back of this book.

The nervous system consists of three main regions:

- The **central nervous system** (CNS), which includes the brain and spinal cord, is protected by the cranium and vertebral column.
- The **peripheral nervous system** (PNS), which includes the neurons outside the CNS—cranial nerves and ganglia and spinal nerves and ganglia—connects the brain and spinal cord with peripheral structures.
- The **autonomic nervous system** (ANS), which has parts in both the CNS and PNS, consists of the neurons that innervate smooth muscle, cardiac muscle, glandular epithelium, or combinations of these tissues.

DEVELOPMENT OF NERVOUS SYSTEM

The nervous system begins during the third week as the **neural plate** and **neural groove** develop on the posterior aspect of the trilaminar embryo (Fig. 16.1A). The nervous system develops from the **neural plate**, a thickened area of embryonic ectoderm (see Fig. 16.1A and B). The notochord and paraxial mesoderm induce the overlying ectoderm to differentiate into the neural plate. *This transformation (neural induction) involves the expression of intercellular proteins, including members of the transforming growth factor-β family (TGF-β), Wnts, sonic hedgehog (SHH), and bone morphogenic proteins (BMPs).* The formation of the **neural folds, neural crest**, and **neural tube** is illustrated in Fig. 16.1B to F. The neural tube differentiates into the CNS, consisting of the brain and spinal cord. The neural crest gives rise to cells that form most of the PNS and ANS.

Neurulation—formation of the neural plate and neural tube—begins during the fourth week (22–23 days) in the region of the fourth to sixth pairs of somites (see Fig. 16.1C). **Fusion of the neural folds** proceeds in a number of areas until only small portions of the neural tube remain open at both ends (Fig. 16.2A and B). At these open sites, the lumen of the neural tube—the **neural canal**—communicates freely with the amniotic cavity (see Fig. 16.2C). The cranial opening—the **rostral neuropore**—closes on approximately the 25th day, and the **caudal neuropore** closes 2 days later (see Fig. 16.2D).

Closure of the neuropores coincides with the establishment of a vascular circulation for the neural tube. *It has been reported that the expression of Snx, Syndecan 4 gene (SDC4), endocytic receptor Lrp2, and van gogh-like 2 (VANGL2) proteins is essential for this process.* The neuroprogenitor cells of the walls of the neural tube proliferate to form the brain and spinal cord (Fig. 16.3). The neural canal forms the ventricular

system of the brain and the central canal of the spinal cord. *The dorsoventral patterning of the neural tube appears to involve the SHH gene,* Pax *genes, BMPs, and dorsalin, a TGF-β.*

DEVELOPMENT OF SPINAL CORD

The primordial spinal cord develops from the neural tube, caudal to the fourth pair of somites, and the caudal eminence (see Fig. 16.3). The lateral walls of the neural tube thicken and gradually reduce the size of the neural canal to a minute **central canal** (Fig. 16.4A to C). Initially, the wall of the neural tube is composed of a thick, pseudostratified, columnar **neuroepithelium** (see Fig. 16.4D).

These neuroepithelial cells constitute the **ventricular zone** (ependymal layer), which gives rise to all neurons and macroglial cells (macroglia) in the spinal cord (Fig. 16.5). Soon, a **marginal zone** composed of the outer parts of the neuroepithelial cells is recognizable (see Fig. 16.4E). This zone gradually becomes the **white matter of the spinal cord** as axons grow into it from nerve cell bodies in the spinal cord, spinal ganglia, and brain.

Some dividing neuroepithelial cells in the ventricular zone differentiate into primordial neurons—**neuroblasts**. These embryonic cells form an **intermediate zone** (mantle layer) between the ventricular and marginal zones. Neuroblasts become neurons as they develop cytoplasmic processes (see Fig. 16.5).

The supporting cells of the CNS—the **glioblasts** (spongioblasts)—differentiate from the neuroepithelial progenitor cells, mainly after neuroblast formation has ceased. The glioblasts (oligodendrocyte progenitor cell) migrate from the ventricular zone into the intermediate and marginal zones. Some glioblasts become **astroblasts** and later **astrocytes**, whereas other glioblasts become oligodendroblasts and eventually **oligodendrocytes** (see Fig. 16.5). When neuroepithelial cells cease producing neuroblasts and glioblasts, they differentiate into ependymal cells, which form the **ependyma** (ependymal epithelium) lining the central canal of the spinal cord.

Microglia (microglial cells), which are scattered throughout the gray and white matter of the spinal cord, are small cells that are derived from mesenchymal cells (see Fig. 16.5). Microglial cells invade the CNS rather late in the fetal period, after it has been penetrated by blood vessels. Microglia originate in the bone marrow and are part of the mononuclear phagocytic cell population.

Proliferation and differentiation of neuroepithelial cells in the developing spinal cord produce thick walls and a thin roof plate and floor plate (see Fig. 16.4B). Differential

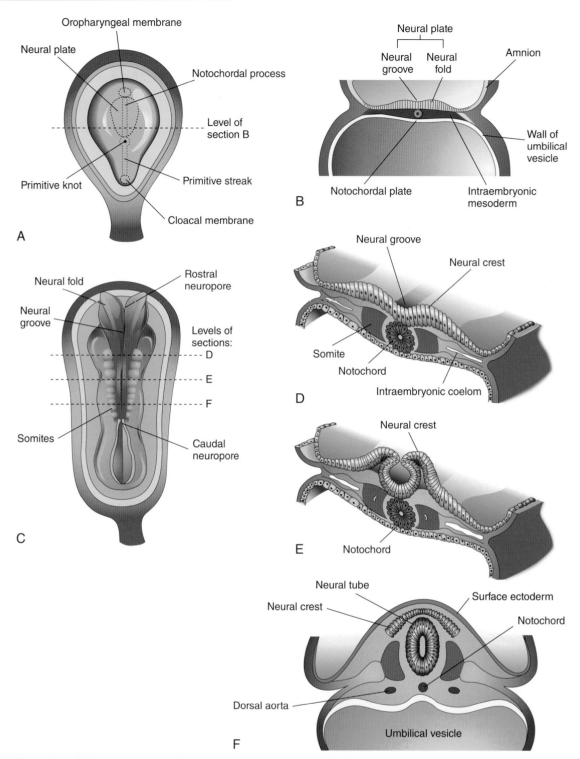

Fig. 16.1   Illustrations of the neural plate and folding of it to form the neural tube. (A) Dorsal view of an embryo of approximately 17 days, exposed by removing the amnion. (B) Transverse section of the embryo showing the neural plate and early development of the neural groove and neural folds. (C) Dorsal view of an embryo of approximately 22 days. The neural folds have fused opposite to the fourth to sixth somites but are open at both ends. (D–F) Transverse sections of this embryo at the levels shown in (C) illustrating the formation of the neural tube and its detachment from the surface ectoderm. Note that some neuroectodermal cells are not included in the neural tube but remain between it and the surface ectoderm as the neural crest.

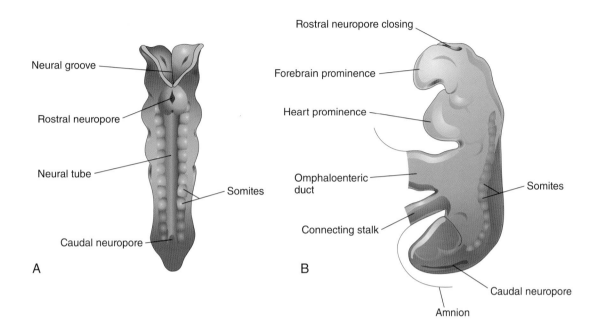

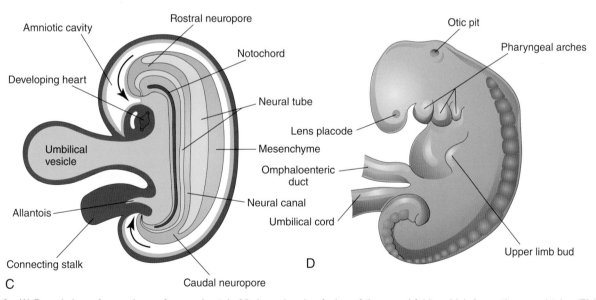

Fig. 16.2   (A) Dorsal view of an embryo of approximately 23 days showing fusion of the neural folds, which forms the neural tube. (B) Lateral view of an embryo of approximately 24 days, showing the forebrain prominence and closing of the rostral neuropore. (C) Diagrammatic sagittal section of the embryo showing the transitory communication of the neural canal with the amniotic cavity *(arrows)*. (D) Lateral view of an embryo of approximately 27 days. Note that the neuropores shown in (B) are closed.

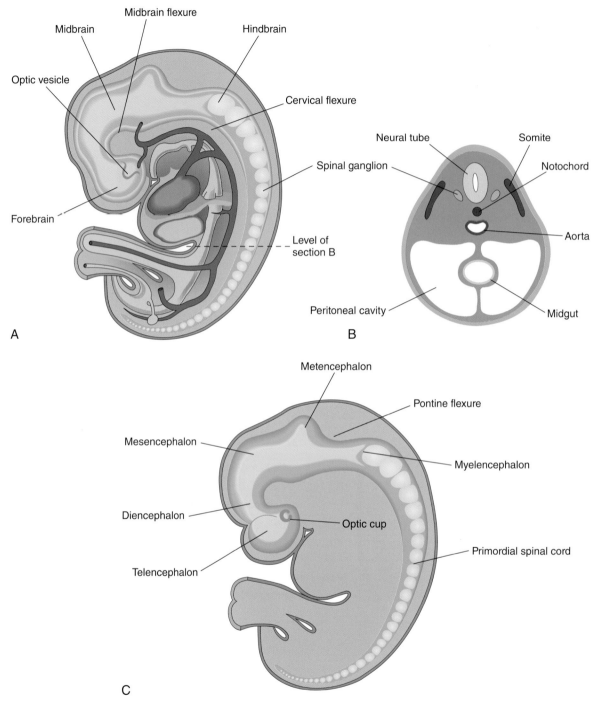

Fig. 16.3 (A) Schematic lateral view of an embryo of approximately 28 days showing the three primary brain vesicles: forebrain, midbrain, and hindbrain. Two flexures demarcate the primary divisions of the brain. (B) Transverse section of the embryo, showing the neural tube that will develop into the spinal cord in this region. The spinal ganglia derived from the neural crest are also shown. (C) Schematic lateral view of the central nervous system of a 6-week embryo showing the secondary brain vesicles and pontine flexure, which occur as the brain grows rapidly.

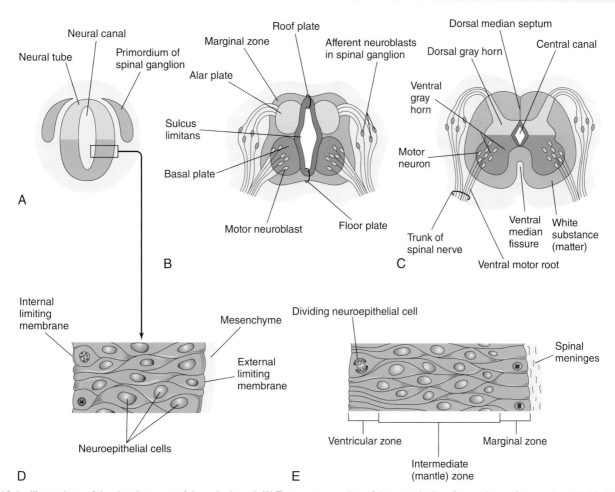

Fig. 16.4   Illustrations of the development of the spinal cord. (A) Transverse section of the neural tube of an embryo of approximately 23 days. (B and C) Similar sections at 6 and 9 weeks, respectively. (D) Section of the wall of the neural tube shown in (A). (E) Section of the wall of the developing spinal cord showing its three zones. (A–C) Note that the neural canal of the neural tube is converted into the central canal of the spinal cord.

thickening of the lateral walls of the spinal cord soon produces a shallow, longitudinal groove on each side, the **sulcus limitans** (Fig. 16.6; see also Fig. 16.4B). This groove separates the dorsal part, the **alar plate**, from the ventral part, the **basal plate**. The alar and basal plates produce longitudinal bulges extending through most of the length of the developing spinal cord. This regional separation is of fundamental importance because the alar and basal plates are later associated with afferent and efferent functions, respectively.

Cell bodies in the alar plates form the **dorsal gray columns** that extend the length of the spinal cord. In transverse sections, these columns are **dorsal gray horns** (Fig. 16.7). Neurons in these columns constitute afferent nuclei, which form the dorsal roots of the spinal nerves. As the alar plates enlarge, the **dorsal median septum** forms.

Cell bodies in the basal plates form the **ventral and lateral gray columns**. n transverse sections of the spinal cord, these columns are the **ventral gray horns** and **lateral gray horns**, respectively. Axons of the ventral horn cells grow out of the spinal cord and form the **ventral roots of the spinal nerves** (see Fig. 16.7). As the basal plates enlarge, they bulge ventrally on each side of the median plane. As this occurs, the **ventral median septum** forms, and a deep longitudinal groove—**the ventral median fissure**—develops on the ventral surface of the cord (see Fig. 16.4C).

DEVELOPMENT OF SPINAL GANGLIA

The unipolar neurons in the **spinal ganglia** (dorsal root ganglia) are derived from neural crest cells (see Fig. 16.7). The peripheral processes of the **spinal ganglion cells** pass through the spinal nerves to sensory endings in somatic or visceral structures (see Fig. 16.7). The central processes enter the spinal cord, constituting the **dorsal roots of the spinal nerves**.

DEVELOPMENT OF SPINAL MENINGES

The meninges develop from cells of the mesenchyme and neural crest cells during days 20 to 35. These cells migrate to surround the neural tube and form the primordial meninges (Fig. 16.8A and B). The external layer of these membranes thickens to form the **dura mater** (see Fig. 16.8A). The internal layer—the **pia mater** and **arachnoid mater (leptomeninges)**—is derived from neural crest cells. Fluid-filled spaces appear within the leptomeninges

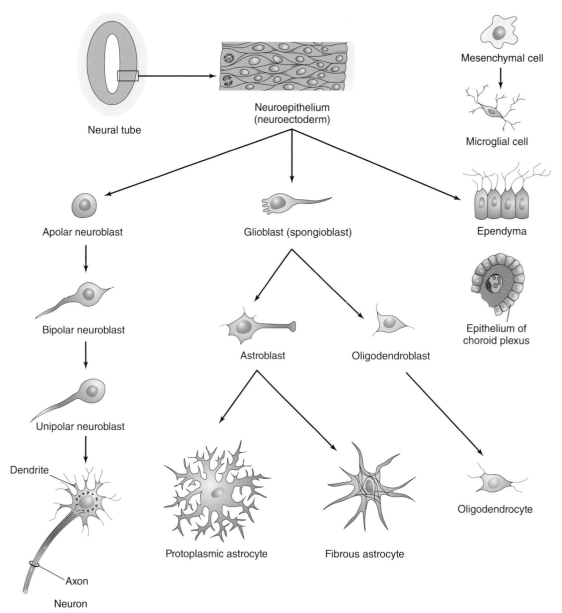

Fig. 16.5 Histogenesis of cells in the central nervous system. After further development, the multipolar neuroblast *(lower left)* becomes a nerve cell or neuron. Neuroepithelial cells give rise to all neurons and macroglial cells. Microglial cells are derived from mesenchymal cells that invade the developing nervous system with blood vessels.

that soon coalesce to form the **subarachnoid space** (Fig. 16.9A). **Cerebrospinal fluid (CSF)** begins to form during the fifth week.

POSITIONAL CHANGES OF SPINAL CORD

The spinal cord in the embryo extends the entire length of the vertebral canal at 8 weeks (see Fig. 16.8A). The spinal nerves pass through the intervertebral foramina opposite to their levels of origin. Because the vertebral column and dura mater grow more rapidly than the spinal cord, this positional relationship to the spinal nerves does not persist. The caudal end of the spinal cord in fetuses gradually comes to lie at relatively higher levels. In 24 weeks, it lies at the level of the first sacral vertebra (see Fig. 16.8B).

The spinal cord in the neonate terminates at the level of the second or third lumbar vertebra (see Fig. 16.8C). In an adult, the spinal cord usually terminates at the inferior border of the first lumbar vertebra (see Fig. 16.8D). As a result, the spinal nerve roots, especially those of the lumbar and sacral segments, run obliquely from the spinal cord to the corresponding level of the vertebral column. The nerve roots inferior to the end of the cord—the **medullary cone (conus medullaris)**—form a sheaf of nerve roots—**cauda equina**—that arises from the lumbosacral enlargement and medullary cone of the spinal cord (see Fig. 16.8C and D).

Although in adults the dura mater and arachnoid mater usually end at the S2 vertebra, the pia mater does not. Distal to the caudal end of the spinal cord, the pia mater forms a long, fibrous thread, the **filum terminale** (terminal filum),

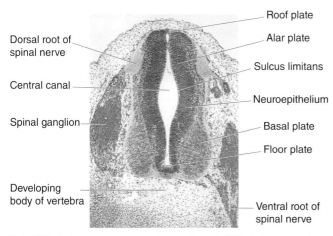

Fig. 16.6 Transverse section of an embryo (×100) at Carnegie stage 16 at approximately 40 days. The ventral root of the spinal nerve is composed of nerve fibers arising from neuroblasts in the basal plate (developing ventral horn of the spinal cord), whereas the dorsal root is formed by nerve processes arising from neuroblasts in the spinal ganglion. From Moore KL, Persaud TVN, Shiota K: *Color atlas of clinical embryology*, ed 2, Philadelphia, 2000, Saunders.

which indicates the original level of the caudal end of the embryonic spinal cord (see Fig. 16.8C and D). This filum extends from the medullary cone to the periosteum of the first coccygeal vertebra (see Fig. 16.8D).

MYELINATION OF NERVE FIBERS

Myelin sheaths surrounding the nerve fibers within the spinal cord begin to form during the late fetal period and continue to form during the first postnatal year. In general, fiber tracts become myelinated at approximately the time they become functional. Motor roots are myelinated before sensory roots. The myelin sheaths are formed by **oligodendrocytes**. The myelin sheaths surrounding the axons of peripheral nerve fibers are formed by the plasma membranes of the **neurolemma (sheath of Schwann cells)**. *Myelination of the nerve fibers is regulated by β_1 integrins and profilin 1 (Pfn1), a protein that plays an essential role in microfilament polymerization.* Neurolemma cells are derived from neural crest cells that migrate peripherally and wrap themselves around the axons of somatic motor neurons and preganglionic autonomic motor neurons as they pass out of the CNS (see Fig. 16.7). These cells also wrap themselves around the central and peripheral processes of the somatic and visceral sensory neurons and around the axons of postsynaptic autonomic motor neurons.

BIRTH DEFECTS OF SPINAL CORD

Most defects result from the failure of fusion of one or more neural arches of the developing vertebrae during the fourth week (Fig. 16.9A). **Neural tube defects (NTDs)** affect the tissues overlying the spinal cord: meninges, neural arches, muscles, and skin (see Fig. 16.9B–D). Birth defects involving the **neural arches** are referred to as **spina bifida**. The term spina bifida denotes nonfusion of the halves of the embryotic neural arches.

Spina Bifida Occulta

This NTD results from the failure of the embryonic halves of the neural arch to grow normally and fuse in the median plane (see Fig. 16.9A). Spina bifida occulta occurs in vertebra L5 or S1 in approximately 10% of otherwise normal people. In its most minor form, the only evidence of its presence may be a small dimple with a tuft of hair arising from it (Fig. 16.10). The cause of localized hypertrichosis is unknown. Spina bifida occulta usually produces no clinical symptoms.

Spina Bifida Cystica

Severe types of spina bifida involve protrusion of the spinal cord and/or meninges through defects resulting from the failure of fusion of one or more neural arches of developing vertebrae during the fourth week (see Fig. 16.9A–D). These severe NTDs are referred to collectively as **spina bifida cystica** because of the cyst-like sac that is associated with these birth defects (Fig. 16.11; see also Fig. 16.9B–D). Spina bifida cystica occurs in approximately 1 in 1000 births. When the sac contains meninges and CSF, the defect is called **spina bifida with meningocele** (see Fig. 16.9B), the most rare form of spina bifida. The spinal cord and spinal roots are in their normal positions, but spinal cord defects may be present. If the spinal cord, nerve roots, or both are included in the sac, the defect is called **spina bifida with meningomyelocele** (2–4:10,000 births) (see Figs. 16.9C and 16.11). Spina bifida with meningomyelocele involving several vertebrae is often associated with partial absence of the brain—**meroencephaly** (Fig. 16.12).

Causes of Neural Tube Defects

Genetic, nutritional, and environmental factors play a role in the production of NTDs. Gene–gene and gene–environmental interactions are likely involved in most cases. Epidemiological studies have shown that folic acid supplements (400 μg daily) taken at least 1 month before conception and continuing through the first trimester reduce the incidence of NTDs (also see www.cdc.gov/ncbddd/folicacid/about.html). Certain drugs increase the risk of NTD. For example, valproic acid, an anticonvulsant, causes NTDs in 1% to 2% of pregnant women if given during the fourth week of development, when the neural folds are fusing.

DEVELOPMENT OF THE BRAIN

The brain begins to develop in the third week when the neural plate and tube are developing from neuroectoderm (see Fig. 16.1). The neural tube, cranial to the fourth pair of somites, develops into the brain. Neural progenitor cells proliferate, migrate, and differentiate to form specific areas of the brain. Even before the neural folds are completely fused, three distinct **primary brain vesicles** are recognizable in the rostral end of the developing neural tube (Fig. 16.13). From rostral to caudal,

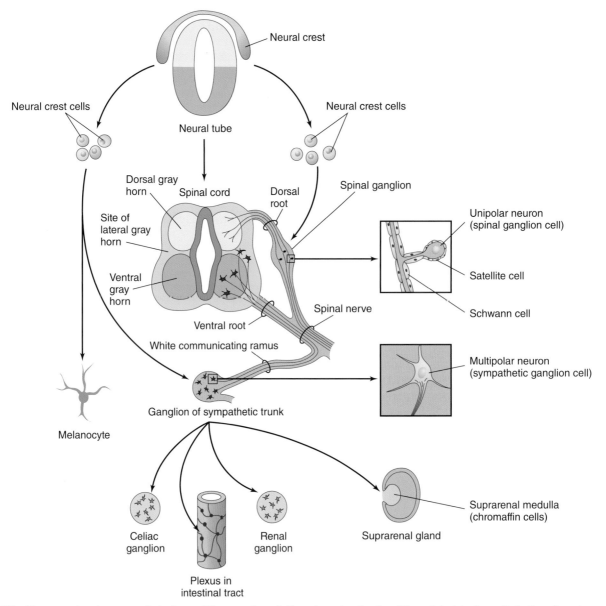

Fig. 16.7 Diagrams showing some derivatives of the neural crest. Neural crest cells also differentiate into the cells in the afferent ganglia of cranial nerves and many other structures. The formation of a spinal nerve is also shown.

these primary brain vesicles form the **forebrain** (prosencephalon), **midbrain** (mesencephalon), and **hindbrain** (rhombencephalon).

During the fifth week, the forebrain partly divides into two **secondary brain vesicles**—the **telencephalon** and **diencephalon**; the midbrain does not divide. The hindbrain partly divides into two vesicles, the **metencephalon** and **myelencephalon**. Consequently, there are five secondary brain vesicles. The development of the brain is closely involved with the surrounding meninges. *Lineage tracing studies show that the meninges of the forebrain are derived from neural crest cells, and that the midbrain and hindbrain meninges originate from both neural crest and mesodermal cells. The transcription factor FoxC1, which has been detected in all three layers of the meninges, appears to play a critical role in their formation.*

BRAIN FLEXURES

The embryonic brain grows rapidly during the fourth week and bends ventrally with the head fold. The bending produces the **midbrain flexure** in the midbrain region and the **cervical flexure** at the junction of the hindbrain and spinal cord (Fig. 16.14A). *A constriction-isthmic organizer is formed between the midbrain and hindbrain, which functions as a signaling center. Wnt, Fgl, and retinoic acid expression, which occur in this region, have been implicated in the morphogenesis and patterning of the adjoining between the midbrain and hindbrain.* Later, unequal growth of these flexures produces the **pontine flexure** in the opposite direction. This flexure results in the thinning of the roof of the hindbrain (see Fig. 16.14C). The **sulcus limitans** extends cranially to the junction of the

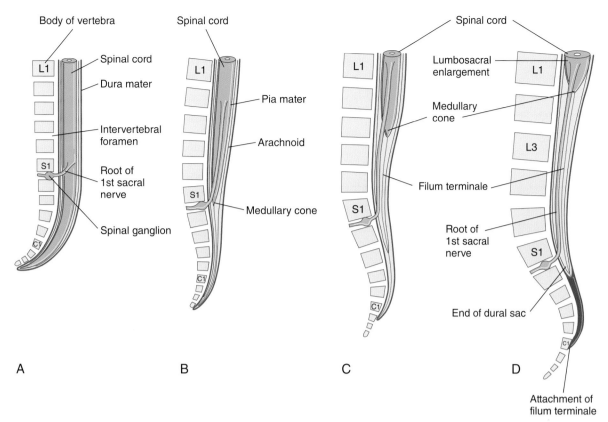

Fig. 16.8 Diagrams showing the position of the caudal end of the spinal cord in relation to the vertebral column and meninges at various stages of development. The increasing inclination of the root of the first sacral nerve is also shown. (A) At 8 weeks. (B) At 24 weeks. (C) Neonate. (D) Adult.

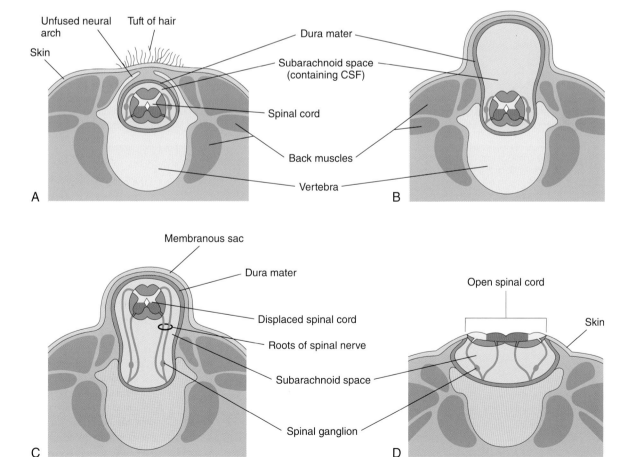

Fig. 16.9 Diagrammatic sketches illustrating various types of spina bifida and the associated defects of the vertebral arches. (A) Spina bifida occulta. Observe the unfused vertebral arch. (B) Spina bifida with meningocele. (C) Spina bifida with meningomyelocele. (D) Spina bifida with myeloschisis. The types shown in (B–D) are referred to collectively as *spina bifida cystica* because of the cyst-like sac that is associated with them. *CSF*, Cerebrospinal fluid.

midbrain and forebrain, and the alar and basal plates are recognizable only in the midbrain and the hindbrain (see Fig. 16.14C).

HINDBRAIN

The **cervical flexure** demarcates the hindbrain from the spinal cord (see Fig. 16.14A). The **pontine flexure** divides the hindbrain into caudal (myelencephalon) and rostral (metencephalon) parts. The myelencephalon becomes the **medulla oblongata**, whereas the metencephalon becomes the **pons** and **cerebellum**. The cavity of the hindbrain becomes the **fourth ventricle** and the **central canal** in the medulla (see Fig. 16.14B and C).

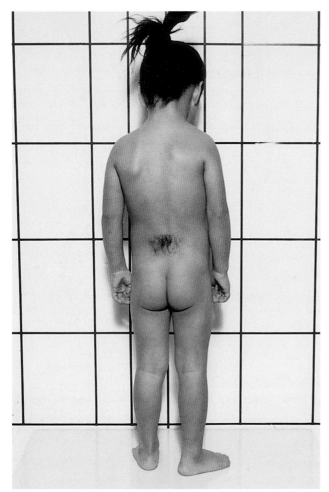

Fig. 16.10 A female child with a tuft of hair covering a small dimple (spinal defect) in the lumbosacral region, indicating the site of a spina bifida occulta. *Courtesy A.E. Chudley, MD, Section of Genetics and Metabolism, Department of Pediatrics and Child Health, Children's Hospital and University of Manitoba, Winnipeg, Manitoba, Canada.*

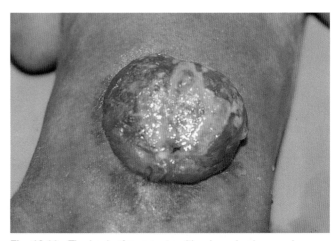

Fig. 16.11 The back of a neonate with a large lumbar meningomyelocele. The neural tube defect is covered with a thin membrane. *Courtesy A.E. Chudley, MD, Section of Genetics and Metabolism, Department of Pediatrics and Child Health, Children's Hospital and University of Manitoba, Winnipeg, Manitoba, Canada.*

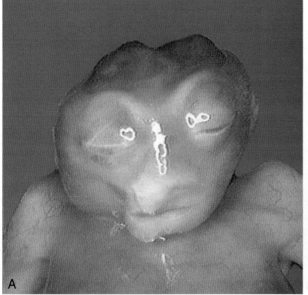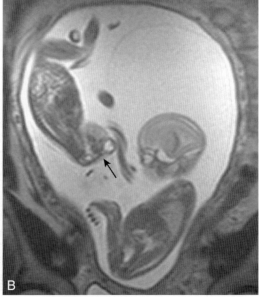

Fig. 16.12 (A) A fetus with meroencephaly. (B) Magnetic resonance image of diamniotic-monochorionic twins, one with meroencephaly. Note the absent calvaria of the abnormal twin *(arrow)* and the amnion of the normal twin. A, *Courtesy Wesley Lee, MD, Division of Fetal Imaging, Department of Obstetrics and Gynecology, William Beaumont Hospital, Royal Oak, Michigan;* B, *Courtesy Deborah Levine, MD, Director of Obstetric and Gynecologic Ultrasound, Beth Israel Deaconess Medical Center, Boston, Massachusetts.*

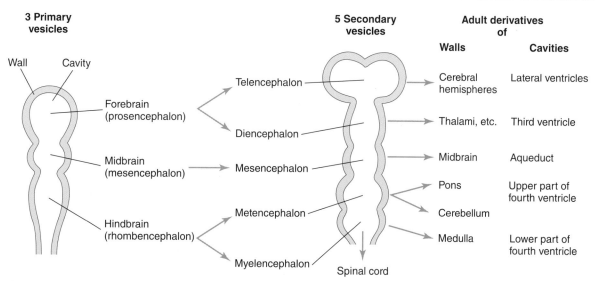

Fig. 16.13 Diagrammatic sketches of the brain vesicles indicating the adult derivatives of their walls and cavities. The rostral part of the third ventricle forms from the cavity of the telencephalon; most of this ventricle is derived from the cavity of the diencephalon.

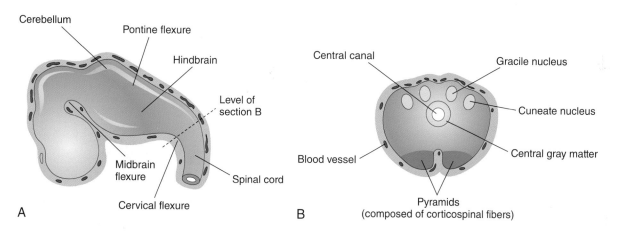

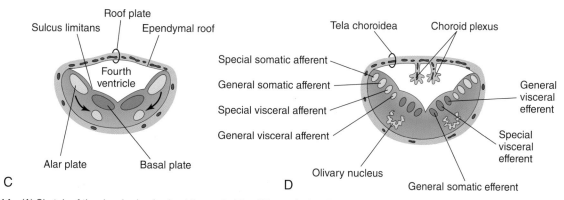

Fig. 16.14 (A) Sketch of the developing brain at the end of the fifth week showing the three primary divisions of the brain and the brain flexures. (B) Transverse section of the caudal part of the myelencephalon (developing closed part of the medulla). (C and D) Similar sections of the rostral part of the myelencephalon (developing open part of the medulla) showing the position and successive stages of differentiation of the alar and basal plates. The *arrows* in (C) show the pathway taken by the neuroblasts from the alar plates to form the olivary nuclei.

MYELENCEPHALON

Neuroblasts from the alar plates in the myelencephalon migrate into the marginal zone and form isolated areas of gray matter: the **gracile nuclei** medially and the **cuneate nuclei** laterally (see Fig. 16.14B). These nuclei are associated with correspondingly named nerve tracts that enter the medulla from the spinal cord. The ventral area of the medulla contains a pair of fiber bundles—**pyramids**—that consist of corticospinal fibers descending from the developing cerebral cortex (see Fig. 16.14B).

The rostral part of the **myelencephalon** is wide and rather flat, especially opposite to the pontine flexure (see Fig. 16.14C and D). As the pontine flexure forms, the walls of the medulla move laterally, and the alar plates come to lie lateral to the basal plates (see Fig. 16.14C). As the positions of the plates change, the motor nuclei generally develop medial to the sensory nuclei.

Neuroblasts in the basal plates of the medulla, like those in the spinal cord, develop into **motor neurons**. The neuroblasts form nuclei groups of nerve cells (nuclei) and organize into three cell columns on each side (see Fig. 16.14D). From medial to lateral, they are as follows:

- The **general somatic efferent**, represented by neurons of the hypoglossal nerve
- The **special visceral efferent**, represented by neurons innervating muscles derived from the pharyngeal arches (see Chapter 10)
- The **general visceral efferent**, represented by some neurons of the vagus and the glossopharyngeal nerves.

Neuroblasts in the alar plates of the medulla form neurons that are arranged in four columns on each side (see Fig. 16.14D). From medial to lateral, the columns are as follows:

- The **general visceral afferent**, receiving impulses from the viscera
- The **special visceral afferent**, receiving taste fibers
- The **general somatic afferent**, receiving impulses from the surface of the head
- The **special somatic afferent**, receiving impulses from the ear.

Some neuroblasts from the alar plates migrate ventrally and form neurons in the **olivary nuclei** (see Fig. 16.14C and D).

METENCEPHALON

The walls of the metencephalon form the pons and cerebellum, and the cavity of the metencephalon forms the superior part of the fourth ventricle (Fig. 16.15A). As in the rostral part of the myelencephalon, the pontine flexure causes divergence of the lateral walls of the pons, which spreads the gray matter on the floor of the fourth ventricle (see Fig. 16.15B).

The cerebellum develops from the dorsal parts of the alar plates (see Fig. 16.15A and B). Initially, the **cerebellar swellings** project into the fourth ventricle (see Fig. 16.15B).

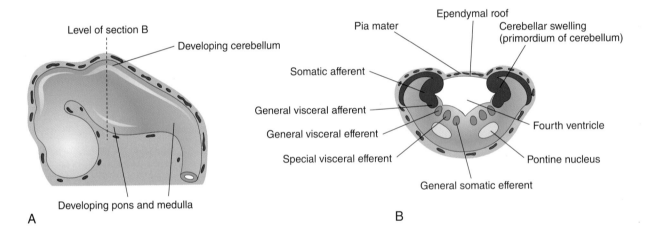

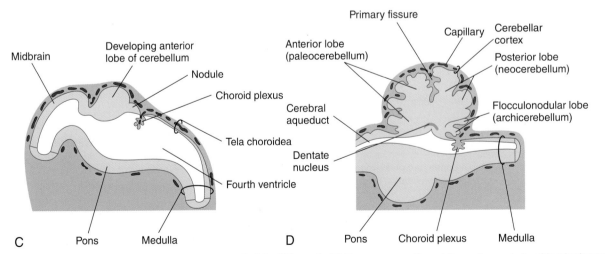

Fig. 16.15 (A) Sketch of the developing brain at the end of the fifth week. (B) Transverse section of the metencephalon (developing pons and cerebellum) showing the derivatives of the alar and basal plates. (C and D) Sagittal sections of the hindbrain at 6 and 17 weeks, respectively, showing successive stages in the development of the pons and cerebellum.

As the swellings enlarge and fuse in the median plane, they overgrow the rostral half of the fourth ventricle and overlap the pons and medulla (see Fig. 16.15D). Some neuroblasts in the intermediate zone of the alar plates migrate to the marginal zone and differentiate into the neurons of the **cerebellar cortex**. Other neuroblasts from these plates give rise to the **central nuclei**, the largest of which is the **dentate nucleus** (see Fig. 16.15D). Cells from the alar plates also give rise to the **pontine nuclei**, the cochlear and vestibular nuclei, and the sensory nuclei of the trigeminal nerve. *The paired box transcription factor Pax6 plays an essential role in the development of the cerebellum.*

Nerve fibers connecting the cerebral and cerebellar cortices with the spinal cord pass through the marginal layer of the ventral region of the metencephalon. This region of the brainstem is the pons, where a robust band of nerve fibers crosses the median plane (see Fig. 16.15C and D).

CHOROID PLEXUSES AND CEREBROSPINAL FLUID

The thin ependymal roof of the fourth ventricle is covered externally by pia mater. This vascular membrane, together with the ependymal roof, forms the **tela choroidea** of the fourth ventricle (see Fig. 16.15C and D). Because of the active proliferation of the pia mater, the tela choroidea invaginates the fourth ventricle, where it differentiates into the **choroid plexus**, infoldings of the choroidal arteries of the pia mater (see Figs. 16.14C and 16.15C and D). Similar choroid plexuses develop in the roof of the third ventricle and in the medial walls of the lateral ventricles.

The choroid plexuses secrete ventricular fluid, which becomes CSF. Various signaling morphogens present in the CSF and choroid plexus are necessary for the development of the brain. The thin roof of the fourth ventricle evaginates in three locations. These outpouchings rupture to form openings, the **median and lateral apertures**. These apertures permit CSF to enter the **subarachnoid space** from the fourth ventricle. Studies have shown that specific neurogenic molecules, such as retinoic acid, control the proliferation and differentiation of neuroprogenitor cells. Thus the epithelium lining the choroid plexus is derived from neuroepithelium (see Fig. 16.5), but the stroma develops from mesenchymal cells.

MIDBRAIN

The midbrain (mesencephalon) undergoes less change than most other parts of the developing brain. The neural canal narrows and becomes the **cerebral aqueduct** (see Fig. 16.15D), a canal that connects the third and fourth ventricles. Neuroblasts migrate from the alar plates of the midbrain into the **tectum**, where they aggregate to form four large groups of neurons—the paired **superior and inferior colliculi** (Fig. 16.16B), which are concerned with visual and auditory reflexes, respectively. Neuroblasts from the basal plates appear to give rise to groups of neurons in the **tegmentum of the midbrain** (red nuclei, nuclei of the third and fourth cranial nerves, and reticular nuclei). The **substantia nigra**, a broad layer of gray matter adjacent to the cerebral peduncle (see Fig. 16.16D and E), may also differentiate from the basal plate, but some authorities believe that it is derived from cells in the alar plate that migrate ventrally.

Fibers growing from the cerebrum form the **cerebral peduncles** anteriorly (see Fig. 16.16B). These peduncles become progressively more prominent as additional descending fiber groups (corticopontine, corticobulbar, and corticospinal) pass through the developing midbrain on their way to the brainstem and spinal cord.

FOREBRAIN

As closure of the rostral neuropore occurs, two lateral outgrowths—**optic vesicles**—appear (see Fig. 16.3A), one on each side of the forebrain. The optic vesicles are the primordia of the retinas and optic nerves (see Chapter 17). A second pair of diverticula soon arises more dorsally and rostrally, representing the **telencephalic vesicles** (see Fig. 16.16C). They are the primordia of the cerebral hemispheres, and their cavities become the **lateral ventricles** (see Fig. 16.19B).

The rostral (anterior) part of the forebrain, including the primordia of the cerebral hemispheres, is the telencephalon; the caudal (posterior) part of the forebrain is the diencephalon. The cavities of the telencephalon and diencephalon contribute to the formation of the **third ventricle** (Fig. 16.17D and E).

DIENCEPHALON

Three swellings develop in the lateral walls of the third ventricle, which later become the **thalamus, hypothalamus**, and **epithalamus** (see Fig. 16.17C–E). The thalamus develops rapidly on each side and bulges into the cavity of the third ventricle, eventually reducing it to a narrow cleft. The hypothalamus arises by the proliferation of neuroblasts in the intermediate zone of the diencephalic walls. A pair of nuclei, the **mammillary bodies**, form pea-sized swellings on the ventral surface of the hypothalamus (see Fig. 16.17C).

The epithalamus develops from the roof and dorsal part of the lateral wall of the diencephalon. Initially, the epithalamic swellings are large, but later they become relatively small (see Fig. 16.17C–E).

The **pineal gland** (pineal body) develops as a median diverticulum of the caudal part of the roof of the diencephalon (see Fig. 16.17D). Proliferation of the cells in its walls soon converts it into a solid, cone-shaped gland.

The **pituitary gland** (hypophysis) is ectodermal in origin (Fig. 16.18 and Table 16.1). It develops from two sources:

- An upgrowth from the ectodermal roof of the stomodeum—the **hypophyseal diverticulum (Rathke pouch)**
- A downgrowth from the neuroectoderm of the diencephalon—the **neurohypophyseal diverticulum**.

This double embryonic origin of the pituitary gland explains why it is composed of two different types of tissue:

- The **adenohypophysis** (glandular part), or anterior lobe, arises from the oral ectoderm.
- The **neurohypophysis** (nervous part), or posterior lobe, arises from the neuroectoderm.

During the third week, a hypophyseal diverticulum projects from the roof of the stomodeum (primordial oral cavity) and lies adjacent to the floor (ventral wall) of the diencephalon (see Fig. 16.18A and B). By the fifth week, this diverticulum has elongated and constricted at its attachment to

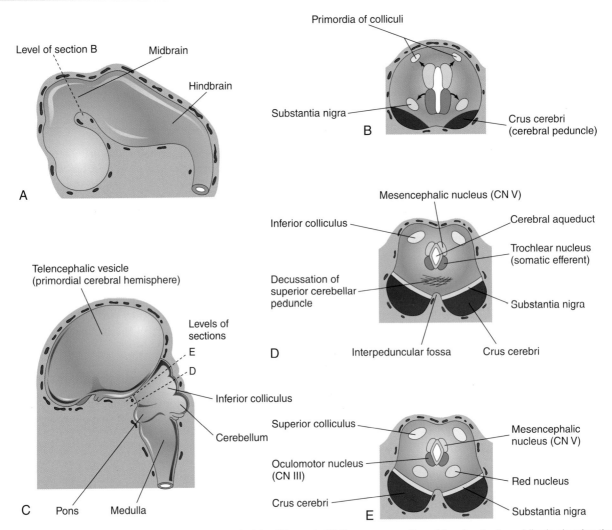

Fig. 16.16   (A) Sketch of the developing brain at the end of the fifth week. (B) Transverse section of the developing midbrain showing the early migration of cells from the basal and alar plates. (C) Sketch of the developing brain at 11 weeks. (D and E) Transverse sections of the developing midbrain at the level of the inferior and superior colliculi, respectively. *CN,* Cranial nerve.

the oral epithelium, giving it a nipple-like appearance (see Fig. 16.18C). By this stage, it has come into contact with the **infundibulum** (derived from the neurohypophyseal diverticulum), a ventral downgrowth of the diencephalon (see Figs. 16.17C and D and 16.18). The stalk of the hypophyseal diverticulum gradually regresses (see Fig. 16.18C–E). The parts of the pituitary gland that develop from the ectoderm of the stomodeum—**pars anterior**, **pars intermedia**, and **pars tuberalis**—form the adenohypophysis (see Table 16.1).

Cells of the anterior wall of the hypophyseal diverticulum proliferate and give rise to the **pars anterior of the pituitary gland**. Later, an extension, the **pars tuberalis**, grows around the **infundibular stem** (see Fig. 16.18F). The extensive proliferation of the anterior wall of the hypophyseal diverticulum reduces its lumen to a narrow cleft (see Fig. 16.18E). Cells in the posterior wall of the hypophyseal diverticulum do not proliferate; they give rise to the thin, poorly defined **pars intermedia** (see Fig. 16.18F). The part of the pituitary gland that develops from the neuroectoderm of the brain (infundibulum) is the neurohypophysis (see Fig. 16.18B–F and Table 16.1). The infundibulum gives rise to the **median eminence, infundibular stem, and pars nervosa**.

Ephrin-β2 and other signaling molecules (e.g., FGF8, BMP4, and WNT5A) from the diencephalon area play an essential role in the formation of the anterior and intermediate lobes of the pituitary gland. The LIM homeobox gene LHX2 appears to control the development of the posterior lobe.

TELENCEPHALON

The telencephalon consists of a median part and two lateral diverticula, the **cerebral vesicles** (Figs. 16.16C and 16.18A). These vesicles are the primordia of the **cerebral hemispheres**, which are identifiable at 7 weeks (Fig. 16.19A). The cavity of the median part of the telencephalon forms the extreme anterior part of the third ventricle. At first, the cerebral hemispheres are in wide communication with the cavity of the third ventricle through the **interventricular foramina** (see Fig. 16.19B). As the cerebral hemispheres expand, they successively cover the diencephalon, midbrain, and hindbrain. The hemispheres eventually meet each other in the midline, flattening their medial surfaces.

The **corpus striatum** appears during the sixth week as a prominent swelling on the floor of each cerebral hemisphere (Fig. 16.20B). The floor of each hemisphere expands

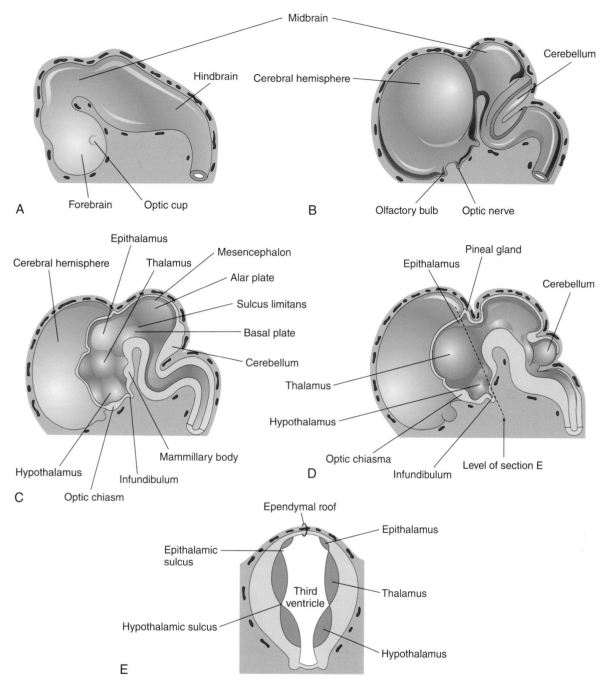

Fig. 16.17 (A) External view of the brain at the end of the fifth week. (B) Similar view at 7 weeks. (C) Median section of this brain showing the medial surface of the forebrain and midbrain. (D) Similar section at 8 weeks. (E) Transverse section of the diencephalon showing the epithalamus dorsally, the thalamus laterally, and the hypothalamus ventrally.

more slowly than its thin cortical walls because it contains the rather large corpus striatum; consequently, the cerebral hemispheres become C-shaped (Fig. 16.21).

The growth and curvature of the hemispheres also affect the shape of the lateral ventricles. They become roughly C-shaped cavities filled with CSF. The caudal end of each cerebral hemisphere turns ventrally and then rostrally, forming the **temporal lobe**; in so doing, it carries with it the ventricle (forming the **temporal horn**) and the choroid fissure (see Fig. 16.21). Here, the thin medial wall of the hemisphere is invaginated along the **choroid fissure**

by the vascular pia mater to form the choroid plexus of the temporal horn of the lateral ventricle (see Figs. 16.20B and 16.21B).

As the cerebral cortex differentiates, fibers passing to and from it pass through the **corpus striatum** and divide it into the **caudate and lentiform nuclei**. This fiber pathway—the **internal capsule** (see Fig. 16.20C)—becomes C-shaped as the hemisphere assumes this form. The **caudate nucleus** becomes elongated and C-shaped, conforming to the outline of the lateral ventricle (see Fig. 16.21A–C). Its pear-shaped head and elongated body lie on the floor of the frontal

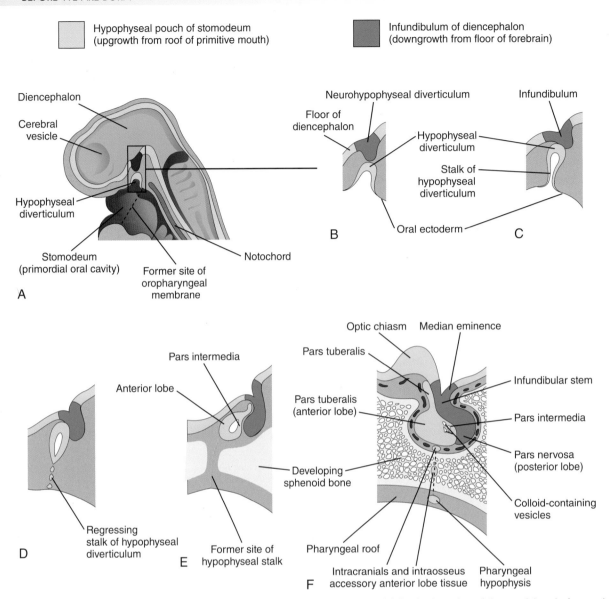

Fig. 16.18 Diagrammatic sketches illustrating the development of the pituitary gland. (A) Sagittal section of the cranial end of an embryo at approximately 36 days showing the hypophyseal diverticulum, an upgrowth from the stomodeum, and the neurohypophyseal diverticulum, a downgrowth from the forebrain. (B–D) Successive stages of the developing pituitary gland. By 8 weeks, the diverticulum loses its connection with the oral cavity and is in close contact with the infundibulum and posterior lobe (neurohypophysis) of the pituitary gland. (E and F) Later stages showing the proliferation of the anterior wall of the hypophyseal diverticulum to form the anterior lobe (adenohypophysis) of the pituitary gland.

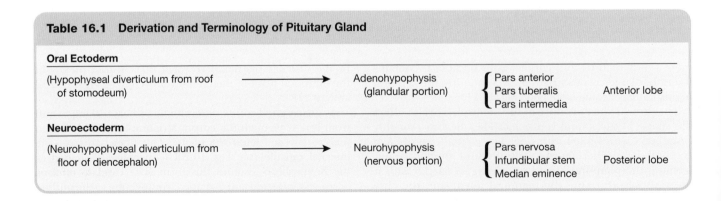

Table 16.1 Derivation and Terminology of Pituitary Gland

Oral Ectoderm

(Hypophyseal diverticulum from roof of stomodeum) → Adenohypophysis (glandular portion) — Pars anterior, Pars tuberalis, Pars intermedia — Anterior lobe

Neuroectoderm

(Neurohypophyseal diverticulum from floor of diencephalon) → Neurohypophysis (nervous portion) — Pars nervosa, Infundibular stem, Median eminence — Posterior lobe

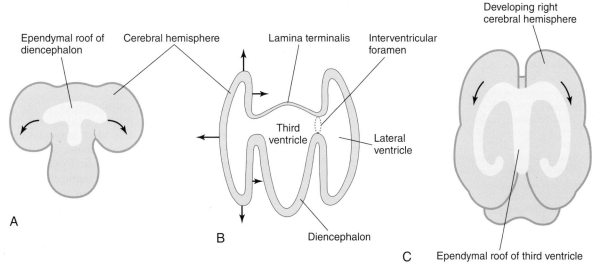

Fig. 16.19 (A) Sketch of the dorsal surface of the forebrain indicating how the ependymal roof of the diencephalon is carried out to the dorso-medial surface of the cerebral hemispheres. (B) Diagrammatic section of the forebrain showing how the developing cerebral hemispheres grow from the lateral walls of the forebrain and expand in all directions until they cover the diencephalon. The rostral wall of the forebrain, the lamina terminalis, is very thin. (C) Sketch of the forebrain showing how the ependymal roof is finally carried into the temporal lobes as a result of the C-shaped growth pattern of the cerebral hemispheres. The *arrows* indicate some of the directions in which the hemispheres expand.

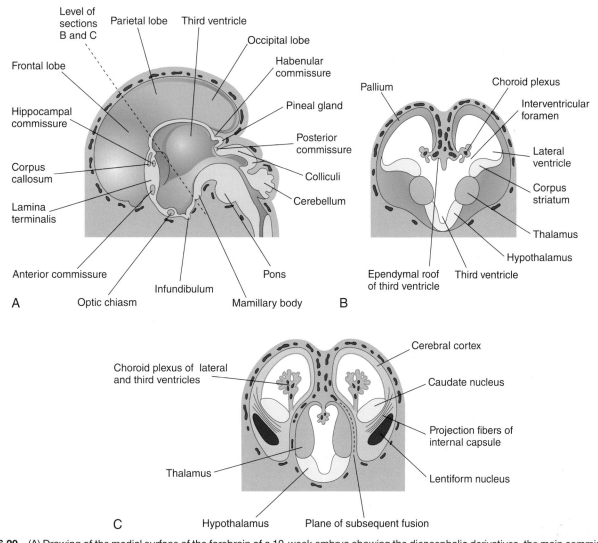

Fig. 16.20 (A) Drawing of the medial surface of the forebrain of a 10-week embryo showing the diencephalic derivatives, the main commissures, and the expanding cerebral hemispheres. (B) Transverse section of the forebrain at the level of the interventricular foramina showing the corpus striatum and choroid plexuses of the lateral ventricles. (C) Similar section at approximately 11 weeks showing division of the corpus striatum into the caudate and lentiform nuclei by the internal capsule. The developing relationship of the cerebral hemispheres to the diencephalon is also illustrated.

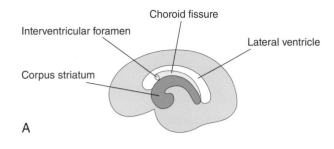

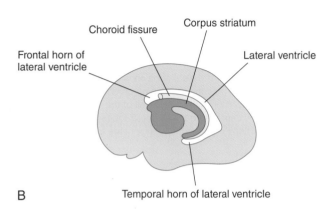

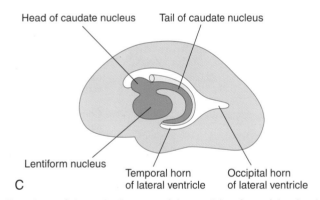

Fig. 16.21 Schematic diagrams of the medial surface of the developing right cerebral hemisphere, showing the development of the lateral ventricle, choroid fissure, and corpus striatum. (A) At 13 weeks. (B) At 21 weeks. (C) At 32 weeks.

horn and the body of the lateral ventricle; its tail makes a U-shaped turn to gain the roof of the temporal horn.

CEREBRAL COMMISSURES

Groups of nerve fibers—**commissures**—connect corresponding areas of the cerebral hemispheres with one another (see Fig. 16.20A). The most important of these commissures crosses the **lamina terminalis**, the rostral (anterior) end of the forebrain. This lamina extends from the roof plate of the diencephalon to the **optic chiasm** (decussation or crossing of the fibers of the optic nerve).

The **anterior commissure** connects the olfactory bulb and related brain areas of one hemisphere with those of the opposite side. The **hippocampal commissure** connects the hippocampal formations. The **corpus callosum**, the largest cerebral commissure, connects the neocortical areas (see Fig. 16.20A). At birth, the corpus callosum extends over the roof of the diencephalon. The rest of the **lamina terminalis** forms the **septum pellucidum**, a thin plate of brain tissue.

The **optic chiasm**, which develops in the ventral part of the lamina terminalis (see Fig. 16.20A), consists of fibers from the medial halves of the retinae, which cross to join the optic tract of the opposite side.

Initially, the surface of the hemispheres is smooth (Fig. 16.22); however, as growth proceeds, **sulci** (grooves between the gyri) and **gyri** (tortuous convolutions) develop (see Fig. 16.22). The sulci and gyri permit a considerable increase in the surface area of the cerebral cortex without requiring an extensive increase in cranial size. At its peak, neurogenesis adds approximately 1,000,000 cells per minute with new synaptic connections occurring at approximately 40,000 per minute. As each cerebral hemisphere grows, the cortex covering the external surface of the corpus striatum grows relatively slowly and is soon overgrown. This buried cortex, hidden from view in the depths of the **lateral sulcus** (fissure) of the cerebral hemisphere, is the **insula** (island).

CONGENITAL ANOMALIES OF BRAIN

Defects of the brain are common—approximately 3 per 1000 births. The most major birth defects, such as meroencephaly and meningoencephalocele, result from the defective closure of the rostral neuropore (**NTDs**) during

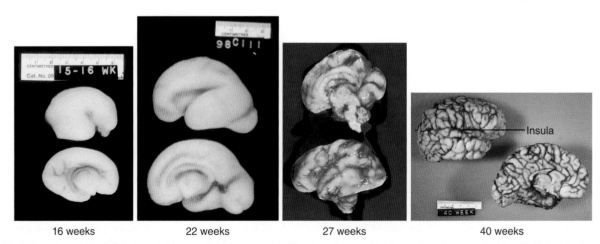

Fig. 16.22 Lateral and medial surfaces of human fetal brains at 16, 22, 27, and 40 weeks' gestation. Courtesy Dr. Marc R. Del Bigio, Department of Pathology [Neuropathology], University of Manitoba and Health Sciences Centre, Winnipeg, Manitoba, Canada.

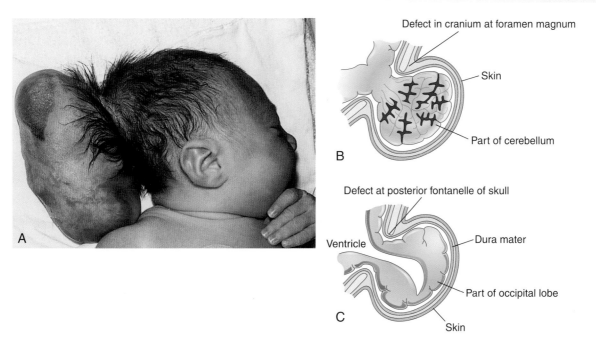

Labels in figure: Defect in cranium at foramen magnum; Skin; Part of cerebellum; B; Defect at posterior fontanelle of skull; Ventricle; Dura mater; Part of occipital lobe; C; Skin

Fig. 16.23 Cranium bifidum (bony defect of cranium) and herniation of the brain and meninges. (A) Infant with a large meningoencephalocele in the occipital area. (B) Meningoencephalocele, consisting of a protrusion of part of the cerebellum that is covered by meninges and skin. (C) Meningohydroencephalocele, consisting of a protrusion of part of the occipital lobe that contains part of the posterior horn of a lateral ventricle. A, Courtesy A.E. Chudley, MD, Section of Genetics and Metabolism, Department of Pediatrics and Child Health, Children's Hospital and University of Manitoba, Winnipeg, Manitoba, Canada.

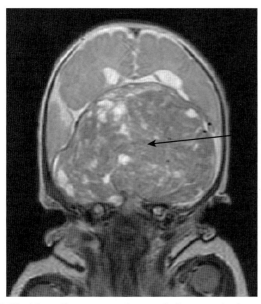

Fig. 16.24 Magnetic resonance image of a large craniopharyngioma *(arrow).* Courtesy Dr. R. Shane Tubbs and Dr. W Jerry Oakes, Children's Hospital, Birmingham, Alabama.

Pharyngeal Hypophysis and Craniopharyngioma

A remnant of the stalk of the hypophyseal diverticulum may persist and form a **pharyngeal hypophysis** in the roof of the oropharynx (see Fig. 16.18E and F). Occasionally, very rare (1:1,000,000) benign tumors—**craniopharyngiomas**, formed from remnants of the stalk—develop in the pharynx or the basisphenoid (posterior part of sphenoid bone), but most often, they form in and/or superior to the sella turcica of the cranium (see Fig. 16.24).

Cranium Bifidum

Defects in the formation of the cranium (skull)—**cranium bifidum**—are often associated with birth defects of the brain, meninges, or both. Defects of the cranium usually involve the median plane of the calvaria. The defect is often in the squamous part of the occipital bone and may include the posterior part of the foramen magnum. When the defect is small, usually only the meninges herniate and the defect is **cranial meningocele**. Cranium bifidum associated with herniation of the brain, meninges, or both occurs in approximately 1 in 2000 births. When the cranial defect is large, the meninges and part of the brain herniate, forming a **meningoencephalocele** (see Fig. 16.23A and B). If the protruding brain contains part of the ventricular system, the defect is a **meningohydroencephalocele** (see Fig. 16.23C).

the fourth week of development (Fig. 16.23A) and involve the overlying tissues (meninges and calvaria). Magnetic resonance imaging (MRI) is often used for evaluation of the fetal brain in pregnancies at risk for fetal defects (Fig. 16.24). The factors causing NTDs are genetic, nutritional, and/or environmental in nature.

Meroencephaly

Meroencephaly is a severe birth defect of the calvaria that results from the failure of the rostral neuropore to close during the fourth week (see Fig. 16.12). As a result, the forebrain, midbrain, most of the hindbrain, and the calvaria are absent. **Meroencephaly** occurs at least once in every 1000 births, and it is two to four times more common in females than in males. Meroencephaly is associated with a multifactorial pattern of inheritance.

Microcephaly

In microcephaly, the calvaria and brain are small, but the face is of normal size. Affected infants usually have cognitive deficits because the cranium and brain are underdeveloped. Microcephaly is the result of altered neurogenesis and a reduction in brain growth. Some cases of **microcephaly** appear to be genetic (autosomal recessive); others are caused by environmental factors such as cytomegalovirus infection in utero (see Chapter 19). Exposure during the fetal period to infectious agents and certain drugs is a contributing factor in some cases.

Hydrocephalus

An infant with hydrocephalus has a significant enlargement of the head, but the face is of normal size. This defect may be associated with cognitive deficits. Hydrocephalus results from impaired circulation and absorption of CSF or, in unusual cases, from increased production of CSF. An excess of CSF is present in the ventricular system of the brain (Fig. 16.25). Impaired circulation of CSF often results from **congenital aqueductal stenosis** (narrow cerebral aqueduct). Blockage of CSF circulation results in dilation of the ventricles proximal to the obstruction and increased pressure on the cerebral hemispheres. This squeezes the brain between the ventricular fluid and calvaria. In infants, the internal pressure results in an accelerated rate of expansion of the brain and calvaria because the fibrous sutures of the calvaria are not fused.

Chiari Malformation

Chiari malformation (CM) is a structural defect of the cerebellum. It is characterized by a tongue-like projection of the medulla and inferior displacement of the cerebellar tonsil through the foramen magnum into the vertebral canal. The posterior cranial fossa is usually abnormally small, thus causing pressure on the cerebellum and brainstem. This condition may lead to a type of noncommunicating hydrocephalus that obstructs the absorption and flow of CSF; as a result, the entire ventricular system is distended. CM can be diagnosed by MRI and, as a result, more cases are detected than in the past.

Several types of CM have been described. In **Type I**, the inferior part of the cerebellum herniates through the foramen magnum. This is the most commonly occurring form, is usually asymptomatic, and is often detected in adolescence or adulthood. In **Type II**, also known as Arnold–Chiari malformation, there is herniation of cerebellar tissue and of the brainstem into the foramen magnum, often accompanied by occipital encephalocele and lumbar myelomeningocele (Fig. 16.26). In **Type III**, a severe and rare form, there is herniation of both the cerebellum and brainstem through the foramen magnum into the vertebral column, with severe neurological consequences. In **Type IV**, the most severe form, the cerebellum is either absent or underdeveloped—these infants do not survive.

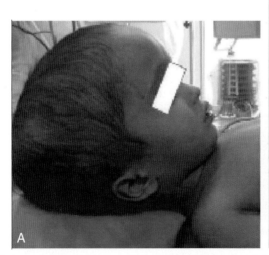
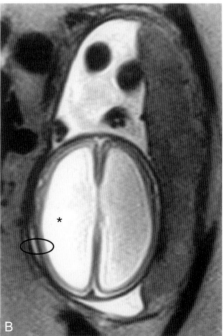

Fig. 16.25   (A) Hydrocephalus with increased head circumference in an infant. (B) Axial magnetic resonance image (transverse section through the brain) of a fetus with X-linked hydrocephalus at approximately 29 weeks' gestation, showing the massively enlarged ventricles *(*)* and thinned cortex *(oval)*. From Rath GP: Pediatric neuroanesthesia. In Prabhakar H, editor: *Essentials of neuroanesthesia,* ed 1, 2017, Academic Press Elsevier, pp 629–641; Courtesy Dr. E.H. Whitby, Magnetic Resonance Imaging Unit, University of Sheffield, United Kingdom.

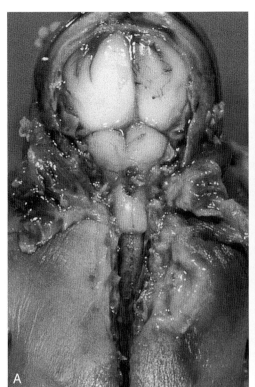
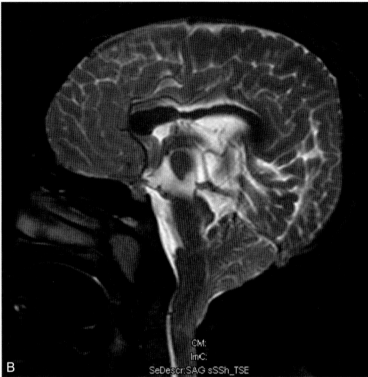

Fig. 16.26 (A) Arnold–Chiari type II malformation in a 23-week fetus. In situ exposure of the hindbrain shows cerebellar tissue well below the level of the foramen magnum *(arrow)*. (B) Midsagittal, T2-weighted MRI of an adolescent with myelomeningocele. By definition, these patients also have a Chiari II malformation as shown here. Note the caudal descent of the cerebellar vermis and brainstem through the foramen magnum. *Courtesy A, Dr. Marc R. Del Bigio, Department of Pathology [Neuropathology], University of Manitoba and Health Sciences Centre, Winnipeg, Manitoba, Canada; B, Courtesy Dr. R. Shane Tubbs, Professor, Chief Scientific Officer and Vice President, Seattle Science Foundation, Washington.*

DEVELOPMENT OF PERIPHERAL NERVOUS SYSTEM

The PNS consists of cranial, spinal, and visceral nerves and cranial, spinal, and autonomic ganglia. All sensory cells (somatic and visceral) of the PNS are derived from neural crest cells. The cell bodies of these sensory cells are located outside the CNS. The cell body of each afferent neuron is closely invested by a capsule of modified Schwann cells—**satellite cells** (see Fig. 16.7), which are derived from neural crest cells. This capsule is continuous with the **neurolemmal sheath of Schwann cells** that surround the axons of afferent neurons.

Neural crest cells in the developing brain migrate to form sensory ganglia only in relation to the trigeminal (CN V), facial (CN VII), vestibulocochlear (CN VIII), glossopharyngeal (CN IX), and vagus (CN X) nerves. Neural crest cells also differentiate into multipolar neurons of the **autonomic ganglia** (see Fig. 16.7), including ganglia of the sympathetic trunks that lie along the sides of the vertebral bodies; collateral, or prevertebral, ganglia in the plexuses of the thorax and abdomen (e.g., cardiac, celiac, and mesenteric plexuses); and parasympathetic, or terminal, ganglia in or near the viscera (e.g., submucosal, or Meissner, plexus).

Cells of the paraganglia—**chromaffin cells**—are also derived from the neural crest. The term **paraganglia** includes several widely scattered groups of cells that are similar in many ways to the medullary cells of the suprarenal glands. The cell groups largely lie retroperitoneally, often in

association with sympathetic ganglia. The **carotid and aortic bodies** also have small islands of chromaffin cells associated with them. These widely scattered groups of chromaffin cells constitute the **chromaffin system**.

SPINAL NERVES

Motor nerve fibers arising from the spinal cord begin to appear at the end of the fourth week (see Fig. 16.4). The nerve fibers arise from cells in the **basal plates** of the developing spinal cord and emerge as a continuous series of rootlets along its ventrolateral surface. The fibers destined for a particular developing muscle group become arranged in a bundle, forming a **ventral nerve root** (see Figs. 16.6 and 16.7). The nerve fibers of the **dorsal nerve root** are derived from neural crest cells that migrate to the dorsolateral aspect of the spinal cord, where they differentiate into the cells of the **spinal ganglion** (see Fig. 16.7).

The central processes of the neurons in the spinal ganglion form a single bundle that grows into the spinal cord, opposite to the apex of the dorsal horn of gray matter (see Fig. 16.4B and C). The distal processes of the spinal ganglion cells grow toward the ventral nerve root and eventually join it to form a **spinal nerve** (see Fig. 16.7).

As the limb buds develop, the nerves from the spinal cord segments opposite to them elongate and grow into the limbs. The nerve fibers are distributed to their muscles, which differentiate from myogenic cells that originate from the somites (see Chapter 15). The skin of the developing limbs is also innervated in a segmental manner.

CRANIAL NERVES

Twelve pairs of cranial nerves form during the fifth and sixth weeks. They are classified into three groups according to their embryological origins.

SOMATIC EFFERENT CRANIAL NERVES

The **trochlear** (CN IV), **abducent** (CN VI), **hypoglossal** (CN XII), and the greater part of the **oculomotor** (CN III) nerves are homologous with the ventral roots of the spinal nerves (Fig. 16.27A). The cells of origin of these nerves are located in the **somatic efferent column** (derived from the basal plates) of the brainstem. Their axons are distributed to the muscles derived from the head myotomes (preotic and occipital) (see Fig. 16.17A).

CN IV arises from nerve cells in the somatic efferent column in the posterior part of the midbrain. Although a motor nerve, CN IV emerges from the brainstem dorsally and passes ventrally to supply the superior oblique muscle of the eye.

CN VI arises from nerve cells in the basal plates of the metencephalon. It passes from its ventral surface to the posterior of the three preotic myotomes from which the lateral rectus muscle of the eye is thought to originate.

CN XII develops by fusion of the ventral root fibers of three or four occipital nerves (see Fig. 16.27A). Sensory roots, corresponding to the dorsal roots of the spinal nerves, are absent. The somatic motor fibers originate from the **hypoglossal nucleus**. These fibers leave the ventrolateral wall of the medulla in several groups—hypoglossal nerve roots—which converge to form the common trunk of CN XII (see Fig. 16.27B). They grow rostrally and eventually innervate the muscles of the tongue, which are derived from the occipital myotomes (see Fig. 16.17A).

CN III supplies the superior, inferior, and medial recti and inferior oblique muscles of the eye.

NERVES OF PHARYNGEAL ARCHES

Cranial nerves V, VII, IX, and X supply the embryonic pharyngeal arches; thus the structures that develop from these arches are innervated by these cranial nerves (see Fig. 16.27A and Table 16.1).

The **trigeminal nerve** (CN V) is the nerve of the first pharyngeal arch, but it has an ophthalmic division that is not a pharyngeal arch component. CN V is the principal sensory nerve for the head. The cells of the large **trigeminal ganglion** are derived from the most anterior part of the neural crest. The central processes of the cells in this ganglion form the large sensory root of CN V, which enters the lateral part of the pons. The peripheral processes of cells in this ganglion separate into three large divisions (ophthalmic, maxillary, and mandibular nerves). Their sensory fibers supply the skin of the face and the lining of the mouth and nose. The motor fibers of CN V arise from cells in the most anterior part of the special visceral efferent column in the metencephalon. These fibers pass to the muscles of mastication and to other muscles that develop in the mandibular prominence of the first pharyngeal arch (see Table 10.1). The mesencephalic nucleus of CN V differentiates from cells in the midbrain.

The **facial nerve** (CN VII) is the nerve of the second pharyngeal arch. It consists mostly of motor fibers that arise principally from a nuclear group in the special visceral efferent

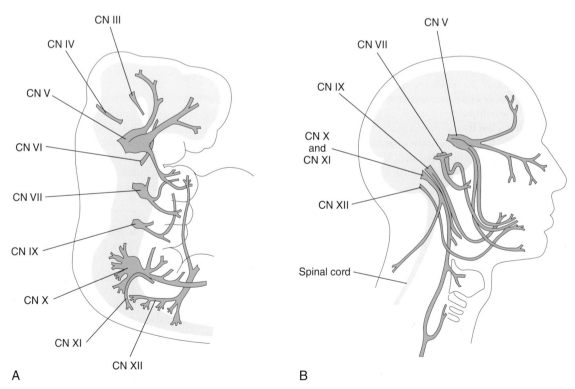

Fig. 16.27   (A) Schematic drawing of a 5-week embryo showing distribution of most of the cranial nerves, especially those supplying the pharyngeal arches. (B) Schematic drawing of the head and neck of an adult showing the general distribution of many of the cranial nerves. *CN*, Cranial nerve.

column in the caudal part of the pons. These fibers are distributed to the muscles of facial expression and to other muscles that develop in the mesenchyme of the second pharyngeal arch (see Table 10.1). The small general visceral efferent component of CN VII terminates in the peripheral autonomic ganglia of the head. The sensory fibers of CN VII arise from the cells of the **geniculate ganglion**. The central processes of these cells enter the pons, and the peripheral processes pass to the greater superficial petrosal nerve and, via the chorda tympani nerve, to the taste buds in the anterior two-thirds of the tongue.

The **glossopharyngeal nerve** (CN IX) is the nerve of the third pharyngeal arch. Its motor fibers arise from the special and, to a lesser extent, the general visceral efferent columns of the anterior part of the myelencephalon. CN IX forms from several rootlets that arise from the medulla just caudal to the developing internal ear. All the fibers from the special visceral efferent column are distributed to the stylopharyngeus muscle, which is derived from the mesenchyme in the third pharyngeal arch (see Table 10.1). The general efferent fibers are distributed to the otic ganglion from which postsynaptic fibers pass to the parotid and posterior lingual glands. The sensory fibers of CN IX are distributed as general sensory and special visceral afferent fibers (taste fibers) to the posterior part of the tongue.

The **vagus nerve** (CN X) is formed by fusion of the nerves of the fourth and sixth pharyngeal arches (see Table 10.1). The nerve of the fourth pharyngeal arch becomes the superior laryngeal nerve, which supplies the cricothyroid muscle and constrictor muscles of the pharynx. The nerve of the sixth pharyngeal arch becomes the recurrent laryngeal nerve, which supplies various laryngeal muscles.

The **spinal accessory nerve** (CN XI) arises from the cranial five or six cervical segments of the spinal cord (see Fig. 16.27A). The fibers of the traditional CN XI root are now considered to be part of CN X. These fibers supply the sternocleidomastoid and trapezius muscles.

SPECIAL SENSORY NERVES

The **olfactory nerve** (CN I) arises from the olfactory organ. The olfactory cells are bipolar neurons that differentiate from cells in the epithelial lining of the primordial nasal sac. The axons of the olfactory cells are collected into 18 to 20 bundles around which the cribriform plate of the ethmoid bone develops. These unmyelinated nerve fibers end in the **olfactory bulb**.

The **optic nerve** (CN II) is formed by more than a million nerve fibers that grow into the brain from neuroblasts in the primordial retina. Because the optic nerve develops from the evaginated wall of the forebrain, it actually represents a fiber tract of the brain. The development of the optic nerve is described in Chapter 17.

The **vestibulocochlear nerve** (CN VIII) consists of two kinds of sensory fibers in two bundles; these fibers are known as the vestibular and cochlear nerves. The **vestibular nerve** originates in the semicircular ducts, and the **cochlear nerve** proceeds from the cochlear duct, in which the **spiral organ**

(of Corti) develops (see Chapter 17). The bipolar neurons of the vestibular nerve have their cell bodies in the **vestibular ganglion**. The central processes of these cells terminate in the vestibular nuclei on the floor of the fourth ventricle. The bipolar neurons of the cochlear nerve have their cell bodies in the **spiral ganglion**. The central processes of these cells end in the ventral and dorsal **cochlear nuclei** in the medulla.

DEVELOPMENT OF AUTONOMIC NERVOUS SYSTEM

Functionally, the ANS can be divided into sympathetic (thoracolumbar) and parasympathetic (craniosacral) parts.

SYMPATHETIC NERVOUS SYSTEM

During the fifth week, neural crest cells in the thoracic region migrate along each side of the spinal cord, where they form paired cellular masses (ganglia) dorsolateral to the aorta (see Fig. 16.7). All these segmentally arranged **sympathetic ganglia** are connected in a bilateral chain by longitudinal nerve fibers. These ganglionated cords—**sympathetic trunks**—are located on each side of the vertebral bodies. Some neural crest cells migrate ventral to the aorta and form neurons in the **preaortic ganglia**, such as the celiac and mesenteric ganglia (see Fig. 16.7). Other neural crest cells migrate to the area of the heart, lungs, and gastrointestinal tract, where they form terminal ganglia in **sympathetic organ plexuses**, located near or within these organs.

After the sympathetic trunks have formed, axons of sympathetic neurons located in the **intermediolateral cell column** (lateral horn) of the thoracolumbar segments of the spinal cord pass through the ventral root of a spinal nerve and a **white ramus communicans** to a paravertebral ganglion (see Fig. 16.7). Here they may synapse with neurons or ascend or descend in the sympathetic trunk to synapse at other levels. Other presynaptic fibers pass through the **paravertebral ganglia** without synapsing, forming splanchnic nerves to the viscera. The postsynaptic fibers course through a **gray communicating branch** (**gray ramus communicans**), passing from a sympathetic ganglion into a spinal nerve; hence, the sympathetic trunks are composed of ascending and descending fibers.

PARASYMPATHETIC NERVOUS SYSTEM

The presynaptic parasympathetic fibers arise from neurons in the nuclei of the brainstem and in the sacral region of the spinal cord. The fibers from the brainstem leave through the oculomotor (CN III), facial (CN VII), glossopharyngeal (CN IX), and vagus (CN X) nerves. The **postsynaptic neurons** are located in the peripheral ganglia or in plexuses near or within the structure being innervated (e.g., pupil of the eye and salivary glands).

CLINICALLY ORIENTED QUESTIONS

1. Are neural tube birth defects hereditary? A female had an infant with spina bifida cystica, and her daughter had an infant with meroencephaly. Is the daughter likely to have another child with a neural tube defect? Can meroencephaly and spina bifida be detected early in fetal life?

2. Some say that pregnant women who are heavy drinkers may have infants who exhibit mental and growth deficiencies. Is this true? There are reports of females who get drunk during pregnancy yet have infants who seem to be normal. Is there a safe threshold for alcohol consumption during pregnancy?

3. A female was told that cigarette smoking during pregnancy probably caused a slight cognitive deficit in her infant. Was the female correctly informed?

4. Do all types of spina bifida cause loss of motor function in the lower limbs? What treatments are there for infants with spina bifida cystica?

The answers to these questions are at the back of this book.

Development of Eyes and Ears

DEVELOPMENT OF EYES AND RELATED STRUCTURES

The eyes are derived from four sources:

- **Neuroectoderm** of the developing brain
- **Surface ectoderm** of the head
- **Mesoderm** between the above layers
- **Neural crest cells** of the prosencephalon and mesencephalon.

Eye development begins when **optic grooves (sulci)** appear in the cranial neural folds (Fig. 17.1A and B) on day 22. As the neural folds fuse, the optic grooves evaginate to form hollow diverticula—**optic vesicles**—that project from the wall of the forebrain into the adjacent mesenchyme (see Fig. 17.1C). Formation of the optic vesicles is induced by the mesenchyme adjacent to the developing brain. As the optic vesicles enlarge, their connections with the forebrain constrict to form hollow **optic stalks** (see Fig. 17.1D).

An inductive signal passes from the optic vesicles and stimulates the surface ectoderm to thicken and form **lens placodes**, the primordia of the lenses (see Fig. 17.1C). The placodes invaginate and sink deep to the surface ectoderm, forming **lens pits** (Fig. 17.2; see also Fig. 17.1D). The edges of the pits approach and fuse to form spherical **lens vesicles** (see Fig. 17.1F and H), which soon lose their connection with the surface ectoderm. *Early eye development results from a series of highly integrated inductive signals, including OTX2, the transcription regulators PAX2, PAX6, and other inducing factors, such as the genes SOX2, PITX2, EFTFs, RAX, LHX2, TBX3, and FGFs.*

As the lens vesicles develop, the optic vesicles invaginate to form double-walled **optic cups** (Figs. 17.1F and 17.2), with the lens becoming infolded by the rim of the optic cup (Fig. 17.3A). By this stage, the lens vesicles have entered the cavities of the optic cups (Fig. 17.4). Linear grooves—**retinal fissures (optic fissures)**—develop on the ventral surface of the optic cups and along the optic stalks (see Figs. 17.1E–H and 17.3A–D). The retinal fissures contain vascular mesenchyme from which the hyaloid blood vessels develop. The **hyaloid artery**, a branch of the ophthalmic artery, supplies the inner layer of the optic cup, the lens vesicle, and the mesenchyme in the optic cup (see Figs. 17.1H and 17.3). As the edges of the retinal fissure fuse, the hyaloid vessels are enclosed within the **primordial optic nerve** (see Fig. 17.3C–F). Distal parts of the hyaloid vessels eventually degenerate, but proximal parts persist as the **central artery** and **vein of the retina** (Fig. 17.5D). *Bone morphogenetic protein (BMP), sonic hedgehog (SHH), and fibroblast growth factor (FGF) are essential for signaling the optical vesicle and closure (PAX2) of the retinal fissure.*

DEVELOPMENT OF RETINA

The retina develops from the walls of the optic cup, an outgrowth of the forebrain (see Figs. 17.1 and 17.2). The walls of the cup develop into two layers of the retina: the outer thin layer becomes the **pigment layer of the retina**, and the thick layer differentiates into the **neural retina**. The two retinal layers are separated by an **intraretinal space** (see Figs. 17.1H and 17.4), which is derived from the cavity of the optic cup. This space gradually disappears as the two layers of the retina loosely fuse (see Fig. 17.5D). Because the optic cup is an outgrowth of the forebrain, the layers of the optic cup are continuous with the wall of the brain (see Fig. 17.1H).

Under the influence of the developing lens, the inner layer of the optic cup proliferates to form a thick **neuroepithelium** (see Fig. 17.4). Subsequently, the cells of this layer differentiate into the neural retina, the light-sensitive region of the retina (see Fig. 17.7). *SHH, Nrl, Lhx2, Six2, PAX2, Pax6, and Rax are eyefield-specific transcription factors involved in retinal neurogenesis.* This region contains **photoreceptors** (rods and cones) and the cell bodies of neurons (e.g., bipolar and ganglion cells). Because the optic vesicle invaginates as it forms the optic cup, the neural retina is "inverted"; that is, light-sensitive parts of the photoreceptor cells are adjacent to the retinal pigment epithelium. As a result, light must pass through the thickest part of the retina before reaching the photoreceptors; however, because the neuroretina is essentially transparent, it does not form a barrier to light.

The axons of the ganglion cells in the superficial layer of the neural retina grow proximally in the wall of the optic stalk to the brain (see Fig. 17.3A). The cavity of the stalk is gradually obliterated as the axons of the ganglion cells form the **optic nerve** (see Fig. 17.3F). *Myelination (formation of a myelin sheath) of the optic nerve fibers begins late in the fetal period.* During the postnatal period, after exposure to light, myelination is completed by the 10th week after birth. *Molecular studies have shown that the homeobox genes PAX6 and OTX2 regulate retinal differentiation and pigment formation, respectively.*

Coloboma

Retinal coloboma is a birth defect that is characterized by a localized gap in the retina, usually inferior to the optic disc. The defect is bilateral in most cases. A typical coloboma results from defective closure of the retinal fissure.

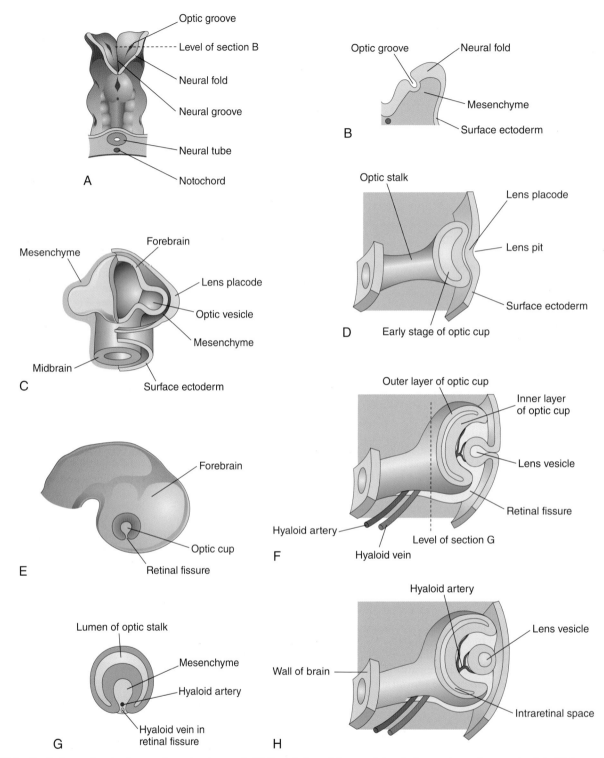

Fig. 17.1 Illustrations of early stages of eye development. (A) Dorsal view of the cranial end of an embryo at approximately 22 days, showing the optic grooves, the first indication of eye development. (B) Transverse section of a neural fold showing the optic groove in it. (C) Schematic drawing of the forebrain of an embryo at approximately 28 days, showing its covering layers of mesenchyme and surface ectoderm. (D, F, and H) Schematic sections of the developing eye, illustrating successive stages in the development of the optic cup and lens vesicle. (E) Lateral view of the brain of an embryo at approximately 32 days, showing the external appearance of the optic cup. (G) Transverse section of the optic stalk, showing the retinal fissure and its contents. Note that the edges of the retinal fissure are growing together, thereby completing the optic cup and enclosing the central artery and vein of the retina in the optic stalk and cup.

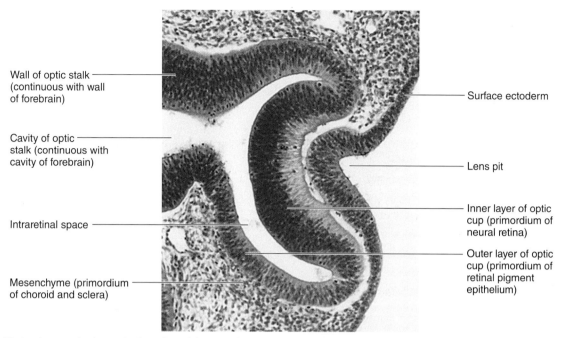

Fig. 17.2 Photomicrograph of a sagittal section of the eye of an embryo (×200) at approximately 32 days. Observe the primordium of the lens (invaginated lens placode), the walls of the optic cup (primordium of retina), and the optic stalk (primordium of the optic nerve). From Moore KL, Persaud TVN, Shiota K: *Color atlas of clinical embryology*, ed 2, Philadelphia, 2000, Saunders.

Labels: Wall of optic stalk (continuous with wall of forebrain); Cavity of optic stalk (continuous with cavity of forebrain); Intraretinal space; Mesenchyme (primordium of choroid and sclera); Surface ectoderm; Lens pit; Inner layer of optic cup (primordium of neural retina); Outer layer of optic cup (primordium of retinal pigment epithelium)

Coloboma of Iris

In infants, this birth defect in the inferior sector of the iris or pupillary margin gives the pupil a keyhole appearance (Fig. 17.6). The coloboma may be limited to the iris, or it may extend deeper and involve the ciliary body and retina. A typical coloboma results from the failure of closure of the retinal fissure during the sixth week. The defect may be genetically determined, or it may be caused by environmental factors. A simple coloboma of the iris is frequently hereditary and is transmitted as an autosomal dominant characteristic.

DEVELOPMENT OF CHOROID AND SCLERA

The mesenchyme surrounding the optic cup differentiates into an inner, vascular layer—the **choroid**—and an outer, fibrous layer—the **sclera** (Fig. 17.7; see also Fig. 17.5C). At the rim of the optic cup, the choroid forms the cores of the **ciliary processes**, consisting chiefly of capillaries supported by delicate connective tissue.

DEVELOPMENT OF CILIARY BODY

The ciliary body is a wedge-shaped extension of the **choroid** (see Fig. 17.5C and D). Its medial surface projects toward the lens, forming **ciliary processes**. The pigmented part of the ciliary epithelium is derived from the outer layer of the optic cup, which is continuous with the retinal pigment epithelium. The **nonvisual retina** is the nonpigmented ciliary epithelium, which represents the anterior prolongation of the neural retina, in which no neural elements develop. The smooth **ciliary muscle** is responsible for focusing the lens

and for the connective tissue in the ciliary body. It develops from the mesenchyme at the edge of the optic cup between the anterior scleral condensation and the ciliary pigment epithelium.

DEVELOPMENT OF IRIS

The iris develops from the rim of the **optic cup**, which grows inward and partially covers the lens (see Fig. 17.5D). The epithelium of the iris represents both layers of the optic cup; it is continuous with the double-layered epithelium of the **ciliary body** and with the retinal pigment epithelium and neural retina. The **stroma** (connective tissue framework) of the iris is derived from neural crest cells that migrate into the iris. The **dilator pupillae** and **sphincter pupillae muscles** of the iris are derived from the neuroectoderm of the optic cup. These smooth muscles result from a transformation of epithelial cells into smooth muscle cells.

DEVELOPMENT OF LENS

The lens develops from the **lens vesicle**, a derivative of the surface ectoderm (see Fig. 17.1F and H). The anterior wall of the lens vesicle becomes the subcapsular **lens epithelium** (see Fig. 17.5C). The nuclei of the tall columnar cells that form the posterior wall of the lens vesicle undergo dissolution. These cells lengthen considerably to form highly transparent epithelial cells, the **primary lens fibers**. As these fibers grow, they gradually obliterate the cavity of the lens vesicle (Fig. 17.8; see also Figs. 17.5A–C and 17.7). The rim of the lens—the **equatorial zone**—is located midway between the anterior and posterior poles of the lens. The cells in the equatorial zone are cuboidal; as they elongate, they lose their nuclei and become **secondary lens fibers** (see Fig. 17.8). These fibers are added to the external sides of

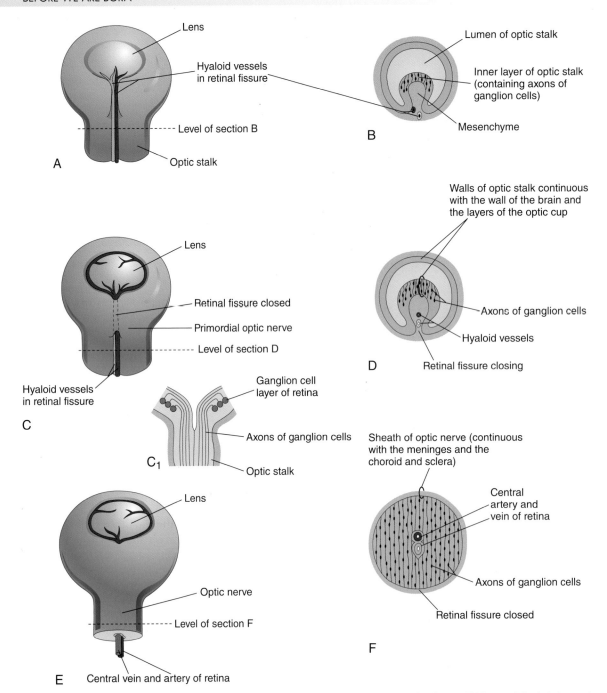

Fig. 17.3 Illustrations of the closure of the retinal fissure and the formation of the optic nerve. (A, C, and E) Views of the inferior surface of the optic cup and optic stalk showing progressive stages in the closure of the retinal fissure. (C_1) Schematic sketch of a longitudinal section of a part of the optic cup and stalk, showing the optic disc and axons of the ganglion cells of the retina growing through the optic stalk to the brain. (B, D, and F) Transverse sections of the optic stalk showing successive stages in the closure of the retinal fissure and the formation of the optic nerve. Note that the lumen of the optic stalk is gradually obliterated as axons of ganglion cells accumulate in the inner layer of the optic stalk as the optic nerve forms.

the primary lens fibers. *Lens formation involves the expression of L-Maf (lens-specific Maf) and other transcription factors in the lens placode and vesicle. The transcription factors Pitx3 and GAT-3 are also essential for the formation of the lens.*

Although secondary lens fibers continue to form during adulthood and the lens increases in diameter as a result, no new primary lens fibers are added. The developing lens is supplied with blood by the distal part of the **hyaloid artery**

(see Figs. 17.4 and 17.5); however, it becomes avascular in the fetal period when this part of the artery degenerates (see Fig. 17.5D). After this, the lens depends on diffusion from the **aqueous humor** in the anterior chamber of the eye (see Fig. 17.5C), which bathes its anterior surface, and from the vitreous humor in other parts. The **lens capsule** is produced by the anterior lens epithelium. The lens capsule represents a greatly thickened basement membrane and has

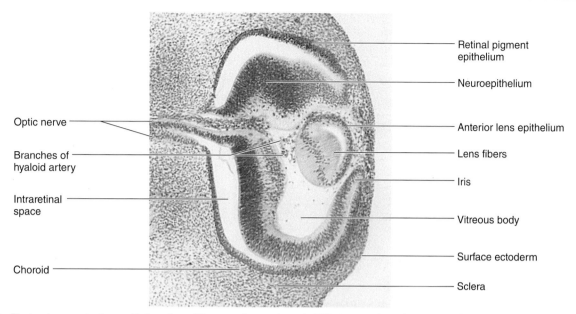

Fig. 17.4 Photomicrograph of a sagittal section of the eye of an embryo (×100) at approximately 44 days. Observe that it is the posterior wall of the lens vesicle that forms the lens fibers. The anterior wall does not change appreciably as it becomes the anterior lens epithelium. From Nishimura H, editor: *Atlas of human prenatal histology*, Tokyo, 1983, Igaku-Shoin.

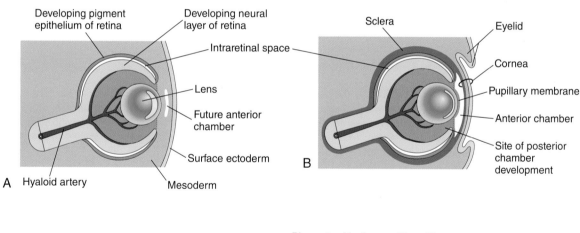

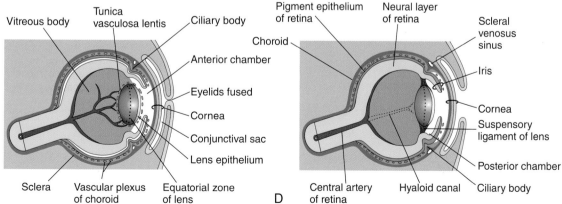

Fig. 17.5 Drawings of sagittal sections of the eye, showing successive developmental stages of the lens, retina, iris, and cornea. (A) At 5 weeks. (B) At 6 weeks. (C) At 20 weeks. (D) Neonate. Note that the retina and optic nerve are formed from the optic cup and optic stalk (Fig. 17.1D).

a lamellar structure. The former site of the **hyaloid artery** is indicated by the **hyaloid canal** in the vitreous body (see Fig. 17.5D); this canal is usually inconspicuous in the living eye. *Drebrin E, an actin-binding protein, regulates the morphogenesis and growth of the lens.*

Persistence of Hyaloid Artery

The distal part of the hyaloid artery normally degenerates as its proximal part becomes the central artery of the retina (see Fig. 17.5C and D). If part of the hyaloid artery persists distally, it may appear as a freely moving, nonfunctional vessel, or a worm-like structure projecting from the optic disc (see Fig. 17.3C), or as a fine strand traversing the vitreous body. In other cases, the hyaloid artery remnant may form a cyst.

The **vitreous body** forms within the cavity of the optic cup (see Figs. 17.4 and 17.5C). It is composed of **vitreous humor**, an avascular mass of transparent, gel-like, intercellular substance.

DEVELOPMENT OF AQUEOUS CHAMBERS

The **anterior chamber of the eye** develops from a cleft-like space that forms in the mesenchyme located between the developing lens and cornea (see Figs. 17.5A–C and 17.8). The **posterior chamber of the eye** develops from a space that forms in the mesenchyme posterior to the developing iris and anterior to the developing lens (see Fig. 17.5D). After the lens is established, it induces the surface ectoderm to develop into the epithelium of the cornea and conjunctiva. When the **pupillary membrane** disappears (see Fig. 17.5B) and the pupil forms, the anterior and posterior chambers

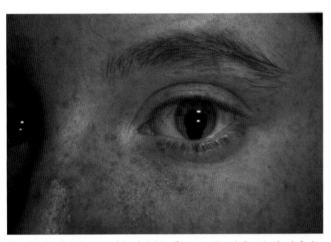

Fig. 17.6 Coloboma of the left iris. Observe the defect in the inferior part of the iris (at the 6 o'clock position). The defect represents failure of fusion of the retinal fissure. From Guercio J, Martyn L: Congenital malformations of the eye and orbit, *Otolaryngol Clin North Am* 40(1):113, 2007.

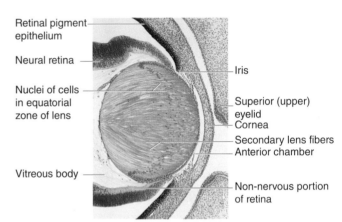

Fig. 17.8 Photomicrograph of a sagittal section of a portion of the developing eye of an embryo at approximately 56 days. Observe that the lens fibers have elongated and obliterated the cavity of the lens vesicle. From Moore KL, Persaud TVN, Shiota K: *Color atlas of clinical embryology*, ed 2, Philadelphia, 2000, Saunders.

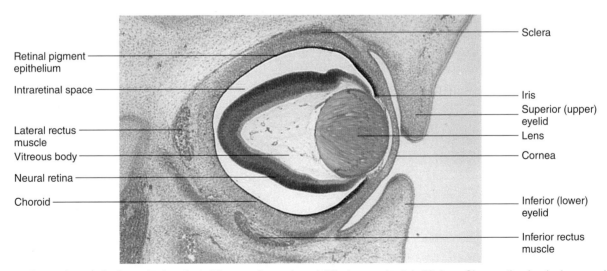

Fig. 17.7 Photomicrograph of a sagittal section of the eye of an embryo (×50) at approximately 56 days. Observe the developing neural retina and pigment layer of the retina. The large intraretinal space disappears when these two layers of the retina fuse. From Moore KL, Persaud TVN, Shiota K: *Color atlas of clinical embryology*, ed 2, Philadelphia, PA, 2000, Saunders.

of the eye communicate with each other through the **scleral venous sinus** (see Fig. 17.5D). This vascular structure encircles the anterior chamber and allows aqueous humor to flow from the anterior chamber to the venous system.

Congenital Glaucoma

Abnormal elevation of intraocular pressure, intraocular tension, occurs in neonates because of an imbalance between the production of aqueous humor and its outflow. This imbalance may result from abnormal development of the **scleral venous sinus** (see Fig. 17.5D). Congenital glaucoma (0.5–1.0:10,000) is usually genetically **heterogeneous**, but the condition may result from a rubella infection in the fetus during early pregnancy (see Fig. 19.16B). It has been shown that the gene *CYP1B1* is responsible for the majority of cases of primary congenital glaucoma.

Congenital Cataracts

In this birth defect (1–15:10,000), the lens is opaque and frequently appears grayish white. Without treatment, blindness results. Many lens opacities are inherited, with dominant transmission being more common than recessive, or sex-linked, transmission. More than 30 genes have been reported in association with primary cataracts. Some congenital cataracts are caused by teratogenic agents—particularly the **rubella virus** (see Fig. 19.16A)—that affect the early development of the lenses. The lenses are vulnerable to rubella and herpes viruses between the fourth and seventh weeks, when primary lens fibers are forming (see Chapter 19).

DEVELOPMENT OF CORNEA

The cornea, induced by the lens vesicle, is formed from three sources:

- External corneal epithelium, derived from **surface ectoderm**
- **Mesenchyme**, derived from mesoderm, which is continuous with the developing sclera
- **Neural crest cells** that migrate from the lip of the optic cup and form the corneal epithelium in addition to the middle stroma layer of collagen-rich extracellular matrix.

DEVELOPMENT OF EYELIDS

The eyelids develop during the sixth week from mesenchyme derived from neural crest cells and from two cutaneous folds of skin that grow over the cornea (see Fig. 17.5B). The eyelids adhere to one another during the eighth week and remain fused until the 26th to 28th weeks (see Fig. 17.5C). The **palpebral conjunctiva** lines the inner surface of the eyelids. The **eyelashes** and **glands** in the eyelids are derived from the surface ectoderm (see Chapter 18). The connective tissue and **tarsal plates (fibrous plates in the eyelids)** develop from mesenchyme in the developing eyelids. The **orbicularis oculi muscle** is derived from the mesenchyme in the second pharyngeal arch (see Chapter 10) and is supplied by CN VII.

Congenital Ptosis of Eyelid

Drooping of the superior eyelids at birth is relatively common. **Ptosis (blepharoptosis)** may result from dystrophy of the **levator palpebrae superioris muscle**. Congenital ptosis occurs more rarely as a result of prenatal injury or **dystrophy (atrophy)** of the superior division of the **oculomotor nerve** (CN III), which supplies this muscle. Congenital ptosis may also be transmitted as an autosomal dominant trait. Severe ptosis can interfere with the development of normal sight and may need to be treated surgically.

Coloboma of Eyelid

This uncommon (1:10,000) birth defect is characterized by a small notch in the superior eyelid; coloboma of the inferior (lower) eyelid is rare. **Palpebral colobomas** appear to result from local developmental disturbances in the formation and growth of the eyelids.

DEVELOPMENT OF LACRIMAL GLANDS

The lacrimal glands are derived from a number of solid buds from the surface ectoderm. The buds branch and canalize to form **lacrimal excretory ducts** and alveoli of the glands. The **lacrimal glands** are small at birth and do not function fully; reflex tearing (such as from crying) does not occur until at least the second month of age, when the lacrimal glands are further developed. *Molecular studies indicate that Fgf10, SOX10, TFAP2, and miR-205 signaling pathways are essential for the development of the lacrimal gland.*

DEVELOPMENT OF EARS

18

The ears are composed of external, middle, and internal anatomic parts. The external and middle parts regulate the transference of sound waves from the exterior to the internal ears, which convert the sound waves into nerve impulses. The internal ears are concerned with both hearing and balance.

DEVELOPMENT OF INTERNAL EARS

The internal ears are the first of the three parts of the ears to develop. Early in the fourth week, a thickening of the surface ectoderm—the **otic placode**—appears on each side of the embryo at the level of the caudal part of the hindbrain (Fig. 17.9A and B). Inductive influences from the notochord and paraxial mesoderm stimulate the surface ectoderm to form the otic placodes. *Inductive signals, including those from the paraxial mesoderm and notochord, stimulate the surface ectoderm to form the placodes (see Fig. 4.9). Placental growth factor–mediated signaling initiates the specification of the otic epibranchial progenitors from sensory precursors in the preplacodal region. Further development of the otic placode involves the protein-coding Pa2G4, transcription factors FoxL1/3, Wnt and Notch pathways, Pax2/8, Mcrs1, Six1, and protein-encoding Dix genes.*

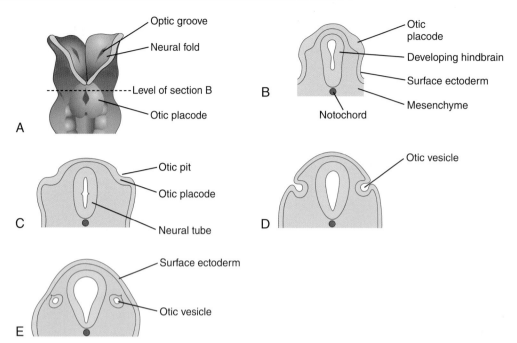

Fig. 17.9   Drawings illustrating early development of the internal ear. (A) Dorsal view of an embryo at approximately 22 days, showing the otic placodes. (B–E) Schematic coronal sections illustrating successive stages in the development of otic vesicles.

Each otic placode invaginates and sinks deep into the surface ectoderm into the underlying mesenchyme, forming an **otic pit** (see Fig. 17.9C). The edges of the pit come together and fuse to form an **otic vesicle** (see Fig. 17.9D and E). The vesicle soon loses its connection with the surface ectoderm, and a diverticulum grows from the vesicle and elongates to form the **endolymphatic duct** and **sac** (Fig. 17.10A–E). Two regions of the otic vesicles are visible:

- Dorsal **utricular** parts, from which the small endolymphatic ducts, utricles, and semicircular ducts arise
- Ventral **saccular** parts, which give rise to the saccules and cochlear ducts.

Three disc-like diverticula grow out from the utricular parts of the **primordial membranous labyrinths**. Soon the central parts of these diverticula fuse and disappear (see Fig. 17.10B–E). The peripheral unfused parts of the diverticula become the **semicircular ducts**, which are attached to the utricle and are later enclosed in the **semicircular canals** of the **bony labyrinth**. Localized dilations, the **ampullae**, develop at one end of each semicircular duct (see Fig. 17.10E). Specialized receptor areas—**cristae ampullares**—differentiate in the ampullae and the utricle and saccule (maculae utricle and sacculi).

From the ventral saccular part of the otic vesicle, a tubular diverticulum—the **cochlear duct**—grows and coils to form the **membranous cochlea** (see Fig. 17.10C–E). A connection of the cochlea with the saccule, the **ductus reuniens**, soon forms. The **spiral organ** differentiates from cells in the wall of the cochlear duct (see Fig. 17.10F–I). Ganglion cells of the **vestibulocochlear nerve** (CN VIII) migrate along the coils of the membranous cochlea and form the **spiral ganglion**. Nerve processes extend from this ganglion to the spiral organ, where they terminate on the bipolar **hair cells**.

Inductive influences from the otic vesicle stimulate the mesenchyme around the vesicle to differentiate into a **cartilaginous otic capsule** (see Fig. 17.10F). The cartilaginous otic capsule later ossifies to form the **bony labyrinth** of the internal ear. *Retinoic acid and transforming growth factor β₁ play a role in modulating epithelial–mesenchymal interaction in the internal ear and directing the formation of the otic capsule.*

As the membranous labyrinth enlarges, vacuoles appear in the cartilaginous otic capsule and soon coalesce to form the **perilymphatic space**. The membranous labyrinth is now suspended in **perilymph**. The perilymphatic space, related to the cochlear duct, develops two divisions, the **scala tympani** and **scala vestibuli** (see Fig. 17.10H and I). The internal ear reaches its adult size and shape by the middle of the fetal period (20–22 weeks), and functional hearing occurs by approximately week 26.

DEVELOPMENT OF MIDDLE EARS

Development of the **tubotympanic recess** (Fig. 17.11B) from the first pharyngeal pouch is described in Chapter 10. The proximal part of the recess forms the **pharyngotympanic tube** (auditory tube). The distal part of the recess expands and becomes the **tympanic cavity** (see Fig. 17.11C), which gradually envelops the **auditory ossicles** (malleus, incus, and stapes), their tendons and ligaments, and the **chorda tympani nerve**. Ossification of the auditory ossicles begins at 16 weeks and is completed by 26 weeks. *Neural crest cells originating from the dorsal hindbrain migrate to specific sites on the first and second pharyngeal arches to form the three auditory ossicles (malleus, incus, and stapes). SHH, FGF, CXCL12, and BMP4 signaling control the formation of the ear ossicles.*

These structures receive a complete epithelial investment that is derived from neural crest cells and the endoderm. The neural crest cells undergo epithelial–mesenchymal

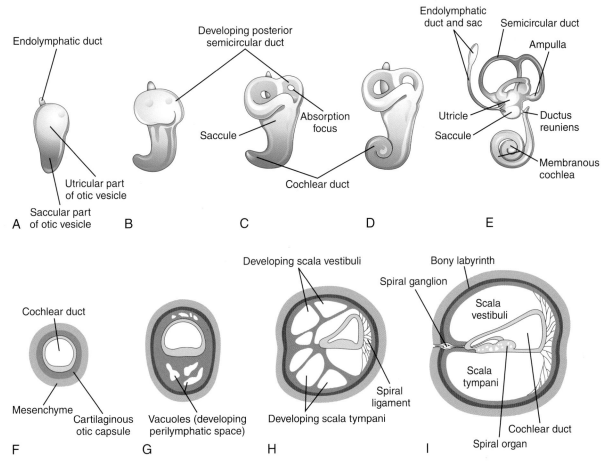

Fig. 17.10 Drawings of the otic vesicles showing the development of the membranous and bony labyrinths of the internal ear. (A–E) Lateral views showing successive stages in the development of the otic vesicle into the membranous labyrinth from the fifth to eighth weeks. (A–D) Diagrammatic sketches illustrating the development of a semicircular duct. (F–I) Sections through the cochlear duct showing successive stages in the development of the spiral organ and the perilymphatic space from the 8th to 20th weeks.

transformation. An epithelial-type organizer, located at the tip of the tubotympanic recess, probably plays a role in the early development of the middle ear cavity through **apoptosis**. Cavitation begins in the third month and is completed by the eighth month. The malleus and the incus develop from the cartilage of the first pharyngeal arch. The stapes has multiple origins. The head and crus are formed from neural crest cells. The outer boundary of the foot plate is mesenchymal in origin, whereas the inner ring is from neural crest cells. The **tensor tympani**, the muscle attached to the malleus, is derived from the mesenchyme in the first pharyngeal arch, and the **stapedius muscle** is derived from the second pharyngeal arch.

During the late fetal period, expansion of the **tympanic cavity** gives rise to the **mastoid antrum**, located in the temporal bone. The antrum is almost adult size at birth; however, *no mastoid cells are present in neonates*. By 5 years of age, the mastoid cells are well developed and produce conic projections of the temporal bones, the **mastoid processes**. The middle ear continues to grow through puberty.

DEVELOPMENT OF EXTERNAL EARS

The **external acoustic meatus** develops from the dorsal part of the first pharyngeal groove. The ectodermal cells at the bottom of this tube proliferate to form a solid epithelial plate, the **meatal plug** (see Fig. 17.11C). Late in the fetal period, the central cells of this plug degenerate, forming a cavity that becomes the internal part of the external acoustic meatus (see Fig. 17.11D).

The primordium of the **tympanic membrane** is the first pharyngeal membrane, which separates the first pharyngeal groove from the first pharyngeal pouch (see Fig. 17.11A). The external covering of the tympanic membrane is derived from the surface ectoderm, whereas its internal lining is derived from the endoderm of the tubotympanic recess.

The **auricle** (pinna), which projects from the side of the head, develops from the mesenchymal proliferations in the first and second pharyngeal arches. Prominences—**auricular hillocks**—surround the first pharyngeal groove (Fig. 17.12A). As the auricle grows, the contribution of the first arch is reduced and forms the tragus (see Fig. 17.12B–D). The **lobule** (earlobe) is the last part of the auricle to develop. *HOXA2 appears to be critical for auricle development.* The auricle obtains its adult structure by 22 weeks. It is initially located at the base of the neck (see Fig. 17.12A and B). As the mandible develops, the auricles assume their normal position at the side of the head as a result of differential growth of the head and neck (see Fig. 17.12C and D).

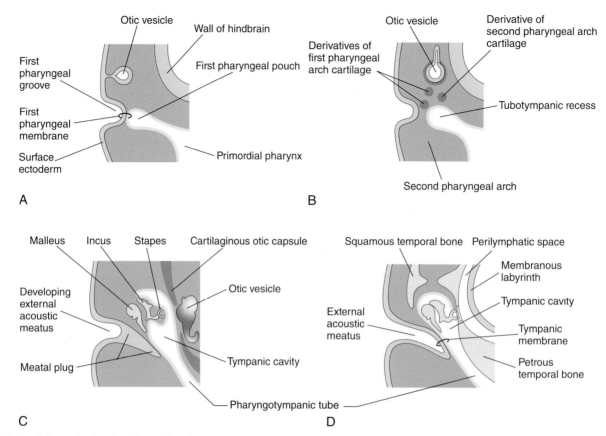

Fig. 17.11 Schematic drawings illustrating development of the external and middle parts of the ear. Observe the relationship of these parts of the ear to the otic vesicle, the primordium of the internal ear. (A) At 4 weeks, illustrating the relation of the otic vesicle to the pharyngeal apparatus. (B) At 5 weeks, showing the tubotympanic recess and pharyngeal arch cartilages. (C) Later stage, showing the tubotympanic recess (future tympanic cavity and mastoid antrum) beginning to envelop the ossicles. (D) Final stage of ear development showing the relationship of the middle ear to the perilymphatic space and external acoustic meatus. Note that the tympanic membrane develops from three germ layers: surface ectoderm, mesenchyme, and endoderm of the tubotympanic recess.

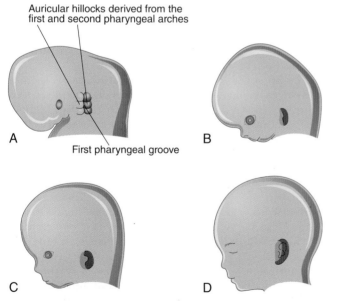

Fig. 17.12 Illustration of the development of the auricle, the part of the external ear that is not within the head. (A) At 6 weeks. Note that three auricular hillocks are located on the first pharyngeal arch and three are on the second arch. (B) At 8 weeks. (C) At 10 weeks. (D) At 32 weeks.

Congenital Hearing Loss

Approximately 3 in every 1000 neonates have significant hearing loss. The deafness may be the result of maldevelopment of the sound-conducting apparatus of the middle and external ears or of the neurosensory structures in the internal ear. Enlargement of the vestibular aqueduct and endolymphatic duct is the most common congenital ear defect in children with hearing loss (Fig. 17.13). This defect is typically bilateral and is an **autosomal recessive condition**. Pathogenic variants (mutations) in the *GJB2* gene are responsible for approximately 50% of nonsyndromic recessive hearing loss.

Half of all nongenetic causes are related to infection. **Fetal cytomegalovirus** is the most common infection causing sensorineural hearing loss. **Rubella infection** during the critical period (fourth week) of development of the internal ear can cause maldevelopment of the spiral organ and deafness.

Congenital fixation of the stapes results in conductive deafness in an otherwise normal ear. Failure of differentiation of the annular ligament, which attaches the base of the stapes to the oval window, results in fixation of the stapes to the bony labyrinth and loss of sound conduction. Congenital deafness may be associated with several other head and neck defects as a part of the **first arch syndrome** (see Fig. 9.14). Abnormalities of the malleus and incus, which occur frequently, are often associated with this syndrome (see Fig. 14.8D).

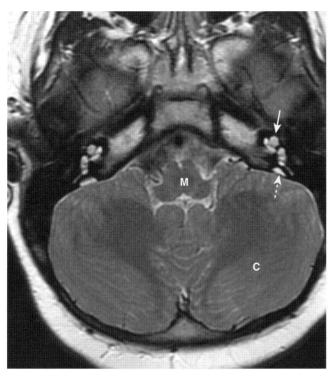

Fig. 17.13 Magnetic resonance image of a 5-year-old child demonstrating bilateral enlargement of the vestibular aqueduct and endolymphatic duct *(dashed arrow)*. Also note the cochlea *(solid arrow)*, the medulla *(M)*, and the cerebellum *(C)*. Courtesy Dr. G. Smyser, Altru Health System, Grand Forks, North Dakota.

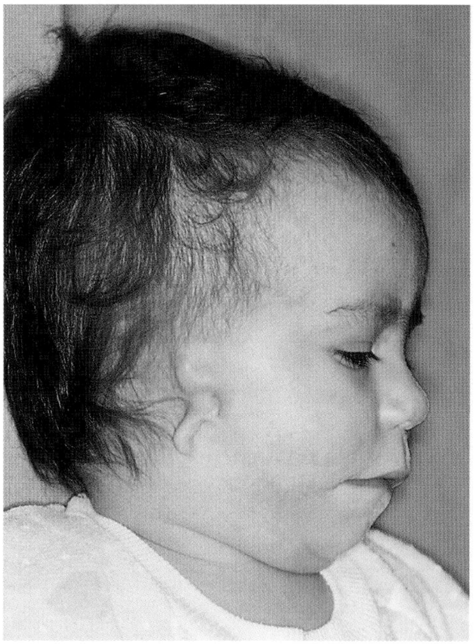

Fig. 17.14 A child with a rudimentary auricle (microtia) and a preauricular tag. She also has several other birth defects. The external acoustic meatus is also absent. Courtesy A.E. Chudley, MD, Section of Genetics and Metabolism, Department of Pediatrics and Child Health, Children's Hospital, University of Manitoba, Winnipeg, Manitoba, Canada.

Auricular Abnormalities

Severe defects of the external ear are rare, but minor deformities are common and may serve as indicators of a specific pattern of congenital defects. For example, the auricles are often low-set and abnormal in shape in infants with **chromosomal syndromes**, such as trisomy 18 (see Chapter 19), and in infants affected by maternal ingestion of certain drugs (e.g., trimethadione).

Accessory Auriculars

Accessory auricles are common (5–10:1000) and may result from the development of **accessory auricular hillocks** (Fig. 17.14). The appendages usually appear anterior to the auricle, more often unilaterally than bilaterally. The appendages, often with narrow pedicles, consist of skin tags, but rarely they may also contain some cartilage (1:25,000).

Microtia

Microtia (a small or rudimentary auricle) results from suppressed mesenchymal proliferation (see Fig. 17.14). This defect (2–3:10,000) often serves as an indicator of associated birth defects, such as an **atresia** of the external acoustic meatus (80% of cases) and abnormalities of the middle ear. The cause can be both genetic and environmental.

Preauricular Sinuses (Ear Pit)

These sinuses located anterior to the auricle usually have pinpoint external openings (see Fig. 10.9D). Some sinuses contain a vestigial cartilaginous mass. These defects are probably related to the abnormal development of the auricular hillocks and defective closure of the dorsal part of the first pharyngeal groove. Preauricular sinuses are familial and are frequently bilateral. These sinuses may be associated with internal defects, such as deafness and kidney malformations.

Congenital Aural Atresia

Atresia of the external acoustic meatus results from failure of the meatal plug to canalize—form a canal (see Fig. 17.11C). Usually, the deep part of the canal is open, but the superficial part is blocked by bone or fibrous tissue. Most cases are associated with the first arch syndrome (see Chapter 10). Often the auricle is also severely affected, and defects of the middle ear, internal ear, or both may be present. Atresia of the external acoustic meatus can occur bilaterally or unilaterally and usually results from autosomal dominant inheritance. Complete absence of the external acoustic meatus is rare (see Fig. 17.14). This defect results from the failure of inward expansion of the first pharyngeal groove and the failure of the meatal plug to disappear.

CLINICALLY ORIENTED QUESTIONS

1. If a woman has rubella during the first trimester of pregnancy, what are the chances that the eyes and ears of the fetus will be affected? What is the most common manifestation of late fetal rubella infection? If a pregnant woman is exposed to rubella, can it be determined whether she is immune to the infection?

2. Is the purposeful exposure of young girls to rubella the best way for a woman to avoid rubella infection during pregnancy? If not, what can be done to provide immunization against rubella infection?

3. It has been reported that deafness and tooth defects occurring during childhood may result from fetal syphilis. Is this true? If so, how could this happen? Can these birth defects be prevented?

4. There are reports that blindness and deafness can result from herpesvirus infections. Is this true? If so, which herpesvirus is involved? What are the affected infant's chances of normal development?

5. It has been reported that methyl mercury exposure in utero can cause mental deficiency, deafness, and blindness. The article cited the eating of contaminated fish as the cause of the abnormalities. How might these birth defects be caused by methyl mercury?

The answers to these questions are at the back of this book.

Integumentary System

The integumentary system consists of the skin and its appendages: sweat glands, nails, hairs, sebaceous glands, and arrector muscles of hairs. The system also includes the mammary glands and teeth.

DEVELOPMENT OF SKIN AND APPENDAGES

The skin consists of two layers (epidermis and dermis) that are derived from two different germ layers (Fig. 18.1): the ectoderm and mesoderm.

- The **epidermis** is a superficial epithelial tissue that is derived from the surface embryonic ectoderm (see Fig. 18.1A).
- The **dermis** is a deep layer composed of dense, irregularly arranged connective tissue that is derived from **mesenchyme** (see Fig. 18.1B–D).

Ectodermal and mesenchymal interactions involve mutual inductive mechanisms. The embryonic skin at 4 to 5 weeks consists of a single layer of surface ectoderm overlying the mesoderm (see Fig. 18.1A).

EPIDERMIS

The cells in the surface ectoderm proliferate and form a layer of squamous epithelium, the **periderm**, and a **basal layer** (see Fig. 18.1B). Cell adhesion proteins and cross-linker proteins play a pivotal role in the development of the epidermis. The cells of the periderm continually undergo **keratinization** and **desquamation** and are replaced by cells arising from the basal layer. Keratinization begins at 19 to 20 weeks. The desquamated (exfoliated) peridermal cells form part of the vernix caseosa, a white, greasy substance, that covers the fetal skin (Fig. 18.2). The vernix protects the developing skin from constant exposure to amniotic fluid containing urine, bile salts, and sloughed cells.

The **basal layer of the epidermis** becomes the **stratum germinativum** (see Fig. 18.1D), which produces new cells that are displaced into the more superficial layers. By 11 weeks, cells from the stratum germinativum have formed an **intermediate layer** (see Fig. 18.1C). Replacement of the peridermal cells continues until approximately the 21st week; thereafter, the **periderm disappears** and the **stratum corneum** forms from the **stratum lucidum** (see Fig. 18.1D).

Proliferation of cells in the **stratum germinativum** also produces **epidermal ridges**, which extend into the developing dermis (see Fig. 18.1C). These ridges begin to appear in embryos at 10 weeks and are permanently established by the 17th week. The pattern of epidermal ridges that develops on the surface of the palms of the hands and the soles of the feet is determined genetically and constitutes the basis for **dermatoglyphics** (examining fingerprints) in medical genetics and criminal investigations. Abnormal chromosome complements can affect the development of ridge patterns.

DERMIS

The dermis develops from mesenchyme underlying the surface ectoderm (see Fig. 18.1A and B). Most of the mesenchyme that differentiates into the connective tissue of the dermis originates from the somatic layer of the lateral mesoderm. Late in the embryonic period, **neural crest cells** migrate into the mesenchyme in the developing dermis and differentiate into **melanoblasts** (see Fig. 18.1B and C). Later, these cells migrate to the **dermoepidermal junction** and differentiate into melanocytes (see Fig. 18.1D). The **melanocytes** begin producing **melanin** before birth and distribute it to the epidermal cells. After birth, increased amounts of melanin are produced in response to ultraviolet light. The relative content of melanin in the melanocytes accounts for the different colors of skin. *Molecular studies indicate that Myosin X (Myo10), SOX10, MITF, DCT and KIT, and the Wnt signaling pathways are essential for melanin formation. Melanocyte-stimulating hormone cell surface receptor and melanosomal P-protein determine the degree of pigmentation by regulating tyrosinase levels and activity.*

By 11 weeks, the mesenchymal cells have begun to produce collagenous and elastic connective tissue fibers (see Fig. 18.1C). As the epidermal ridges form, the dermis projects into the epidermis, forming **dermal papillae**. Capillary loops develop in some of the **dermal ridges** and provide nourishment for the epidermis. Sensory nerve endings form in other ridges. The developing **afferent nerve fibers** apparently play an important role in the spatial and temporal sequence of dermal ridge formation.

The blood vessels in the dermis differentiate from the mesenchyme. As the skin grows, new capillaries grow out of the primordial vessels. Some capillaries acquire muscular coats through the differentiation of myoblasts developing in the surrounding mesenchyme, and they become arterioles, arteries, venules, and veins. By the end of the first trimester, the blood supply of the fetal dermis is well established.

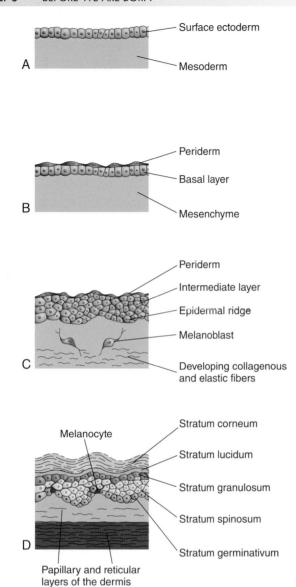

Fig. 18.1 Illustrations of the successive stages of skin development. (A) At 4 weeks. (B) At 7 weeks. (C) At 11 weeks. The cells of the periderm continually undergo keratinization and desquamation. Exfoliated peridermal cells form part of the vernix caseosa. (D) Neonate. Note the melanocytes in the basal layer of the epidermis and the way their processes extend between the epidermal cells to supply them with melanin.

Disorders of Keratinization

Ichthyosis is a general term for a group of skin disorders resulting from **excessive keratinization** (keratin formation). The skin is characterized by dryness and scaling, which may involve the entire body surface (Fig. 18.3). **Harlequin ichthyosis** results from an extremely rare keratinizing disorder that is inherited as an autosomal recessive trait and is caused by a pathogenic variant (mutation) in the *ABCA12* gene. The skin is markedly thickened, ridged, and cracked. Most of the affected neonates require intensive care, and even so, 70% die early. A "**collodion baby**" (prevalence 1:200,000) is covered by a thick, taut membrane that resembles collodion or parchment. This membrane cracks with the first respiratory efforts and begins to fall off in large sheets. Complete shedding of membranes may take several weeks, occasionally leaving normal-appearing skin.

Angiomas of Skin

These vascular anomalies are defects in which transitory and/or surplus blood or lymphatic vessels persist. Those composed of blood vessels may be mainly arterial, venous, or **cavernous** angiomas. Similar lesions that are composed of lymphatics are called **cystic lymphangiomas**, or **cystic hygromas**. True angiomas are benign tumors of endothelial cells, usually composed of solid or hollow cords; the hollow cords contain blood.

Nevus flammeus denotes a flat, pink, or red, flame-like blotch that often appears on the posterior surface of the neck. A **port-wine stain hemangioma** is a larger, darker angioma than a nevus flammeus and is nearly always anterior or lateral on the face, neck, or both.

Albinism

In **generalized (oculocutaneous) albinism**, an autosomal recessive condition (1:20,000), the skin, hair, and retina lack pigment; however, the iris usually shows some pigmentation. There are eight known subtypes of albinism. Albinism occurs when the melanocytes do not produce melanin because of a lack of the enzyme tyrosinase. In *localized albinism*—**piebaldism**—an autosomal dominant trait, there is a lack of melanin in patches of skin, hair, or both.

DEVELOPMENT OF GLANDS

The glands of the skin include sebaceous glands, eccrine and apocrine sweat glands, and mammary glands. They are derived from the epidermis and grow into the dermis (see Fig. 18.2).

SEBACEOUS GLANDS

Most sebaceous glands develop as buds from the sides of the developing **epidermal root sheaths** of the hair follicles (see Fig. 18.2). The buds grow into the surrounding connective tissue and branch to form the primordia of the **alveoli** (hollow sacs) and their associated ducts. The central cells of the alveoli break down, forming sebum, an oily secretion. Sebum is released into the hair follicle and passes to the surface of the skin. It mixes with desquamated peridermal cells to form **vernix caseosa**. Sebaceous glands, independent of the hair follicles (e.g., in the glans penis and labia minora), develop in a similar manner as buds from the epidermis that invade the dermis.

SWEAT GLANDS

Eccrine sweat glands develop as **cellular buds** into the underlying mesenchyme (see Fig. 18.2). As a bud elongates, its end coils to form the primordium of the secretory part of the gland. The epithelial attachment of the developing gland to the epidermis forms the **primordium of the sweat duct**. The central cells of the primordial ducts degenerate, forming a lumen. The peripheral cells of the secretory part of the gland differentiate into *myoepithelial* and *secretory cells* (see Fig. 18.2). The **myoepithelial cells** are believed to be specialized smooth muscle cells that assist in expelling sweat from the glands. Eccrine sweat glands begin to function shortly after birth.

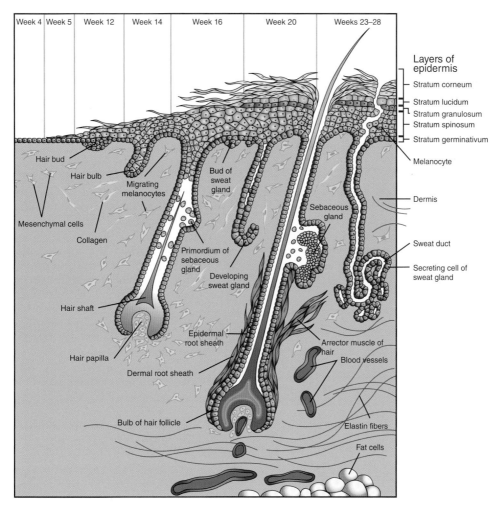

Fig. 18.2 Drawing of the successive stages in the development of hairs, sebaceous glands, and arrector muscles of hair. Note that the sebaceous gland develops as an outgrowth from the side of the hair follicle.

Apocrine sweat glands develop from downgrowths of the stratum germinativum of the epidermis that give rise to the hair follicles (see Fig. 18.2). As a result, the ducts of these glands open into the upper part of the hair follicles, superficial to the openings of the sebaceous glands. These glands are mostly confined to the axillary, pubic, and perineal regions and the areolae surrounding the nipples. Secretion from these glands does not begin until puberty.

DEVELOPMENT OF MAMMARY GLANDS

Mammary glands are modified and highly specialized types of sweat glands. **Mammary buds** begin to develop during the sixth week as solid downgrowths of the epidermis into the underlying mesenchyme (Fig. 18.4C). These changes occur in response to an inductive influence from the mesenchyme. The mammary buds develop from **mammary crests**, which are thickened strips of ectoderm extending from the axillary to the inguinal regions (see Fig. 18.4A). The **mammary crests** appear during the fourth week but normally persist only in the pectoral area where the breasts develop (see Fig. 18.4B). Each primary mammary bud soon gives rise to several secondary mammary buds that develop into the **lactiferous ducts** and their branches (see Fig. 18.4D and E). Canalization of these buds is induced by maternal

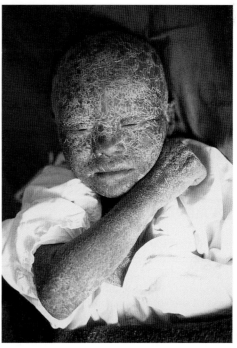

Fig. 18.3 A child with severe keratinization of the skin (ichthyosis) from the time of birth. This particular defect has an autosomal dominant inheritance pattern. Courtesy Dr. Joao Carlos Fernandas Rodrigues, Servico de Dermatologia, Hospital de Desterro, Lisbon, Portugal.

sex hormones entering the fetal circulation. This process continues until late gestation and, by term, 15 to 20 lactiferous ducts have formed. The fibrous connective tissue and fat of the mammary gland develop from the surrounding mesenchyme.

During the late fetal period, the epidermis at the site of origin of the **primordial mammary gland** becomes depressed, forming a shallow **mammary pit** (see Fig. 18.4C and E). The nipples are poorly formed and depressed in neonates. Soon after birth, the nipples usually rise from the mammary pits because of the proliferation of the surrounding connective tissue of the **areola** (see Fig. 18.4F). The mammary glands develop similarly and are of the same structure in both sexes. In females, the glands enlarge rapidly during puberty, mainly because of fat and other connective tissue development in the breasts under the influence of estradiol. Growth of the duct and lobe systems also occurs because of the increased levels of circulating **estrogen** and progesterone.

Gynecomastia

Excessive development of male mammary tissue is termed gynecomastia and occurs in most male neonates because of stimulation of the mammary glands by maternal sex hormones. This effect disappears in a few weeks. During mid-puberty, approximately two-thirds of males have varying degrees of temporary (6–24 months in duration) **hyperplasia** of the breasts. Approximately 80% of males with **Klinefelter syndrome** have gynecomastia (see Fig. 19.7).

Supernumerary Breasts and Nipples

An extra breast **(polymastia)** or nipple **(polythelia)** is an inheritable condition that occurs in approximately 0.2% to 5.6% of the female population. **Supernumerary nipples** are also relatively common in males; they are often mistaken for moles. Polythelia is often found in association with other congenital defects, including renal and urinary tract anomalies. Less commonly, **supernumerary breasts** or nipples appear in the axillary or abdominal regions of females. In these positions, the nipples or breasts arise from extra mammary buds that develop along the mammary crests (see Fig. 18.4A and B).

DEVELOPMENT OF HAIRS

Hairs begin to develop during the 9th to 12th weeks, but they do not become easily recognizable until approximately the 20th week (see Fig. 18.2). Hairs are first recognizable on the eyebrows, upper lip, and chin. A hair follicle begins as a proliferation of the stratum germinativum of the epidermis and extends into the underlying dermis. The **hair bud** soon becomes a club-shaped hair bulb. The epithelial cells of the hair bulb constitute the **germinal matrix**, which later produces the hair. The hair bulb is soon invaginated by a small mesenchymal **hair papilla** (see Fig. 18.2). The peripheral cells of the developing hair follicle form the **epidermal root sheath**, and the surrounding mesenchymal cells differentiate into the **dermal root sheath**. As cells in the germinal matrix proliferate, they are pushed toward the surface, where they **keratinize** to form **hair shafts**. The hair grows through the epidermis on the eyebrows and the upper lip by the end of the 12th week.

The first hairs—lanugo—are fine, soft, and lightly pigmented. Lanugo begins to appear toward the end of the 12th week and is plentiful by 17 to 20 weeks. These hairs help hold the vernix on the skin. Lanugo is replaced during the perinatal period by coarser hairs that persist over most of the body. In the axillary and pubic regions, the lanugo is replaced at puberty by even coarser **terminal hairs**. In males, similar coarse hairs also appear on the face and often on the chest.

Melanoblasts migrate into the hair bulbs and differentiate into melanocytes. The melanin produced by these cells is transferred to the hair-forming cells in the germinal matrix several weeks before birth. The relative content of melanin accounts for different hair colors. **Arrector muscles of hairs**, small bundles of smooth muscle fibers, differentiate from the mesenchyme surrounding the hair follicle and attach to the dermal root sheath and the papillary layer of the dermis (see Fig. 18.2). The arrector muscles are poorly developed in the hairs of the axilla and in certain parts of the face. The hairs forming the eyebrows and eyelashes have no arrector muscles.

DEVELOPMENT OF NAILS

Toenails and fingernails begin to develop at the tips of the digits (fingers and toes) at approximately 10 weeks (Fig. 18.5). Development of the **fingernails** precedes that of the **toenails** by approximately 4 weeks. The primordia of the nails appear as thickened areas, or fields, of the epidermis at the tip of each digit. Later, these **nail fields** migrate onto the dorsal surface (see Fig. 18.5A), carrying their innervation from the ventral surface. The nail fields are surrounded laterally and proximally by folds of epidermis—**nail folds**.

Cells from the proximal nail fold grow over the nail field and keratinize to form the **nail plate** (see Fig. 18.5B). At first, the developing nail is covered by superficial layers of epidermis, the **eponychium** (see Fig. 18.5C). These layers degenerate, exposing the nail, except at its base, where it persists as the **cuticle**. The skin under the free margin of the nail is the **hyponychium** (see Fig. 18.5C). The fingernails reach the fingertips at approximately 32 weeks; the toenails reach the toe tips at approximately 36 weeks.

DEVELOPMENT OF TEETH

Two sets of teeth normally develop: the primary dentition, or **deciduous teeth**, and the secondary dentition, or **permanent teeth**. Teeth develop from the oral ectoderm, mesenchyme, and neural crest cells. The **enamel** is derived from the ectoderm of the oral cavity; all other tissues differentiate from the surrounding mesenchyme and neural crest cells. *Sonic hedgehog signaling is essential for the initiation of tooth development and, with Wnt/β-catenin pathway, regulates many stages of tooth development.*

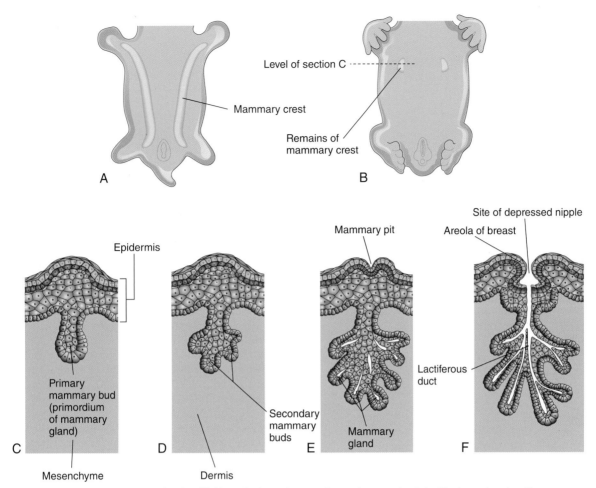

Fig. 18.4 Development of mammary glands. (A) Ventral view of an embryo at approximately 28 days showing the mammary crests. (B) Similar view at 6 weeks showing the remains of these crests. (C) Transverse section of a mammary crest at the site of a developing mammary gland. (D–F) Similar sections showing successive stages of breast development between the 12th week and birth.

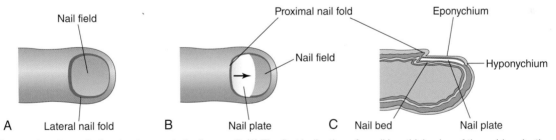

Fig. 18.5 Successive stages in the development of a fingernail. (A) The first indication of a nail is a thickening of the epidermis, the nail field, at the tip of the finger. (B) As the nail plate develops, it slowly grows toward the tip of the finger. (C) The fingernail normally reaches the end of the digit by 32 weeks.

Odontogenesis (tooth development) is initiated by the inductive influence of the **neural crest–induced mesenchyme** on the overlying ectoderm. The first tooth buds appear in the anterior mandibular region; later tooth development occurs in the anterior maxillary region and progresses posteriorly in both jaws. Tooth development continues for years after birth (Table 18.1). The first indication of tooth development is a thickening of the oral epithelium, a derivative of the surface ectoderm seen during the sixth week. These U-shaped bands—**dental laminae**—follow the curves of the primordial jaws (Figs. 18.6A and 18.7A).

BUD STAGE OF TOOTH DEVELOPMENT

Each dental lamina (see Fig. 18.6A) develops 10 centers of proliferation from which **tooth buds** grow into the underlying mesenchyme (see Figs. 18.6B and 18.7B). These buds develop into the **deciduous teeth**, which are shed during childhood (see Table 18.1). There are 10 tooth buds in each jaw, one for each deciduous tooth. The tooth buds for the **permanent teeth** begin to appear at approximately 10 weeks from deep continuations of the dental laminae (see Fig. 18.7D). The permanent molars have no deciduous predecessors; they develop as buds from posterior extensions of the **dental laminae**. The tooth buds for the permanent teeth appear at different times, mostly during the fetal period. The buds for the second and third permanent molars develop after birth.

CAP STAGE OF TOOTH DEVELOPMENT

As each tooth bud is invaginated by mesenchyme—the **primordium of the dental papilla and dental follicle**—the bud becomes cap-shaped (see Fig. 18.7C). The ectodermal part of the developing tooth, the **enamel organ**, eventually produces **enamel**. The internal part of each cap-shaped tooth, the **dental papilla**, is the primordium of the dental pulp. Together, the dental papilla and enamel organ form the

tooth germ (primordial tooth). The outer cell layer of the enamel organ is the **outer enamel epithelium**, whereas the inner cell layer lining the papilla is the **inner enamel epithelium** (see Fig. 18.7D).

The central core of loosely arranged cells between the layers of enamel epithelium is the **enamel reticulum (stellate reticulum)** (see Fig. 18.7E). As the enamel organ and dental papilla develop, the mesenchyme surrounding the developing tooth condenses to form the **dental sac**, a vascularized capsular structure (see Fig. 18.7E). The dental sac is the primordium of the **cement** and **periodontal ligament**. The cement is the bone-like, rigid connective tissue covering the root of the tooth. The periodontal ligament is derived from neural crest cells. It is a specialized vascular connective tissue that surrounds the root of the tooth, separating it from and attaching it to the **alveolar bone** (see Fig. 18.7G).

BELL STAGE OF TOOTH DEVELOPMENT

As the enamel organ differentiates, the developing tooth becomes bell-shaped (Fig. 18.8; see also Fig. 18.7D). The mesenchymal cells in the dental papilla adjacent to the inner enamel epithelium differentiate into **odontoblasts**, which produce **predentin** and deposit it adjacent to the epithelium. Later, the predentin calcifies and becomes **dentin**. As the dentin thickens, the odontoblasts regress toward the center of the dental papilla; however, their cytoplasmic processes—**odontoblastic processes**—remain embedded in dentin (see Fig. 18.7F and I). Enamel is the hardest tissue in the body. It overlies the yellowish dentin, the second hardest tissue in the body, and protects it from being fractured.

Cells of the inner enamel epithelium differentiate into **ameloblasts**, which produce enamel in the form of prisms (rods) over the dentin. As the enamel increases, the ameloblasts regress toward the outer enamel epithelium. The **root of the tooth** begins to develop after dentin and enamel formation are well advanced. The inner and outer enamel epithelia come together at the neck of the tooth, where they form a fold, the **epithelial root sheath** (see Fig. 18.7F). This sheath grows into the mesenchyme and initiates root formation. The odontoblasts adjacent to the epithelial root sheath form dentin that is continuous with that of the crown. As the dentin increases, it reduces the pulp cavity to a narrow **root canal** through which the vessels and nerves pass. The

Table 18.1   The Order and Usual Time of Eruption of Teeth and the Time of Shedding of Deciduous Teeth

Tooth	Usual Eruption Time	Shedding Time
Deciduous		
Medial incisor	6–8 mo	6–7 yr
Lateral incisor	8–10 mo	7–8 yr
Canine	16–20 mo	10–12 yr
First molar	12–16 mo	9–11 yr
Second molar	20–24 mo	10–12 yr
Permanent		
Medial incisor	7–8 yr	
Lateral incisor	8–9 yr	
Canine	10–12 yr	
First premolar	10–11 yr	
Second premolar	11–12 yr	
First molar	6–7 yr	
Second molar	12 yr	
Third molar	13–25 yr	

Data from Moore KL, Dalley AF, Agur AMR: *Clinically oriented anatomy*, ed 6, Baltimore, MD, 2010, Williams & Wilkins.

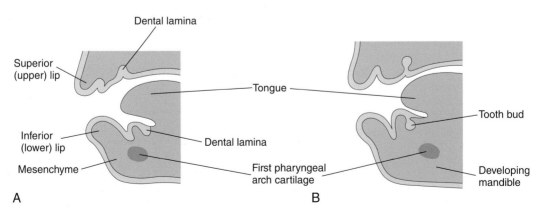

Fig. 18.6 Sketches of sagittal sections through the developing jaws, illustrating early development of the teeth. (A) Early in the sixth week, showing the dental laminae. (B) Later in the sixth week, showing tooth buds arising from the laminae.

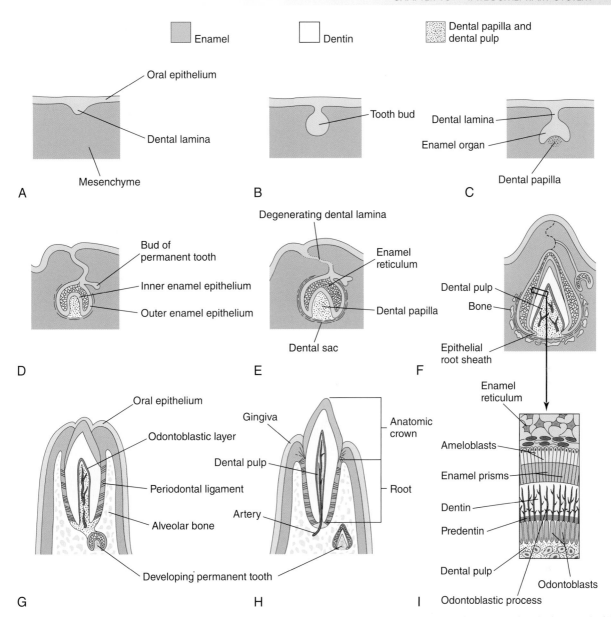

Fig. 18.7 Schematic drawing of sagittal sections illustrating successive stages in the development and eruption of an incisor tooth. (A) At 6 weeks, showing the dental lamina. (B) At 7 weeks, showing the tooth bud developing from the dental lamina. (C) At 8 weeks, showing the cap stage of tooth development. (D) At 10 weeks, showing the early bell stage of a deciduous tooth and the bud stage of a permanent tooth. (E) At 14 weeks, showing the advanced bell stage of tooth development. Note that the connection (dental lamina) of the tooth to the oral epithelium is degenerating. (F) At 28 weeks, showing the enamel and dentin layers. (G) At 6 months postnatally, showing early tooth eruption. (H) At 18 months postnatally, showing a fully erupted deciduous incisor tooth. The incisor tooth now has a well-developed crown. (I) Section through a developing tooth, showing ameloblasts (enamel producers) and odontoblasts (dentin producers).

inner cells of the dental sac differentiate into **cemento-blasts**, which produce cement that is restricted to the root. Cement is deposited over the dentin of the root and meets the enamel at the neck of the tooth.

As the teeth develop and the jaws ossify, the outer cells of the dental sac also become active in bone formation. Each tooth soon becomes surrounded by bone, except over its crown. The tooth is held in its **alveolus** (bony socket) by the strong **periodontal ligament**, a derivative of the dental sac (see Fig. 18.7G and H). Some fibers of this ligament are embedded in the cement of the root; other fibers are embedded in the bony wall of the alveolus. The periodontal ligament is located between the cement of the root and the bony alveolus.

TOOTH ERUPTION

As the **deciduous teeth** develop, they begin a continuous slow movement toward the oral cavity (see Fig. 18.7F and G). The **mandibular teeth** usually erupt before the maxillary teeth, and teeth of females usually erupt sooner. A child's dentition contains **20 deciduous teeth**. As the root of the tooth grows, its crown gradually erupts through the oral epithelium. The part of the oral mucosa around the erupted crown becomes the **gingiva**. Usually, eruption of the deciduous teeth occurs between 6 and 24 months after birth (see Table 18.1). The mandibular medial incisors—or **central incisors**—usually erupt 6 to 8 months after birth,

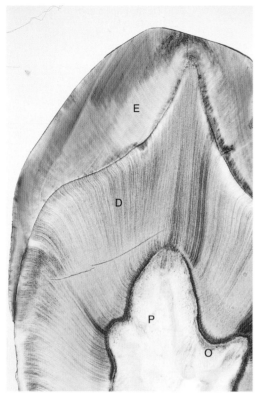

Fig. 18.8 Photomicrograph of a section of the crown and neck of a tooth (×17). Observe the enamel *(E)*, dentin *(D)*, dental pulp *(P)*, and odontoblasts *(O)*. From Gartner LP, Hiatt JL: *Color textbook of histology*, ed 2, Philadelphia, PA, 2001, Saunders.

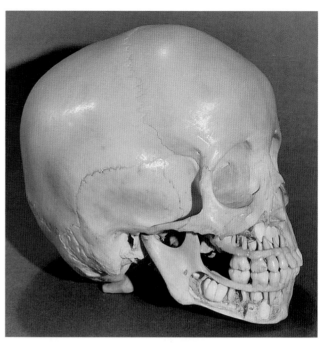

Fig. 18.9 Cranium of a 4-year-old child. Bone has been removed from the jaws to show the relation of the developing permanent teeth to the erupted deciduous teeth.

but this process may not begin until 12 or 13 months in some children. Despite this, all 20 deciduous teeth are usually present by the end of the second year in healthy children.

The **permanent teeth** develop in a manner similar to that described for deciduous teeth. As a permanent tooth grows, the root of the corresponding deciduous tooth is gradually resorbed by **osteoclasts**. Consequently, when the deciduous tooth is shed, it consists only of the crown and the cervical, or uppermost, part of the root. The permanent teeth usually begin to erupt during the 6th year and continue to appear until early adulthood (Fig. 18.9; see also Table 18.1).

Enamel Hypoplasia

Defective enamel formation causes pits, fissures, or both in the enamel of teeth (Fig. 18.10). These defects result from temporary disturbances in enamel formation. Various factors may injure ameloblasts (source of enamel), such as nutritional deficiency, tetracycline therapy, and infectious diseases. **Rickets** arising during the critical period of permanent tooth development (6–12 weeks) is the most common cause of enamel hypoplasia.

Variations of Tooth Shape

Abnormally shaped teeth are relatively common. Occasionally there are spherical masses of enamel—**enamel pearls**—attached to the tooth (see Fig. 18.10E). They are formed by **aberrant groups of ameloblasts**. In other cases, the maxillary lateral incisor teeth may have a slender, tapered shape (peg-shaped incisors). **Congenital syphilis** affects the differentiation of the permanent teeth, resulting in incisors with central notches.

Numeric Abnormalities of Teeth

One or more **supernumerary teeth** may develop, or the normal number of teeth may not form (see Fig. 18.10D). Supernumerary teeth usually develop in the area of the maxillary incisors and may disrupt the position and eruption of normal teeth. The extra teeth commonly erupt posterior to the normal teeth. In **partial anodontia**, one or more teeth are absent. Congenital absence of one or more teeth (**tooth agenesis**) is often a familial trait. In **total anodontia**, no teeth develop; this very rare condition is usually associated with **congenital ectodermal dysplasia**.

Macrodontia (a single large tooth) is a condition caused by the union of two adjacent tooth germs. The crowns of the two teeth can be partially or completely fused. The same applies to roots. Occasionally, a tooth bud divides or two buds partially fuse to form fused teeth. This condition is commonly observed in the mandibular incisors of the primary dentition, but it can also occur in the permanent dentition.

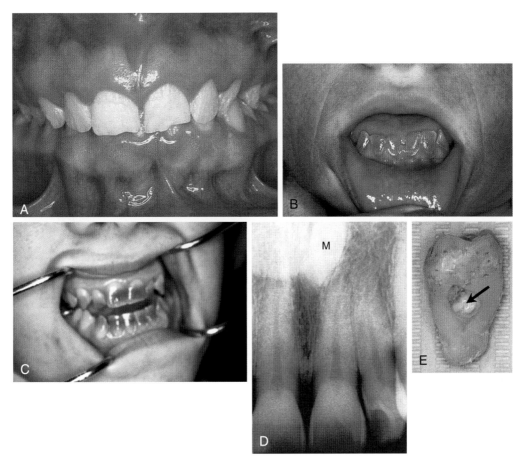

Fig. 18.10   Common tooth anomalies. (A) Amelogenesis imperfecta. (B) Dentinogenesis imperfecta. (C) Tetracycline-stained teeth. (D) Midline supernumerary tooth (*M*, mesiodens), located near the root apex of the central incisor. (E) Molar tooth with an enamel pearl *(arrow)*. A, Courtesy Dr. Cleghorn B, Faculty of Dentistry, Dalhousie University, Halifax, Nova Scotia, Canada; B to D, Courtesy Dr. Steve Ahing, Faculty of Dentistry, University of Manitoba, Winnipeg, Manitoba, Canada.

Amelogenesis Imperfecta

In amelogenesis imperfecta, the tooth enamel is soft and friable because of **hypocalcification** and the teeth are yellow to brown in color (see Fig. 18.10A). Pathogenic variants (mutational defects) of AMELX, ENAM, MMP20, KLK4, and other genes that encode for enamel, dentin, and mineralization are likely involved. The teeth are covered with only a thin layer of abnormally formed enamel through which the color of the underlying dentin is visible, giving the teeth a darkened appearance. This rare autosomal dominant condition affects approximately 1 in 700 (in Sweden) to 1 in 12,000 children (in the United States).

Dentinogenesis Imperfecta

Dentinogenesis imperfecta is relatively common in Caucasian children (see Fig. 18.10B). In affected children, the teeth are brown to gray-blue, with an opalescent sheen. This is caused by the failure of the odontoblasts to differentiate normally, producing poorly calcified dentin. Both deciduous and permanent teeth are usually involved. The enamel tends to wear down rapidly, exposing the dentin. This defect is inherited as an autosomal dominant trait, most commonly involving chromosome 4q21.

Discolored Teeth

Foreign substances discolor the teeth if they are incorporated into the developing enamel and dentin. The hemolysis associated with **hemolytic disease** of the neonate (see Chapter 8) may produce blue to black discoloration of the teeth. The critical period of risk is from approximately 14 weeks of fetal life to the 10th postnatal month for deciduous teeth, and from approximately 14 weeks of fetal life to the 16th postnatal year for permanent teeth. *All tetracyclines are extensively incorporated into the teeth* and produce brownish-yellow discoloration (mottling) and enamel hypoplasia because they interfere with the metabolic processes of the ameloblasts (see Fig. 18.10C). The enamel is completely formed on all but the third molars by approximately 8 years of age. For this reason, tetracyclines should not be administered to pregnant women or to children younger than 8 years.

CLINICALLY ORIENTED QUESTIONS

1. A neonate was reportedly born without skin. Is this possible? If so, could such an infant survive?

2. A dark-skinned person presented with patches of white skin on the face, chest, and limbs. He even had a white forelock. What is this condition called, and what is its developmental basis? Is there any treatment for these skin defects?

3. Some males have enlarged breasts at birth. Is this an indication of abnormal sex development?

4. A girl developed a breast in the axilla during puberty. She also had an extra nipple on her chest. What is the embryological basis for these birth defects?

5. A neonate was born with two teeth. Would they be normal teeth? Is this a common occurrence? Are they usually extracted?

The answers to these questions are at the back of this book.

Human Birth Defects 19

Birth defects are developmental disorders (congenital anomalies) present at birth and are the leading cause of infant mortality. Globally, approximately to 6% of children are born annually with a birth defect. Birth defects may be structural, functional, metabolic, or behavioral. Babies born with isolated or multiple congenital anomalies are usually evaluated by a clinical geneticist so that a diagnosis can be determined. Genetic counseling is an important component of the clinical investigation and follow-up for the families. There are four clinically significant types of birth defects:

- **Malformation:** A morphological defect of an organ, part of an organ, or larger region of the body resulting from an intrinsically abnormal developmental process
- **Disruption:** A morphological defect of an organ, part of an organ, or larger region of the body resulting from the extrinsic breakdown of, or an interference with, an originally normal developmental process
- **Deformation:** An abnormal form, shape, or position of a part of the body caused by mechanical force
- **Dysplasia:** An abnormal organization of cells into tissue(s) and its morphological result(s)—a process and consequence of dyshistogenesis.

Other descriptive terms are used to describe infants with multiple defects including, and these have evolved to express causation and pathogenesis: **polytopic field defect, sequence, syndrome, and association**.

TERATOLOGY: STUDY OF ABNORMAL DEVELOPMENT

Teratology is the branch of science that studies the causes, mechanisms, and patterns of abnormal development. A fundamental concept in teratology is that certain stages of embryonic development are more vulnerable to disruption than others (see Fig. 19.11).

More than 20% of infant deaths in North America are attributable to birth defects. Major structural anomalies are observed in approximately 3% of neonates. Additional defects may only be detected after birth. The incidence of birth defects approaches 6% in 2-year-old infants and 8% in 5-year-old children.

The causes of birth defects may be due to **genetic factors**, such as chromosomal abnormalities, and **environmental factors**, such as drugs. However, many common defects are the result of **multifactorial inheritance;** that is, they are caused by genetic and environmental factors acting together; epigenetic mechanisms may also be involved. For 50% to 60%

of birth defects, the etiology is unknown (Fig. 19.1). Birth defects may be single or involve multiple organ systems and are of major or minor clinical significance.

Single minor defects are present in approximately 14% of neonates. Some of these defects are of no serious medical significance, but they may indicate the presence of associated major defects. For example, the presence of a single umbilical artery alerts a clinician to the possible presence of cardiovascular and renal anomalies.

Major defects are much more common in early embryos (10%–15%), but most of these embryos abort spontaneously during the first 6 weeks. **Chromosomal abnormalities** are present in more than 50% to 60% of spontaneously aborted embryos.

BIRTH DEFECTS CAUSED BY GENETIC FACTORS

Numerically, *genetic factors are the most important cause of birth defects.* Pathogenic variants (mutations) in genes are common causes of birth defects. It has been estimated that they cause approximately one-third of all defects (see Fig. 19.1). Persons with chromosomal abnormalities usually have characteristic phenotypes, such as the physical characteristics of individuals with Down syndrome (trisomy 21) (see Fig. 19.4). A process as complex as mitosis or meiosis can occasionally result in chromosomal aberrations, which are present in 6% to 7% of zygotes. The changes may affect the sex chromosomes, the autosomes, or both. Many early embryos never undergo normal cleavage to become blastocysts.

NUMERICAL CHROMOSOMAL ABNORMALITIES

The chromosomes in somatic (body) cells are normally paired. The **homologous chromosomes** making up a pair are homologs. Normal females have 22 pairs of autosomes plus two X chromosomes, whereas normal males have 22 pairs of autosomes plus one X and one Y chromosome. Numerical aberrations of chromosomes (aneuploidy) usually result from **nondisjunction**, an error in cell division in which a chromosome pair or two chromatids of a chromosome do not disjoin during mitosis or meiosis. As a result, the chromosome pair or chromatids pass to one daughter cell, whereas the other cell receives neither (Fig. 19.2). Nondisjunction may occur during maternal or paternal gametogenesis (see Chapter 2). Other mechanisms that result in aneuploidy include reverse segregation and precocious separation of sister chromatids.

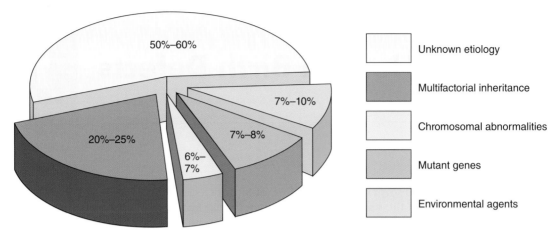

Fig. 19.1 Graphic illustration of the causes of human birth defects. Note that the causes of most defects are unknown and that 20% to 25% of them are caused by a combination of genetic and environmental factors (multifactorial inheritance).

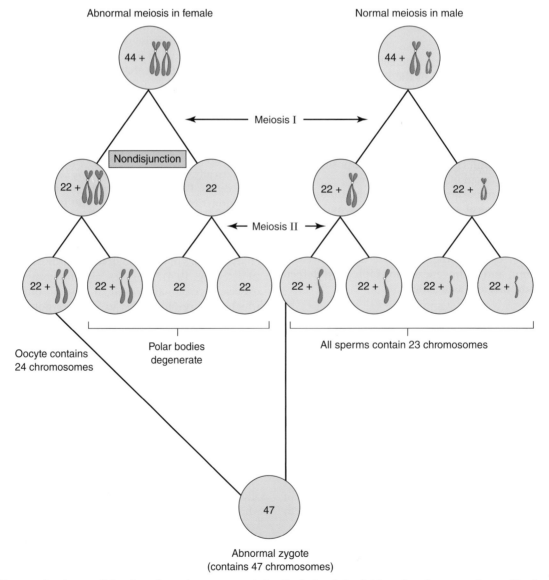

Fig. 19.2 Diagram showing nondisjunction of sex chromosomes during the first meiotic division of a primary oocyte, resulting in an abnormal oocyte with 24 chromosomes. Subsequent fertilization by a normal sperm produces a zygote with 47 chromosomes—aneuploidy—a deviation from the human diploid number of 46.

Inactivation of Genes

During embryogenesis, one of the two X chromosomes in female somatic cells is randomly inactivated and appears as a mass of **sex chromatin**. Inactivation of the genes on one X chromosome in the somatic cells of female embryos occurs early in embryonic development.

X-inactivation is important clinically because it means that each cell from a carrier of an X-linked disease has the pathogenic variant (mutation) associated with the disease, either on the active X chromosome or on the inactivated X chromosome that is represented by sex chromatin. Skewed X-inactivation in monozygotic twins is one reason given for discordance in a variety of birth defects. The genetic basis for discordance is that one twin preferentially expresses the paternal X and the other, the maternal X. Certain autosomal genes can also be inactivated (silenced) due to methylation (epigenetic effects).

Turner Syndrome (Monosomy X)

Only about 1% of female embryos with monosomy X survive. The most frequent chromosome constitution is 45,X; however, almost 50% have other X chromosome anomalies. The incidence of 45,X—or **Turner syndrome**—in neonates is approximately 1 in 8000 live births. The **phenotype** of Turner syndrome is female (Fig. 19.3). Phenotype refers to the morphological characteristics of an individual, as determined by the genotype and environment in which it is expressed. Secondary sexual characteristics do not develop completely in 90% of girls with Turner syndrome, necessitating hormone replacement therapy.

The monosomy X chromosomal abnormality is the most common cytogenetic abnormality observed in live-born neonates and in fetuses that abort spontaneously; it accounts for approximately 18% of all spontaneous abortions caused by chromosomal abnormalities. In approximately 75% of cases, it is the paternal X chromosome that is missing.

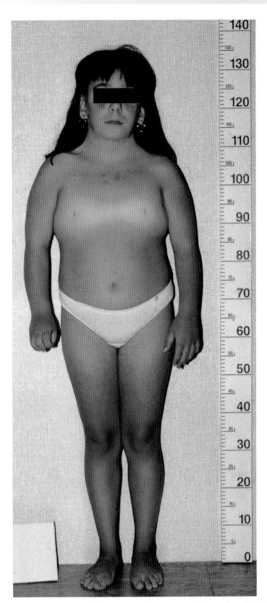

Fig. 19.3 Turner syndrome in a 14-year-old girl. Note the classic features of the syndrome: short stature; webbed neck; absence of sexual maturation; broad chest with widely spaced nipples; and lymphedema swelling of the hands and feet. *Courtesy Dr. F. Antoniazzi and Dr. V. Fanos, Department of Pediatrics, University of Verona, Verona, Italy.*

Aneuploidy and Polyploidy

Changes in chromosome number result in either aneuploidy or polyploidy. **Aneuploidy** is any deviation from the diploid number of 46 chromosomes, that is, not an exact multiple of the haploid number of 23 (e.g., 45 or 47). The principal cause of aneuploidy is nondisjunction during cell division (see Fig. 19.2), resulting in an unequal distribution of one pair of homologous chromosomes to the daughter cells. One cell has two chromosomes and the other has neither chromosome of the pair. As a result, the embryo's cells may be hypodiploid (e.g., 45,X, or Turner syndrome) (see Fig. 19.3) or hyperdiploid, usually 47, as in trisomy 21 or Down syndrome (Fig. 19.4). Embryos with **monosomy**—missing a chromosome—usually die.

TRISOMY

If three chromosomes of one type are present instead of the usual pair, the abnormality is called **trisomy**. Trisomies are the most common abnormalities of chromosome number. The usual cause of this numerical error is meiotic nondisjunction of chromosomes (see Fig. 19.2), resulting in a gamete with 24 instead of 23 chromosomes and, subsequently, a zygote with 47 chromosomes.

Trisomy of autosomes is associated mainly with three syndromes (Table 19.1):

- Trisomy 21 or Down syndrome (see Fig. 19.4)
- Trisomy 18 or Edwards syndrome (Fig. 19.5)
- Trisomy 13 or Patau syndrome (Fig. 19.6).

Table 19.1   Trisomy of Autosomes

Chromosomal Aberration/Syndrome	Incidence	Usual Morphological Characteristics	Figures
Trisomy 21 (Down syndrome)[a]	1:800	Intellectual disability; brachycephaly; flat nasal bridge; upward slant to palpebral fissures; protruding tongue; simian crease; clinodactyly of fifth digit; congenital heart defects	19.4
Trisomy 18 (Edwards syndrome)[b]	1:8,000	Neurocognitive impairment; prominent occiput; short sternum; ventricular septal defect; micrognathia; low-set, malformed ears; flexed digits; hypoplastic nails; rocker-bottom feet	19.5
Trisomy 13 (Patau syndrome)[b]	1:25,000	Neurocognitive impairment; severe central nervous system malformations; sloping forehead; malformed ears; scalp defects; microphthalmia; bilateral cleft lip or palate; polydactyly; posterior prominence of heels	19.6

[a]The incidence of trisomy 21 at fertilization is greater than that at birth; however, 75% of affected embryos are spontaneously aborted and at least 20% are stillborn.
[b]Infants with this syndrome rarely survive beyond 6 months of age.

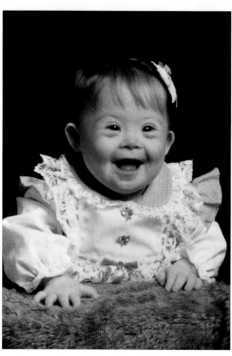

Fig. 19.4   A child with Down syndrome (trisomy 21). Note the round face, up-slanted palpebral fissures, and short digits with incurving of the fifth digit (clinodactyly). Courtesy A.E. Chudley, MD, Section of Genetics and Metabolism, Department of Pediatrics and Child Health, Children's Hospital and University of Manitoba, Winnipeg, Manitoba, Canada.

Table 19.2   Incidence of Down Syndrome in Neonates

Maternal Age (Yr)	Incidence
20–24	1:1400
25–29	1:1100
30–34	1:700
35	1:350
37	1:225
39	1:140
41	1:85
43	1:50
45+	1:25

Mosaicism

Mosaicism occurs when an individual has at least two cell lines with two or more different genotypes (genetic constitutions). Either the autosomes or sex chromosomes may be involved. Usually, the birth defects are less serious than in persons with monosomy or trisomy (e.g., features of the Turner syndrome are not as evident in 45,X/46,XX mosaicism as in the usual 45,X genotype). **Mosaicism** usually results from nondisjunction during early cleavage of the zygote (see Chapter 3). Mosaicism resulting from loss of a chromosome by anaphase lagging also occurs; the chromosomes separate normally, but one of them is delayed in its migration and is eventually lost.

Infants with trisomy 13 and trisomy 18 have multiple anomalies and severe neurodevelopmental disorders. These life-limiting disorders typically result in a 1-year survival of 6% to 12%. More than 50% of **trisomic embryos** spontaneously abort early. Trisomy of the autosomes occurs with increasing frequency as maternal age increases (Table 19.2). The incidence of trisomy 21 syndrome in the United States is estimated to be 1:800 live births. Molecular and pathophysiological studies of the different phenotypes of trisomy 21 suggest that this condition is a disorder of gene expression dysregulation.

Trisomy of the sex chromosomes is a common condition (Table 19.3); however, because no characteristic physical findings are seen in infants or children, this defect is not usually detected before puberty (Fig. 19.7). The diagnosis is best established by chromosomal and molecular analysis.

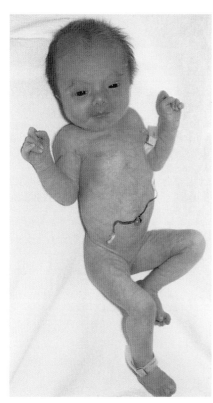

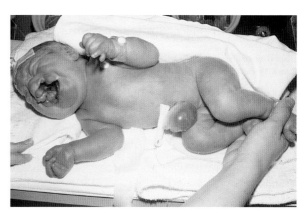

Fig. 19.6   Female neonate with trisomy 13. Note the bilateral cleft lip; low-set, malformed ears; and polydactyly (extra digits). A small omphalocele (herniation of viscera into the umbilical cord) is also present. Courtesy A.E. Chudley, MD, Section of Genetics and Metabolism, Department of Pediatrics and Child Health, Children's Hospital and University of Manitoba, Winnipeg, Manitoba, Canada.

Fig. 19.5   Female neonate with trisomy 18. Note the growth retardation, clenched fists with characteristic positioning of the fingers (second and fifth digits overlapping the third and fourth), short sternum, and narrow pelvis. Courtesy A.E. Chudley, MD, Section of Genetics and Metabolism, Department of Pediatrics and Child Health, Children's Hospital and University of Manitoba, Winnipeg, Manitoba, Canada.

Triploidy and Tetraploidy

The most common type of polyploidy is **triploidy** (69 chromosomes). Triploid fetuses have severe intrauterine growth restriction (IUGR), with a disproportionately small trunk and other defects. Most often, triploidy results when an oocyte is fertilized by two sperms **(dispermy)** almost simultaneously. Triploidy may also result if the second polar body does not separate from the oocyte during the second meiotic division (see Chapter 2). Triploidy occurs in approximately 2% of embryos but most of them abort spontaneously. Triploid fetuses account for approximately 20% of chromosomally abnormal spontaneous abortions. Doubling of the diploid chromosome number to 92 **(tetraploidy)** probably occurs during the first cleavage division. Division of this abnormal zygote would subsequently result in an embryo with cells containing 92 chromosomes. **Tetraploid embryos** abort very early; often, all that is recovered is an empty chorionic sac (blighted embryo).

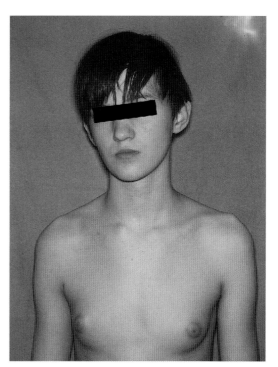

Fig. 19.7   A teenage boy with Klinefelter syndrome (XXY trisomy). Note the presence of developed breasts; approximately 40% of males with this syndrome have gynecomastia (excessive development of the male mammary glands) and small testes. Courtesy Children's Hospital and University of Manitoba, Winnipeg, Manitoba, Canada.

STRUCTURAL CHROMOSOMAL ABNORMALITIES

Most abnormalities of chromosome structure result from **chromosome breakage**, followed by reconstitution in an abnormal combination (Fig. 19.8). Chromosome breakage may be induced by various environmental factors, such as irradiation, drugs, chemicals, and viruses. The resulting abnormality in chromosome structure depends on what happens to the broken pieces. The only two aberrations of chromosome structure that are likely to be transmitted from parent to child are structural rearrangements, such as inversion and translocation.

Table 19.3   Trisomy of Sex Chromosomes

Chromosome Complement[a]	Sex	Incidence	Usual Characteristics
47,XXX	Female	1:1000	Normal appearance; usually fertile; 15%–25% have an increased risk of developmental delays and learning disabilities
47,XXY	Male	1:1000	Klinefelter syndrome; small testes; hyalinization of seminiferous tubules; aspermatogenesis; often tall, with disproportionately long lower limbs; intelligence is less than in normal siblings; gynecomastia is approximately 40%
47,XYY	Male	1:1000	Normal appearance, usually tall, and behavioral problems

Data from Nussbaum RL, McInnes RR, Willard HF: *Thompson & Thompson genetics in medicine*, ed 8, Philadelphia, PA, 2015, Saunders.
[a]The number designates the total number of chromosomes, including the sex chromosomes (shown after the comma).

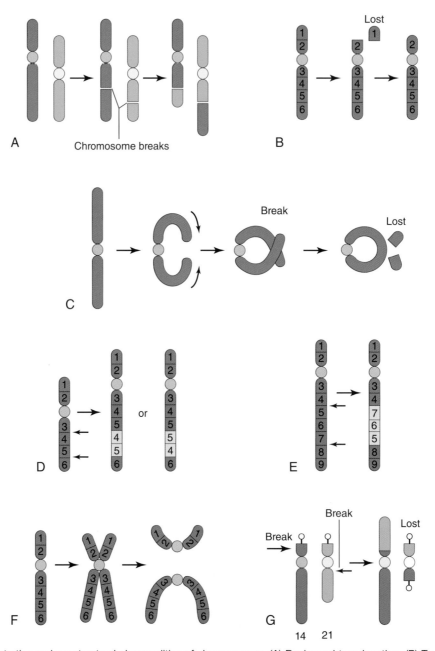

Fig. 19.8   Diagrams illustrating various structural abnormalities of chromosomes. (A) Reciprocal translocation. (B) Terminal deletion. (C) Ring chromosome. (D) Duplication. (E) Paracentric inversion. (F) Isochromosome. (G) Robertsonian translocation. *Arrows* indicate how the structural abnormalities are produced. Modified from Nussbaum RL, McInnes RR, Willard HE: *Thomson & Thompson genetics in medicine*, ed 6, Philadelphia, PA, 2004, Saunders.

INVERSION

Inversion is a chromosomal aberration in which a segment of a chromosome is reversed. Paracentric inversion is confined to a single arm of the chromosome (see Fig. 19.8E), whereas pericentric inversion involves both arms and includes the centromere. Carriers of pericentric inversions are at risk for having offspring with birth defects because of unequal crossing over and malsegregation at meiosis.

TRANSLOCATION

Translocation is the transfer of a piece of one chromosome to a nonhomologous chromosome. If two nonhomologous chromosomes exchange pieces, it is called a **reciprocal translocation** (see Fig. 19.8A). Translocation does not necessarily cause abnormal development. Persons with a **Robertsonian translocation** (the most common structural chromosomal abnormality in the general public) between chromosome 21 and chromosome 14, for example (see Fig. 19.8G), are phenotypically normal. Such persons are called **balanced translocation carriers**. They have a tendency, independent of age, to produce germ cells with an abnormal translocation chromosome. Between 3% and 4% of persons with Down syndrome have trisomy due to the extra chromosome 21 being attached to another chromosome.

DELETION

When a chromosome breaks, a portion of it may be lost (see Fig. 19.8B). A partial terminal deletion from the short arm of chromosome 5 causes **cri du chat syndrome**. Affected neonates have a weak, cat-like cry at birth; microcephaly (small neurocranium); hypertelorism (wide-set eyes); low-set ears; micrognathia (a small jaw); global developmental delays; and congenital heart disease.

A **ring chromosome** is a type of deletion chromosome from which both ends have been lost and the broken ends have rejoined to form a ring-shaped chromosome (see Fig. 19.8C). **Ring chromosomes** are very rare, but they have been found for all chromosomes. These abnormal chromosomes have been described in persons with Turner syndrome, trisomy 18, and other abnormalities.

DUPLICATIONS

Duplications may be manifested as a duplicated part of a chromosome located within a chromosome (see Fig. 19.8D), as a duplicated part attached to a chromosome, or as a separate fragment. Duplications are more common than deletions, and they are less harmful because no loss of genetic material occurs. Duplication may involve part of a gene, a whole gene, or a series of genes.

ISOCHROMOSOMES

The abnormality resulting in **isochromosomes** occurs when the centromere divides transversely instead of longitudinally (see Fig. 19.8F). An isochromosome is a chromosome in which one arm is missing and the other is duplicated. It appears to be the most common structural abnormality of the X chromosome. Persons with this chromosomal abnormality are often short in stature and have other stigmata of Turner syndrome. These characteristics are related to the loss of an arm of an X chromosome.

Molecular Cytogenetics

Methods for merging classic cytogenetics with **DNA technology** have facilitated precise definitions of chromosome abnormalities, location, and origins, including unbalanced translocations, accessory or marker chromosomes, and **gene mapping**. One approach to chromosome identification is based on **fluorescent in situ hybridization (FISH)**, in which chromosome-specific **DNA probes** adhere to complementary regions located on specific chromosomes. FISH techniques applied to interphase cells may soon obviate the need to culture cells for specific chromosome analysis, as in the case of prenatal diagnosis of fetal trisomies.

Comparative genomic hybridization (CGH) can detect and map changes in specific regions of the genome. **Microarray-based CGH** (array comparative genomic hybridization), also referred to as chromosomal microarray analysis, has been used to identify genomic rearrangements and changes in copy number in individuals who were previously considered to have cognitive deficiency or multiple birth defects of unknown origin despite normal test results from traditional chromosome or gene analysis. A chromosome **single-nucleotide polymorphism array** is a more refined genetic test that is able to detect very small changes in a person's chromosomes and has replaced the use of CGH in clinical practice.

Noninvasive prenatal testing is available clinically in some jurisdictions for the detection of certain aneuploidies. Advances in genomic sequencing (GS) technology using whole exome sequencing and whole GS have further defined smaller regions of genomic rearrangements (deletions/duplications) and changes at the base-pair level. These technologies have transformed the ability to diagnose individuals with suspected genetic disorders. Genetic counseling is indicated at the pre- and posttest stage for families considering sequencing. Rapid trio-based (proband and both parents) GS of neonates in the intensive care unit has dramatically impacted the time to diagnosis, care, and management of these babies.

BIRTH DEFECTS CAUSED BY PATHOGENIC VARIANTS IN GENES

Exome sequencing and genome sequencing have identified the genetic cause of numerous different single-gene disorders with birth defects. A **pathogenic (disease-causing) variant**, usually involving a loss or change in the function of a gene, is a permanent change in the sequence of genomic DNA. Variants can be classified as pathogenic, likely pathogenic, benign, or a variant of unknown significance. Pathogenic variants can be inherited from a parent or be the result of a new change (de novo).

The mutation rate can be increased by a number of environmental agents, such as large doses of radiation. Birth defects resulting from gene mutations are inherited according to **Mendelian laws** (the laws of inheritance of single-gene traits that form the basis of the science of genetics); consequently, predictions can be made about the probability of their occurrence in the affected person's children and other relatives.

An example of an autosomal dominant disorder that can be inherited or de novo is inherited **achondroplasia**—abnormality in the conversion of cartilage to bone (Fig. 19.9)—which results from a mutation of the complementary DNA

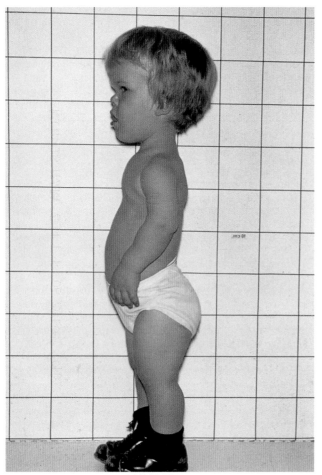

Fig. 19.9 A young boy with achondroplasia. Note the short stature, short limbs and fingers, normal length of the trunk, relatively large head, prominent forehead, and depressed nasal bridge. Courtesy A.E. Chudley AE, MD, Section of Genetics and Metabolism, Department of Pediatrics and Child Health, Children's Hospital and University of Manitoba, Winnipeg, Manitoba, Canada.

in the fibroblast growth factor receptor 3 gene on chromosome 4p. Other birth defects are attributable to autosomal recessive inheritance. Autosomal recessive genes manifest themselves only when homozygous; as a consequence, many carriers of these genes (heterozygous persons) are not identified.

Fragile X syndrome is the most commonly known inherited cause of intellectual disability. Autism spectrum disorders and attention deficit hyperactivity disorder are also prevalent in this condition (Fig. 19.10). Fragile X syndrome occurs in 1 of 4000 male births. Diagnosis of this syndrome can be confirmed by chromosome analysis showing the full expansion (>200 triplet repeats of CGG nucleotides) in a specific region of the FMR1 gene.

Several genetic disorders are caused by the expansion of trinucleotides (combination of three adjacent nucleotides) in specific genes. Examples include myotonic dystrophy type 1, Huntington disease, spinobulbar atrophy (Kennedy syndrome), and Friedreich ataxia.

The **human genome** comprises an estimated 25,000 to 31,000 protein-coding genes per haploid set or 3 billion base pairs; the exact number remains unsettled. Because of the **Human Genome Project** and international research collaboration, many disease-causing and birth defect-causing mutations in genes have been and will continue to be identified. Understanding the cause of birth defects will require an improvement in our understanding of gene expression during early development.

Most genes that are expressed in a cell are expressed in a wide variety of cells. These **housekeeping genes** are involved in basic cellular metabolic functions, such as nucleic acid and protein synthesis, cytoskeleton and organelle biogenesis, and nutrient transport and mechanisms. The **specialty genes** are expressed at specific times in specific cells and define the hundreds of different cell types that make up the human organism. An essential aspect of developmental biology is the regulation of gene expression. Regulation is often achieved by transcription factors, which bind to regulatory or promoter elements of specific genes.

Genomic imprinting is an epigenetic process in which the allele inherited from the mother or father is marked by methylation (imprinted), silencing the gene and allowing expression of the nonimprinted gene from the other parent. When imprinting occurs, only the paternal or maternal allele (any one of a series of two or more different genes) of a gene is active in the offspring. The sex of the transmitting parent, therefore, influences expression or nonexpression of certain genes.

BIRTH DEFECTS CAUSED BY ENVIRONMENTAL FACTORS

Although the embryo is well protected in the uterus, certain environmental agents—**teratogens**—may cause developmental disruptions after maternal exposure to them (Table 19.4). A teratogen is any agent that can produce a birth defect or increase the incidence of a defect in a population. Environmental factors, such as infections and drugs, may simulate genetic conditions, such as when two or more children of normal parents are affected. The important principle to remember is that not everything that is familial is genetic.

The cells, tissues, and organs of an embryo are most sensitive to teratogenic agents during periods of rapid differentiation (Fig. 19.11). Because molecular signaling and embryonic induction precede morphological differentiation, the period during which structures are sensitive to interference by teratogens often precedes the stage of their visible development.

Rapid progress in molecular biology is providing additional information on the genetic control of differentiation and the cascade of molecular signals and factors controlling gene expression and pattern formation. Researchers are now directing increasing attention to the molecular mechanisms of abnormal development in an attempt to understand better the pathogenesis of birth defects.

PRINCIPLES OF TERATOGENESIS

When considering the possible teratogenicity of an agent, such as a drug or a chemical, three factors are important to consider:

- Critical periods of development (see Fig. 19.11)
- Dose of the drug or chemical
- Genotype (genetic constitution) of the embryo.

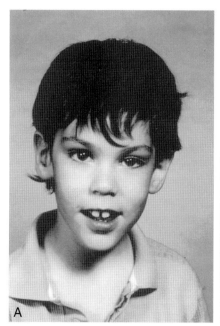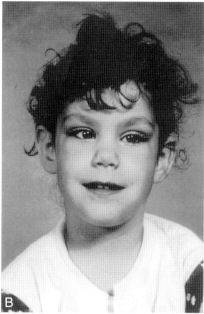

Fig. 19.10   Fragile X syndrome. (A) An 8-year-old boy with this syndrome exhibiting a relatively normal appearance, with a long face and prominent ears. He also has significant cognitive impairment. (B) His 6-year-old sister also has this syndrome. She has a mild learning disability and similar features of long face and prominent ears. Note the strabismus (crossed right eye). Although an X-linked disorder, female carriers sometimes express the disorder. *Courtesy A.E. Chudley, MD, Section of Genetics and Metabolism, Department of Pediatrics and Child Health, Children's Hospital and University of Manitoba, Winnipeg, Manitoba, Canada.*

CRITICAL PERIODS OF HUMAN DEVELOPMENT

An embryo's susceptibility to a teratogen depends on its stage of development when an agent, such as a drug, is present. The most **critical period** in development is when cell differentiation and morphogenesis are at their peak. For example, the most critical period for brain development is from 3 to 16 weeks (see Fig. 19.11), but its development may be disrupted by teratogens after this time because the brain is differentiating and growing rapidly at birth.

Tooth development continues long after birth; hence, the development of the permanent teeth may be disrupted by tetracyclines from 18 weeks prenatal to 16 years of age. The **skeletal system** has a prolonged critical period of development, extending into childhood; hence, the growth of skeletal tissues provides a good gauge of general growth.

Environmental disturbances during the first 2 weeks after fertilization may interfere with cleavage of the zygote and implantation of the blastocyst, which may cause early death and spontaneous abortion of the embryo (see Fig. 19.11).

Development of the embryo is most easily disrupted when the tissues and organs are forming (see Fig. 19.11). During this **organogenetic period (fourth to eighth weeks)**, teratogenic agents may induce major birth defects. Physiological defects—minor morphological defects of the external ear, for example—and functional disturbances, such as limitation of mental development, are likely to result from disruption of development during the fetal period. Each part, tissue, and organ of an embryo has a critical period during which its development may be disrupted (see Fig. 19.11). The type of birth defect produced depends on which parts, tissues, and organs are most susceptible at the time the teratogen is active.

Embryological timetables, such as the one in Fig. 19.11, are helpful when considering the cause of birth defects.

However, it is incorrect to assume that defects always result from a single event occurring during the critical period of development or that it is possible to determine from these timetables the day on which a defect was produced. What is known is that the teratogen would have to disrupt the development of the tissue, part, or organ before the end of the critical period.

HUMAN TERATOGENS

Awareness that certain agents can disrupt prenatal development offers the opportunity to prevent some birth defects. For example, when made aware of the harmful effects of drugs, alcohol, cigarette smoking (nicotine), environmental chemicals, and viruses, most pregnant women will avoid exposure to these teratogenic agents.

Drugs vary considerably in their teratogenicity. Some teratogens, such as thalidomide, cause severe disruption of development if administered during the organogenetic period of certain parts (e.g., the limbs) of the embryo (see Fig. 19.15). Other teratogens cause mental and growth restrictions of embryos (see Table 19.4). Despite this, less than 2% of birth defects are caused by drugs and chemicals. Only a few drugs have been positively implicated as human teratogenic agents, but new agents continue to be identified. It is best to avoid using all medications during the first trimester unless a strong medical reason exists for their use.

CIGARETTE SMOKING

Maternal smoking during pregnancy is a well-established cause of **IUGR**. Despite warnings that cigarette smoking is harmful to the embryo/fetus, more than 25% of females

Table 19.4   Some Teratogens Known to Cause Human Birth Defects

Agents	Most Common Congenital Birth Defects
Drugs	
Alcohol	Fetal alcohol syndrome; IUGR; mental deficiency; microcephaly; ocular defects; joint abnormalities; short palpebral fissures; fetal alcohol spectrum disorders; cognitive and neurobehavioral disturbances
Androgens and high doses of progestogens	Varying degree of masculinization of female fetuses; ambiguous external genitalia (labial fusion and clitoral hypertrophy)
Cocaine	IUGR; prematurity; microcephaly; cerebral infarction; urogenital defects; neurobehavioral disturbances
Diethylstilbestrol	Abnormalities of uterus and vagina; cervical erosion and ridges
Isotretinoin (13-*cis*-retinoic acid)	Craniofacial abnormalities; neural tube defects such as spina bifida cystica; cardiovascular defects; cleft palate; thymic aplasia
Lithium carbonate	Various birth defects, usually involving the heart and great vessels
Methotrexate	IUGR; multiple birth defects, especially skeletal (involving the face, cranium, limbs, and vertebral column) and renal
Misoprostol	Abnormal development of the limbs; ocular defects; cranial nerve defects; autism spectrum disorders
Phenytoin (Dilantin)	Fetal hydantoin syndrome; IUGR; microcephaly; mental deficiency; ridged metopic suture; inner epicanthal folds; eyelid ptosis; broad, depressed nasal bridge; phalangeal hypoplasia
Tetracycline	Stained teeth; hypoplasia of enamel
Thalidomide	Abnormal development of the limbs: meromelia (partial absence of limb) and amelia (complete absence of limb); facial defects; systemic defects (e.g., cardiac and kidney defects and ocular anomalies)
Trimethadione	Developmental delay; V-shaped eyebrows; low-set ears; cleft lip and/or palate
Valproic acid	Craniofacial defects; neural tube defects; often hydrocephalus; heart and skeletal defects; poor postnatal cognitive development
Warfarin	Nasal hypoplasia; stippled epiphyses; hypoplastic phalanges; eye defects; mental deficiency
Chemicals	
Methyl mercury	Cerebral atrophy; spasticity; seizures; mental deficiency
Polychlorinated biphenyls	IUGR; skin discoloration
Infections	
Cytomegalovirus	Microcephaly; chorioretinitis; sensorineural loss; delayed psychomotor and mental development; hepatosplenomegaly; hydrocephaly; cerebral palsy; brain (periventricular) calcification
SARS-CoV-2 virus	Spontaneous abortion, stillbirth, preterm birth, fetal growth restriction, low birth weight
Hepatitis B virus	Preterm birth; fetal macrosomia
Herpes simplex virus	Skin vesicles and scarring; chorioretinitis; hepatomegaly; thrombocytopenia; petechiae; hemolytic anemia; hydranencephaly
Human parvovirus B19	Fetal anemia; nonimmune hydrops fetalis; fetal death
Rubella virus	IUGR; postnatal growth retardation; cardiac and great vessel abnormalities; microcephaly; sensorineural deafness; cataract; microphthalmos; glaucoma; pigmented retinopathy; mental deficiency; neonatal bleeding; hepatosplenomegaly; osteopathy; tooth defects
Zika virus	Microcephaly, arthrogryposis, sensorineural hearing loss, swallowing difficulties, hypertonia, neurodevelopmental disorders, failure to thrive.
Toxoplasma gondii	Microcephaly; mental deficiency; microphthalmia; hydrocephaly; chorioretinitis; cerebral calcifications; hearing loss; neurological disturbances
Treponema pallidum	Hydrocephalus; congenital deafness; mental deficiency; abnormal teeth and bones
Varicella virus	Cutaneous scars (dermatome distribution); neurological defects (e.g., limb paresis, hydrocephaly, seizures); cataracts; microphthalmia; Horner syndrome; optic atrophy; nystagmus; chorioretinitis; microcephaly; mental deficiency; skeletal defects (e.g., hypoplasia of limbs, fingers, and toes); urogenital defects
High Levels of Ionizing Radiation	Microcephaly; mental deficiency; skeletal defects; growth retardation; cataracts

IUGR, Intrauterine growth restriction; *SARS-CoV-2,* severe acute respiratory syndrome coronavirus 2.

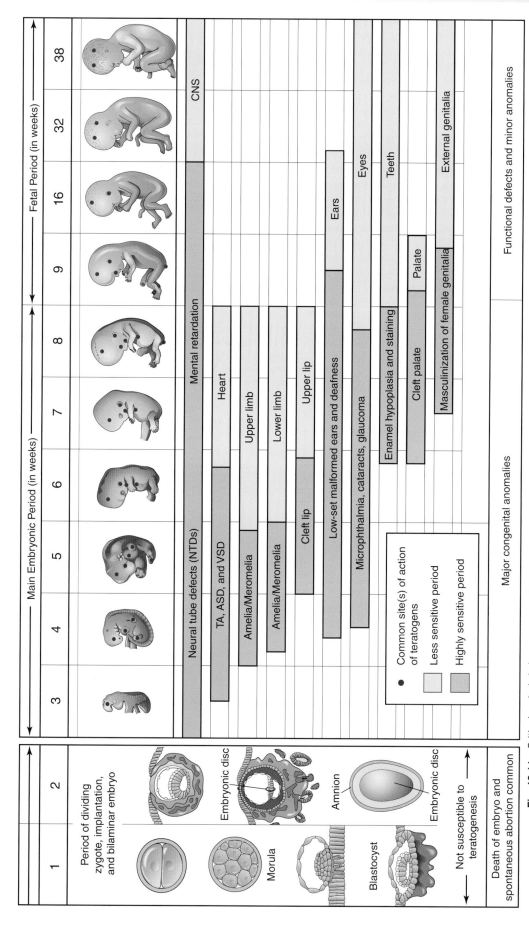

Fig. 19.11 Critical periods in human prenatal development. During the first 2 weeks, the embryo is not usually susceptible to teratogens. At this point, a teratogen damages all or most of the cells, resulting in the death of the cells, or damages only a few cells, allowing the conceptus to recover and the embryo to develop without birth defects. The purple areas denote highly sensitive periods, when major defects may be produced (e.g., amelia, absence of limbs). The green sections indicate stages that are less sensitive to teratogens, when minor birth defects may be induced. *ASD*, Atrial septal defect; *CNS*, central nervous system; *TA*, truncus arteriosus; *VSD*, ventricular septal defect.

continue to smoke during pregnancy. In heavy cigarette smokers (>20 per day), premature delivery is twice as frequent as in mothers who do not smoke. In addition, the infants of smokers weigh less than normal.

A population-based case–control study revealed that conotruncal and atrioventricular septal defects occur more frequently in infants of mothers who smoke during the first trimester of pregnancy. Compared with infants of nonsmokers, a higher incidence of cleft lip and cleft palate has been reported in the offspring of females who smoke during pregnancy. Nicotine constricts the uterine blood vessels, thereby causing a decrease in uterine blood flow and reducing the supply of oxygen and nutrients available to the embryo or fetus from the maternal blood in the intervillous space of the placenta. High levels of **carboxyhemoglobin**, resulting from cigarette smoking, appear in the maternal and fetal blood and may alter the capacity of the blood to transport oxygen. As a result, chronic fetal hypoxia (decrease in the oxygen level to below normal) may occur, affecting fetal growth and development.

ALCOHOL

In the Americas, alcohol use disorder affects approximately 3% of females of childbearing age while approximately 11% use alcohol during pregnancy. Both moderate and high levels of alcohol intake during early pregnancy may result in alterations in the growth and morphogenesis of the fetus; the greater the intake, the more severe the signs. Infants born to mothers who are chronic alcohol users exhibit a specific pattern of defects, including prenatal and postnatal growth retardation, cognitive deficiency, and other defects (Fig. 19.12). This specific pattern of defects in affected infants and children is called **fetal alcohol syndrome** (FAS), and it is present in 1 to 2 infants per 1000 live births, but the prevalence of FAS is related to population studies.

Even moderate maternal alcohol consumption (e.g., 1–2 oz daily) may produce **partial FAS**—children with behavioral problems and cognitive impairment, for example—especially if the drinking is associated with malnutrition. Binge drinking (heavy consumption of alcohol for 1–3 days) during pregnancy is very likely to produce FASs.

The preferred term for the range of prenatal alcohol effects is **fetal alcohol spectrum disorder (FASD)**. Alcohol-related neurodevelopmental disorder is an FASD that results in cognitive and behavioral changes but without the facial features seen with other FASDs. The prevalence of FASD in the general population may be as high as 1%. Because the susceptible period of brain development spans the major part of gestation, **the safest advice is total abstinence from alcohol while trying to get pregnant and during pregnancy**, as there is no known safe amount or safe time. Moreover, there is a higher risk of sudden infant death syndrome associated with concurrent alcohol drinking and cigarette smoking during pregnancy.

ANDROGENS AND PROGESTOGENS

Androgens and progestogens may affect the female fetus, producing masculinization of the external genitalia (Fig. 19.13). The medications that should be avoided typically contain progestins, ethisterone, or norethisterone. However, progestin exposure during the critical period of development is also associated with an increased prevalence of cardiovascular defects, and exposure of male fetuses during this period may double the incidence of hypospadias in the offspring (see Fig. 13.26).

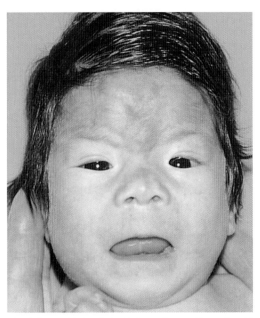

Fig. 19.12 Infant with fetal alcohol syndrome. Note the thin upper lip, short palpebral fissures, flat nasal bridge, short nose, and elongated and poorly formed philtrum (vertical groove in the median part of the upper lip). Severe maternal alcohol abuse is believed to be the most common environmental cause of mental deficiency. Courtesy A.E. Chudley, MD, Section of Genetics and Metabolism, Department of Pediatrics and Child Health, Children's Hospital and University of Manitoba, Winnipeg, Manitoba, Canada.

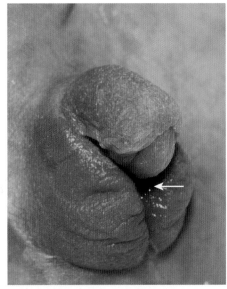

Fig. 19.13 Masculinized external genitalia of a female infant with a 46,XX chromosome constitution. Observe the enlarged clitoris and fused labia majora. The *arrow* indicates the single orifice of a urogenital sinus. The virilization (mature masculine characteristics in a female) was caused by excessive androgens produced by the suprarenal glands during the fetal period (congenital adrenal hyperplasia). Courtesy Dr. Heather Dean, Department of Pediatrics and Child Health and University of Manitoba, Winnipeg, Manitoba, Canada.

Oral contraceptives containing progestogens and estrogens, when taken during the early stages of an unrecognized pregnancy, are believed to be teratogenic agents. Many infants of mothers who took progestogen–estrogen birth control pills during the critical period of development have been found to exhibit the VACTERL syndrome—*v*ertebral, *a*nal, *c*ardiac, *t*racheal, esophageal, *r*enal, and *l*imb anomalies.

ANTIBIOTICS

Tetracyclines cross the placental membrane and are deposited in the embryo's bones and teeth at sites of active calcification. As little as 1 g daily of tetracycline during the third trimester of pregnancy can produce yellow staining of the deciduous teeth. Tetracycline therapy during the fourth to ninth months of pregnancy may also cause tooth defects (e.g., enamel hypoplasia) and diminished growth of the long bones (see Fig. 18.10). More than 30 cases of hearing deficit and CN VIII damage have been reported in infants exposed to **streptomycin** derivatives in utero. By contrast, **penicillin** has been used extensively during pregnancy and appears to be harmless to the embryo/fetus.

ANTICOAGULANTS

All anticoagulants except heparin, a glycosaminoglycan, cross the placental membrane and may cause hemorrhage in the embryo/fetus. **Warfarin**, an anticoagulant that acts as an antagonist of vitamin K, is definitely a teratogen. The period of greatest sensitivity is 6 to 12 weeks after fertilization. Second- and third-trimester exposure may result in mental deficiency, optic nerve atrophy, and microcephaly. Heparin does not cross the placental membrane and so is the drug of choice for pregnant women requiring anticoagulant therapy.

ANTICONVULSANTS

Epilepsy affects approximately 1 in 200 pregnant women, and these women require treatment with an anticonvulsant. Of the anticonvulsant drugs available, **phenytoin** has been definitively identified as a teratogen. **Fetal hydantoin syndrome** occurs in 5% to 10% of children born to mothers treated with phenytoins or hydantoin anticonvulsants (Fig. 19.14).

The use of **valproic acid** (an anticonvulsant) in pregnant women has led to a pattern of birth defects consisting of poorer postnatal cognitive development and craniofacial, heart, and limb defects. There is also an increased risk of neural tube defects. **Phenobarbital** is considered to be a safe antiepileptic drug for use during pregnancy.

ANTINEOPLASTIC AGENTS

Tumor-inhibiting chemicals are highly teratogenic. This is not surprising because these agents inhibit mitosis in rapidly dividing cells. It is recommended that they be avoided, especially during the first trimester of pregnancy. **Methotrexate**, a folic acid antagonist and a derivative of aminopterin, is a known potent teratogen that produces major congenital defects.

ANTIHYPERTENSIVE MEDICATIONS

Exposure of the fetus to **angiotensin-converting enzyme inhibitors** and **AT1 blockers,** used as antihypertensive agents, has fetotoxic potential and can cause oligohydramnios, fetal death, long-lasting hypoplasia of the bones of the calvaria, IUGR, renal dysfunction, and fetal death.

RETINOIC ACID (VITAMIN A)

Retinoic acid is a metabolite of vitamin A. **Isotretinoin** (13-*cis*-retinoic acid), used for the oral treatment of severe cystic acne, is teratogenic in humans, even at very low doses. The critical period for exposure appears to be from the third to the fifth week (5–7 weeks after the last normal

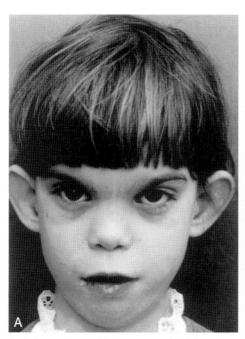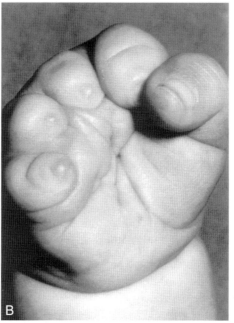

Fig. 19.14 Fetal hydantoin syndrome. (A) This young girl has a learning disability. Note the unusual ears, the wide spacing of the eyes, the epicanthal folds, the short nose, and the long philtrum. Her mother has epilepsy and took phenytoin (Dilantin) throughout her pregnancy. (B) Right hand of an infant with severe digital hypoplasia (short fingers), born to a mother who took phenytoin (Dilantin) throughout her pregnancy. A, Courtesy A.E. Chudley, MD, Section of Genetics and Metabolism, Department of Pediatrics and Child Health, Children's Hospital and University of Manitoba, Winnipeg, Manitoba, Canada; B, From Chodirker BN, Chudley AE, Persaud TVN: Possible prenatal hydantoin effect in child born to a nonepileptic mother, *Am J Med Genet* 27:373, 1987.

menstrual period). The risk of spontaneous abortion and birth defects after exposure to excessive **retinoic acid** is high. Postnatal follow-up studies of children exposed to isotretinoin in utero showed significant neuropsychological impairment. Vitamin A is a valuable and necessary nutrient during pregnancy, but long-term exposure to large doses of vitamin A is unwise because of insufficient evidence to rule out a teratogenic risk.

ANALGESICS

Acetylsalicylic acid, or **aspirin**, is the most commonly ingested drug during pregnancy. Large doses are potentially harmful to the embryo/fetus. Low-dose aspirin has been used to prevent or delay the onset of preeclampsia, preterm birth, and early pregnancy loss. Follow-up studies indicate that low doses appear not to be teratogenic.

Acetaminophen (paracetamol), a common, over-the-counter medication, is widely used for the treatment of headache, fever, pain, and symptoms of the common cold. Clinical trials suggest that large doses of analgesics may be harmful to the embryo or fetus. Nonsteroidal antiinflammatory drugs used after 20 weeks may cause rare but serious defects of the fetal renal system and oligohydramnios. Using after 30 weeks may also cause premature closure of the ductus arteriosus.

THYROID DRUGS

Iodides readily cross the placental membrane and interfere with thyroxin production. They may also cause thyroid enlargement and other anomalies such as arrested physical and cognitive development and dystrophy of bones and soft tissue. Maternal iodine deficiency may cause **congenital iodine deficiency**, which may present with growth deficiency and intellectual disability. The administration of antithyroid drugs for the treatment of maternal thyroid disorders may cause **congenital goiter** if the dose administered exceeds that required to control the disease.

TRANQUILIZERS

Thalidomide is a potent teratogen. Nearly 12,000 neonates had birth defects caused by this drug. Originally intended as a tranquilizer, it has been used to treat various disorders including morning sickness. The characteristic presenting feature is **meromelia** (including phocomelia) (Fig. 19.15). It has been well established clinically that the period when thalidomide causes congenital defects is from 20 to 36 days after fertilization. *Thalidomide is absolutely contraindicated in females of childbearing age.*

PSYCHOTROPIC DRUGS

Lithium is the drug of choice for long-term maintenance therapy in patients with bipolar disorder. It has been known to cause birth defects, mainly of the heart and great vessels, in neonates born to mothers given the drug early in pregnancy.

Benzodiazepines are psychoactive drugs that are frequently prescribed for pregnant women. These drugs include diazepam and oxazepam, which readily cross the placental membrane (see Fig. 8.7). The use of these drugs during the first trimester of pregnancy is associated with transient withdrawal symptoms and craniofacial defects in neonates. **Selective serotonin reuptake inhibitors** are used to treat depression. Use of these drugs by the mother during pregnancy has been shown to slightly increase the risk of atrial and septal defects,

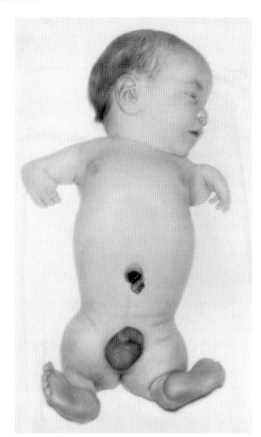

Fig. 19.15 Male neonate with malformed limbs (meromelia—congenital absence of parts of the limbs) caused by maternal ingestion of thalidomide during the critical period of limb development. From Moore KL: The vulnerable embryo: causes of malformation in man, *Manitoba Med Rev* 43:306, 1963.

persistent pulmonary hypertension, have impacts on the brain functional networks (hyperconnectivity of the auditory network) and result in neurobehavioral disturbances including autism spectrum disorder.

ILLICIT DRUGS

Cocaine is one of the most commonly abused illicit drugs in North America, and its increasing use by females of childbearing age is of major concern. Many reports deal with the prenatal effects of cocaine; these include spontaneous abortion, prematurity, and diverse birth defects in their infants.

Methadone, used for the treatment of heroin addiction, is considered a "behavioral teratogen," as is heroin. Infants of narcotic-dependent females have lower birth weights, and infants of females receiving maintenance methadone therapy have been found to have central nervous system dysfunction and smaller head circumferences than nonexposed infants. There is also concern about the long-term postnatal developmental effects of methadone.

Cannabinoids consumed by the pregnant mother can cross the placental barrier and directly affect the fetus through G-protein-coupled cannabinoid receptors (CB1 and CB2). They can adversely affect fetal growth and can cause neurological deficits and immunological impairment in the offspring.

Methamphetamine is a potent CNS stimulant and its effects on pregnancy and the embryo/fetus are less well studied. Use of the drug during pregnancy increases the risk of small-for-gestational age and low birth weight and appears to increase the risk for neurodevelopmental abnormalities.

Neonatal Abstinence Syndrome (NAS)

NAS results in neonates exposed to opioids in utero. Symptoms may include fever, diarrhea, and feeding and sleeping disturbances. Therapy typically requires opioid monotherapy..

ENVIRONMENTAL CHEMICALS AS TERATOGENS

There has been increasing concern about the possible teratogenicity of environmental, industrial, and agricultural chemicals, pollutants, and food additives. Most of these chemicals have not been positively implicated as teratogens in humans. A systematic review and meta-analysis of epidemiological reports showed that in the United States and other populations, there is a significant association between the occurrence of specific congenital heart defects (atrial septal defect, coarctation of the aorta, tetralogy of Fallot) in the offspring and pregnant women who were exposed to polluted air (ozone, carbon dioxide, carbon monoxide, and heat particulate material).

ORGANIC MERCURY

Infants of mothers whose main diet during pregnancy consists of fish containing abnormally high levels of organic mercury acquire fetal **Minamata disease**—neurological and behavioral disturbances resembling those associated with cerebral palsy. **Methyl mercury** is a teratogen that causes cerebral atrophy, spasticity, seizures, and intellectual disability.

LEAD

Lead is abundantly present in the workplace and the environment. The lead passes the placental membrane and accumulates in fetal tissues. Prenatal exposure to lead is associated with an increased incidence of abortions, fetal defects, IUGR, and functional deficits.

POLYCHLORINATED BIPHENYLS

Polychlorinated biphenyls (PCBs) are teratogenic chemicals that produce IUGR and skin discoloration in fetuses exposed to these agents. The main dietary source of PCBs in North America is probably sport fish caught in contaminated waters.

INFECTIOUS AGENTS AS TERATOGENS

CYTOMEGALOVIRUS

Cytomegalovirus (CMV) is the most common viral infection of the fetus, occurring in approximately 1% of neonates. Most pregnancies end in spontaneous abortion when the infection occurs during the first trimester. It is the leading cause of congenital infection with morbidity at birth. Neonates infected during the early fetal period usually show no clinical signs and are identified through screening programs. CMV infection later in pregnancy may result in severe birth defects: developmental delay, IUGR, microphthalmia, chorioretinitis, blindness, microcephaly, cerebral calcification, cognitive deficiency, deafness, cerebral palsy, and hepatosplenomegaly (enlargement of the liver and spleen). Of particular concern are cases of asymptomatic CMV infection, which are often associated with audiological, neurological, and neurobehavioral disturbances in infancy. Detection of congenital CMV infection in an infant at the time of birth, or shortly thereafter, is critical for the clinical management and care of the future development of the child.

RUBELLA

Rubella infection is a worldwide problem that can cause severe illness, epidemics, and birth defects in pregnant women. The **rubella virus** crosses the placental membrane and infects the embryo/fetus. In cases of primary maternal infection during the first trimester of pregnancy, the overall risk of embryonic or fetal infection is approximately 20%. The clinical features of **congenital rubella syndrome** are cataracts, congenital glaucoma, cardiac defects, and deafness (Fig. 19.16). The earlier in pregnancy that maternal rubella infection occurs, the greater is the danger that the embryo will be impacted.

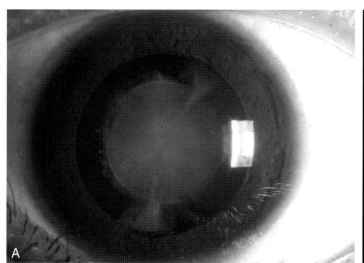
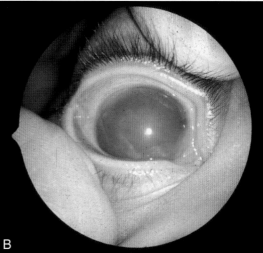

Fig. 19.16 (A) Typical appearance of a congenital cataract that may have been caused by the rubella virus. Cardiac defects and deafness are other congenital defects common to this infection. (B) Clouding of the cornea caused by congenital glaucoma. Corneal clouding may also result from infection, trauma, or metabolic disorders. *From Guercio J, Martyn L: Congenital malformations of the eye and orbit, Otolaryngol Clin North Am* 40:113, 2007.

HERPES SIMPLEX VIRUS

Maternal infection with **herpes simplex virus** in early pregnancy increases the spontaneous abortion rate threefold. Infection after the 20th week is associated with an increased rate of prematurity and birth defects (e.g., microcephaly and mental deficiency). Infection of the fetus with herpes simplex virus usually occurs very late in pregnancy, probably most often during delivery.

VARICELLA

Varicella (chickenpox) and **herpes zoster** (shingles) are caused by the same virus, **varicella-zoster virus**, which is highly infectious. There is convincing evidence that maternal varicella infection during the first 4 months of pregnancy causes several birth defects (muscle atrophy and mental deficiency). There is a 20% incidence of these or other defects when the infection occurs during the critical period of development (see Fig. 19.11).

HUMAN IMMUNODEFICIENCY VIRUS

HIV is the retrovirus that causes **AIDS**. Infection of pregnant women with HIV is associated with serious health problems in the fetus. There are conflicting reports on in utero infection with HIV and fetal outcome. Some adverse perinatal effects included preterm birth, intrauterine growth retardation, low birth weight, and infant mortality, Transmission of the HIV virus to the fetus can occur during pregnancy, labor, or delivery.

ZIKA VIRUS

Pregnant women infected with the Zika virus gave birth to babies with microcephaly and severe neurological abnormalities. In 2015 the first case of Zika embryopathy was reported in Brazil, and there have been outbreaks in other countries, including Western (Yap Island) and South Pacific (French Polynesia) South America, Central America, and the Caribbean.

Zika virus is transmitted by the *Aedes* mosquito locally to humans. In most cases, a causal relationship was established between prenatal Zika infection and the birth of babies with low birth weight for gestational age, microcephaly, and other anomalies. The transmission of the virus to the fetus is vertical. The Centers for Disease Control (CDC) concluded from their assessment of the situation that pregnant women infected with the Zika virus have an increased risk of spontaneous abortion and giving birth to a child of low birth weight for gestational age with microcephaly, cerebral calcification, ventriculomegaly, and ocular defects. The CDC did observe that many females infected with the Zika virus gave birth to healthy babies indicating that other genetic factors may be at play. There is no vaccine available for the treatment of Zika infection.

SARS-COV-2 VIRUS

The **coronavirus disease (COVID-19)** caused mounting deaths and a public health pandemic response worldwide. An area of special concern is the neonatal outcome of children born to mothers who had been infected with COVID-19 during pregnancy. Several studies indicated an increased risk of pregnancy complications, which included preeclampsia, miscarriage, stillbirth, preterm birth, fetal growth restriction, and possibly later neurodevelopmental problems. It was reported that SARS-CoV-2 was transmitted to the fetus in utero, not during or after birth. The neonates tested positive for the virus and coronavirus particles were found in the fetal cells of the placenta.

TOXOPLASMOSIS

Maternal infection with the intracellular parasite ***Toxoplasma gondii*** is usually through one of the following routes:

- Eating raw or poorly cooked meat (usually pork or lamb containing *Toxoplasma* cysts)
- Close contact with infected domestic animals (usually cats) or infected soil.

The *T. gondii* organism crosses the placental membrane and infects the fetus, causing destructive changes in the brain that result in cognitive deficiency and other birth defects. Mothers of infants with birth defects are often unaware of having had **toxoplasmosis**. Because animals (cats, dogs, rabbits, and other domestic and wild animals) may be infected with this parasite, pregnant women should avoid contact with them. In addition, unpasteurized milk should be avoided.

CONGENITAL SYPHILIS

Syphilis is increasing in its prevalence in many countries, and pregnant women are consequently often affected. From 2013 to 2018 in the United States, congenital syphilis increased from 362 to 1306 cases (including 128 infant deaths and stillbirths). ***Treponema pallidum***, the small, spiral microorganism that causes syphilis, rapidly crosses the placental membrane as early as 6 to 8 weeks of development. The fetus can become infected at any stage of the disease or at any stage of pregnancy. **Primary maternal infections** (acquired during pregnancy and untreated) nearly always cause serious fetal infection and birth defects. However, adequate treatment of the mother kills the organism. If the mother remains untreated, only 20% of women will deliver a normal neonate. **Secondary maternal infections** (acquired before pregnancy) can also result in congenital syphilis and similar fetal outcomes.

RADIATION AS A TERATOGEN

Exposure to **high levels of ionizing radiation** may injure embryonic cells, resulting in cell death, chromosomal injury, mental deficiency, and deficient physical growth. The severity of the embryonic damage is related to the absorbed dose, the dose rate, and the stage of embryonic or fetal development when the exposure occurs. Accidental exposure of pregnant women to radiation is a common cause of anxiety.

No conclusive proof exists that human congenital defects have been caused by diagnostic levels of radiation (<10,000 millirads [mrad]). Scattered radiation from a radiographic examination of a part of the body that is not near the uterus (e.g., thorax, sinuses, and teeth) produces a dose of only a few millirads, which is not teratogenic to the embryo. The recommended limit of maternal exposure of the whole body to radiation from all sources is 500 mrad (0.005 Gy) for the entire gestational period. Magnetic resonance imaging does not use ionizing radiation and poses no known risk.

MATERNAL FACTORS AS TERATOGENS

Pregestational diabetes mellitus is a major public health problem. In the United States more than 60 million females of reproductive age are affected. An estimated 4% of pregnant women worldwide have diabetes. During pregnancy, poorly controlled **diabetes mellitus** in the mother with persisting hyperglycemia and ketosis, particularly during embryogenesis, is associated with a two- to threefold higher incidence of birth defects. Neonates of a diabetic mother are usually large (**macrosomia**). The common defects include holoprosencephaly (failure of the forebrain to divide into hemispheres), meroencephaly (partial absence of the brain), sacral agenesis, vertebral defects, congenital heart defects, and limb defects or vascular disruption.

If left untreated, females who are homozygous for phenylalanine hydroxylase deficiency—**phenylketonuria**—and those with **hyperphenylalaninemia** are at increased risk for having offspring with **microcephaly** (abnormal smallness of the head), cardiac defects, mental deficiency, and IUGR. The congenital defects can be prevented if the mother with phenylketonuria follows a phenylalanine-restricted diet before and during pregnancy.

PATERNAL FACTORS AS TERATOGENS

Few studies have considered the effects of paternal factors on neonatal outcomes. A recent systematic review and meta-analysis showed that the age of the father is a risk factor for the occurrence of birth defects.

MECHANICAL FACTORS AS TERATOGENS

Clubfoot and congenital dislocation of the hip may be caused by mechanical forces, particularly in a malformed uterus. Such birth defects may be caused by any factor that restricts the mobility of the fetus, thereby causing prolonged compression in an abnormal posture. A significantly reduced quantity of amniotic fluid (oligohydramnios) may result in mechanically induced deformation of the limbs, such as hyperextension of the knee. **Intrauterine amputations** or other defects caused by local constriction during fetal growth may result from **amniotic bands** (see Fig. 8.14), rings formed as a result of rupture of the amnion during early pregnancy.

BIRTH DEFECTS CAUSED BY MULTIFACTORIAL INHERITANCE

Many common birth defects (e.g., cleft lip, with or without cleft palate) have familial distributions consistent with multifactorial inheritance (see Fig. 19.1). Multifactorial inheritance may be represented by a model in which one's "liability" for a disorder is a continuous variable determined by a combination of genetic and environmental factors, with a developmental threshold dividing individuals with the defect from those without it. Multifactorial traits are often single major defects, such as cleft lip, isolated cleft palate, and neural tube defects. Some of these defects may also occur as part of the phenotype in syndromes determined by single-gene inheritance, chromosomal abnormality, or an environmental teratogen. The recurrence risks used for genetic counseling of families having birth defects that have been determined by multifactorial inheritance are empirical risks based on the frequency of the defect in the general population and in different categories of relatives. In individual families, such estimates may be inaccurate because they are usually averages for the population rather than precise probabilities for the individual family.

GENETIC COUNSELING

For families who have a child with a congenital malformation, or multiple anomalies, a detailed physical examination by a clinical geneticist is an important part of the clinical workup. The genetics session typically also involves obtaining a detailed three-generation family history (often obtained by a genetic counselor) and ordering of other investigations, including genetic testing, if indicated. Genetic counseling is a communication process designed to educate, support, and assist individuals in making informed choices, adapting to a new diagnosis, or the susceptibility risk of a genetic disorder. The complexity of different types of results that can be generated, the potential impact on extended family members, and the risk of incidental findings in addition to privacy and insurance implications justify why pre- and posttest genetic counseling is recommended for all families considering genetic sequencing.

CLINICALLY ORIENTED QUESTIONS

1. If a pregnant woman takes aspirin in normal doses, will it cause congenital birth defects?

2. In a female with a substance abuse disorder, will her child show signs of drug addiction?

3. Are all drugs tested for teratogenicity before they are marketed? If the answer is "yes," why are these teratogens still sold?

4. Is cigarette smoking during pregnancy harmful to the embryo or fetus? If the answer is "yes," would refraining from inhaling cigarette smoke be safer?

5. Are any drugs safe to take during pregnancy? If so, what are they?

The answers to these questions are at the back of this book.

The Cellular and Molecular Basis of Development

Jeffrey T. Wigle | David D. Eisenstat

During embryonic development, undifferentiated precursor cells differentiate and organize into the complex structures found in functional adult tissues. This process requires cells to integrate many different cues, both intrinsic and extrinsic, for development to occur properly. These cues control the proliferation, differentiation, and migration of cells to determine the final size and shape of the developing organs. Disruption of these signaling pathways can result in human developmental disorders and birth defects. Interestingly, these key developmental signaling pathways may also be co-opted in the adult by diseases such as cancer.

Although there are diverse changes that occur during embryogenesis, the differentiation of many different cell types is regulated through a relatively restricted set of molecular signaling pathways:

- **Intercellular communication:** Development involves the interaction of a cell with its neighboring cell either directly (gap junctions) or indirectly (cell adhesion molecules).
- **Morphogens:** These are diffusible molecules that specify which cell type will be generated at a specific anatomic location. Morphogens also direct the migration of cells and their processes to their final destination. These include retinoic acid, transforming growth factor-β (TGF-β)/bone morphogenetic proteins (BMPs), and the hedgehog and Wnt protein families (Table 20.1 for gene and protein nomenclature).
- **Hedgehog:** The hedgehog signaling pathway in human cells is localized to a structure called the *primary cilium*. Disruption of the components of the hedgehog pathway results in a set of diseases termed *ciliopathies*.
- **Receptor tyrosine kinases (RTKs):** Many growth factors signal by binding to and activating membrane-bound RTKs. These kinases are essential for the regulation of cellular proliferation, apoptosis, and migration.
- **Notch–Delta:** This pathway often specifies the fate of precursor cells.
- **Transcription factors:** This set of evolutionarily conserved proteins activates or represses downstream genes that are essential for a number of cellular processes. Many transcription factors are members of the homeobox or helix–loop–helix families. Their activity can be regulated by all of the other pathways described in this chapter.
- **Epigenetics:** Epigenetics relates to the heritable properties of gene function that do not occur as a result of changes of the DNA code. Examples of epigenetic modifications are DNA methylation, histone modifications, and microRNAs.
- **Stem cells:** Stem cells in the embryo can give rise to all cells and tissues in the developing organism. Adult stem cells maintain tissues in the mature organism. These types of stem cells and induced pluripotent stem cells (iPSCs) are potential sources of cells for regeneration and/or repair of injured or degenerating cells and organs.

INTERCELLULAR COMMUNICATION

Cells can communicate with each other in several different ways.

GAP JUNCTIONS

Gap junctions are channels that permit ions and small molecules (<1 kDa) to directly pass from one cell to another—gap junctional intercellular communication (GJIC). However, large proteins and nucleic acids cannot transfer through gap junctions. Gap junctions are made from hemichannels present on the surface of each cell known as **connexons**. Each connexon is made up of six *connexin* molecules that form a hexamer. In early development, gap junctions are usually open, permitting exchange of small molecules in relatively large regions. However, as development proceeds, GJIC is more restricted with the establishment of boundaries, such as in the **rhombomeres**, transient structures of the developing hindbrain. Gap junctions are particularly important for electrical coupling in the heart and brain. Mutations of specific connexin molecules are associated with human diseases (e.g., mutation of *CX43* is associated with atherosclerosis).

CELL ADHESION MOLECULES

Cell adhesion molecules have large extracellular domains that interact with extracellular matrix components or adhesion molecules in neighboring cells. These molecules often contain a transmembrane segment and a short cytoplasmic domain, which regulates intracellular signaling cascades. Examples of cell adhesion molecules are the cadherins, a family of proteins that have important roles during embryonic development.

Cadherins are critical for embryonic morphogenesis, as they regulate the separation of cell layers (endothelial and epidermal), cell migration, cell sorting, establishment of well-defined boundaries, synaptic connections, and the growth cones of neurons. These roles result from cadherins

Table 20.1   International Nomenclature Standards for Genes and Proteins

Gene	Human	Italics, all letters capitalized	*PAX6*
	Mouse	Italics, first letter capitalized	*Pax6*
Protein	Human	Roman, all letters capitalized	PAX6
	Mouse	Roman, all letters capitalized	PAX6

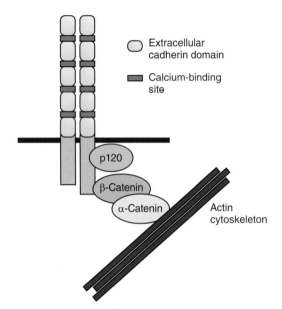

Fig. 20.1   Structure of cadherin. The cadherin extracellular domain contains four calcium-binding sites and five repeated domains called *extracellular cadherin domains*. Each cadherin molecule forms a homodimer. In the intracellular domain, cadherin binds directly to p120-catenin and to β-catenin, which binds to α-catenin. This complex links the cadherin molecules to the actin cytoskeleton.

mediating the interaction between the cell and its extracellular milieu (both neighboring cells and extracellular matrix). Cadherins were originally classified by their site of expression; for example, E-cadherin is highly expressed in epithelial cells, whereas N-cadherin is highly expressed in neural cells.

A typical cadherin molecule has a large extracellular domain, a transmembrane domain, and an intracellular tail (Fig. 20.1). The extracellular domain contains five extracellular repeats and four Ca²⁺-binding sites. Cadherins form dimers that interact with cadherin dimers in adjacent cells. These complexes are found clustered in **adherens junctions**, which result in the formation of a tight barrier between epithelial or endothelial cells. Via its intracellular domain, cadherin binds to p120-catenin, β-catenin, and α-catenin. These proteins connect cadherin to the cytoskeleton. E-cadherin expression is lost as epithelial cells transition to mesenchymal cells—**epithelial-to-mesenchymal transition** (EMT). EMT is required for the formation of neural crest cells during development, and the same process also occurs during tumor development.

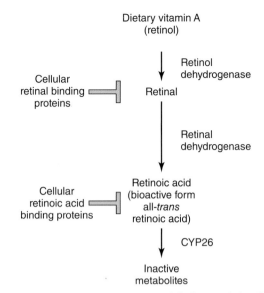

Fig. 20.2   Regulation of retinoic acid metabolism and signaling. Dietary retinol (vitamin A) is converted to retinal via the action of retinol dehydrogenases. The concentration of free retinal is controlled by the action of cellular retinal-binding proteins. Similarly, retinal is converted to retinoic acid by retinal dehydrogenases, and its free level is modulated by sequestration by cellular retinoic acid–binding proteins and degradation by CYP26. The bioactive form of retinoic acid is all-*trans* retinoic acid.

MORPHOGENS

Extrinsic signaling by morphogens guides the differentiation and migration of cells during development, determining the morphology and function of developing tissues and organs (see Chapter 6). Many morphogens are found in concentration gradients in the embryo. Different morphogens can be expressed in opposing gradients in the dorsoventral (DV), anteroposterior (AP), and mediolateral (ML) axes. The fate of a specific cell can be determined by its location along these different gradients. Cells can also be attracted or repelled by morphogens, depending on the set of receptors expressed on the cell surface.

RETINOIC ACID

The AP axis of the embryo is crucial for determining the correct location for structures such as limbs and for the patterning of the nervous system. For decades, it has been clinically evident that alterations in the level of vitamin A (retinol) in the maternal diet (excessive or insufficient amounts) can lead to the development of congenital malformations (see Chapter 19). The bioactive form of vitamin A is retinoic acid is formed by enzymatic oxidation by retinol aldehyde dehydrogenase and subsequently retinal aldehyde dehydrogenase. Free levels of retinoic acid can be modulated by cellular retinoic acid–binding proteins that sequester retinoic acid. Retinoic acid can also be actively degraded into inactive metabolites by enzymes such as CYP26 (Fig. 20.2).

Normally, retinoic acid acts to "posteriorize" the body plan, and either excessive retinoic acid or inhibition of its degradation leads to a truncated body axis where structures have a more posterior nature. In contrast, insufficient retinoic acid or defects in the enzymes (e.g., retinal aldehyde dehydrogenase) will lead to a more "anteriorized" structure. At the molecular level, retinoic acid binds to its receptors (transcription factors) inside the cell, and their activation will regulate the expression of downstream genes. Hox genes are crucial targets of retinoic acid receptors in development. Because of their profound influence on early development, retinoids are powerful teratogens, especially during the first trimester. Retinoids are sometimes used in the oncology clinic for differentiation therapy of specific leukemias (acute promyelocytic leukemia) and the childhood solid tumor neuroblastoma.

TRANSFORMING GROWTH FACTOR-β/BONE MORPHOGENETIC PROTEIN

Members of the TGF-β superfamily include TGF-β, BMPs, and activin. These molecules contribute to the establishment of DV patterning, cell fate decisions, and formation of specific organs and systems, including the kidneys, nervous system, skeleton, and blood. In humans, there are three different forms of TGF-β (isoforms TGF-β_1, TGF-β_2, and TGF-β_3).

Binding of these ligands to transmembrane kinase receptors results in the phosphorylation of intracellular receptor–associated Smad proteins (R-Smads) (Fig. 20.3). The Smad proteins are a large family of intercellular proteins that are divided into three classes: receptor-activated (R-Smads), common-partner Smads (co-Smads [e.g., Smad4]), and inhibitory Smads (I-Smads). R-Smad/Smad4 complexes regulate target gene transcription by interacting with other proteins or as transcription factors by directly binding to DNA. The diversity of TGF-β ligand, receptor, and R-Smad combinations contributes to particular developmental and cell-specific processes, often in combination with other signaling pathways.

SONIC HEDGEHOG

Sonic hedgehog (SHH) was the first mammalian ortholog of the *Drosophila* gene hedgehog to be identified. SHH and other related proteins, such as desert hedgehog and Indian hedgehog, are secreted morphogens critical for early patterning, cell migration, and differentiation of many cell types and organ systems. Cells have variable thresholds for response to the secreted SHH signal. The primary receptor for SHH is Patched (PTCH in human, PTC family in mouse), a transmembrane domain protein. In the absence of SHH, Patched inhibits the transmembrane domain, G-protein–linked protein called Smoothened (Smo). This results in inhibition of downstream signaling to the nucleus. However, in the presence of SHH, PTC inhibition is blocked and downstream events follow, including transcriptional activation of target genes, such as *Ptc-1*, *Engrailed*, and others (Fig. 20.4).

Posttranslational modification of SHH protein affects its association with the cell membrane, formation of SHH multimers, and the movement of SHH, which, in turn, alters its tissue distribution and concentration gradients.

The role of SHH in patterning the vertebrate ventral neural tube is one of its best-studied activities. SHH is secreted at high levels by the notochord, and therefore the concentration of SHH is highest in the floor plate of the neural tube and lowest in the roof plate, where members of the TGF-β family are highly expressed. The cell fates of ventral interneuron classes and motor neurons are determined by the relative SHH concentrations in the tissue and other factors.

The understanding of the requirement of SHH pathway signaling for many developmental processes has been enhanced by the discovery of human mutations of members of the SHH pathway. In addition, corresponding phenotypes of genetically modified mice, in which members of the SHH pathway are either inactivated (loss of function/knockout) or overexpressed (gain of function), have also added to this knowledge. Mutations of *SHH* and *PTCH* have been associated with holoprosencephaly in humans, a congenital brain defect resulting in the fusion of the two cerebral hemispheres, dorsalization of forebrain structures, and anophthalmia or cyclopia (see Chapter 17). In sheep, this same defect has been associated with in utero exposure to the teratogen cyclopamine, which disrupts SHH signaling (see Fig. 20.4). **Gorlin syndrome**, often due to germline *PTCH* mutations, is a constellation of congenital malformations mostly affecting the epidermis, craniofacial structures, and nervous system. Mutations of the *GLI3* gene, encoding a zinc finger that mediates SHH signaling, are associated with autosomal dominant polydactyly syndromes.

In vertebrates, the SHH signaling pathway is closely linked to **primary cilia** (see Fig. 20.4, inset) and their constituent intraflagellar transport (IFT) and basal body proteins. Primary cilia are sometimes referred to as **nonmotile cilia**.

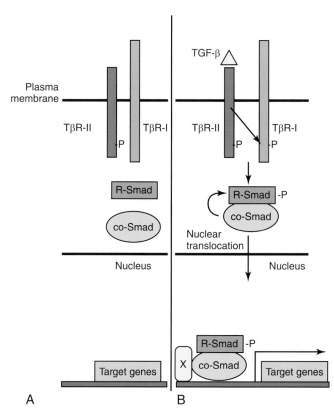

Fig. 20.3 Transforming growth factor-β (TGF-β)/Smad signaling pathway. (A) The type II TGF-β receptor subunit (TβR-II) is constitutively active. (B) On binding of ligand to TβR-II, a type I TGF-β receptor subunit (TβR-I) is recruited to form a heterodimeric receptor complex, and the TβR-I kinase domain is transphosphorylated (-P). Signaling from the activated receptor complex phosphorylates R-Smads, which then bind to a co-Smad, translocate from the cytoplasm to the nucleus, and activate gene transcription with cofactor(s).

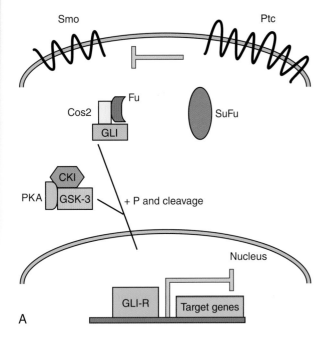

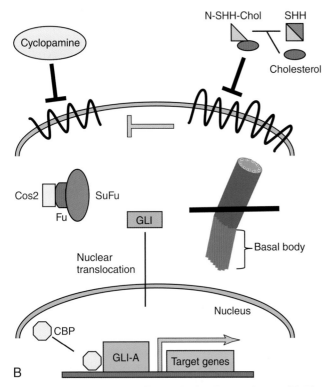

Fig. 20.4 Sonic hedgehog/Patched signaling pathway. (A) The Patched (Ptc) receptor inhibits signaling from the Smoothened (Smo) receptor. In a complex with Costal-2 (Cos2) and Fused (Fu), GLI is modified to become a transcriptional repressor, GLI-R. (B) Sonic hedgehog (SHH) is cleaved, and cholesterol is added to its *N*-terminus (N-SHH-Chol). This modified SHH ligand inhibits the Ptc receptor, permitting Smo signaling, and ultimately activated GLI (GLI-A) translocates to the nucleus to activate target genes with CBP. In vertebrates, SHH signaling takes place in the primary cilia *(inset).CBP*, Cyclic AMP–binding protein; *CKI*, casein kinase I; *GSK-3*, glycogen synthase kinase 3; *P*, phosphate group; *PKA*, protein kinase A; *SuFu*, suppressor of Fused.

IFT proteins act upstream of the GLI activator (GLI-A) and repressor (GLI-R) proteins and are necessary for their production. Mutations involving genes encoding basal body proteins, such as *KIAA0586* (formerly *TALPID3*) and oral-facial-digital syndrome 1 *(OFD1)*, affect SHH signaling in knockout mice. A group of human cilia–related diseases called **ciliopathies** results from disruption of primary cilia function and includes rare genetic diseases and more common disorders such as autosomal recessive polycystic kidney disease. Over 40 ciliopathies have been described to date involving up to 200 genes. Although there may be some overlap (as with many congenital heart defects and left–right asymmetries), diseases of primary, nonmotile cilia are usually distinguished from disorders affecting motile cilia (found in sperm and in epithelial cells lining the airways, ventricles of the brain, and oviducts). Manifestations of diseases affecting motile cilia include hydrocephalus, lung infections, and infertility.

WNT/β-CATENIN PATHWAY

The Wnt-secreted glycoproteins are vertebrate orthologs of the *Drosophila* gene Wingless. Similar to the other morphogens, the 19 Wnt family members control several processes during development, including establishment of cell polarity, proliferation, apoptosis, cell fate specification, and migration. Wnt signaling is a very complex process; three Wnt signaling pathways have been elucidated to date. Only the classic or "canonical" β-catenin-dependent pathway is discussed here (Fig. 20.5). Specific Wnts bind to 1 of 10 Frizzled (Fzd) seven-transmembrane domain cell surface receptors and with low-density, lipoprotein receptor–related proteins 5 and 6 (LRP5/LRP6) coreceptors, thereby activating downstream intracellular signaling events. In the absence of Wnt binding, cytoplasmic β-catenin is phosphorylated by glycogen synthase kinase 3 (GSK-3) and targeted for degradation. In the presence of Wnts, GSK-3 is inactivated and β-catenin is not phosphorylated and accumulates in the cytoplasm. β-catenin then translocates to the nucleus, where it activates target gene transcription in a complex with T-cell factor (TCF) transcription factors. β-Catenin/TCF target genes include vascular endothelial growth factor *(VEGF)* and matrix metalloproteinases.

Dysregulated Wnt signaling is a prominent feature in many developmental disorders, such as **Williams–Beuren syndrome** (heart, neurodevelopmental, and facial defects), and in cancer. *LRP5* mutations are found in the *osteoporosis-pseudoglioma syndrome* (congenital blindness and juvenile osteoporosis). Similar to the SHH pathway, canonical Wnt pathway mutations have been described in children with **medulloblastoma**, a common pediatric malignant brain tumor.

RECEPTOR TYROSINE KINASES

COMMON FEATURES

Growth factors, such as insulin, epidermal growth factor, nerve growth factor and other neurotrophins, and members of the platelet-derived growth factor family, bind to

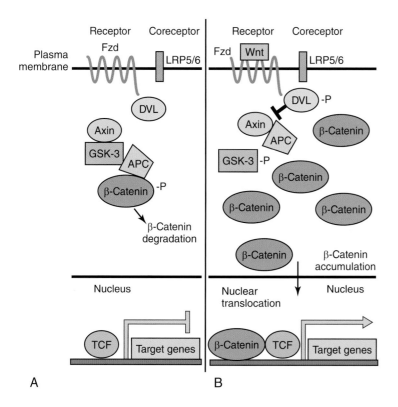

Fig. 20.5 Wnt/β-catenin canonical signaling pathway. (A) In the absence of Wnt ligand binding to Frizzled (Fzd) receptor, β-catenin is phosphorylated (-P) by a multiprotein complex and targeted for degradation. Target gene expression is repressed by T-cell factor (TCF). (B) When Wnt binds to the Fzd receptor, LRP coreceptors are recruited, Disheveled (DVL) is phosphorylated, and β-catenin then accumulates in the cytoplasm. Some β-catenin enters the nucleus to activate target gene transcription. *APC,* Adenomatous polyposis coli; *GSK-3,* glycogen synthase kinase 3; *LRP,* lipoprotein receptor–related protein.

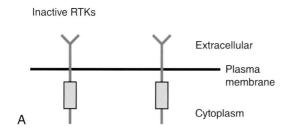

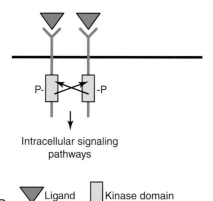

Fig. 20.6 Receptor tyrosine kinase (RTK) signaling. (A) In the absence of ligand, the receptors are monomers and are inactive. (B) On binding of ligand, the receptors dimerize and transphosphorylation occurs, which activates downstream signaling cascades. *P,* Phosphorylated.

cell surface transmembrane receptors found on target cells. These receptors, members of the RTK superfamily, have three domains: (1) an extracellular ligand–binding domain, (2) a transmembrane domain, and (3) an intracellular kinase domain (Fig. 20.6). They are found as monomers in their unbound state but dimerize on ligand binding. This process of dimerization brings the two intracellular kinase domains into close proximity such that one kinase domain can phosphorylate and activate the other receptor (transphosphorylation), which is required to fully activate the receptors. In turn, this initiates a series of intracellular signaling cascades. An inactivating mutation of one receptor subunit kinase domain results in the abolishment of signaling; such a mutation in the kinase domain of the VEGF receptor 3 *(VEGFR-3)* results in the autosomal dominantly inherited lymphatic disorder called **Milroy disease**.

REGULATION OF ANGIOGENESIS BY RECEPTOR TYROSINE KINASES

Growth factors generally promote cellular proliferation, migration, and survival (i.e., they are antiapoptotic). During embryogenesis, signaling through RTKs is crucial for normal development and affects many different processes, such as the growth of new blood vessels (see Chapter 5), cellular migration, and neuronal axonal guidance.

Endothelial cells are derived from a progenitor cell (the hemangioblast) that can give rise to both the hematopoietic cell lineage and endothelial cells. The early endothelial cells proliferate and eventually coalesce to form the first primitive blood vessels. This process is termed **vasculogenesis** (see Chapter 5). After the first blood vessels are formed, they undergo intensive remodeling into the mature blood vessels in a process called **angiogenesis**. This maturation process involves the recruitment of vascular smooth muscle cells stabilize the vessels. Vasculogenesis and angiogenesis are both dependent on the function of two distinct RTK classes, members of the VEGF and Tie receptor families. VEGF-A was shown to be essential for endothelial and blood cell development; VEGF-A knockout mice fail to develop blood or endothelial cells and die at early embryonic stages. A related molecule, VEGF-C, was shown to be crucial for the development of lymphatic endothelial cells. VEGF-A signals through three receptors, VEGFR-1, VEGFR-2, and VEGFR-3, expressed by endothelial cells.

The process of angiogenic refinement depends on the function of the angiopoietin/Tie2 signaling pathway. Tie2 is an RTK that is specifically expressed by endothelial cells, and angiopoietin 1 and angiopoietin 2 are ligands that are expressed by the surrounding vascular smooth muscle cells. This represents a paracrine signaling system in which receptor and ligand are expressed in adjacent cells.

Normal signaling pathways in the embryo can be co-opted reused by disease processes, such as cancer. In tumors, both the VEGF/VEGFR-2 and angiopoietin/Tie2 signaling pathways are co-opted to stimulate growth of new blood vessels, which in turn stimulate their growth and metastasis. Chromosomal recombination events involving RTKs and different partners can result in the formation of **oncoproteins** that drive the development of different types of cancer such as anaplastic large cell lymphomas, acute myeloid leukemia, and 8p11 myeloproliferative syndrome. The chromosomal fusion events generate a protein that contains the intracellular kinase domain of the RTK and an oligomerization domain of another protein. These fusion proteins cluster via the oligomerization domains, resulting in RTK activation and downstream signaling. RTKs such as platelet-derived growth factor receptor, fibroblast growth factor receptor, and anaplastic lymphoma kinase are involved in chromosomal recombinations that lead to the generation of oncoproteins.

NOTCH–DELTA PATHWAY

The Notch signaling pathway is integral for cell fate determination, including maintenance of stem cell niches, proliferation, apoptosis, and differentiation. These processes are essential for all aspects of organ development the through the regulation of lateral and inductive cell–cell signaling. Notch proteins are single transmembrane receptors that interact with membrane-bound Notch ligands (e.g., Delta-like ligands and serrate-like ligands [Jagged]) on adjacent cells (Fig. 20.7). Ligand-receptor binding triggers proteolytic events leading to the release of the Notch intracellular domain (NICD). When the NICD translocates to the nucleus, a series of intranuclear events culminates in the induction of expression of a transcription factor that maintains the progenitor state of the cell.

Lateral inhibition ensures the correct number of two distinct cell types from a population of cells with equivalent developmental potential. In the initial cell–cell interaction, Notch receptor signaling maintains one cell as an uncommitted progenitor. The adjacent cell maintains a reduced level of Notch signaling and undergoes differentiation. Inductive signaling with other surrounding cells expressing morphogens may overcome a cell's commitment to a default fate and lead to an alternative cell fate. Understanding the

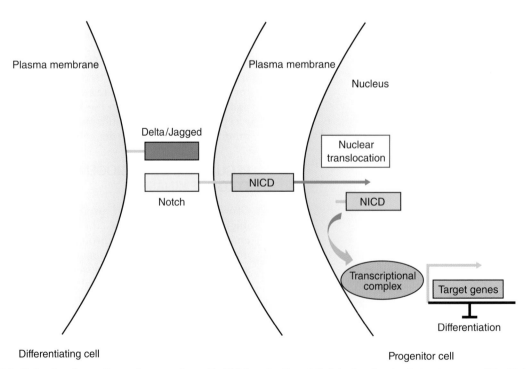

Fig. 20.7 Notch–Delta signaling pathway. In progenitor cells *(right)*, activation of Notch signaling leads to cleavage of the Notch intracellular domain (NICD). NICD translocates to the nucleus, binds to a transcriptional complex, and activates target genes, such as the bHLH gene *Hes1*, which inhibit differentiation. In differentiating cells *(left)*, Notch signaling is not active.

function of the Notch–Delta signaling pathway in mammalian development has been assisted by loss-of-function studies in the mouse. The findings that mutations in Jagged1 are associated with **Alagille syndrome** (arteriohepatic dysplasia), with liver, kidney, cardiovascular, ocular, and skeletal malformations, and that *NOTCH-3* gene mutations are found in CADASIL (*c*erebral *a*utosomal *d*ominant *a*rteriopathy with *s*ubcortical *i*nfarcts and *l*eukoencephalopathy), an adult vascular degenerative disease with a tendency to early-age onset of stroke-like events, support the importance of the Notch signaling pathway in embryonic and postnatal development, respectively.

TRANSCRIPTION FACTORS

Transcription factors belong to a large class of proteins that regulate the expression of many target genes, either through activation or repression mechanisms. Typically, a transcription factor will bind to specific nucleotide sequences in the promoter/enhancer regions of target genes and regulate the rate of transcription of its target genes via interacting with accessory proteins. Transcription factors can either activate or repress target gene transcription depending on the cell in which they are expressed, the specific promoter, the chromatin context, and the developmental stage. Some transcription factors do not need to bind to DNA to regulate transcription; they may bind to other transcription factors already bound to the promoter DNA, thereby regulating transcription, or bind to and sequester other transcription factors from their target genes, thus repressing their transcription. The transcription factor superfamily is composed of many different classes of proteins. Three examples of this diverse family of proteins are described: Hox/Homeobox, Pax, and basic helix–loop–helix (bHLH) transcription factors.

HOX/HOMEOBOX PROTEINS

The *Hox* genes were first discovered in the fruit fly, *Drosophila melanogaster*. The order of the Hox genes along the AP axis is faithfully reproduced in their organization at the level of the chromosome. Mutations in these genes of the HOM-C complex lead to dramatic phenotypes (homeotic transformation) such as the Antennapedia gene, in which legs instead of antennae sprout from the head of the fruit fly. In humans, the order of the *Hox* genes along the AP axis and chromosomal location is conserved as well. Defects in *HOXA1* have been shown to impair human neural development, and mutations in *HOXA13* and *HOXD13* result in limb malformations.

All of the *Hox* genes contain a 180–base pair sequence, the homeobox, which encodes a 60–amino acid homeodomain composed of three α-helices. The third (recognition) helix binds to DNA sites that contain one or more binding motifs in the promoters of their target genes. The homeodomain is highly conserved across evolution, whereas other regions of the protein are not as well conserved. Mutations in the DNA-binding region of the homeobox gene *NKX2.5* are associated with **cardiac atrial septal defects** (see Chapter 14), and mutations in *ARX* are associated with the central nervous system malformation syndrome known as **lissencephaly**.

PAX GENES

The *Pax* genes all contain conserved bipartite DNA-binding motifs called the Pax (or paired) domain, and most Pax family members also contain a homeodomain. PAX proteins have been shown to both activate and repress transcription of target genes. The *D. melanogaster* ortholog of *Pax6*, eyeless, was shown to be essential for eye development because homozygous mutant flies had no eyes. Eyeless shares a high degree of sequence conservation with its human ortholog *PAX6* and is associated with ocular malformations such as **aniridia** (absence of the iris) and **Peters anomaly**. In human eye diseases, the level of *PAX6* expression seems to be crucial because patients with only one functional copy (haploinsufficiency) have ocular defects, and patients without *PAX6* function are anophthalmic. This concept of haploinsufficiency is a recurring theme for many different transcription factors and corresponding human malformations.

PAX3 and *PAX7* encode both homeodomain and Pax DNA-binding domains. The human childhood cancer alveolar rhabdomyosarcoma results from a translocation that results in the formation of a chimeric protein wherein PAX3 or PAX7 (including both DNA domains) is fused to the strong activating domains of the Forkhead family transcription factor FOXO1. The autosomal dominant human disease Waardenburg syndrome type I results from mutations in the *PAX3* gene. Patients with this syndrome have hearing deficits, ocular defects (dystopia canthorum), and pigmentation abnormalities best typified by a white forelock.

BASIC HELIX–LOOP–HELIX TRANSCRIPTION FACTORS

The *bHLH* genes are a class of transcription factors that regulate cell fate determination and differentiation in many different tissues during development. At a molecular level, bHLH proteins contain a basic (positively charged) DNA-binding region that is followed by two α-helices that are separated by a loop. The α-helices have a hydrophilic and a hydrophobic side (amphipathic). The hydrophobic side of the helix is a motif for protein–protein interactions between different members of the bHLH family. This domain is the most conserved region of the bHLH proteins across different species. bHLH proteins often bind other bHLHs (heterodimerize) to regulate transcription. These heterodimers are composed of tissue-specific bHLH proteins bound to ubiquitously expressed bHLH proteins. The powerful prodifferentiation effect of bHLH genes can be repressed by several different mechanisms. For example, inhibitor of differentiation (Id) proteins are HLH proteins that lack the basic DNA-binding motif. When Id proteins heterodimerize with specific bHLH proteins, they prevent binding of these bHLH proteins to their target gene promoter sequences (called E-boxes).

Growth factors, which tend to inhibit differentiation, increase the level of Id proteins that sequester bHLH proteins from their target promoters. In addition, growth factors can stimulate the phosphorylation of the DNA-binding domain of bHLH proteins, which inhibits their ability to bind to DNA. *bHLH* genes are crucial for the development of tissues such as muscle *(MyoD/Myogenin)* and neurons *(NeuroD/Neurogenin)* in humans. *MyoD* expression was shown to be sufficient to transdifferentiate several different cell lines into muscle cells, demonstrating that it is a master regulator of muscle differentiation. Studies of knockout mice confirmed that *MyoD* and another bHLH, *Myf5*, are crucial for the differentiation of precursor cells into primitive muscle cells (myoblasts). Similarly, *Mash1/Ascl1* and *Neurogenin1* are proneural genes that regulate the formation of neuroblasts from the neuroepithelium. Mouse models have shown that these genes are crucial for the specification of different subpopulations of precursors in the developing central nervous system. For example, *Mash1/Ascl1* knockout mice have defects in forebrain development, whereas *Neurogenin1* knockout mice have defects in cranial sensory ganglia and ventral spinal cord neurons. Muscle and neuronal differentiation are controlled by a cascade of bHLH genes that function at early and late stages of cellular differentiation. In addition, both differentiation pathways are inhibited via signaling through the Notch pathway.

EPIGENETICS

Epigenetics refers to inherited modifications that affect gene expression as a result of mechanisms other than changes in the DNA sequence. Examples include DNA methylation, microRNAs, and chromatin modifications, such as acetylation, methylation, and phosphorylation of histones. These epigenetic marks (*epigenetic code*) are regulated by classes of enzymes that: (1) recognize the epigenetic marks (*readers*), (2) add epigenetic markers to DNA or histones (*writers*), or (3) remove these epigenetics marks (*erasers*). Disorders of chromatin remodeling include Rett, Rubinstein-Taybi, and alpha-thalassemia/X-linked mental retardation syndromes.

DNA METHYLATION

DNA is methylated at cytosine residues by DNA methyltransferases at CpG sites—where cytosine and guanine nucleotides are directly paired. CpG islands are DNA regions with high concentrations of CpG sites and are often located in the proximal promoter regions of genes. DNA methylation at CpG sites, in general, leads to reduced gene expression or gene silencing, whereas DNA hypomethylation at CpG sites leads to gene overexpression. Silencing of tumor suppressor genes or overexpression of oncogenes may lead to cancer. Proteins, such as methyl-CpG-binding protein 2 (MECP2), which is mutated in the neurodevelopmental disorder Rett syndrome, function as *"readers"* by binding to methylated DNA and subsequently assembling protein complexes that repress gene expression.

HISTONE MODIFICATIONS

Histones are the positively charged nuclear proteins around which genomic DNA is coiled to tightly pack it within the nucleus. Modification of these proteins is a common pathway by which transcription factors regulate the activity of their target promoters. Examples of histone modifications include phosphorylation, ubiquitination (also known as ubiquitylation), sumoylation, acetylation, and methylation. The latter two modifications are discussed here in more depth.

HISTONE ACETYLATION

DNA is less tightly bound to acetylated histones, thus allowing for more open access of transcription factors and other

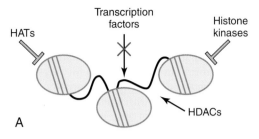
Transcriptionally inactive chromatin

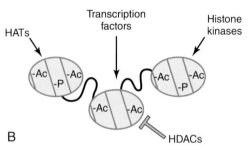
Transcriptionally active chromatin

Fig. 20.8 Histone modifications alter transcriptional properties of chromatin. (A) In areas of transcriptionally inactive chromatin, the DNA is tightly bound to the histone cores. The histones are not acetylated or phosphorylated. Histone deacetylases (HDACs) are active, whereas histone acetyl transferases (HATs) and histone kinases are inactive. (B) In areas of transcriptionally active chromatin, the DNA is not as tightly bound to the histone cores. The histone proteins are acetylated (Ac) and phosphorylated (-P). HDACs are inactive, whereas HATs and histone kinases are active.

proteins to the promoters of their target genes. Histone acetylation status is controlled by genes that add acetyl groups (histone transferase, a *writer*) or remove acetyl groups (histone deacetylase, an *eraser*) (Fig. 20.8). Phosphorylation of histones also leads to an opening of the chromatin structure and activation of gene transcription. These epigenetic marks are recognized (read) by both bromodomain proteins and pleckstrin homology domain proteins.

HISTONE METHYLATION

Histone methyltransferases, or *writers*, catalyze the addition of a methyl group to lysine residues on histone tails. This modification is removed by histone demethylases, or *erasers*. In contrast to histone acetylation, methylation of histones can result in (1) the addition of 1, 2, or 3 methyl groups to an individual lysine residue and (2) either the activation or repression of gene expression depending on the particular lysine residue that is modified. For example, trimethylation of lysine 9 or lysine 27 on histone 3 (H3K9me3, H3K27me3) is associated with repressed promoters, whereas trimethylation of lysine 4 on histone 3 (H3K4me3) is associated with active promoters. Histone methylation status is *read* by a large number of different classes of proteins. Mutations of histone modification *readers, writers, and erasers* can lead to diseases such as neurodevelopmental disorders and cancer. Recent identification of mutations in the genes encoding histone variants H3.3 and H3.1, especially H3 K27M and H3 G34R/V, have contributed to our understanding of pediatric high-grade gliomas, especially diffuse midline gliomas incorporating diffuse intrinsic pontine gliomas.

MICRORNAS

MicroRNAs (miRNA or miRs) are highly conserved, short (22-nucleotide), noncoding RNAs that act posttranscriptionally to silence RNA. The biogenesis of miRNAs is complex and a highly regulated process. After export to the cytoplasm, pre-miRNAs require a ribonuclease known as *Dicer* to become processed into mature miRNA duplexes. One miRNA strand is included in the RNA-induced silencing complex.

miRNAs target more than one-half of the genes expressed during development, and each miRNA may specifically target hundreds of genes. Although they are not considered as a classic epigenetic means to modify gene expression, such as DNA methylation and histone modifications, miRNAs also modify gene expression without changing DNA sequence.

Many diseases associated with miRNA dysregulation, including developmental syndromes and cancer, are included in the miR2Disease online database (http://www.mir2disease.org/). Specific miRNAs associated with cancer are called **oncomirs**. Germline mutations of *DICER1* are associated with a familial tumor predisposition syndrome that includes several rare cancers such as pleuropulmonary blastoma, cystic nephroma, and medulloepithelioma.

STEM CELLS: DIFFERENTIATION VERSUS PLURIPOTENCY

Stem cells have the property of self-renewal through symmetric or asymmetric cell divisions, and under specific conditions in the embryo and adult, can give rise to all of the differentiated cell types in the body (totipotent or pluripotent). Several types of stem cell populations have been characterized: **embryonic stem cells** (ESCs), **adult stem cells**, and **cancer stem cells** (CSCs). ESCs, derived from the inner cell mass of the blastula, are **pluripotent** and can give rise to all differentiated cell types from the ectoderm, endoderm, and mesoderm, the primary germ layers (see Chapter 5) but do not contribute to extraembryonic tissues. ESCs express several transcription factors, such as SOX2 and OCT-4, which repress differentiation.

Adult stem cells are found in relative abundance in differentiated tissues and organs that undergo rapid regeneration, such as the bone marrow, hair follicles, and intestinal mucosal epithelium. However, there are "nests" of adult stem cells in many other tissues, including those that have been previously considered nonregenerative, such as the central nervous system and retina; these stem cell populations are small and located in the subventricular zone and ciliary margins, respectively. Hematopoietic stem cells derived from bone marrow, peripheral blood, and umbilical cord sources are now routinely used to treat primary immunodeficiencies and various inherited metabolic disorders and as a "rescue" strategy after marrow-destroying cancer treatments.

CSCs are under intense study since it has become evident through the study of leukemias and solid tumors (e.g., colorectal cancer, malignant gliomas) that a small population of these cells, identified by various cell surface markers (e.g., CD133 in solid tumors), are often resistant to cancer treatments such as radiation or chemotherapy. Investigators are focusing their efforts on eradicating the CSC population, in addition to standard therapies, to increase cure rates.

It is possible to harness the power of stem cells to repair degenerative disorders such as Parkinson disease and tissues severely damaged by ischemia (stroke) and trauma (spinal cord injury). However, researchers have been limited by the available sources of stem cells from the embryo or adult. Hence, there has been tremendous interest in dedifferentiating somatic cells such as epithelial cells and fibroblasts from adults into **induced pluripotent stem cells** (iPSCs). Recent studies have identified several key master transcription factors (Fig. 20.9), such as OCT3/4, SOX2, and KLF4, or Nanog, that can reprogram differentiated cells into pluripotent cells. A key step in this reprogramming event is the rewriting of the epigenetic code of the donor cells.

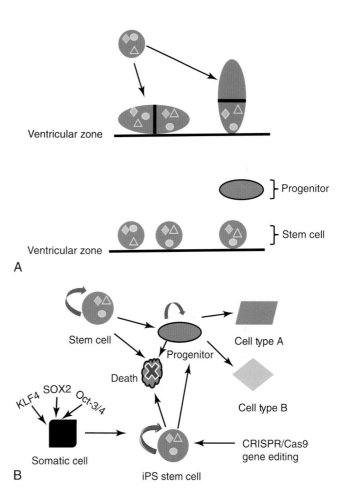

Fig. 20.9 Neural stem cells and induced pluripotent stem cells (*iPS*). (A) Adult or embryonic stem cells can divide *symmetrically*, giving rise to two equivalent daughter stem cells (vertical cell division; the plane of mitosis is perpendicular to the ventricular surface) or *asymmetrically*, giving rise to a daughter stem cell and a nervous system progenitor cell (horizontal cell division; the plane of mitosis is parallel to the ventricular surface). In this example, the progenitor cell does not retain the nuclear or cytoplasmic factors (colored geometric shapes) that remain in the stem cell; however, the progenitor cell expresses new proteins (e.g., receptor tyrosine kinases) in its plasma membrane. (B) Stem cells and *iPS* have the capacity for self-renewal, cell death, and becoming progenitors. Progenitor cells have a more limited capacity for self-renewal, but they can also differentiate into various cell types or undergo cell death. Adult, differentiated somatic cells, such as skin fibroblasts, can be reprogrammed into iPS cells with the introduction of the master transcription factors SOX2, OCT3/4 (now called POU5F1), or KLF4.

These iPSC can be manipulated using nonviral means of gene delivery and have the potential to treat the majority of human diseases in which cell regeneration may restore structure and/or function. In addition, iPSC from human patients can be differentiated into different lineages in vitro (e.g., cardiomyocytes, neural cells, and lung epithelial cells) to model the pathogenesis of human developmental disorders such as cystic fibrosis in a manner that facilitates screening of potential drug candidates. The application of the newly discovered CRISPR/*Cas* gene-editing technology (refer to the following section) has raised the possibility of deriving patient-specific iPSC, correcting the genetic defect in vitro, differentiating the cells into the required lineage, and then returning the corrected cells to the patient (see Fig. 20.9).

A recent advance in iPSC technologies has been the evolution of iPSC-derived tissue **organoids**, including heart, kidney, and specific regions of the brain. These three-dimensional (3D) structures are self-organizing and highly reproducible. Tissue organoids permit the study of spatial organization and cell–cell interactions ex vivo, complementing studies using humans or intact model organisms, such as mice or zebrafish. Furthermore, tissue organoids can be used to model human disease and enable high-throughput drug compounds or functional genomic screens.

GENE EDITING

The study of embryonic development in mice has been enhanced by the development of technologies to specifically inactivate (knockout) or ectopically express genes of interest. However, this technology has not been amenable for use in human cells or to alter gene expression in patients. This has led to the development of new approaches to specifically alter genomic DNA sequence (gene editing) in vitro and in vivo such as the **C**lustered **R**egularly **I**nterspaced **S**hort **P**alindromic **R**epeats (CRISPR)/*Cas9* endonuclease system, which is easy to use, modular in design, highly specific, and being widely implemented. The CRISPR/*Cas9* system was discovered as a bacterial immune response to viral infections. The technology has been simplified to involve a single guide RNA that contains a 20-bp sequence, which is complementary to the target genomic sequence, and a double-stranded section that is bound by Cas9 and localizes the nuclease to the correct genomic location (Fig. 20.10). The genomic DNA at the target site must contain a protospacer adjacent motif sequence that is located at the 3′-end sequence targeted by the guide RNA, which is used by Cas9 to bind DNA and to cleave it. The specific double-strand break in genomic DNA can either be repaired by nonhomologous end joining (NHEJ) or by homology-directed repair (HDR). NHEJ results in deletions that can result in missense mutations (frameshift/stop) being introduced. In contrast, HDR with the appropriate template can be used to correct genetic defects, introduce a putative disease-causing mutation, or incorporate a reporter gene into a specific locus. A nuclease related to Cas9, Cas12, allows for large-scale functional genetic screens since Cas12 can effectively knockout two different targets in a cell since it can use multiple guide RNAs encoded in single transcript. This ability to knockout two genes in a cell allows for the identification

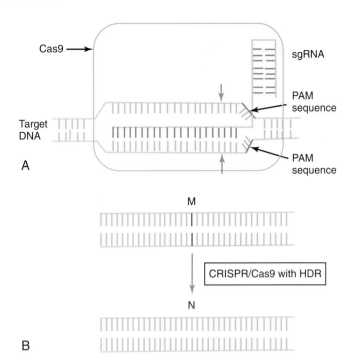

Fig. 20.10 Overview of the CRISPR/Cas9 gene-editing system. (A) This editing system is modular and composed of a single-stranded guide RNA (sgRNA) that has a region complementary to the target sequence in the genomic DNA and a stem structure that is required to localize the endonuclease Cas9, which cleaves both strands of the target DNA sequence. For DNA cleavage by Cas9 to occur, a protospacer adjacent motif (PAM) sequence is required adjacent to the region to be cleaved (*blue arrows*). (B) The resulting double-strand break can be repaired by nonhomologous end joining (NHEJ) or by homology-directed repair (HDR). NHEJ results in deletions that can result in loss-of-function mutations. In contrast, HDR enables specific editing of a target sequence such as the conversion of a mutant allele (M) to the normal allele (N).

of functional interactions between genes with respect to a given cellular output such as survival or proliferation. The uptake of this gene-editing technology has been rapid; it has already been used to correct genetic defects in vivo in mice and ex vivo in humans and has enhanced the ability to model human developmental diseases in vitro. The therapeutic potential of this technology is very promising as it allows, for the first time, our ability to specifically alter the human genome, either ex vivo or in vivo, to correct genetic defects.

SUMMARY OF COMMON SIGNALING PATHWAYS USED DURING DEVELOPMENT

- There are marked differences among the various signaling pathways, but they share many common features: ligands, membrane-bound receptors and coreceptors, intracellular signaling domains, adapters, and effector molecules.
- Signaling pathways are co-opted at various times during development for stem cell renewal, cell proliferation, migration, apoptosis, and differentiation.
- Pathways have "default" settings that result in generation or maintenance of one cell fate rather than another.

- Many genes and signaling pathways are highly conserved throughout evolution.
- Knowledge of gene function has been acquired by reverse genetics using model systems with loss- or gain-of-function transgenic approaches. As well, much insight has been gained by forward genetics that begins with the description of abnormal phenotypes arising spontaneously in mice and humans and then subsequent identification of the mutant gene.

- There is evidence of cross-talk among pathways. This communication among various signaling pathways facilitates our understanding of the far-reaching consequences of single gene mutations that result in malformation syndromes affecting the development of multiple organ systems or in cancers.

Bibliography and Suggested Reading

Chapter 1

Corsini NS, Knoblich JA: Human organoids: new strategies and methods for analyzing human development and disease, *Cell* 185:2756, 2022.

Craft AM, Johnson M: From stem cells to human development: a distinctly human perspective on early embryology, cellular differentiation and translational research, *Development* 144(1):12–16, 2017. https://doi.org/10.1242/dev.142778

Gasser R: *Atlas of human embryos*, Hagerstown, MD, 1975, Harper & Row.

Gasser R: *The virtual human embryo project (VHE)*, Baltimore, MD, 2012, NICHD (see also The Endowment for Human Development Project, Inc. [EHD] 2018).

Jirásel JE: *An atlas of human prenatal developmental mechanics: anatomy and staging*, London, 2004, Taylor & Francis.

Lovell-Badge R, Anthony E, Barker RA, et al: ISSCR guidelines for stem cell research and clinical translation: the 2021 update, *Stem Cell Reports* 16(6):1398–1408, 2021. https://doi.org/10.1016/jstemcr.2021.05.012

O'Rahilly R, Müller F: *Developmental stages in human embryos (Publication 637)*, Washington, DC, 1987, Carnegie Institution of Washington.

Rossant J: Why study human embryo development?, Dev Biol. 2024 May;509:43-50. https://doi.10.1016/j.ydbio.2024.02.001. Epub 2024 Feb 5. PMID: 38325560.

Rugg-Gunn PJ, Moris N, Tam PPL: Technical challenges of studying early human development, *Development* 150(11):dev201797, 2023. https://doi.org/10.1242/dev.201797. Epub 2023 Jun 1. PMID: 37260362.10163788

Stern CD: Reflections on the past, present and future of developmental biology, *Dev Biol* 488:30–34, 2022.

Streeter GL, et al: Developmental horizons in human embryos: description of age group XI, 13 to 20 somites, and age group XII, 21 to 29 somites. *Contributions to embryology*, vol 30; 1942 pp 211–245.

Yamada S, Samtani RR, Lee ES, et al: Developmental atlas of the early first trimester embryo, *Dev Dyn* 239(6):1585–1595, 2010. https://doi.org/10.1002/dvdy.22316

Chapter 2

Agarwal A, Sharma RK, Gupta S, et al: Sperm vitality and necrozoospermia: diagnosis, management, and results of a global survey of clinical practice, *World J Men's Health* 40:228–242, 2022.

Cameron S: The normal menstrual cycle. In Magowan BA, Owen P, Thomson A, editors: *Clinical obstetrics & gynaecology*, ed 3, Philadelphia, 2014, Saunders.

Khatun A, Rahman MS, Pang MG: Clinical assessment of the male fertility, *Obstet Gynecol Sci* 61(2):179–191, 2018. https://doi.org/10.5468/ogs.2018.61.2.179

Tüttelmann F, Ruckert C, Röpke A: Disorders of spermatogenesis: perspectives for novel genetic diagnostics after 20 years of unchanged routine, *Med Genet* 30(1):12–20, 2018. https://doi.org/10.1007/s11825-018-0181-7

Wei Y, Wang J, Qu R, Zhang W, et al: Genetic mechanisms of fertilization failure and early embryonic arrest: a comprehensive review, Hum Reprod Update., 2024 Jan 3;30(1):48–80. https://doi.10.1093/humupd/dmad026. PMID: 37758324.

World Health Organization. WHO Laboratory Manual for the Examination and Processing of Human Semen. 6th ed. Geneva: World Health Organization; 2021.

Chapter 3

Coticchio G, Langella C, Sturmey R, Pennetta F, Borini A: The enigmatic morula: mechanisms of development, cell fate determination, self-correction and implication for ART, *Human Reprod Update* 25:422, 2019.

Georgadaki K, Khoury N, Spandios DA, Zoumpourlis V: The molecular basis of fertilization (review), *Int J Mol Med* 38(4):979–986, 2016. https://doi.org/10.3892/ijmm.2016.2723

Herbert M, Choudhary M, Zander-Fox D: Assisted reproductive technologies at the nexus of fertility treatment and disease prevention, *Science* 380(6641):164–167, 2023 Apr 14. http://doi.org/10.1126/science.adh 0073. Epub 2023 Apr 13. PMID: 37053308.

Kolle S, Hughes B, Steele H: Early embryo-maternal communication in the oviduct, *Mol Reprod Dev*.1–13, 2020. https://doi.org/10.1002/mrd.23352

Litscher ES, Wasserman PM: Zona pellucida genes and proteins and human fertility, *Trends Dev Biol* 13:21, 2020.

Plaisier M: Decidualisation and angiogenesis, *Best Pract Res Clin Obstet Gynaecol* 25(3):259–271, 2011. https://doi.org/10.1016/j.bpobgyn.2010.10.011

Rock J, Hertig AT: The human conceptus during the first two weeks of gestation, *Am J Obstet Gynecol* 55(1):6–17, 1948.

Simpson JL: Birth defects and assisted reproductive technology, *Semin Fetal Neonatal Med* 19(3):177–182, 2014. https://doi.org/10.1016/j.siny.2014.01.001

Chapter 4

Hendriks E, Rosenberg R, Prine L: Ectopic pregnancy: diagnosis and management, *Am Fam Physician* 101(10):599–606, 2020.

Gauster M, Moser G, Wernitznig S, Kupper N, Huppertz B: Early human trophoblast development: from morphology to function, *Cell Mol Life Sci* 79(6):345, 2022. https://doi.org/10.1007/s00018-022-04377-0

Hertig AT, Rock J, Adams EC: A description of 34 human ova within the first seventeen days of development, *Am J Anat* 98:435–493, 1956.

Kirk E, Bottomley C, Bourne T: Diagnosing ectopic pregnancy and current concepts in the management of pregnancy of unknown location, *Hum Reprod Update* 20(2):250–261, 2014. https://doi.org/10.1093/humupd/dmt047

Luckett WP: Origin and differentiation of the yolk sac and extraembryonic mesoderm in presomite human and rhesus monkey embryos, *Am J Anat* 152(1):59–97, 1978. https://doi.org/10.1002/aja.1001520106

Muter J, Lynch VJ, McCoy RC, Brosens JJ: Human embryo implantation, *Development* 150(10):dev201507, 2023 May 15. https://doi.org/10.1242/dev.201507. Epub 2023 May 31. PMID: 37254877.oted

Quenby S, Brosens JJ: Human implantation: a tale of mutual maternal and fetal attraction, *Biol Reprod* 88(3):81, 2013. https://doi.org/10.1095/biolreprod.113.108886

Zorn AM, Wells JM: Vertebrate endoderm development and organ formation, *Annu Rev Cell Dev Biol* 25:221–251, 2009. https://doi.org/10.1146/annurev.cellbio.042308.113344

Chapter 5

Betz C, Lenard A, Belting HG, Affolter M: Cell behaviors and dynamics during angiogenesis, *Development* 143(13):2249–2260, 2016. https://doi.org/10.1242/dev.135616

Dawes JHP, Kelsh RN: Cell fate decisions in the neural crest, from pigment to neural development, *Int J Mol Sci* 22:13531, 2021.

Dias AS, de Almeida I, Belmonte JM: Somites without a clock, *Science* 343(6172):791–795, 2014. https://doi.org/10.1126/science.1247575

Jagannathan-Bogdan M, Zon LI: Hematopoiesis, *Development* 140(12):2463–2467, 2013. https://doi.org/10.1242/dev.083147

Männer J: When does the human embryonic heart start beating? A review of contemporary and historical sources of knowledge about the onset of blood circulation in man, *J Cardiovasc Dev Dis* 9(6):187, 2022.10.3390/jcdd9060187 PMID: 35735816; PMCID: PMC9225347

Mukhopadhyay M: Resolving human gastrulation, *Nat Methods* 19:34, 2022. https://doi.org/10.1038/s41592-021-01384-0

Ramesh T, Nagula SV, Tardieu GG, Saker E, Shoja M, et al: Update on the notochord including its embryology, molecular development, and pathology: a primer for the clinician, *Cureus* 9(4):e1137, 2017. https://doi.org/10.7759/cureus.1137

Savage P: Gestational trophoblastic disease. In Magowan BA, Owen P, Thomson A, editors: *Clinical obstetrics & gynaecology*, ed 3, Philadelphia, 2014, Saunders.

Tata M, Ruhrberg C: Cross-talk of neural progenitors and blood vessels in the developing brain, *Neuronal Signal* 2(1):NS20170139, 2018. https://doi.org/10.1042/NS20170139

Yoon HM, Byeon SJ, Hwang JY, Kim JR, Jung AY, Lee JS, Yoon HK, Cho YA: Sacrococcygeal teratomas in newborns: a comprehensive review for the radiologists, *Acta Radiol* 59(2):236–246, 2018. https://doi.org/10.1177/0284185117710680

Chapter 6

Butt K, Lim K: Determination of gestational age by ultrasound, *J Obstet Gynaecol* 36(2):171–181, 2014. https://doi.org/10.1016/S1701-2163(15)30664-2

de Bakker BS, de Jong KH, Hagoort J, de Bree K, Besselink CT, de Kanter FE, et al: An interactive three-dimensional digital atlas and quantitative database of human development, *Science* 354(6315):2016. https://doi.org/10.1126/science.aag0053. pii: aag0053.

FitzPatrick DR: Human embryogenesis. In Magowan BA, Owen P, Thomson A, editors: *Clinical obstetrics & gynaecology*, ed 3, Philadelphia, 2014, Saunders.

Gasser R: *Virtual human embryo DREM project*, Bethesda, MD, 2012, NIH.

Jirásel JE: *An atlas of human prenatal developmental mechanics: anatomy and staging*, London, 2004, Taylor & Francis.

O'Rahilly R, Müller F: *Development stages in human embryos (Publication 637)*, Washington, DC, 1987, Carnegie Institution of Washington.

Pechriggl E, Blumer M, Tubbs RS, Olewnik Ł, Konschake M, Fortélny R, et al: Embryology of the abdominal wall and associated malformations-a review. Front Surg, published 07 July 2022 9:891896. https://doi.org/10.3389/fsurg.2022.891896

Persaud TVN, Hay JC: Normal embryonic and fetal development. In Reece EA, Hobbins JC, editors: *Clinical obstetrics: the fetus and mother*, ed 3, Oxford, 2006, Blackwell Publishing.

Pooh RK, Shiota K, Kurjak A: Imaging of the human embryo with magnetic resonance imaging microscopy and high-resolution transvaginal 3-dimensional sonography: human embryology in the 21st century, *Am J Obstet Gynecol* 204(1):77.e1–77.e16, 2011. https://doi.org/10.1016/j.ajog.2010.07.028

Rossant J: Why study human embryo development?, Dev Biol. 2024 May;509:43–50. https://doi.10.1016/j.ydbio.2024.02.001. Epub 2024 Feb 5. PMID: 38325560.

Steding G: *The anatomy of the human embryo: a scanning electron-microscopic atlas*, Basel, 2009, Karger.

Yamada S, Samtani RR, Lee ES, Lockett E, Uwabe C, Shiota K, Anderson SA, Lo CW: Developmental atlas of the early first trimester embryo, *Dev Dyn* 239(6):1585–1595, 2010. https://doi.org/10.1002/dvdy.22316

Chapter 7

American College of Obstetricians and Gynecologists' Committee on Obstetric Practice: Methods for estimating the due date; Committee opinion 700. Obstet Gynecol 129:e150,2017.

Butt K, Lim K: Determination of gestational age by ultrasound, *J Obstet Gynaecol* 36(2):171–181, 2014. https://doi.org/10.1016/S1701-2163(15)30664-2

David AL, Spencer RN: Clinical assessment of fetal wellbeing and fetal safety indications, *J Clin Pharmacol* 62(Suppl 1):567–578, 2022. https://doi.org/10.1002/jcph.2126

Huang H, Wang Y, Zhang M, Lin N, An G, He D, Chen M, et al: Diagnostic accuracy and value of chromosomal microarray analysis for chromosomal abnormalities in prenatal detection: a prospective clinical study, *Medicine (Baltimore)* 100(20):e25999, 2021.

Jirásel JE: *An atlas of human prenatal developmental mechanics: anatomy and staging*, London, 2004, Taylor & Francis.

Whitworth M, Bricker L, Neilson JP, Dowswell T: Ultrasound for fetal assessment in early pregnancy, *Cochrane Database Syst Rev*(4): CD007058, 2010. https://doi.org/10.1002/14651858.CD007058.pub2

Chapter 8

Alecsandru D, García-Velasco JA: Immunology and human reproduction, *Curr Opin Obstet Gynecol* 27(3):231–234, 2015. https://doi.org/10.1097/GCO.0000000000000174

Bakhsh H, Alenizy H, Alenazi S, Alnasser S, Alanazi N, Alsowinea M, Alharbi L, Alfaifi B: Amniotic fluid disorders and the effects on prenatal outcome: a retrospective cohort study, *BMC Pregnancy Childbirth* 21:75, 2021. https://doi.org/10.1186/s12884-021-03549-3

Banks CL: Labour. In Magowan BA, Owen P, Thomson A, editors: *Clinical obstetrics & gynaecology*, ed 3, Philadelphia, 2014, Saunders.

Burton GJ, Jauniaux E: The human placenta: new perspectives on its formation and function during early pregnancy, *Proc Biol Sci* 290(1997):20230191, 2023 Apr 26. https://doi.org/10.1098/rspb.2023.0191. Epub 2023 Apr 19. PMID: 37072047; PMCID: PMC10113033

Chakraborty C, Gleeson LM, McKinnon T, Lala PK: Regulation of human trophoblast migration and invasiveness, *Can J Physiol Pharmacol* 80(2):116–124, 2002.

Chen Y, Siriwardena D, Penfold C, Pavlinek A, Boroviak TE: An integrated atlas of human placental development delineates essential regulators of trophoblast stem cells, *Development* 149(13):dev 200171, 2022 Jul 1. https://doi.org/10.1242/dev.200171

Cindrova-Davies T, Sferruzzi-Perri AN: Human placental development and function, *Semin Cell Dev Biol* 138:83–93, 2022. https://doi.org/10.1016/j.semcdb.2022.03.009

Collins JH: Umbilical cord accidents: human studies, *Semin Perinatol* 26(1):79–82, 2002.

Dashe JS, Hoffman BL: Ultrasound evaluation of the placenta, membranes and umbilical cord. Ultrasound evaluation of normal fetal anatomy. In Norton ME, editor: *Callen's ultrasonography in obstetrics and gynecology*, ed 6, Philadelphia, 2017, Elsevier.

Gibson J: Multiple pregnancy. In Magowan BA, Owen P, Thomson A, editors: *Clinical obstetrics & gynaecology*, ed 3, Philadelphia, 2014, Saunders.

Jabrane-Ferrat N, Siewiera J: The up side of decidual natural killer cells: new developments in immunology of pregnancy, *Immunology* 141(4):490–497, 2014. https://doi.org/10.1111/imm.12218

Knöfler M, Pollheimer J: Human placental trophoblast invasion and differentiation: a particular focus on Wnt signaling, *Front Genet* 4:190, 2013. https://doi.org/10.3389/fgene.2013.00190

Lala N, Girish GV, Cloutier-Bosworth A, Lala PK: Mechanisms in decorin regulation of vascular endothelial growth factor-induced human trophoblast migration and acquisition of endothelial phenotype, *Biol Reprod* 87(3):59, 2012. https://doi.org/10.1095/biolreprod.111.097881

Lala PK, Chatterjee-Hasrouni S, Kearns M, Montgomery B, Colavincenzo V: Immunobiology of the feto-maternal interface, *Immunol Rev* 75:87–116, 1983.

Lala PK, Kearns M, Colavincenzo V: Cells of the fetomaternal interface: their role in the maintenance of viviparous pregnancy, *Am J Anat* 170(3):501–517, 1984. https://doi.org/10.1002/aja.1001700321

Lala PK, Nandi P: Mechanisms of trophoblast migration, endometrial angiogenesis in preeclampsia: the role of decorin, *Cell Adh Migr* 10(1–2):111–125, 2016. https://doi.org/10.1080/19336918.2015.1106669

Magann EF, Sandin AI: Amniotic fluid volume in fetal health and disease. In Norton ME, editor: *Callen's ultrasonography in obstetrics and gynecology*, ed 6, Philadelphia, 2017, Elsevier.

Masselli G, Gualdi G: MR imaging of the placenta: what a radiologist should know, *Abdom Imaging* 38(3):573–587, 2013. https://doi.org/10.1007/s00261-012-9929-8

Redline RW: Placental pathology. In Martin RJ, Fanaroff AA, Walsh MC, editors: *Fanaroff and Martin's neonatal-perinatal medicine: diseases of the fetus and infant*, ed 9, Philadelphia, 2011, Mosby.

van der Schot AM, Sikkel E, Spaanderman MEA, Vandenbussche FPHA: Computer-assisted fetal laser surgery in the treatment of twin-to-twin transfusion syndrome: recent trends and prospects, *Prenat Diagn* 42(10):1225–1234, 2022 Sep. https://doi.org/10.1002/pd.6225

Chapter 9

Antounians L, Zani A: Beyond the diaphragm and the lung: a multisystem approach to understanding congenital diaphragmatic hernia,

Pediatr Surg Int 39(1):194, 2023 May 9. https://doi.org/10.1007/s00383-023-05471-5. PMID: 37160490.

Ariza L, Carmona R, Cañete A, Cano E, Muñoz-Chápuli R: Coelomic epithelium-derived cells in visceral morphogenesis, *Dev Dyn* 245(3):307–322, 2016. https://doi.org/10.1002/dvdy.24373

Badillo A, Gingalewski C: Congenital diaphragmatic hernia: treatment and outcomes, *Semin Perinatol* 38(2):92–96, 2014.

Brosens E, Peters NCJ, van Weelden KS, Bendixen C, Brouwer RWW, Sleutels F, et al: Unraveling the genetics of congenital diaphragmatic hernia: an ongoing challenge, *Front Pediatr* 9:800915, 2022 Feb 3. https://doi.org/10.3389/fped.2021.800915

Cannata G, Caporilli C, Grassi F, Perrone S, Esposito S: Management of congenital diaphragmatic hernia (CDH): role of molecular genetics, *Int J Mol Sci* 22(12):6353, 2021. https://doi.org/10.3390/ijms22126353 Published 2021 Jun 14

Clugston RD, Zhang W, Alvarez S, de Lera AR, Greer JJ: Understanding abnormal retinoid signaling as a causative mechanism in congenital diaphragmatic hernia, *Am J Respir Cell Mol Biol* 42(3):276–285, 2010. https://doi.org/10.1165/rcmb.2009-0076OC

Donahoe PK, Longoni M, High FA: Polygenic causes of congenital diaphragmatic hernia produce common lung pathologies, *Am J Pathol* 186(10):2532–2543, 2016. https://doi.org/10.1016/j.ajpath.2016.07.006

Knowles MR, Zariwala M, Leigh M: Primary ciliary dyskinesia, *Clin Chest Med* 37(3):449–461, 2016. https://doi.org/10.1016/j.ccm.2016.04.008

Koo CW, Johnson TF, Gierada DS, White DB, Blackmon S, Matsumoto JM, et al: The breadth of the diaphragm: updates in embryogenesis and role of imaging, *Br J Radiol* 91(1088), 2018 Jul. https://doi.org/10.1259/bjr.20170600 20170600

Oh T, Chan S, Kieffer S: Fetal outcomes of prenatally diagnosed congenital diaphragmatic hernia: nine years of clinical experience in a Canadian tertiary hospital, *J Obstet Gynaecol Can* 38(1):17–22, 2016. https://doi.org/10.1016/j.jogc.2015.10.006

Oluyomi-Obi T, Kuret V, Puligandla P, Lodha A, Lee-Robertson H, Lee K, et al: Antenatal predictors of outcome in prenatally diagnosed congenital diaphragmatic hernia (CDH), *J Pediatr Surg* 52(5):881–888, 2017. https://doi.org/10.1016/j.jpedsurg.2016.12.008

Pechriggl E, Blumer M, Tubbs RS, Olewnik Ł, Konschake M, Fortélny R, et al: Embryology of the abdominal wall and associated malformations-a review. Front Surg, published 07 July 2022;9:891896. https://doi.org/10.3389/fsurg.2022.891896

Slavotinek AM: The genetics of common disorders—congenital diaphragmatic hernia, *Eur J Med Genet* 57(8):418–423, 2014. https://doi.org/10.1016/j.ejmg.2014.04.012

Wells LJ, et al: Development of the human diaphragm and pleural sacs *Contributions to embryology*, vol 35; 1954, pp 107–134.

Chapter 10

Bajaj Y, Ifeacho S, Tweedie D, Jephson CG, Albert DM, Cochrane LA, et al: Branchial anomalies in children, *Int J Pediatr Otorhinolaryngol* 75(8):1020–1023, 2011. https://doi.org/10.1016/j.ijporl.2011.05.008

Berkovitz BKB, Holland GR, Moxham B: *Oral anatomy, histology, and embryology*, ed 4, Philadelphia, 2018, Elsevier.

Cordes M, Coerper S, Kuwert T, Schmidkonz C: Ultrasound imaging of cervical anatomic variants, *Curr Med Imaging* 17:966, 2021.

de Paula F, Teshima THN, Hsieh R, Souza MM, Nico MMS, Lourenco SV: Overview of human salivary glands: highlights of morphology and developing processes, *Anat Rec* 300:1180, 2017.

Fabik J, Psutkova V, Machon O: The mandibular and hyoid arches-from molecular patterning to shaping bone and cartilage, *Int J Mol Sci* 22(14):7529, 2021 Jul 14. https://doi.org/10.3390/ijms22147529

Hinrichsen K: The early development of morphology and patterns of the face in the human embryo, *Adv Anat Embryol Cell Biol* 98:1–79, 1985.

Jones KL, Jones MC, Campo MD: *Smith's recognizable patterns of human malformation*, ed 7, Philadelphia, 2013, Saunders.

Khan MI, Cs P, Srinath NM: Genetic factors in nonsyndromic orofacial clefts, *Glob Med Genet* 7(4):101–108, 2020 Dec. https://doi.org/10.1055/s-0041-1722951

Martinelli M, Palmieri A, Carinci F, Scapoli L: Non-syndromic cleft palate: An overview on human genetic and environmental risk factors, Front Cell Dev Biol 8:592271, 2020.

Mueller DT, Callanan VP: Congenital malformations of the oral cavity, *Otolaryngol Clin North Am* 40(1):141–160, 2007. https://doi.org/10.1016/j.otc.2006.10.007

Nanci A: *Ten Cate's oral histology: development, structure, and function*, ed 8, Philadelphia, 2012, Mosby.

Parada C, Han D, Chai Y: Molecular and cellular regulatory mechanisms of tongue myogenesis, *J Dent Res* 91(6):528–535, 2012. https://doi.org/10.1177/0022034511434055

Rice DPC: Craniofacial anomalies: from development to molecular pathogenesis, *Curr Mol Med* 5(7):699–722, 2005. https://doi.org/10.2174/156652405774641043

Sweat YY, Sweat M, Mansaray M, Cao H, Eliason S, Adeyemo WL, et al: Six2 regulates PAX9 expression, palatogenesis and craniofacial bone formation, *Dev Biol* 458:246, 2020.

Waldhausen JHT: Branchial cleft and arch anomalies in children, *Semin Pediatr Surg* 15(2):64–69, 2006. https://doi.org/10.1053/j.sempedsurg.2006.02.002

Yatzey KE: DiGeorge syndrome, Tbx1, and retinoic acid signaling come full circle, *Circ Res* 106(4):630–632, 2010. https://doi.org/10.1161/CIRCRESAHA.109.215319

Chapter 11

Berman DR, Treadwell MC: Ultrasound evaluation of fetal thorax. In Norton ME, editor: *Callen's ultrasonography in obstetrics and gynecology* ed 6, Philadelphia, 2017, Elsevier.

Brown E, James K: The lung primordium an outpunching from the foregut! Evidence-based dogma or myth? *J Pediatr Surg* 44(3):607–615, 2009. https://doi.org/10.1016/j.jpedsurg.2008.09.012

Gowen CW Jr: Fetal and neonatal medicine (respiratory diseases of the newborn). In Marcdante KJ, Kliegman RM, editors: *Nelson essentials of pediatrics* ed 7, Philadelphia, 2015, Saunders.

Herriges M, Morrisey EE: Lung development: orchestrating the generation and regeneration of a complex organ, *Development* 141(3):502–513, 2014. https://doi.org/10.1242/dev.098186

Jobe AH: Lung development and maturation. In Martin RJ, Fanaroff AA, Walsh MC, editors: *Fanaroff and Martin's neonatal-perinatal medicine: diseases of the fetus and infant*, ed 9, Philadelphia, 2011, Mosby.

Moghieb A, Clair G, Mitchell HD, Kitzmiller J, Zink EM, Kim YM, et al: Time-resolved proteome profiling of normal lung development, *Am J Physiol Lung Cell Mol Physiol* 315(1):L11–L24, 2018. https://doi.org/10.1152/ajplung.00316.2017

Morrisey EE, Cardoso WV, Lane RH, Rabinovitch M, Abman SH, Ai X, et al: Molecular determinants of lung development, *Ann Am Thorac Soc* 10(2):S12–S16, 2013. https://doi.org/10.1513/AnnalsATS.201207-036OT

O'Rahilly R, Boyden E: The timing and sequence of events in the development of the human respiratory system during the embryonic period proper, *Z Anat Entwicklungsgesch* 141(3):237–250, 1973.

Perin S, McCann CJ, Borrelli O, De Coppi P, Thapar N: Update on foregut molecular embryology and role of regenerative medicine therapies, *Front Pediatr* 5:91, 2017 Apr 28. https://doi.org/10.3389/fped.2017.00091

Sardesai S, Biniwale M, Wertheimer F, Garingo A, Ramanathan R: Evolution of surfactant therapy for respiratory distress syndrome: past, present, and future, *Pediatr Res* 81(1-2):240–248, 2017 Jan. https://doi.org/10.1038/pr.2016.203

Warburton D, El-Hashash A, Carraro G, Tiozzo C, Sala F, Rogers O, et al: Lung organogenesis, *Curr Top Dev Biol* 90:73–158, 2010. https://doi.org/10.1016/S0070-2153(10)90003-3

Wells LJ, Boyden EA: The development of the bronchopulmonary segments in human embryos of horizons XVII to XIX, *Am J Anat* 95(2):163–201, 1954. https://doi.org/10.1002/aja.1000950202

Zepp JA, Morrisey EE: Cellular crosstalk in the development and regeneration of the respiratory system, *Nat Rev Mol Cell Biol* 20:551, 2019. https://doi.org/10.1038/s41580-019-0141-3

Chapter 12

Bastidas-Ponce A, Scheibner K, Lickert L: Cellular and molecular mechanisms coordinating pancreas development, *Development* 144(16):2873–2888, 2017. https://doi.org/10.1242/dev.140756

Belo J, Krishnamurthy M, Oakie A, Wang R: The role of SOX9 transcription factor in pancreatic and duodenal development, *Stem Cells Dev* 22(22):2935–2943, 2013. https://doi.org/10.1089/scd.2013.0106

DeLaForest A, Di Furio F, Jing R, et al: HNF4A Regulates the formation of hepatic progenitor cells from human iPSC-Derived Endoderm by Facilitating Efficient recruitment of RNA Pol II, Genes (Basel). 2018 Dec 28;10(1):21. https://doi.10.3390/genes10010021. PMID: 30597922; PMCID: PMC6356828.

Keplinger KM, Bloomston M: Anatomy and embryology of the biliary tract, *Surg Clin North Am* 94:203–217, 2014.

Khanna K, Sharma S, Pabalan N, Singh N, Gupta DK: A review of genetic factors contributing to the etiopathogenesis of anorectal malformations, *Pediatr Surg Int* 34:9, 2018.

Klein M, Varga I: Hirschsprung's disease-recent understanding of embryonic aspects, etiopathogenesis and future treatment avenues, *Medicina (Kaunas)*, 56(11):611, 2020 Nov 13. http://doi.org/10.3390/medicina 56110611

Klezovitch O, Vasioukhin V: Your gut is right to turn left, *Dev Cell* 26(6):553–554, 2013. https://doi.org/10.1016/j.devcel.2013.08.018

Kluth D, Fiegel HC, Metzger R: Embryology of the hindgut, *Semin Pediatr Surg* 20(3):152–160, 2011. https://doi.org/10.1053/j.sempedsurg.2011.03.002

Kostouros A, Koliarakis I, Natsis K, Spandidos DA, Tsatsakis A, Tsiaoussis J: Large intestine embryogenesis: molecular pathways and related disorders (review), *Int J Mol Med* 46:27, 2020.

Kruepunga N, Hikspoors JPJM, Hülsman CJM, Mommen GMC, Köhler SE, Lamers WH: Development of extrinsic innervation in the abdominal intestines of human embryos. *J Anat* 237:655, 2020.

Ledbetter DJ: Gastroschisis and omphalocele, *Surg Clin North Am* 86(2):249–260, 2006. https://doi.org/10.1016/j.suc.2005.12.003

Metzger R, Metzger U, Fiegel HC, Kluth D: Embryology of the midgut, *Semin Pediatr Surg* 20(3):145–151, 2011. https://doi.org/10.1053/j.sempedsurg.2011.03.005

Nadel A: The fetal gastrointestinal tract and abdominal wall. In Norton ME, Scoutt LM, Feldstein VA, editors: *Callen's ultrasonography in obstetrics and gynecology*, ed 6, Philadelphia, 2017, Elsevier.

Nagy N, Goldstein AM: Enteric nervous system development: a crest cell's journey from neural tube to colon, *Semin Cell Dev Biol* 66:94–106, 2017. https://doi.org/10.1016/j.semcdb.2017.01.006

Naik-Mathuria B, Olutoye OO: Foregut abnormalities, *Surg Clin North Am* 86(2):261–284, 2006. https://doi.org/10.1016/j.suc.2005.12.011

Soffers JH, Hikspoors JP, Mekonen HK, Koehler SE, Lamers WH: The growth pattern of the human intestine and its mesentery, *Dev Biol* 15:31, 2015. https://doi.org/10.1186/s12861-015-0081-x

Vakili K, Pomfret EA: Biliary anatomy and embryology, *Surg Clin North Am* 88(6):1159–1174, 2008. https://doi.org/10.1016/j.suc.2008.07.001

van den Brink GR: Hedgehog signaling in development and homeostasis of the gastrointestinal tract, *Physiol Rev* 87(4):1343–1375, 2007. https://doi.org/10.1152/physrev.00054.2006

Van der Putte SCJ: The development of the human anorectum, *Anat Rec* 292(7):951–954, 2009. https://doi.org/10.1002/ar.20914

Zorn AM: Development of the digestive system, *Semin Cell Dev Biol* 66:1–2, 2017. https://doi.org/10.1016/j.semcdb.2017.05.015

Chapter 13

Ali MAA, Maalman RS-U, Dankar YO: Ambiguous genitalia: clinical management of adult female with male assigned gender: case report, *J Med Case Rep* 15:362, 2021.

Amândio AR, Lopez-Delisle L, Bolt CC, Mascrez B, Duboule D: A complex regulatory landscape involved in the development of mammalian external genitals, *eLife*, 9:e52962, 2020. https://doi.org/10.7554/eLife.52962

Budhwar S, Singh V, Verma P, et al: Fertilization failure and gamete health: Is there a link? Front Biosci (Schol Ed). 2017 Jun 1;9(3):395-419. https://doi.10.2741/s494. PMID: 28410126.

Creighton S: Disorders of sex development. In Magowan BA, Owen P, Thomson A, editors: *Clinical obstetrics & gynaecology*, ed 3, Philadelphia, 2014, Saunders.

Davies R, Davies L, Alleemudder D, MacDougall J: Differences of sexual development and their clinical implications, *Obstet Gynaecol* 22:257, 2020.

Gates RL, Shelton J, Diefenbach KA, Arnold M, St Peter SD, Renaud EJ, et al: Management of the undescended testis in children: an American Pediatric Surgical Association Outcomes and Evidence Based Practice Committee Systematic Review, *J Pediatr Surg* 57:1293, 2022.

Gulas E, Wysiadecki G, Szymański J, Majos A, Stefańczyk L, Topol M, Polguj M: Morphological and clinical aspects of the occurrence of accessory (multiple) renal arteries, *Arch Med Sci* 14(2):442–453, 2018 Mar. https://doi.org/10.5114/aoms.2015.55203

Haynes JH: Inguinal and scrotal disorders, *Surg Clin North Am* 86(2):371–381, 2006. https://doi.org/10.1016/j.suc.2005.12.005

Kollin C, Ritzén EM: Cryptorchidism: a clinical perspective, *Pediatr Endocrinol Rev* 11(Suppl 2):240–250, 2014.

Kutney K, Konczal L, Kaminski B, Uli N: Challenges in the diagnosis and management of disorders of sex development, *Birth Defects Res C Embryo Today* 108(4):293–308, 2016. https://doi.org/10.1002/bdrc.21147

Odiba AO, Dick JM: Fetal genitourinary tract. In Norton ME, editor: *Callen's ultrasonography in obstetrics and gynecology*, ed 6, Philadelphia, 2017, Elsevier.

Overland MR, Li Y, Derpinghaus A, et al.: Development of the human ovary: fetal through pubertal ovarian morphology, folliculogenesis, and expression of cellular differentiation markers. https://doi.org/10.1016/j.diff.2022.10.005

Persaud TVN: Embryology of the female genital tract and gonads. In Copeland LJ, Jarrell J, editors: *Textbook of gynecology*, ed 2, Philadelphia, 2000, Saunders.

Rodprasert W, Virtanen HE, Toppari J: Cryptorchidism and puberty. Front Endocrinol (Lausanne). 2024 Mar 12;15:1347435. https://doi.10.3389/fendo.2024.1347435. PMID: 38532895.

Svingen T, Koopman P: Building the mammalian testis: origins, differentiation, and assembly of the component cell populations, *Genes Dev* 27(22):2409–2426, 2013. https://doi.org/10.1101/gad.228080.113

Virtanen HE, Toppari J: Embryology and physiology of testicular development and descent, *Pediatr Endocrinol Rev* 11(Suppl 2):206–213, 2014.

Woo LL, Thomas JC, Brock JW: Cloacal exstrophy: a comprehensive review of an uncommon problem, *J Pediatr Urol* 6(2):102–111, 2010. https://doi.org/10.1016/j.jpurol.2009.09.011

Chapter 14

Adams SM, Good MW, DeFranco GM: Sudden infant death syndrome, *Am Fam Physician* 79(10):870–874, 2009.

Annabi MR, Makaryus AN: *Embryology, atrioventricular septum*, Treasure Island, FL, 2018, StatPearls Publishing.

Ashworth M, Chapter 3, Development of the heart. In *Pathology of heart disease in the fetus, infant and child: autopsy, surgical and molecular pathology*, 2019, Cambridge University Press: Cambridge, pp. 53–74. http://doi.org/10.1017/9781316337073.003.

Dyer LA, Kirby ML: The role of secondary heart field in cardiac development, *Dev Dyn* 336(2):137–144, 2009. https://doi.org/10.1016/j.ydbio.2009.10.009

El Robrini N, Etchevers HC, Ryckebüsch L, Faure E, Eudes N, Niederreither K, Zaffran S, Bertrand N: Cardiac outflow morphogenesis depends on effects of retinoic acid signaling on multiple cell lineages, *Dev Dyn* 245(3):388–401, 2016. https://doi.org/10.1002/dvdy.24357

Hildreth V, Anderson RH, Henderson DJ: Autonomic innervation of the developing heart: origins and function, *Clin Anat* 22(1):36–46, 2009. https://doi.org/10.1002/ca.20695

Horsthuis T, Christoffels VM, Anderson RH, Moorman AF: Can recent insights into cardiac development improve our understanding of congenitally malformed hearts? *Clin Anat* 22(1):4–20, 2009. https://doi.org/10.1002/ca.20723

International Society of Ultrasound in Obstetrics and Gynecology, Carvalho JS, Allan LD, Chaoui R, Copel JA, DeVore GR, et al: ISUOG Practice Guidelines (updated): sonographic screening examination of the fetal heart, *Ultrasound Obstet Gynecol* 41(3):348–359, 2013. http://doi.org/10.1002/uog.12403.

Kamedia Y: Hoxa3 and signaling molecules involved in aortic arch patterning and remodeling, *Cell Tissue Res* 336(2):165–178, 2010. https://doi.org/10.1007/s00441-009-0760-7

Kodo K, Yamagishi H: A decade of advances in the molecular embryology and genetics underlying congenital heart defects, *Circ J* 75(10):2296–2304, 2011.

Loukas M, Groat C, Khangura R, Owens DG, Anderson RH: The normal and abnormal anatomy of the coronary arteries, *Clin Anat* 22(1):114–128, 2009. https://doi.org/10.1002/ca.20761

Loukas M, Bilinsky S, Bilinsky E, el-Sedfy A, Anderson RH: Cardiac veins: a review of the literature, *Clin Anat* 22(1):129–145, 2009. https://doi.org/10.1002/ca.20745

Männer J.: When does the human embryonic heart start beating? A review of contemporary and historical sources of knowledge about eh onset of blood circulation in man. J Cardiovasc Dev Dis. 9:187, 2022.

Morris SA, Ayres NA, Espinoza J, Maskatia SA, Lee W: Sonographic evaluation of the fetal heart. In Norton ME, editor: *Callen's ultrasonography in obstetrics and gynecology*, ed 6, Philadelphia, 2017, Elsevier.

Quijada P, Trembley MA, Small EM: The role of epicardium during heart development and repair, *Circ Res* 126:377, 2020.

Sethi N, Miller S, Hill KD: Prenatal diagnosis, management, and treatment of fetal cardiac disease, *Neoreviews* 24(5):e285–e299, 2023 May 1. https://doi.org/10.1542/neo.24-5-e285. PMID: 37122058

Škorić-Milosavljević D, Tadros R, Bosada FM, Tessadori F, van Weerd JH, Woudstra OI, et al: Common genetic variants contribute to risk of transposition of the great arteries, *Circ Res* 130(2):166–180, 2022 Jan 21. https://doi.org/10.1161/CIRCRESAHA.120.317107

Steele RE, Sanders R, Phillips HM, Bamforth SD: PAX genes in cardiovascular develop, *Int J Mol Sci* 23(14):7713, 2022. https://doi.org/10.3390/ijms23147713

Stoller JZ, Epstein JA: Cardiac neural crest, *Semin Cell Dev Biol* 16(6):704–715, 2005. https://doi.org/10.1016/j.semcdb.2005.06.004

Watanabe M, Schaefer KS: Cardiac embryology. In Martin RJ, Fanaroff AA, Walsh MC, editors: *Fanaroff and Martin's neonatal-perinatal medicine: diseases of the fetus and infant*, ed 9, Philadelphia, 2011, Mosby.

Zaffran S, Kelly RG: New developments in the second heart field, *Differentiation* 84(1):17–24, 2012. https://doi.org/10.1016/j.diff.2012.03.003

Chapter 15

Andreescu N, Sharma A, Mihailescu A, Zimbru CG, David VL, Horhat R, et al: Chest wall deformities and their possible associations with different genetic syndromes, *Eur Rev Med Pharmacol Sci* 26(14):5107–5114, 2022.

Applebaum M, Kalcheim C: Mechanisms of myogenic specification and patterning, *Results Probl Cell Differ* 56:77–98, 2015. https://doi.org/10.1007/978-3-662-44608

Berenguer M, Duester G: Role of retinoic acid signaling, FGF signaling and meis genes in control of limb development, *Biomolecules* 11:80, 2021. https://doi.org/10.3390/biom11010080

Buckingham M, Rigby PWJ: Gene regulatory networks and transcriptional mechanisms that control myogenesis, *Dev Cell* 28(3):225–238, 2014. https://doi.org/10.1016/j.devcel.2013.12.020

Chang KZ, Likes K, Davis K, Demos J, Freischlag JA: The significance of cervical ribs in thoracic outlet syndrome, *J Vasc Surg* 57(3):771–775, 2013. https://doi.org/10.1016/j.jvs.2012.08.110

Cohen MM: Jr: Perspectives on craniosynostosis: sutural biology, some well-known syndromes, and some unusual syndromes, *J Craniofac Surg* 20(Suppl 1):646–651, 2009. https://doi.org/10.1097/SCS.0b013e318193d48d

Cole P, Kaufman Y, Hatef DA, Hollier LH Jr: Embryology of the hand and upper extremity, *J Craniofac Surg* 20(4):992–995, 2009. https://doi.org/10.1097/SCS.0b013e3181abb18e

Dias MS, Samson T, Rizk EB, Governale LS, Richtsmeier JT: Identifying the misshapen head: craniosynostosis and related disorders, *Pediatrics* 146(3), 2020 Sep. https://doi.org/10.1542/peds.2020-015511 e202001 5511

Etich J, Leßmeier L, Rehberg M, Sill H, Zaucke F, Netzer C, Semler O: Osteogenesis imperfecta-pathophysiology and therapeutic options, *Mol Cell Pediatr* 7(1):9, 2020 Aug 14. https://doi.org/10.1186/s40348-020-00101-9

Galea GL, Zein MR, Allen S, Francis-West P: Making and shaping endochondral and intramembranous bones, *Dev Dyn* 250(3):414–449, 2021 Mar. https://doi.org/10.1002/dvdy.278

Gandhi M, Rac MWF, McKinney J: Radial ray malformation, Fetal Anomalies Consult Series #2. B16-18, *Am J Obstet Gynecol*, 2019. https://www.smfm.org/publications/283-smfm-fetal-anomalies-consult-series-2-extremities

Gillgrass TJ, Welbury RR: Craniofacial growth and development. In Welbury RR, Duggal MS, Hosey MT, editors: *Paediatric dentistry*, ed 4, Oxford, UK, 2014, Oxford University Press.

Hall BK: *Bones and cartilage: developmental skeletal biology*, ed 2, Philadelphia, 2015, Elsevier Academic Press.

Hernandez-Andre E, Yeo L, Gonçalves LF: Fetal musculoskeletal system. In Norton ME, editor: *Callen's ultrasonography in obstetrics and gynecology*, ed 6, Philadelphia, 2017, Elsevier.

Hinrichsen KV, Jacob HJ, Jacob M, Brand-Saberi B, Christ B, Grim M: Principles of ontogenesis of leg and foot in man, *Ann Anat* 176(2):121–130, 1994.

Ippolito E, Gorgolinin G: Clubfoot pathology in fetus and pathogenesis. A new pathogenetic theory based on pathology, image findings,

and biomechanics – a narrative review. Ann Transl Med 9(13):1095, 2021.

Kang SG, Kang JK: Current and future perspectives in craniosynostosis, *J Korean Neurosurg Soc* 59(3):247–249, 2016. https://doi.org/10.3340/jkns.2016.59.3.247

Kowalczyk B, Feluś J: Arthrogryposis: an update on clinical aspects, etiology, and treatment strategies, *Arch Med Sci* 12:10, 2016.

Laquerriere A, Jaber D, Abiusi E, Maluenda J, Mejlachowicz D, Vivanti A, et al: Phenotypic spectrum and genomics of undiagnosed arthrogryposis multiplex congenita, *J Med Genet* 59(6):559–567, 2022 Jun. https://doi.org/10.1136/jmedgenet-2020-107595

Liao J, Huang Y, Wang Q, Chen S, Zhang C, Wang D, et al: Gene regulatory network from cranial neural crest cells to osteoblast differentiation and calvarial bone development, *Cell Mol Life Sci* 79(3):158, 2022 Feb 27. https://doi.org/10.1007/s00018-022-04208-2

Liu RE: Musculoskeletal disorders in neonates. In Martin RJ, Fanaroff AA, Walsh MC, editors: *Fanaroff and Martin's neonatal-perinatal medicine: diseases of the fetus and infant, current therapy in neonatal-perinatal medicine*, ed 10, Philadelphia, 2015, Saunders.

Longobardi L, Li T, Tagliafierro L, Temple JD, Willcockson HH, Ye P, Esposito A, Xu F, Spagnoli A: Synovial joints: from development to homeostasis, *Curr Osteoporos Rep* 13(1):41–51, 2015. https://doi.org/10.1007/s11914-014-0247-7

Ma L, Yu X: Arthrogryposis multiplex congenita: classification, diagnosis, perioperative care, and anesthesia, *Front Med* 11(1):48–52, 2017. https://doi.org/10.1007/s11684-017-0500-4

Montero JA, Lorda-Diez CI, Sanchez-Fernandez C, Hurle JM: Cell death in the developing vertebrate limb: a locally regulated mechanism contributing to musculoskeletal tissue morphogenesis and differentiation, *Dev Dyn* 250(9):1236–1247, 2021 Sep. https://doi.org/10.1002/dvdy.237

Newton AH, Williams SM, Major AT, Smith CA: Cell lineage specification and signalling pathway use development of the lateral plate mesoderm and forelimb mesenchyme, *Development* 149(18), 2022 September 15. http://doi.org/10.1242/dev 200702

O'Rahilly R, Gardner E: The timing and sequence of events in the development of the limbs in the human embryo, *Anat Embryol (Berl)* 148(1):1–23, 1975.

Payumo AY, McQuade LE, Walker WJ, Yamazoe S, Chen JK: Tbx16 regulates hox gene activation in mesodermal progenitor cells, *Nat Chem Biol* 12(9):694–701, 2016. https://doi.org/10.1038/nchembio.2124

Plotkin LI, Bruzzaniti A: Molecular signaling in bone cells: regulation of cell differentiation and survival, *Adv Protein Chem Struct Biol* 16:237–281, 2019. https://doi.org/10.1016/bs.apcsb.2019.01.002

Powel JE, Sham CE, Spiliopoulos M, Ferreira CR, Rosenthal E, Sinkovskaya ES, et al: Genetics of non-isolated hemivertebra-a systematic review of fetal, neonatal, and infant cases, *Clin Genet* 102(3), July 2022. https://doi.org/10.1111/cge.14188

Towers M, Tickle C: Generation of pattern and form in the developing limb, *Int J Dev Biol* 53(5–6):805–812, 2009. https://doi.org/10.1387/ijdb.072499mt

Chapter 16

Azahraa Haddad F, Qaisi I, Joudeh N, Dajani H, Jumah F, Elmashala A, et al: The newer classifications of the Chiari malformations with clarifications: an anatomical review, *Clin Anat* 31(3):314–322, 2018. https://doi.org/10.1002/ca.23051

Blessing M, Gllagher ER: Epidemiology, generics, and pathophysiology of craniosynostosis. *Oral maxillofacial surg Clin N Am.* 34:341, 2022

Briscoe J: On the growth and form of the vertebrate neural tube, *Mech Dev* 145(Suppl):S1, 2017. https://doi.org/10.1016/j.mod.2017.04.513

Brown RE: Overview of CNS organization and development. In Eisenstat DD, Goldowitz D, Oberlander TF, Yager JY, editors: *Neurodevelopmental pediatrics*, Cham, 2023, Springer. https://doi.org/10.1007/978-3-031-20792-1-1

Catala M, Kubis N: Gross anatomy and development of the peripheral nervous system. In Said G, Krarup C, editors: *Handbook of clinical neurology*, Amsterdam, 2013, Elsevier B.V.

Dawes JHP, Kelsh RN: Cell fate decisions in the neural crest, from pigment cell to neural development, *Int J Mol Sci* 22(24):13531, 2021 Dec 16. https://doi.org/10.3390/ijms222413531

de Bakker BS, de Jong KH, Hagoort J, de Bree K, Besselink CT, de Kanter FE, et al: An interactive three-dimensional digital atlas and quantitative database of human development, *Science* 354(6315): 2016. https://doi.org/10.1126/science.aag0053. pii: aag0053.

Fenton LZ: Imaging of congenital malformations of the brain, *Clin Perinatol* 49:587, 2022.

Garcia-Bonilla M, McAllister JP, Limbrick DD: Genetics and molecular pathogenesis of human hydrocephalus, *Neurology India* 69:268–274, 2021. https://digitalcommons.wustl.edu/open_access_pubs/11215

Gressens P, Hüppi PS: Normal and abnormal brain development. In Martin RJ, Fanaroff AA, Walsh MC, editors: *Fanaroff and Martin's neonatal-perinatal medicine: diseases of the fetus and infant*, ed 10, Philadelphia, 2014, Mosby.

Guimaraes CVA, Dahmoush HM: Fetal brain anatomy. *Neuroimaging Clin N Am.* 2022.

Haines DE: *Neuroanatomy atlas in clinical context: structures, sections, systems, and syndromes*, ed 10, Baltimore, MD, 2019, Wolters Kluwer.

Hata T: Recent advances in 3D/4D ultrasound in obstetrics, *Donald School J Ultrasound Obstet Gynecol* 16(2):95–106, 2022.

Kaplan KM, Spivak JM, Bendo JA: Embryology of the spine and associated congenital abnormalities, *Spine J* 5:564, 2005.

Kinsman SL, Johnson MV: Congenital anomalies of the central nervous system. In Kliegman RM, Johnson MV, St Geme JWIII, Schor NF, editors: *Nelson textbook of pediatrics*, ed 20, Philadelphia, 2016, Elsevier.

O'Rahilly R, Müller F: *Embryonic human brain: an atlas of developmental stages*, ed 2, New York, 1999, Wiley-Liss.

Osterhues A, Ali NS, Michels KB: The role of folic acid fortification in neural tube defects: a review, *Crit Rev Food Sci Nutr* 53(11):1180–1190, 2013. https://doi.org/10.1080/10408398.2011.575966

Scott-Solomon E, Boehm E, Kuruvilla R: The sympathetic nervous system in development and disease, *Nat Rev Neurosci* 22:685, 2021.

Tata M, Ruhrberg C: Cross-talk of neural progenitors and blood vessels in the developing brain, *Neuronal Signal* 2(1), 2018.10.1042/NS20170139

Ten Donkelaar HT, Lammens M: Development of the human cerebellum and its disorders, *Clin Perinatol* 36(3):513–530, 2009. https://doi.org/10.1016/j.clp.2009.06.001

White C, Milla SS, Maloney JA, Neuberger I: Imaging of congenital spine malformations, *Clin Perinatol* 49:623, 2022.

Zhan J, Dinov ID, Li J, Zhang Z, Hobel S, Shi Y, et al: Spatial-temporal atlas of human fetal brain development during the early second trimester, *Neuroimage* 82:115–126, 2013. https://doi.org/10.1016/j.neuroimage.2013.05.063

Chapter 17

Ankamreddy H, Koo H, Lee YJ, Bok J: CXCL12 is required for stirrup-shaped stapes formation during mammalian middle ear development, *Dev Dyn* 249:1117, 2020.

Anthwal N, Thompson H: The development of the mammalian outer and middle ear, *J Anat* 228, 2015.10.1111/joa.12344

Barishak YR: *Embryology of the eye and its adnexa*, ed 2, Basel, 2001, Karger.

Bauer PW, MacDonald CB, Melhem ER: Congenital inner ear malformation, *Am J Otol* 19(5):669–670, 1998.

Cardozo MJ, Sánchez-Bustamante E, Bovolenta P: Optic cup morphogenesis across species and related inborn human eye defects, *Development* 150(2):dev200399, 2023 Jan 15. https://doi.org/10.1242/dev.200399. Epub 2023 Jan 30. PMID: 36714981

Casey MA, Lusk S, Kwan KM: Build me up optic cup: intrinsic and extrinsic mechanisms of vertebrate eye morphogenesis, *Dev Biol* 476:128, 2021.

Dash P, Rout JP, Panigrahi PK: Clinical patterns of congenital ocular anomalies in the pediatric age group (0 to 5 years) and its association with various demographic parameters, *Indian J Ophthalmol* 70:944, 2022.

FitzPatrick DR, van Heyningen V: Developmental eye disorders, *Curr Opin Genet Dev* 15(3):348–353, 2005. https://doi.org/10.1016/j.gde.2005.04.013

Garg A, Zhang X: Lacrimal gland development: from signaling interactions to regenerative medicine, *Dev. Dyn.* 246:970–980, 2017. https://doi.org/10.1002/dvdy.24551

Ghada MWF: Ear embryology, *Glob J Oto* 4(1):555627, 2017. https://doi.org/10.19080/GJO.2017.04.555627003

Guercio JR, Martyn LJ: Congenital malformations of the eye and orbit, *Otolaryngol Clin North Am* 40(1):113–140, 2007. https://doi.org/10.1016/j.otc.2006.11.013

Jones KL, Jones MC, del Campo M: *Smith's recognizable patterns of human malformation*, ed 7, Philadelphia, 2013, Saunders.

O'Rahilly R: The prenatal development of the human eye, *Exp Eye Res* 21(2):93–112, 1975.

Porter CJW, Tan ST: Congenital auricular anomalies: topographic anatomy, embryology, classification, and treatment strategies, *Plast Reconstr Surg* 115(6):1701–1712, 2005. https://doi.org/10.1097/01.PRS.0000161454.08384.0A

Thompson H, Ohazama A, Sharpe PT, Tucker AS: The origin of the stapes and relationship to the otic capsule and oval window, *Dev Dyn* 241(9):1396–1404, 2012. https://doi.org/10.1002/dvdy.23831

Williams AL, Bohnsack BL: Review. Neural crest derivatives in ocular development: discerning the eye of the storm, *Birth Defects Res C Embryo Today* 105(2):87–95, 2015. https://doi.org/10.1002/bdrc.21095

Chapter 18

Chiu YE: Dermatology. In Marcdante KJ, Kliegman KJ, editors: *Nelson essentials of pediatrics*, ed 7, Philadelphia, 2015, Saunders.

Crawford PJM, Aldred MJ: Anomalies of tooth formation and eruption. In Welbury RR, Duggal MS, Hosey MT, editors: *Paediatric dentistry*, ed 4, Oxford, UK, 2014, Oxford University Press.

Foulds H: Developmental defects of enamel and caries in primary teeth, *Evid Based Dent* 18(3):72–73, 2017. https://doi.org/10.1038/sj.ebd.6401252

Gillgrass TS, Welbery R: Craniofacial growth and development. In Welbury RR, Duggal MS, Hosey MT, editors: *Paediatric dentistry*, ed 4, Oxford, UK, 2014, Oxford University Press.

Harryparsad A, Rahman L, Bunn BK: Amelogenesis imperfecta: a diagnostic and pathological review with case illustration, *SADJ* 68(9):404–407, 2013.

Inman JL, Robertson C, Mott JD, Bissell MJ: Mammary gland development: cell fate specification, stem cells and the microenvironment, *Development* 142(6):1028–1042, 2015. https://doi.org/10.1242/dev.087643

Kawasaki M, Porntaveetus T, Kawasaki K, Oommen S, Otsuka-Tanaka Y, Hishinuma M, et al: R-spondins/Lgrs expression in tooth development, *Dev Dyn* 243(6):844–851, 2014. https://doi.org/10.1002/dvdy.24124

Kliegman RR, Stanton B, Geme J, editors: *Nelson textbook of pediatrics*, ed 20, Philadelphia, 2016, Elsevier.

Little H, Kamat D, Sivaswamy L: Common neurocutaneous syndromes, *Pediatr Ann* 44(11):496–504, 2015. https://doi.org/10.3928/00904481-20151112-11

Nanci A: *Ten Cate's oral histology: development, structure, and function*, ed 9, Philadelphia, 2018, Mosby.

Paller AS, Mancini AJ: *Hurwitz clinical pediatric dermatology: a textbook of skin disorders of childhood and adolescence*, ed 3, Philadelphia, 2006, Saunders.

Papagerakis P, Mitsiadis T: Development and structure of teeth and periodontal tissues. In Rosen CJ, editor: *Primer on the metabolic bone diseases and disorders of mineral metabolism*, ed 8, New York, 2013, John Wiley & Sons.

Seppala M, Fraser GJ, Birjandi AA, Xavier GM, Cobourne MT: Sonic hedgehog signaling and development of the dentition, *J Dev Biol* 5(2):6, 2017. https://doi.org/10.3390/jdb5020006

Smolinski KN, Yan AC: Hemangiomas of infancy: clinical and biological characteristics, *Clin Pediatr (Phila)* 44(9):747–766, 2005. https://doi.org/10.1177/000992280504400902

Som PM, Laitman JT, Mak K: Embryology and anatomy of the skin, its appendages, and physiologic changes in the head and neck, *Neurographics* 7(5):390–415, 2017. https://doi.org/10.3174/ng.9170210

Chapter 19

ACOG, SMFM: *Joint statement on WHO recommendations regarding COVID-19 vaccines and pregnant individuals*, Washington, DC, January 27, 2021

Alves C, Franco RR: Prader-Willi syndrome: endocrine manifestations and management, *Arch Endocrinol Metab* 64:223, 2020.

Antonarakis SE, Skotko BG, Rafii MS, Strydom A, Pape SE, Bianchi DW, Sherman SL, Reeves RH: Down syndrome, *Nat Rev Dis Primers* 6(1):9, 2020 Feb 6. https://doi.org/10.1038/s41572-019-0143-7

Auriti C, De Rose DU, Santisi A, Martini L, Piersigilli F, Bersani I, Ronchetti MP, Caforio L: Pregnancy and viral infections: mechanisms of fetal damage, diagnosis and prevention of neonatal adverse outcomes from cytomegalovirus to SARS-CoV-2 and Zika virus, *Biochim Biophys Acta Mol Basis Dis* 1867(10):166198, 2021. https://doi.org/10.1016/j.bbadis.2021.166198

Bandoli G, Chambers CD, Wells A, Palmsten K: Prenatal antidepressant use and risk of adverse neonatal outcomes, *Pediatrics* 146(1), 2020 e20192493. https://doi.org/10.1542/peds.2019-2493

Bandoli G, Palmsten K, Chambers C: Acetaminophen use in pregnancy: examining prevalence, timing, and indication of use in a prospective birth cohort, *Paediatr Perinat Epidemiol* 34:237, 2020.

Bekkar B, Pacheco S, Basu R, DeNicola N: Association of Air Pollution and Heat Exposure With Preterm Birth, Low Birth Weight, and Stillbirth in the US: A Systematic Review, *JAMA Netw Open* 3(6), 2020 Jun 1.10.1001/jamanetworkopen.2020.8243 e208243

Banerjee J, Mullins E, Townson J, Playle R, Shaw C, Kirby N, et al: Pregnancy and neonatal outcomes in COVID-19: study protocol for a global registry of women with suspected or confirmed SARS-CoV-2 infection in pregnancy and their neonates, understanding natural history to guide treatment and prevention, *BMJ Open* 11(1), 2021.10.1136/bmjopen-2020-041247 e041247.

Bowen VB, McDonald R, Grey JA, Kimball A, Torrone EA: High congenital syphilis case count among U.S. infants born in 2020, *N Engl J Med* 385:1144, 2021.

Briggs GG, Freeman RK, Towers CV, Forinash AB: *Brigg's drugs in pregnancy and lactation*. In *A reference guide to fetal and neonatal risk*, ed 12, Philadelphia, 2021, Wolters Kluwer.

Denomme MM, McCallie BR, Haywood ME, et al: Paternal aging impacts expression and epigenetic markers as early as the first embryonic tissue lineage differentiation. Hum Genomics, 2024 Mar 26;18(1):32. https://doi.10.1186/s40246-024-00599-4. PMID: 38532526; PMCID: PMC10964547.

Fang Y, Wang Y, Peng M, Xu J, Fan Z, Liu C, Zhao K, Zhang H: Effect of paternal age on offspring birth defects: a systematic review and meta-analysis, *Aging* 12:25373, 2020.

Elliott AJ, Kinney HC, Haynes RL, Dempers JD, Wright C, Fifer WP, et al: Concurrent prenatal drinking and smoking increases risk for SIDS: Safe Passage Study report, *EClinicalMedicine* 19:100247, 2020 Jan 20. https://doi.org/10.1016/j.eclinm.2019.100247

Ezer B, Rencuzogullari E: The Future of the teratogenicity testing. Methods Mol Biol. 2024;2753:143-150. https://doi.10.1007/978-1-0716-3625-1_5. PMID: 38285336.

Hamułka J, Zielińska MA, Chądzyńska K: The combined effects of alcohol and tobacco use during pregnancy on birth outcomes, *Rocz Panstw Zakl Hig* 69(1):45–54, 2018.

Honein MA: Recognizing the global impact of Zika virus infection during pregnancy, *N Engl J Med* 378(11):1055–1056, 2018. https://doi.org/10.1056/NEJMe1801398

Hu CY, Huang K, Fang Y, Yang XJ, Ding K, Jiang W, et al: Maternal air pollution exposure and congenital heart defects in offspring: a systematic review and meta-analysis, *Chemosphere* 253:126668, 2020.10.1016/j.chemosphere.2020.126668 ISSN 0045-6535

Levy PA, Marion RW: Human genetics and dysmorphology. In Marcdante KJ, Kliegman KJ, editors: *Nelson essentials of pediatrics* ed 7, Philadelphia, 2015, Saunders.

Luke B, Brown MB, Wantman E, Forestieri NE, Browne ML, Fisher SC, et al: The risk of birth defects with conception by ART, *Hum Reprod* 36:116, 2021.

Rasmussen SA: Human teratogens update 2011: can we ensure safety during pregnancy? *Birth Defects Res A Clin Mol Teratol* 94(3):123–128, 2012. https://doi.org/10.1002/bdra.22887

Reece AS, Hulse GK: Patterns of cannabis- and substance-related congenital general anomalies in Europe: a geospatiotemporal and causal inferential study, *Pediatr Rep* 15(1):69–118, 2023 Feb 7.10.3390/pediatric15010009 PMID: 36810339; PMCID: PMC9944887

Simpson JL: Birth defects and assisted reproductive technology, *Semin Fetal Neonatal Med* 19(3):177–182, 2014. https://doi.org/10.1016/j.siny.2014.01.001

Turnpenny P, Ellard S, Cleaver R: *Emery's elements of medical genetics and genomics*, ed 16, Philadelphia, 2020, Elsevier.

Valladares DA, Rasmussen SA: An update on teratogens for pediatric healthcare providers, *Curr Opin Pediatr* 34:565, 2022.

World Health Organization: *International statistical classification of diseases and related health problems*, ed 11, 2019. https://icd.who.int/

Chapter 20

Alvarez-Buylla A, Ihrie RA: Sonic hedgehog signaling in the postnatal brain, *Semin Cell Dev Biol* 33:105, 2014.

Amakye D, Jagani Z, Dorsch M: Unraveling the therapeutic potential of the hedgehog pathway in cancer, *Nat Med* 19:1410, 2013.

Andersson ER, Lendahl U: Therapeutic modulation of notch signalling—are we there yet? *Nat Rev Drug Discov* 13:357, 2014.

Anzalone AV, Koblan LW, Liu DR: Genome editing with CRISPR–Cas nucleases, base editors, transposases and prime editors, *Nat Biotech* 38:824, 2020.

Aster JC: In brief: notch signalling in health and disease, *J Pathol* 232(1), 2014.

Bahubeshi A, Tischkowitz M, Foulkes WD: miRNA processing and human cancer: DICER1 cuts the mustard, *Sci Transl Med* 3(111):ps46, 2011.

Barriga EH, Mayor R: Embryonic cell-cell adhesion: a key player in collective neural crest migration, *Curr Top Dev Biol* 112:301, 2015.

Beets K, Huylebroeck D, Moya IM, et al: Robustness in angiogenesis: notch and BMP shaping waves, *Trends Genet* 29:140, 2013.

Benoit YD, Guezguez B, Boyd AL, et al: Molecular pathways: epigenetic modulation of Wnt/glycogen synthase kinase-3 signaling to target human cancer stem cells, *Clin Cancer Res* 20:5372, 2014.

Berdasco M, Esteller M: Genetic syndromes caused by mutations in epigenetic genes, *Hum Genet* 132:359, 2013.

Berindan-Neagoe I, Monroig Pdel C, Pasculli B, et al: MicroRNAome genome: a treasure for cancer diagnosis and therapy, *CA Cancer J Clin* 64:311, 2014.

Blake JA, Ziman MR: *Pax* genes: regulators of lineage specification and progenitor cell maintenance, *Development* 141:737, 2014.

Brafman D, Willert K: Wnt/β-catenin signaling during early vertebrate neural development, *Dev Neurobiol* 77:1239, 2017.

Capper D, Jones DTW, Sill M, et al: DNA methylation-based classification of central nervous system tumours, *Nature* 555(7697):469–474, 2018.

Castro DS, Guillemot F: Old and new functions of proneural factors revealed by the genome-wide characterization of their transcriptional targets, *Cell Cycle* 10:4026, 2011.

Christ A, Herzog K, Willnow TE: LRP2, an auxiliary receptor that controls sonic hedgehog signaling in development and disease, *Dev Dyn* 245:569, 2016.

Corsini NS, Knoblich JA: Human organoids: new strategies and methods for analyzing human development and disease, *Cell* 185(15):2756–2769, 2022.

Cuneo MJ, Mittag T: Oncogenic signaling of RTK fusions becomes more granular, *Mol Cell* 81:2504, 2021.

De Robertis EM: Spemann's organizer and the self-regulation of embryonic fields, *Mech Dev* 126:925, 2009.

Dekanty A, Milán M: The interplay between morphogens and tissue growth, *EMBO Rep* 12:1003, 2011.

Dhanak D, Jackson P: Development and classes of epigenetic drugs for cancer, *Biochem Biophys Res Commun* 455:58, 2014.

Doudna JA, Charpentier E: Genome editing. The new frontier of genome engineering with CRISPR-Cas9, *Science* 346(6213), 2014. 1258096

Dubey A, Rose RE, Jones DR, Saint-Jeannet JP: Generating retinoic acid gradients by local degradation during craniofacial development: one cell's cue is another cell's poison, *Genesis* 56(2), 2018, e23091.

Gaarenstroom T, Hill CS: TGF-β signaling to chromatin: how smads regulate transcription during self-renewal and differentiation, *Semin Cell Dev Biol* 32:107, 2014.

Giannotta M, Trani M, Dejana E: VE-cadherin and endothelial adherens junctions: active guardians of vascular integrity, *Dev Cell* 26:441, 2013.

Goldman D: Regeneration, morphogenesis and self-organization, *Development* 141:2745, 2014.

Gier RA, Budinich KA, Evitt NH, et al: High-performance CRISPR-Cas12a genome editing for combinatorial genetic screening, *Nature Comm* 11:3455, 2020.

Guillot C, Lecuit T: Mechanics of epithelial tissue homeostasis and morphogenesis, *Science* 340:1185, 2013.

Gutierrez-Mazariegos J, Theodosiou M, Campo-Paysaa F, et al: Vitamin a: a multifunctional tool for development, *Semin Cell Dev Biol* 22:603, 2011.

Hendriks WJ, Pulido R: Protein tyrosine phosphatase variants in human hereditary disorders and disease susceptibilities, *Biochim Biophys Acta* 1832:1673, 2013.

Hori K, Sen A, Artavanis-Tsakonas S: Notch signaling at a glance, *J Cell Sci* 126(Pt 10):2135, 2013.

Imayoshi I, Kageyama R: bHLH factors in self-renewal, multipotency, and fate choice of neural progenitor cells, *Neuron* 82:9, 2014.

Inoue H, Nagata N, Kurokawa H, et al: iPS cells: a game changer for future medicine, *EMBO J* 33:409, 2014.

Izzi L, Lévesque M, Morin S, et al: Boc and gas1 each form distinct shh receptor complexes with ptch1 and are required for Shh-mediated cell proliferation, *Dev Cell* 20:788, 2011.

Jiang Q, Wang Y, Hao Y, et al: miR2Disease: a manually curated database for microRNA deregulation in human disease, *Nucleic Acids Res* 37:D98, 2009.

Kaya-Okur HS, Wu SJ, Codomo CA, et al: CUT&Tag for efficient epigenomic profiling of small samples and single cells, *Nat Commun* 10(1):1930, 2019.

Kim W, Kim M, Jho EH: Wnt/β-catenin signalling: from plasma membrane to nucleus, *Biochem J* 450:9, 2013.

Kotini M, Mayor R: Connexins in migration during development and cancer, *Dev Biol* 401:143, 2015.

Lam EW, Brosens JJ, Gomes AR, et al: Forkhead box proteins: tuning forks for transcriptional harmony, *Nat Rev Cancer* 13:482, 2013.

Lamouille S, Xu J, Derynck R: Molecular mechanisms of epithelial-mesenchymal transition, *Nat Rev Mol Cell Biol* 15:178, 2014.

Lancaster MA, Corsini NS, Wolfinger S, et al: Guided self-organization and cortical plate formation in human brain organoids, *Nat Biotechnol* 35(7):659–666, 2017.

Le Dréau G, Martí E: The multiple activities of BMPs during spinal cord development, *Cell Mol Life Sci* 70:4293, 2013.

Leung RF, George AM, Roussel EM, et al: Genetic regulation of vertebrate forebrain development by homeobox genes, *Front Neurosci* 16, 2022, 843794

Li CG, Eccles MR: PAX genes in cancer; friends or foes? *Front Genet* 3:6, 2012.

Lien WH, Fuchs E: Wnt some lose some: transcriptional governance of stem cells by Wnt/β-catenin signaling, *Genes Dev* 28:1517, 2014.

Lim J, Thiery JP: Epithelial-mesenchymal transitions: insights from development, *Development* 139:3471, 2012.

Lowe EK, Cuomo C, Voronov D, Arnone MI: Using ATAC-seq and RNA-seq to increase resolution in GRN connectivity, *Methods Cell Biol* 151:115–126, 2019.

MacGrogan D, Luxán G, de la Pompa JL: Genetic and functional genomics approaches targeting the notch pathway in cardiac development and congenital heart disease, *Brief Funct Genomics* 13:15, 2014.

Mackay A, Burford A, Carvalho D, et al: Integrated molecular meta-analysis of 1,000 pediatric high-grade and diffuse intrinsic pontine glioma, *Cancer Cell* 32(4):520, 2017.

Mallo M, Alonso CR: The regulation of *Hox* gene expression during animal development, *Development* 140:3951, 2013.

Mallo M, Wellik DM, Deschamps J: *Hox* genes and regional patterning of the vertebrate body plan, *Dev Biol* 344:7, 2010.

Manoranjan B, Venugopal C, McFarlane N, et al: Medulloblastoma stem cells: where development and cancer cross pathways, *Pediatr Res* 71(Pt 2):516, 2012.

Mašek J, Andersson ER: The developmental biology of genetic notch disorders, *Development* 144:1743, 2017.

Maze I, Noh KM, Soshnev AA, et al: Every amino acid matters: essential contributions of histone variants to mammalian development and disease, *Nat Rev Genet* 15:259, 2014.

Meijer DH, Kane MF, Mehta S, et al: Separated at birth? The functional and molecular divergence of OLIG1 and OLIG2, *Nat Rev Neurosci* 13:819, 2012.

Mo JS, Park HW, Guan KL: The hippo signaling pathway in stem cell biology and cancer, *EMBO Rep* 15:642, 2014.

Neben CL, Lo M, Jura N, Klein OD: Feedback regulation of RTK signaling in development, *Dev Biol*:71–89, 2017.

Nelson KN, Peiris MN, Meyer AN, et al: Receptor tyrosine kinases: translocation partners in hematopoietic disorders, *Trends Mol Med* 23:59, 2017.

O'Brien P, Morin P Jr, Ouellette RJ, et al: The *Pax-5* gene: a pluripotent regulator of b-cell differentiation and cancer disease, *Cancer Res* 71:7345, 2011.

Park KM, Gerecht S: Harnessing developmental processes for vascular engineering and regeneration, *Development* 141:2760, 2014.

Pignatti E, Zeller R, Zuniga A: To BMP or not to BMP during vertebrate limb bud development, *Semin Cell Dev Biol* 32:119, 2014.

Rao A, Barkley D, França GS, Yanai I: Exploring tissue architecture using spatial transcriptomics, *Nature* 596(7871):211–220, 2021.

Reiter JF, Leroux MR: Genes and molecular pathways underpinning ciliopathies, *Nat Rev Mol Cell Biol* 18(9):533, 2017.

Rhinn M, Dollé P: Retinoic acid signalling during development, *Development* 139:843, 2012.

Roussel MF, Robinson GW: Role of MYC in medulloblastoma, *Cold Spring Harb Perspect Med* 3(11):a014308, 2013.

Salma M, Andrieu-Soler C, Deleuze V, Soler E: High-throughput methods for the analysis of transcription factors and chromatin modifications: low input, single cell and spatial genomic technologies, *Blood Cells Mol Dis* 101, 2023. 102745

Sánchez Alvarado A, Yamanaka S: Rethinking differentiation: stem cells, regeneration, and plasticity, *Cell* 157:110, 2014.

Scadden DT: Nice neighborhood: emerging concepts of the stem cell niche, *Cell* 157:41, 2014.

Schlessinger J: Receptor tyrosine kinases: legacy of the first two decades, *Cold Spring Harb Perspect Biol* 6(3), 2014, a008912

Shah N, Sukumar S: The hox genes and their roles in oncogenesis, *Nat Rev Cancer* 10:361, 2010.

Shashikant T, Ettensohn CA: Genome-wide analysis of chromatin accessibility using ATAC-seq, *Methods Cell Biol* 151:219–235, 2019.

Shearer KD, Stoney PN, Morgan PJ, et al: A vitamin for the brain, *Trends Neurosci* 35:733, 2012.

Sotomayor M, Gaudet R, Corey DP: Sorting out a promiscuous superfamily: towards cadherin connectomics, *Trends Cell Biol* 24:524, 2014.

Steffen PA, Ringrose L: What are memories made of? How polycomb and trithorax proteins mediate epigenetic memory, *Nat Rev Mol Cell Biol* 15:340, 2014.

Tee WW, Reinberg D: Chromatin features and the epigenetic regulation of pluripotency states in ESCs, *Development* 141:2376, 2014.

Thompson JA, Ziman M: Pax genes during neural development and their potential role in neuroregeneration, *Prog Neurobiol* 95:334, 2014.

Torres-Padilla ME, Chambers I: Transcription factor heterogeneity in pluripotent stem cells: a stochastic advantage, *Development* 141:2173, 2014.

Vanan MI, Underhill DA, Eisenstat DD: Targeting epigenetic pathways in the treatment of pediatric diffuse (high grade) gliomas, *Neurotherapeutics* 14:274–283, 2017.

Verstraete K, Savvides SN: Extracellular assembly and activation principles of oncogenic class III receptor tyrosine kinases, *Nat Rev Cancer* 12:753, 2012.

Wilkinson G, Dennis D, Schuurmans C: Proneural genes in neocortical development, *Neuroscience* 253:256, 2013.

Willaredt MA, Tasouri E, Tucker KL: Primary cilia and forebrain development, *Mech Dev* 130:373, 2013.

Wu MY, Hill CS: Tgf-beta superfamily signaling in embryonic development and homeostasis, *Dev Cell* 16:329, 2009.

Yan F, Powell DR, Curtis DJ, Wong NC: From reads to insight: a hitchhiker's guide to ATAC-seq data analysis, *Genome Biol* 21(1):22, 2020.

Yang Y, Oliver G: Development of the mammalian lymphatic vasculature, *J Clin Invest* 124:888, 2014.

Zagozewski JL, Zhang Q, Pinto VI, et al: The role of homeobox genes in retinal development and disease, *Dev Biol* 393:195, 2014.

Appendix: Answers to Clinically Oriented Questions

CHAPTER 1

1. Health-care professionals are expected to give evidence-based answers to the questions people ask, such as "When does the baby's heart start to beat?" "When does it move its limbs?" "When is the embryo most at risk for effects from alcohol?" For prenatal diagnosis and any medical treatment before birth, physicians—especially family doctors, obstetricians, and pediatricians—need to know how the embryo and fetus develop and also what might cause developmental defects. Moreover, research in embryology supports the application of stem cells for the treatment of certain chronic diseases.

2. Physicians date pregnancies from the first day of the last normal menstrual period because this date is usually remembered by women. It is not possible to detect the precise time of ovulation or fertilization except in cases of in vitro fertilization. Laboratory tests and ultrasound imaging can be performed to detect when ovulation is likely to occur and when pregnancy has occurred.

CHAPTER 2

1. Pregnant women do not menstruate, even though there may be some bleeding at the usual time of menstruation. This blood may be leaking from the intervillous space of the placenta because of the partial separation of the placenta from the endometrium of the uterine wall. Because there is no shedding of endometrium, this blood is not menstrual fluid; it is maternal blood that escaped from the intervillous space of the placenta.

2. It depends on when she forgot to take the oral contraceptive. If it was at midcycle, ovulation may occur and pregnancy could result. Taking two doses the next day would not prevent ovulation.

3. Coitus interruptus refers to the withdrawal of the penis from the vagina before ejaculation occurs. This method is not reliable. Often, a few sperms are expelled from the penis with the secretions of the auxiliary sex glands (e.g., seminal glands) before ejaculation occurs. One of these sperms may fertilize the oocyte.

4. Spermatogenesis refers to the complete process of sperm formation. Spermiogenesis is the transformation of a spermatid into a sperm. Therefore spermiogenesis is the final stage of spermatogenesis.

5. A copper-releasing intrauterine device (IUD) may inhibit the capacitation of sperms and their transport through the uterus to the fertilization site in the uterine tube; in

this case, it would be a contraceptive device. A hormone-releasing IUD (e.g., levonorgestrel) may cause changes that alter the morphological features of the endometrium; as a result, the blastocyst does not implant. In this case, the hormonal IUD could be called a "contra-implantation" device.

CHAPTER 3

1. The ovarian and menstrual cycles typically cease between 48 and 55 years of age, with the average age being 51 years. Menopause results from the gradual cessation of gonadotropin production by the pituitary gland; however, it does not mean that the ovaries have exhausted their supply of oocytes. The risk of Down syndrome (trisomy 21) and other trisomies is increased in the children of women who are 39 years or older (see Table 19.2). Sperm fertility decreases after the age of 45 years, although sperm production continues until old age. Advanced paternal age (>44 years old) has been shown to increase the risk of chromosomal defects and subsequent congenital anomalies, including cardiovascular defects and achondroplasia (see Chapter 19).

2. Considerable research on new contraceptive methods is being conducted, including the development of oral contraceptives for men. This research includes experimental work on hormonal and nonhormonal prevention of spermatogenesis and stimulation of immune responses to sperms. Arresting the development of millions of sperms on a continuous basis has proven much more difficult than arresting the monthly development of a single oocyte. The results of molecular approaches, such as retinoic acid receptor alpha or cyclin-dependent kinase inhibitors, may eventually provide a safe and reversible male contraceptive.

3. It is not known whether polar bodies are ever fertilized; however, it has been suggested that dispermic chimeras result from the fusion of a fertilized oocyte with a fertilized polar body. Chimeras are rare individuals who are composed of a mixture of cells from two zygotes. More likely, dispermic chimeras result from the fusion of dizygotic twin zygotes early in development. Dizygotic twins are derived from two zygotes. If a polar body were fertilized and remained separate from the normal zygote, it could form an embryo.

4. The most common cause of spontaneous abortion during the first week is chromosomal abnormality, which results from nondisjunction (see Chapter 2). Failure of the syncytiotrophoblast to produce an adequate amount

of human chorionic gonadotropin to maintain the corpus luteum in the ovary could also result in early spontaneous abortion.

5. Mitosis is the usual process of cell reproduction that results in the formation of daughter cells in the zygote. Cleavage is the series of mitotic cell divisions of the zygote. This process results in the formation of daughter cells—blastomeres. The expressions *cleavage division* and *mitotic division* have the same meaning when referring to the dividing zygote.

6. The nutritional requirements of the dividing zygote are not great. The nutrients are derived mainly from the secretions of the uterine tubes.

7. Yes. One of the blastomeres could be removed, and a Y chromosome could be identified by molecular techniques (see Chapter 7). This technique could be made available to couples with a family history of sex-linked genetic diseases (e.g., hemophilia, muscular dystrophy), and to women who have already given birth to a child with such a disease and are reluctant to have more children. In these cases, only female embryos developing in vitro would be transferred to the uterus.

CHAPTER 4

1. Implantation bleeding refers to the loss of small amounts of blood from the implantation site of a blastocyst that occurs a few days after the expected time of menstruation. Women unfamiliar with this possible occurrence may misinterpret the bleeding as a light menstrual flow. In such cases, they may give the physician the wrong date for their last normal menstrual period. This blood is not menstrual fluid; it is blood from the intervillous space of the developing placenta. Blood loss could also result from the rupture of chorionic arteries, veins, or both (see Chapter 8).

2. Drugs or other agents may cause early abortion of an embryo, but they do not cause birth defects if taken during the first 2 weeks. A drug or other agent either damages all the embryonic cells, killing the embryo, or injures only a few cells, in which case the embryo recovers to develop normally.

3. Intrauterine devices are typically very effective at preventing pregnancy by altering sperm capacitation or motility or by altering the morphological features of the endometrium. However, an intrauterine device does not physically block a sperm from entering the uterine tube and fertilizing an oocyte, if one is present. Although the endometrium could be hostile to implantation, a blastocyst could develop and implant in the uterine tube (i.e., ectopic tubal pregnancy). If fertilization occurs in a woman who is using an intrauterine device, the risk of an ectopic pregnancy is approximately 5%.

4. Abdominal pregnancies are very uncommon. In most cases, it is believed to result from a tubal ectopic pregnancy. The embryo spontaneously aborts from the ruptured uterine tube and enters the peritoneal cavity. The risk of severe maternal bleeding and fetal mortality is high in cases of abdominal pregnancy. However, if the diagnosis is made late in pregnancy and the patient (mother) is free of symptoms, the pregnancy may be allowed to continue until the viability of the fetus is ensured, at which time it would be delivered by cesarean section.

CHAPTER 5

1. Yes, certain drugs can produce birth defects if administered during the third week (see Chapter 19). For instance, antineoplastic agents (chemotherapy or antitumor drugs) can produce severe skeletal and neural tube defects in the embryo, such as acrania and meroencephaly (partial absence of the brain), if administered during the third week.

2. Yes, risks to the mother aged 40 years or older and the embryo are increased. The most common risks are birth defects associated with chromosomal abnormalities, such as trisomy 21 and trisomy 13 (see Chapter 19); however, women older than 40 years may have normal children. Advanced maternal age is a predisposing factor for certain medical conditions. For example, preeclampsia, a hypertensive disorder of pregnancy characterized by increased blood pressure and edema, occurs more frequently in older pregnant women than in younger ones. Advanced maternal age is also associated with a significantly increased risk for the embryo or fetus.

CHAPTER 6

1. By the end of the eighth week, embryos and early fetuses appear similar. The name change is arbitrarily made to indicate that a new *fetal* phase of development (rapid growth and differentiation) has begun and that the most critical period of *embryonic* development has been completed.

2. There are different opinions when an embryo becomes a human being because opinions are often affected by religious and personal views. The scientific answer is that the embryo is a human being from the time of fertilization because of its human chromosomal constitution. The zygote is the beginning of a developing human. Some people consider that the embryo becomes human only after birth.

3. No, it cannot. *During the embryonic period*, more similarities than differences exist in the external genitalia (see Chapter 13). It is impossible to tell by ultrasound examination whether the primordial sexual organ (genital tubercle at 5 weeks and phallus at 7 weeks) will become a penis or a clitoris. Sex differences are not clear until the *early fetal period* (10th–12th week). Fluorescence *in situ hybridization* (FISH) of embryonic cells obtained during amniocentesis can show the chromosomal sex of the embryo (see Chapter 7).

CHAPTER 7

1. Ultrasound examinations have shown that mature embryos (8 weeks) and young fetuses (9 weeks) show spontaneous movements, such as twitching (sudden jerking movements) of the trunk and limbs. Although the

fetus begins to move its back and limbs during the 12th week, the mother cannot feel the fetus move until the 16th–20th week. Women who have had several children usually detect this movement, called *quickening*, sooner than women who are pregnant for the first time because they know what fetal movements feel like. Quickening is often perceived as a faint flutter or a quivering motion.

2. Folic acid supplementation before conception and during early pregnancy is effective in reducing the incidence of neural tube defects (e.g., spina bifida). It has been shown that the risk of having a child with a neural tube defect is significantly lower when a vitamin supplement containing 400 mg of folic acid is consumed daily. However, no consensus exists that vitamins are helpful in preventing these defects in most at-risk pregnancies.

3. Direct injury to the fetus from the needle during amniocentesis is very uncommon when ultrasound guidance is used to locate the position of the fetus and monitor needle insertion. The risk of inducing an abortion is slight (approximately 0.5%) in second-trimester pregnancies. Maternal or fetal infection is also an uncommon complication.

CHAPTER 8

1. A stillbirth is the birth of a fetus that was dead before delivery, weighs at least 500 g, and is at least 20 weeks old. The incidence of having a stillborn infant is approximately three times greater among mothers older than 40 years than among women aged 20–30 years. More male fetuses than female fetuses are stillborn. The reason for this is unknown.

2. Sometimes the umbilical cord is abnormally long and wraps around part of the fetus, such as the neck or a limb. This cord accident may obstruct the flow of high-oxygen blood in the umbilical vein to the fetus and in the umbilical arteries from the fetus to the placenta. If this obstruction causes the fetus to receive insufficient oxygen and nutrients, then the fetus is likely to die. A true knot in the umbilical cord, formed when the fetus passes through a loop in the cord, also obstructs blood flow through the cord. Prolapse of the umbilical cord into the cervix at the level of a presenting part (often the head) may also be considered a cord accident. This creates pressure on the cord and prevents the fetus from receiving adequate oxygen. Entanglement of the cord around the fetus can also cause birth defects (e.g., absence of a forearm).

3. Most over-the-counter pregnancy tests are based on the detection of relatively large amounts of human chorionic gonadotropin in the woman's urine. The results of such tests are positive for a short time (approximately 1 week) after the first missed menstrual period (after embryo implantation). Human chorionic gonadotropin is produced by the syncytiotrophoblast of the chorion. These tests usually give an accurate diagnosis of pregnancy; however, a physician should be consulted as soon as possible to confirm pregnancy because some tumors (choriocarcinomas) also produce this hormone.

4. The "bag of water" is a colloquial term for the amniotic sac, which contains amniotic fluid (largely composed of water). Sometimes the amniochorionic sac ruptures before labor begins, allowing fluid to escape. Premature rupture of the membranes is the most common event leading to premature labor and birth. Premature rupture of the membranes may complicate the birth process, or it may allow a vaginal infection to spread to the fetus. Sometimes sterile saline is infused into the uterus by way of a catheter—*amnioinfusion*—to alleviate fetal distress.

5. Fetal distress is synonymous with fetal hypoxia, indicating decreased oxygenation to the fetus as a result of a general decrease in maternal oxygen content in the blood, decreased oxygen-carrying capacity, or diminished blood flow. Fetal distress exists when the fetal heart rate is less than 100 beats per minute. Pressure on the umbilical cord may also cause fetal distress secondary to impairment of the blood supply to the fetus in approximately 1 in 200 deliveries. In these cases, the fetal body compresses the umbilical cord as it passes through the cervix and vagina.

6. The incidence of dizygotic twins increases with maternal age. This twinning is an autosomal recessive trait that is carried by the daughters of mothers of twins; hence, dizygotic twinning is hereditary. Monozygotic twinning, on the other hand, is a random occurrence that is not genetically controlled.

CHAPTER 9

1. Yes, it is. When a neonate is born with a congenital diaphragmatic hernia (CDH), part of its stomach and liver may enter the thorax (chest); however, this is uncommon. Usually, the abnormally placed viscera are the intestines. The viscera enter the thorax through a posterolateral defect in the diaphragm, usually on the left side.

2. CDH occurs in 1 in 3000 neonates. A neonate with a CDH may survive; however, the mortality rate approximately 30–50% and even higher when other abnormalities are present. Treatment must be given immediately. A feeding tube is inserted into the stomach, and the air and the gastric contents are aspirated with continuous suction. Intubation of the airway, mechanical ventilation, and stabilization of the neonate are critical until surgery can be performed. The displaced viscera are replaced in the abdominal cavity, and the defect in the diaphragm is surgically repaired. Infants with large diaphragmatic hernias who are operated on within 24 hours after birth have survival rates of 40%–70%. Intrauterine surgical repair of a CDH has been attempted; however, this intervention carries considerable risk to the fetus and mother. The developing use of minimally invasive surgical techniques may reduce this risk.

3. It depends on the degree of herniation of the abdominal viscera. With a moderate hernia, the lungs may be mature but small. With a severe degree of herniation, lung development is impaired. Most infants with a CDH die, but not because of the defect in the diaphragm or viscera in the thorax; they die because the lung on the affected side is hypoplastic (underdeveloped).

4. Yes, it is possible to have a small CDH and not be aware of it. Some small hernias may remain asymptomatic into adulthood and may be discovered only during routine

radiographic or ultrasound examination of the thorax. The lung on the affected side would probably develop normally because there would be little or no pressure on it during prenatal development.

CHAPTER 10

1. All embryos have grooves in their upper lips where the maxillary prominences meet the merged medial nasal prominences; however, normal embryos do not have cleft lips. When lip development is abnormal, the tissue in the floor of the labial groove breaks down, forming a cleft lip.
2. The risk in this case is the same as in the general population, approximately 1 in 1000.
3. Although environmental factors may be involved, it is reasonable to assume that the son's cleft lip and cleft palate were hereditary and recessive in their expression. This would mean that the father also carried a concealed gene for cleft lip and that his family genetics were equally responsible for the son's anomalies.
4. Minor anomalies of the auricle of the external ear are common, and usually they are of no serious medical or cosmetic consequence. Approximately 14% of neonates have minor birth defects; less than 1% of them have other defects. The child's abnormal ears could be considered pharyngeal (branchial) arch anomalies because the six small auricular hillocks (swellings) of the first two pairs of pharyngeal arches contribute to the auricles; however, such minor abnormalities of ear shape would not be normally classified in this way.

CHAPTER 11

1. Multiple stimuli initiate breathing at birth. Slapping the buttocks used to be a common physical stimulus; however, this stimulus is usually unnecessary. Under normal circumstances, the neonate's breathing begins promptly, which suggests that it is a reflex response to the sensory stimuli of exposure to air and touching. The changes in blood gases after interruption of the placental circulation, such as the decrease in oxygen tension and pH and the increase in partial pressure of carbon dioxide, are also important in stimulating breathing.
2. Hyaline membrane disease, another name for respiratory distress syndrome (RDS), occurs after the onset of breathing in infants with immature lungs and a deficiency of pulmonary surfactant. The incidence of RDS is approximately 1% of all live births, and it is the leading cause of death in newborn infants. It occurs mainly in infants who are born prematurely. RDS is caused mainly by surfactant deficiency.
3. A 22-week fetus is viable and, if born prematurely and given special care in a neonatal intensive care unit, may survive. The chances of survival, however, are poor for infants who weigh less than 600 g because the lungs are immature and incapable of adequate alveolar–capillary gas exchange. Furthermore, the fetus's brain is not usually differentiated sufficiently to permit regular respiration. Administration of exogenous surfactant (surfactant

replacement therapy) reduces the severity of RDS and neonatal mortality.

CHAPTER 12

1. Undoubtedly, the infant has congenital hypertrophic pyloric stenosis, a diffuse hypertrophy (enlargement), and hyperplasia of smooth muscle in the pyloric part of the stomach. This condition produces a hard palpable mass; however, it is a benign enlargement and is definitely not a malignant tumor. The muscular enlargement causes narrowing of the exit canal (pyloric canal). In response to the outflow obstruction and vigorous peristalsis, the vomiting is projectile, as in the case of the infant described. Surgical relief of the pyloric obstruction is the usual treatment. The cause of pyloric stenosis is not known; however, it is believed to have a multifactorial pattern of inheritance (i.e., genetic and environmental factors arc probably involved).
2. It is true that infants with trisomy 21 (Down syndrome) have an increased incidence of duodenal atresia. They are also more likely to have an imperforate anus and other birth defects (e.g., atrial septal defects). These birth defects are likely caused by their abnormal chromosomal constitution (i.e., three instead of two copies of chromosome 21). Duodenal atresia can be corrected surgically by bypassing the pyloric obstruction (duodenoduodenostomy).
3. In very uncommon cases, when the intestines return to the abdomen after physiological umbilical herniation, they may rotate in a clockwise direction rather than in the usual counterclockwise manner. As a result, the cecum and appendix are located on the left side, a condition called *situs inversus abdominis*. A left-sided cecum and appendix can also result from a mobile cecum. If the cecum is not fixed to the posterior abdominal wall during the fetal period, the cecum and appendix are freely movable and could migrate to the left side.
4. Undoubtedly, the individual described had an ileal (Meckel) diverticulum, a finger-like outpouching of the ileum. This common anomaly is sometimes referred to as a second appendix, which is a misnomer. An ileal diverticulum produces symptoms that are similar to those of appendicitis. It is also possible, although rare, that the person had a duplication of the cecum, which would result in two appendices.
5. Hirschsprung disease, or congenital megacolon, is the most common cause of obstruction of the descending colon in newborn infants. The cause of the condition is the failure of the migration of neural crest cells into the wall of the intestine. The neural crest cells normally form neurons, so there is a deficiency of the nerve cells that innervate the muscular wall of the bowel—congenital aganglionosis. When the bowel wall collapses, obstruction occurs and constipation results. Bowel distention and perforation may also occur.
6. If the infant had an umbilico-ileal fistula, the abnormal canal connecting the ileum and the umbilicus could permit the passage of the contents of the ileum to the umbilicus. This occurrence would be an important diagnostic clue to the presence of this canal. The fistula results from

the persistence of the intraabdominal part of the omphaloenteric duct.

CHAPTER 13

1. Most people with a horseshoe kidney have no urinary problems. The abnormal position of the fused kidneys is usually discovered postmortem or during diagnostic imaging procedures. Nothing needs to be done with the abnormal kidney unless the person has an uncontrolled infection of the urinary tract. In some cases, the urologist may divide the kidney into two parts and fix them in positions that do not result in urinary stagnation.

2. His developing kidneys probably fused during the sixth to eighth weeks as they "migrated" from the pelvis. The fused kidneys then ascended toward the normal position on one side or the other. Usually, no problems are associated with fused kidneys; however, surgeons must be conscious of the possibility of this condition and recognize it for what it is. This abnormality is called *crossed renal ectopia*.

3. Affected individuals have both ovarian and testicular tissue. Although spermatogenesis is uncommon, ovulation is not. Pregnancy and childbirth have been observed in a few patients; however, this is very unusual.

4. By 48 hours after birth, a genetic sex assignment can be made in most cases. Karyotyping (chromosomal staining, visualization, and counting) from whole blood lymphocytes is conducted, as well as identification of the *SRY* gene (sex-determining region of the Y chromosome) by either FISH or polymerase chain reaction amplification. Hormone studies may also be required. Based on a number of factors and test results, the medical team may suggest a gender for the neonate, however there are many complex considerations.

5. Virilization (masculinization) of a female fetus as a result of congenital adrenal hyperplasia is the most common cause of ambiguous external genitalia. In other cases, androgens enter the fetal circulation after maternal ingestion of androgenic hormones. In unusual cases, these hormones are produced by a tumor on one of the mother's suprarenal glands. Partial or complete fusion of the urogenital folds or labioscrotal swellings is the result of exposure to androgens before the 12th week of development. Clitoral enlargement occurs after this point; however, androgens do not cause sexual ambiguity because the other external genitalia are fully formed by this time.

CHAPTER 14

1. Heart murmurs are sounds transmitted to the thoracic wall by the turbulence of blood in the heart or great arteries. Loud murmurs often represent stenosis of one of the semilunar valves (aortic or pulmonary valve). A ventricular septal defect or a patent oval foramen (foramen ovale) may also produce a murmur.

2. Congenital heart defects (CHDs) are common. They occur in 6–8 in 1000 newborn infants and represent approximately 10% of all congenital anomalies. Ventricular septal defects are the most common type of heart anomaly. They occur more frequently in males than in females, but the reason for this is unknown. Some CHDs are caused by single-gene or chromosomal mechanisms; others result from exposure to teratogens such as the rubella virus.

3. The cause of most congenital anomalies of the cardiovascular system is unknown. In approximately 8% of children with heart disease, a genetic basis is clear. Most of these anomalies are associated with obvious chromosomal abnormalities (e.g., trisomy 21) and deletion of parts of chromosomes. Trisomy 21 (Down syndrome) is associated with congenital heart disease in 50% of cases. Maternal ingestion of drugs, such as antimetabolites and warfarin (an anticoagulant), has been shown to be associated with a high incidence of cardiac defects. Heavy consumption of alcohol during pregnancy may cause heart defects.

4. Several viral infections are associated with congenital cardiac defects; however, only rubella virus (German measles) is known to cause cardiovascular disease (e.g., patent ductus arteriosus). Rubeola (common measles) does not cause cardiovascular defects. Rubella virus vaccine is available and is effective in preventing the development of rubella infection in a woman who has not had the disease and is planning to have a child. It will subsequently prevent rubella syndrome from developing in her infant as well. Because of the potential hazard of the vaccine to the embryo, the vaccine is given only if there is assurance that there is no likelihood of pregnancy for the next 2 months.

5. This anomaly is called transposition of the great arteries because the positions of the great vessels (aorta and pulmonary trunk) are reversed. Survival after birth depends on mixing between the pulmonary and systemic circulations (e.g., through an atrial septal defect—patent oval foramen). Transposition of the great arteries occurs in slightly more than 1 in 5000 live births and is more common in males (by almost 2 to 1). Relatively few infants with this severe cardiac anomaly die during the first months of life. Nowadays, corrective surgery can be performed on those who survive. Initially, an atrial septal defect may be created to increase mixing between the systemic and pulmonary circulations (atrial switch operation). Later, an arterial switch operation (reversing the aorta and the pulmonary trunk) can be performed. However, more commonly, a baffle (a device used to restrain the flow of blood) is inserted into the atrium to divert systemic venous blood through the mitral valve, left ventricle, and pulmonary artery to the lungs and to divert pulmonary venous blood through the tricuspid valve, right ventricle, and aorta. This physiologically corrects the circulation.

6. Very likely, one twin has dextrocardia, which is usually of no clinical significance. The heart is simply displaced to the right. In the individual described, the heart presents a mirror image of the normal cardiac structure. This occurs during the fourth week of development, when the heart tube rotates to the left rather than to the right. Dextrocardia is a rare anomaly, relatively more common in monozygotic twins.

CHAPTER 15

1. An accessory rib associated with the seventh cervical vertebra is of clinical importance because it may compress the subclavian artery, the brachial plexus, or both, producing symptoms of artery and nerve compression. The most common type of accessory rib is a lumbar rib, but it usually causes no problems.

2. A hemivertebra can produce lateral curvature of the vertebral column (scoliosis). A hemivertebra is composed of one half of a body, a pedicle, and a lamina. This anomaly occurs when mesenchymal cells from the sclerotomes on one side do not form the primordium of half of a vertebra. As a result, more growth centers are found on one side of the vertebral column; this imbalance causes the vertebral column to bend laterally.

3. The cranial sutures allow the brain to develop and increase in size. Craniosynostosis indicates premature closure of one or more of the cranial sutures. This developmental abnormality results in changes in the shape of the skull, which may lead to increased intracranial pressure. Scaphocephaly or dolichocephaly—a long, narrow cranium—results from premature closure of the sagittal suture. This type of craniosynostosis accounts for approximately 50% of cases of premature closure of cranial sutures and is more commonly seen in males.

4. The features of Klippel–Feil syndrome are a short neck, a low hairline, and restricted neck movements. In most cases, cervical vertebral bodies are fused before birth and fewer than normal cervical vertebrae are present.

5. Prune belly syndrome results from the partial or complete absence of the abdominal musculature. Usually the abdominal wall is thin. This syndrome is usually associated with malformations of the urinary tract, especially the urinary bladder (e.g., exstrophy of the bladder). In males, almost all patients have cryptorchidism (failure of one or both testes to descend into the scrotum).

6. Absence of the sternocostal part of the left pectoralis major muscle is usually the cause of an abnormally low nipple and areola. Despite its numerous and important actions, absence of all or part of the pectoralis major muscle usually causes no disability. The actions of other muscles associated with the shoulder joint compensate for the partial absence of this muscle.

7. The girl has a prominent sternocleidomastoid muscle. This muscle attaches the mastoid process to the clavicle and sternum; hence, continued growth of the side of the neck results in tilting and rotation of the head. This relatively common condition—congenital torticollis (wry neck)—may occur because of an injury to the muscle during birth. Stretching and tearing of some muscle fibers may have occurred during delivery, resulting in bleeding into the muscle. Over several weeks, necrosis of some fibers occurs and the blood is replaced by fibrous tissue. This results in shortening of the muscle and pulling of the child's head to one side. If the condition is not corrected, the shortened muscle could also distort the shape of the face on the affected side.

8. The young athlete probably had an accessory soleus muscle. It is present in approximately 3% of people. This anomaly probably results from the splitting of the primordium of the soleus muscle into two parts.

9. The ingestion of drugs did not cause the child's short limbs. The infant has a skeletal disorder known as achondroplasia. This type of short-limbed dwarfism has an incidence of 1 in 10,000 and shows an autosomal dominant inheritance. Approximately 80% of affected infants are born to normal parents and, presumably, the condition results from new mutations (changes in the genetic material) in the parents' germ cells. Most people with achondroplasia have normal intelligence and lead normal lives within their physical capabilities. If the parents of an achondroplastic child have more children, the risk of having another child with this condition is slightly higher than the risk in the general population; however, the risk for the achondroplastic person's own children is 50%.

10. Brachydactyly (very short fingers) is an autosomal dominant trait. If the woman (likely bb) marries the brachydactylous man (likely Bb), the risk is 50% for a brachydactylous child and 50% for a normal child. It would be best for them to discuss their obvious concern with a medical geneticist.

11. Bendectin (now marketed as Diclegis), an antinauseant mixture of doxylamine succinate and pyridoxine hydrochloride, does not produce limb defects in human embryos. Several epidemiological studies have not shown an increased risk of birth defects after exposure to Bendectin or its separate ingredients during early pregnancy. In the case described, the mother took the drug more than 3 weeks after the end of the critical period of limb development (24–36 days after fertilization). Most limb reduction defects have a genetic basis.

12. Cutaneous syndactyly is the most common type of limb anomaly. It varies from cutaneous webbing between the digits to synostosis (union of the phalanges, the bones of the digits). This anomaly occurs when separate digital rays do not form in the fourth week or when the tissue between the developing digits does not undergo apoptosis. Simple cutaneous syndactyly is easy to correct surgically.

13. The most common type of talipes is *talipes equinovarus*, occurring in approximately 1 in 1000 newborn infants, twice as frequently in males. In this deformity, the soles of the feet are turned medially, and the feet are plantar flexed. The feet are fixed in the tiptoe position, resembling the foot of a horse (Latin *equinus*, horse).

CHAPTER 16

1. Neural tube defects (NTDs) have a multifactorial inheritance pattern. Although only a few environmental factors have been shown to be directly related (such as folic acid), studies indicate that there are also genetic components. After the birth of one child with an NTD, the risk of a subsequent child having an NTD is much higher. The recurrence risk in the United Kingdom, where NTDs are common (7.6 per 1000 in South Wales and 8.6 per 1000

in Northern Ireland), is approximately 1 in 25. NTDs can be detected prenatally by a combination of ultrasound scanning and measurement of levels of alpha-fetoprotein in the amniotic fluid and maternal serum.

2. Intellectual disability and growth restriction are the most serious complications of fetal alcohol syndrome. Currently, no safe threshold for alcohol consumption during pregnancy is known. Physicians recommend complete abstinence from alcohol during pregnancy.

3. No conclusive evidence indicates that maternal smoking affects the mental development of a fetus; however, cigarette smoking compromises the oxygen supply to the fetus because blood flow to the placenta is decreased during smoking. Now that it is well established that heavy maternal smoking seriously affects the physical growth of the fetus and is a major cause of intrauterine growth restriction, and it is not wise for mothers to smoke during pregnancy. The reduced oxygen supply to the brain could affect fetal intellectual development, even though the effect may be undetectable. Not smoking gives the fetus the best chance for normal development.

4. Most laypeople use the term *spina bifida* in a general way. They are unaware that the common type, spina bifida occulta, is usually clinically insignificant. It is an isolated finding in up to 20% of radiographically examined vertebral columns. Most people are unaware that they have this vertebral defect because it produces no symptoms unless it is associated with a neural tube defect or an abnormality of the spinal nerve roots. Various types of spina bifida cystica are of clinical significance. Meningomyelocele is a more severe defect than meningocele because neural tissue is included in the lesion. Because of this, the function of the abdominal and limb muscles may be affected. Meningoceles are usually covered with skin, and motor function in the limbs is usually normal unless associated developmental defects of the spinal cord or brain are present. Management of infants with spina bifida cystica is complex and involves several medical and surgical specialties. Spinal meningocele is easier to correct surgically than spinal meningomyelocele, and the prognosis is also better.

CHAPTER 17

1. The chance of significant damage to an embryo or fetus after a rubella infection depends primarily on the timing of the viral infection. In cases of primary maternal infection during the first trimester of pregnancy, the overall risk of embryonic or fetal infection is approximately 20%. It is estimated that approximately 50% of such pregnancies end in spontaneous abortion, stillbirth, or birth defects (deafness, cataract, glaucoma, and intellectual disability). When infection occurs at the end of the first trimester, the probability of birth defects is only slightly higher than that for an uncomplicated pregnancy. Certain infections occurring late in the first trimester, however, may result in severe eye infections (e.g., chorioretinitis), which may affect visual development. Deafness is the most common manifestation of late fetal rubella infection (i.e., during the second and third trimesters). If a pregnant woman is exposed to rubella, an antibody test can be performed. If she is determined to be immune, she can be reassured that her embryo or fetus will not be affected by the virus. Preventive measures are essential for the protection of the embryo. It is especially important for girls to obtain immunity to rubella (e.g., by active immunization) before they reach childbearing age.

2. The purposeful exposure of young girls to rubella (German measles) is not recommended. Although complications resulting from such infections are uncommon, neuritis and arthritis (inflammation of the nerves and joints, respectively) occasionally occur. Encephalitis (inflammation of the brain) occurs in approximately 1 in 6000 cases. Rubella infection is often subclinical (difficult to detect), yet children with such infections represent an exposure risk to pregnant women. There is a chance of injury to embryos because the danger period is greatest when the eyes and ears are developing. This occurs early enough in pregnancy that some women might be unaware that they are pregnant. A much better way of providing immunization against rubella is the administration of live virus vaccine to children older than 15 months and to nonpregnant postpubertal females who can be reasonably relied on not to become pregnant within 3 months of immunization.

3. Congenital syphilis (fetal syphilis) results from transplacental transmission of the microorganism *Treponema pallidum*. Transfer of this microorganism from untreated pregnant women may occur throughout pregnancy; however, it usually takes place during the last trimester. Deafness and tooth deformities commonly develop in these children. These birth defects can be prevented by treating the mother early in pregnancy. The microorganism that causes syphilis is very sensitive to penicillin, an antibiotic that does not harm the fetus.

4. Several viruses in the herpesvirus family can cause fetal blindness and deafness during infancy. Cytomegalovirus can cross the placenta, be transmitted to the infant during birth, and be passed to the infant in breast milk. Herpes simplex viruses (usually type 2, or genital herpes) are usually transmitted just before or during birth. The chances of normal development in infected infants are not good. Infants exposed earlier in pregnancy may have microcephaly, seizures, deafness, and blindness; there is a 50% risk of death from disseminated disease in the neonate.

5. Methyl mercury is teratogenic (causing birth defects) in human embryos, especially in the developing brain. Because the eyes and internal ears develop as outgrowths of the brain, it is understandable that their development is also affected. Besides the methyl mercury that passes from the mother to the embryo or fetus through the placenta, the neonate may receive additional methyl mercury from breast milk. Sources of methyl mercury include fish from contaminated water, flour made from methyl mercury–treated seed grain, and meat from animals raised on contaminated food.

CHAPTER 18

1. Congenital absence of the skin is very uncommon. Patches of skin may be absent, most often from the scalp or sometimes from the trunk and limbs. Affected infants

usually survive because healing of the lesions is uneventful and takes 1–2 months. A hairless scar persists. The cause of congenital absence of hair, termed *aplasia cutis congenita*, is usually unknown. Most cases are sporadic; however, several well-documented pedigrees show autosomal dominant transmission of this skin defect.

2. The white patches of skin on a dark-skinned person result from partial albinism (piebaldism). This defect, which also affects light-skinned people, is inherited in an autosomal recessive manner. Ultrastructural studies show an absence of melanocytes in the depigmented areas of the skin. Presumably, the cause is a defect in the differentiation of melanoblasts resulting from gene mutation. These skin and hair defects are not amenable to treatment; however, they can be covered with cosmetics and hair dyes.

3. The breasts, including the mammary glands within them, of males and females are similar at birth. Slight breast enlargement in a neonate is common and results from stimulation by maternal hormones that enter the infant's blood through the placenta. Therefore enlarged breasts are a normal occurrence in young male infants and do not indicate abnormal sex development.

4. An extra breast (polymastia) or nipple (polythelia) is common. The axillary breast may enlarge during puberty, or it may not be noticed until pregnancy occurs. The embryological basis of extra breasts and nipples is the presence of mammary crests (ridges) that extend from the axillary to the inguinal regions. Usually, only one pair of breasts develops; however, breasts can develop anywhere along the mammary crests. The extra breast or nipple is usually just superior or inferior to the normal breast. An axillary breast or nipple is very uncommon.

5. Teeth that are present at birth are termed *natal teeth* and are observed in approximately 1 in 2000 newborn infants. Usually, two mandibular medial (central) incisors are present. The presence of natal teeth usually suggests that an early eruption of other teeth may occur. Often, they fall out on their own. Because there is a danger that they may be aspirated, natal teeth are sometimes extracted.

CHAPTER 19

1. No evidence indicates that the occasional use of aspirin in recommended therapeutic dosages is harmful during pregnancy; however, large doses at subtoxic levels (e.g., for rheumatoid arthritis) have not been proven to be harmless to the embryo and fetus. Pregnant women should discuss the use of over-the-counter medications with their physicians.

2. A woman with a substance abuse disorder (e.g., opioids) and takes them during pregnancy is almost certain to give birth to a child who shows signs of drug addiction.

The fetus's chances of survival until birth, however, are not good; mortality and premature birth rates are high among fetuses of drug-addicted mothers.

3. All drugs prescribed in North America are tested for teratogenicity before they are marketed. The thalidomide tragedy clearly showed the need for improved methods for detecting potential human teratogens. Thalidomide was not found to be teratogenic in pregnant mice and rats—yet it is a potent teratogen in humans during the fourth to sixth weeks of pregnancy. Because it is unethical to test the effects of drugs on human embryos, no way exists to guarantee that some drugs that may be human teratogens will not be marketed. Human teratological evaluation depends on retrospective epidemiological studies and reports of astute physicians. This is the way that the teratogenicity of thalidomide was detected. Most new drugs contain a disclaimer in the accompanying package insert, such as, "This drug has not been proven safe for pregnant women." Some drugs may be used if, in the opinion of the physician, the potential benefits outweigh the possible hazards. All known teratogenic drugs that may be taken by a pregnant woman are available only on prescription from a physician.

4. Cigarette smoking during pregnancy is harmful to embryos and fetuses. Its most adverse effect is intrauterine growth restriction. Women who stop smoking during the first half of pregnancy have infants with birth weights closer to the birth weights of infants of nonsmokers. Decreased placental blood flow, believed to be a nicotine-mediated effect, is believed to cause decreased intrauterine blood flow. Babies born to mothers who smoke during pregnancy are more likely to have birth defects, such as cleft lip and cleft palate, compared with mothers who do not smoke. The growth of the fetus of a woman who smokes but does not inhale is still endangered because nicotine, carbon monoxide, and other harmful substances are also absorbed into the maternal bloodstream through the mucous membranes of the mouth and throat. These substances are then transferred to the embryos or fetuses through the placenta. Smoking in any manner during pregnancy is not advisable.

5. Most drugs do not cause birth defects in human embryos and fetuses; however, a pregnant woman should take only drugs that are essential and are recommended by her physician. A pregnant woman with a severe lower respiratory infection, for example, would be unwise to refuse drugs recommended by her physician to cure her illness; her health and that of her embryo or fetus could be endangered by the infection. Most drugs, including sulfonamides, meclizine, penicillin, and antihistamines, are considered safe drugs. Similarly, local anesthetic agents, killed vaccines, and salicylates (e.g., aspirin) in low doses are not known to cause birth defects.

Index

Page numbers followed by "*f*" indicate figures, "*t*" indicate tables, and "*b*" indicate boxes.

Implantation, of blastocyst *(Continued)*
 inhibition of, 31*b*
 sites of, 29–31, 30*f*, 31*f*
In vitro fertilization, 24*f*, 25*b*
Incisor teeth, 274*t*, 275*f*, 276*b*
Indifferent gonad, 161
 adult derivatives and vestigial remains
  of, 150*t*
Induced pluripotent stem cells, 305–306, 305*f*
Inductions, 47–49
Infection, fetal, 72
Infectious agents
 placental transport of, 71–72
 as teratogens, 288*t*, 293–294
Inferior
 mesenteric artery, 83
Inferior, as descriptive term, 4*f*
Inferior colliculi, 245, 246*f*
Inferior mesenteric artery, 83, 141
Inferior parathyroid glands, 95
Inferior rectal nerve, 142
Inferior vena cava, 87*f*, 88*f*
 development of, 175, 177*f*
 hepatic segment of, 177*f*
 postrenal segment, 177*f*
 prerenal segment, 177*f*
 renal segment, 177*f*
 valves of, 187*f*
Infundibular stem, 246
Infundibular stenosis, 197*b*
Infundibulum, 245–246, 247*f*
 of uterine tube, 16
Inguinal canals, development of, 170
Inguinal hernia, congenital, 173*b*, 173*f*
Insula, 250
Insulin
 in fetal growth, 61
 pancreatic development, 130–133
Integumentary system, 269–278
Intercalated discs, 223–224
Intercellular communication, 297–298
Intercostal arteries, 176, 213
Intermediate layer, in skin development,
 269, 270*f*
Intermediate mesenchyme, metanephric
 mass of, 147, 148*f*
Intermediate zone, 233
Intermediolateral cell column, 255
Internal hernia, 140*b*
Internal os, 5, 75*f*
Intersegmental arteries, 176, 176*f*, 213, 214*f*
Interventricular foramina, 184*f*, 189*f*, 246, 249*f*
Interventricular septum
 membranous, 188, 191*f*
 muscular, 183, 190*f*
 primordial, 184*f*, 190*f*
Intervertebral (IV) discs, 213, 214*f*
Intervillous space, 42, 43*f*, 66*f*, 69*f*
 maternal blood in, 290
Interzonal mesenchyme, 211
Intestines, 77*f*
 atresia of, 126*b*, 130*f*, 141*b*
 fixation of, 136, 137*f*
 herniation of, 89*b*, 136*b*
 mesenteries of, 137*f*
 stenosis of, 141*b*
 volvulus, 140*b*
Intracytoplasmic sperm injection, 25*b*
Intraembryonic coelom, 83, 84*f*, 86*f*
 development of, 36, 39*f*
 embryonic folding and, 84*f*
Intraembryonic mesoderm, 209, 210*f*

Intramembranous bone formation, 209
Intraocular tension, 263*b*
Intraretinal space, 257, 258*f*
Intrauterine amputations, 295
Intrauterine device, and implantation, 31*b*
Intrauterine growth restriction (IUGR), 69–70
 alcohol, consumption of, 61
 cigarette smoking and, 287–290
 teratogens causing, 288*t*
 triploidy and, 283*b*
Inversion, chromosomal, 285
Iodides, as teratogens, 292
Iodine deficiency, congenital, 292
Ionizing radiation, as teratogen, 288*t*, 294
Iris
 in albinism, 270*b*
 coloboma of, 259*b*, 262*f*
 development of, 259, 261*f*
Iron, placental transport of, 71*f*
Ischemia, of spiral arteries, menstrual cycle, 16
Isochromosomes, 284*f*
Isotretinoin, as teratogen, 288*t*, 291–292

J
Jaundice, 130*b*
Joints
 cartilaginous, 211, 213*f*
 costovertebral, 214*f*, 215
 development of, 211, 213*f*
 fibrous, 211, 213*f*
 neurocentral, 214*f*
 synovial, 211, 213*f*
Joint cavity, 211
Jugular lymph sacs, 206, 207*f*
Jugular vein, 207*f*

K
Keratinization, 76, 269, 270*f*
 disorders of, 270*b*, 271*f*
Kidney(s)
 blood supply, changes in, 148–157
 congenital anomalies of, 150*b*, 156*f*
 development of, 147–159
  molecular aspects of, 154*f*
 discoid, 156*f*
 double, 156*f*
 ectopic, 154, 156*f*
 fused, 155*b*, 156*f*
 horseshoe, 155*b*, 157*f*
 lobulation of, 147–148
 malrotation of, 154*b*
 pelvic, 156*f*
 positional changes of, 148, 155*f*
 supernumerary, 155*b*, 156*f*
Klinefelter syndrome, 272*b*, 283*f*, 284*t*
Klippel–Feil syndrome, 215*b*
Kupffer cells, hepatic, 127–129

L
Labia majora, 5, 8*f*, 150*t*, 166–170
Labia minora, 5, 8*f*, 150*t*, 166–170
Labioscrotal swellings, 150*t*, 166–170
Labor
 definition, 72–74
 factors triggering, 72–74
 stages of, 74
Lacrimal excretory ducts, 263
Lacrimal glands, development of, 263
Lacrimal sac, 106–107
Lacunae, 27–28, 28*f*
Lacunar networks, 28–29, 28*f*, 67–68

Lamina terminalis, 249*f*, 250
Lanugo, 57, 272
Laryngeal atresia, 117*b*
Laryngeal cartilage, 117
Laryngeal inlet, primordial, 117
Laryngeal lumen, temporary occlusion of, 117
Laryngeal muscles, 117
Laryngeal nerves, recurrent, 200–202, 200*f*
Laryngeal ventricles, 117
Laryngotracheal diverticulum, 117, 118*f*
Laryngotracheal groove, 117, 118*f*
Laryngotracheal tube, 117
Larynx
 development of, 117, 119*f*
 recanalization of, 117
Last normal menstrual period (LNMP), 57
Late neonatal period, 63
Lateral body walls, muscular ingrowth
 from, 87, 88*f*
Lateral cervical sinuses, 96*b*
Lateral folds, of embryo, 45, 47*f*, 48*f*
Lateral gray horns, 237
Lateral inhibition, in Notch–Delta pathway,
 302–303
Lateral mesoderm, 175
Lateral palatine processes, 110
Lateral sulcus, 250
Lateral thoracic wall, 87*f*
Lead, as teratogen, 293
Left-sided colon, 139*b*
Lens, development of, 259–262, 261*f*
Lens epithelium, 261*f*
 anterior, 261*f*
 subcapsular, 259–260
Lens fiber, 262*f*
 primary, 259–260
 secondary, 259–260
Lens pits, 257, 258*f*
Lens placodes, 50–51, 54*f*, 257, 258*f*
Lens vesicles, 257, 258*f*
Lesser omentum, 130
Levator palpebrae superioris muscle, 263*b*
Lewis, Edward B., 1
Ligament(s)
 abdominal, 206
 broad, 164
 falciform, 130
 hepatoduodenal, 130
 hepatogastric, 130
 ovarian, 150*t*
 periodontal, 274, 275*f*
 round
  of liver, 205
  of uterus, 150*t*
 umbilical
  medial, 178
  median, 157
Ligamentum arteriosum, 200–202, 200*f*, 206
Ligamentum venosum, 205–206
Limb(s)
 anomalies of, 230*b*
 blood supply of, 227–231, 227*f*
 cutaneous innervation of, 225–227
 dermatomal pattern of, 226*f*
 development of
  early stages of, 224, 225*f*, 226*f*
  final stages of, 224–225, 226*f*
 muscles, 222*f*, 223
 plexuses, 225, 226*f*
Limb buds, 224
 lower, 50–51, 51*f*, 224
 upper, 50–51, 54*f*, 224